JANE REEDY

THE BOOKS OF F. MATTHIAS ALEXANDER

MAN'S SUPREME INHERITANCE

CONSTRUCTIVE CONSCIOUS CONTROL OF THE INDIVIDUAL

THE USE OF THE SELF

THE UNIVERSAL CONSTANT IN LIVING

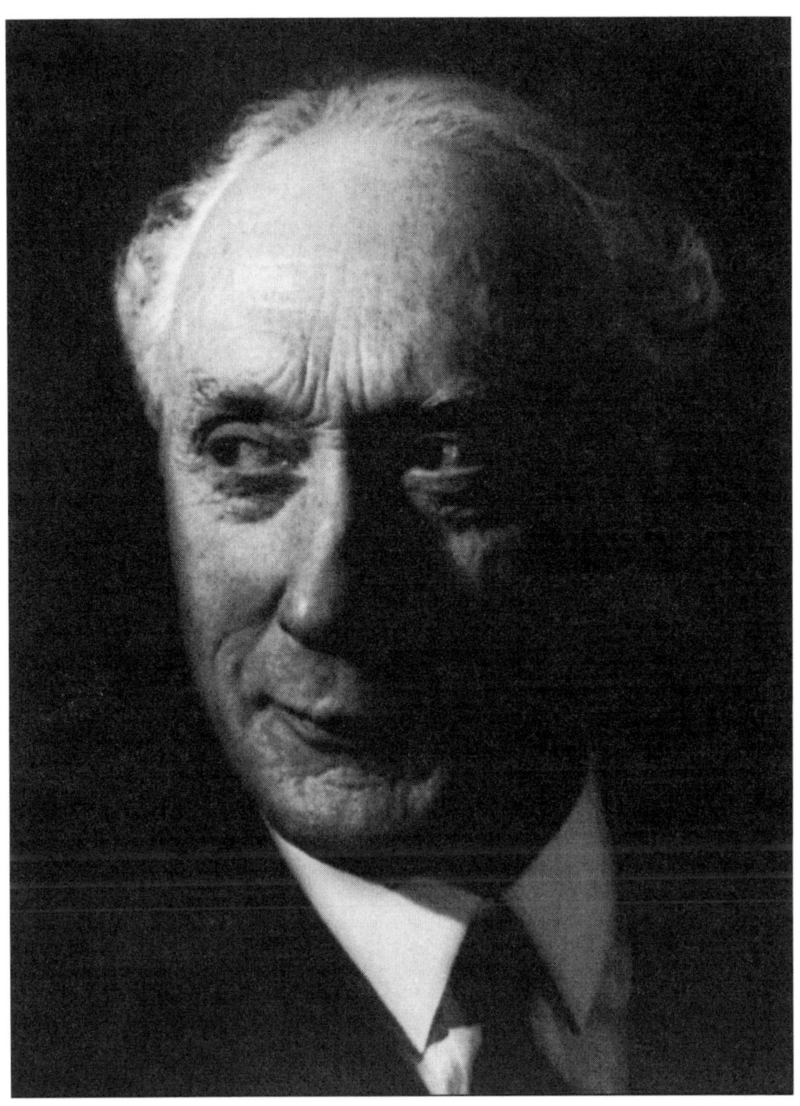

Photograph of F. Matthias Alexander courtesy of Marjory Barlow.

THE BOOKS OF
F. MATTHIAS ALEXANDER

MAN'S SUPREME
INHERITANCE

CONSTRUCTIVE CONSCIOUS CONTROL
OF THE INDIVIDUAL

THE USE OF THE SELF

THE UNIVERSAL CONSTANT
IN LIVING

IRDEAT
New York, N.Y.

Man's Supreme Inheritance, The Use of Self and *The Universal Constant in Living* are each being printed here as first published by E. P. Dutton & Co., Inc. *Constructive Conscious Control of the Individual* appears here as printed by E. P. Dutton & Co, Inc. in 1942.

This 1997 edition is published by
IRDEAT
74 MacDougal Street
New York, New York 10012
with the permission of Dutton Signet,
a division of Penguin Books USA Inc.

ISBN 0-9658446-0-9

Printed in the United States of America

TABLE OF CONTENTS

MAN'S SUPREME INHERITANCE

Conscious Guidance and Control in Relation to Human Evolution in Civilization

With an Introductory Word By
PROFESSOR JOHN DEWEY

PREFACE TO FIRST EDITION
(London, 1910)

AMONG my intimates I once numbered a boatman known as Old Sol, or to his familiars just Sol, without the courtesy title, for he was not notably old. I could not say whether his name was an abbreviated form of Solomon or not, nor if it were, whether the longer name was baptismal or conferred in later years as a tribute to his undoubted wisdom. I have thought it possible that the name was not an abbreviation at all, but it was certainly descriptive of my friend's habit of optimism in regard to the weather. For the cockney oarsman who doubtfully contemplated the weather conditions on the upper Thames, Sol was unwavering in his encouragement. His certainty that the weather would clear and the sun come out was so inspiring that the pale-faced Londoner cheerfully faced the most unpromising outlook, and started out on his uncertain course upstream, buoyed with a beautiful confidence in Old Sol's infallibility. But for me and for his other intimates, regular clients whose custom was not dependent on the chances of a fine week-end, Sol had another method. In answer to the usual question, "Well, Sol, what's it going to do?" he would first look up into the sky, then step to the edge of the landing-stage and study as much of the horizon as was within his limit of vision. After this careful survey he would deliver his opinion judicially, and I rarely found him at fault in his prophecy.

Facing my critics, lay and professional, I wish at the outset to disclaim the methods by which Sol invigorated the casual amateur. I am not prophesying unlimited sunshine for every one, without regard to conditions. In this book no mention will be found of royal roads, panaceas, or grand specifics. I have attempted rather to treat every reader as Sol treated his intimates. I have looked into the sky and made a careful survey of the horizon. It is true that I have seen an ideal and the promise of its fulfilment, but by deductions have been drawn with patient care from signs which I have studied with diligence; if I am an optimist, it is because I see the promise of fair weather, and not because I wish to delude the unwary. And with this I will lay down my metaphor and come to a practical statement.

I know that I shall be regarded in many quarters as a revolutionary and a heretic, for my theory and practice, though founded on a principle as old as the life of man, are not in accord with, nor even a development of, the tradition which still obtains. But in thus rejecting tradition I am, happily, sustained by something more than an unproved theory. Moreover, on this firm ground I do not stand alone. Though my theory may appear revolutionary and heretical, it is shared by men of attainment in science and medicine. On a small scale I have made many converts, and in now making appeal to a wider circle I am upheld by the knowledge that what I have to say can no longer be classed as an isolated opinion.

Not that I should have hesitated to come forward now, even if I had been without support. During the past thirteen years I have built up a practice in London which has reached the bounds of my capacity. This work has not been done by any advancement of a wavering hypothesis. I have had cases brought to me as the result of the failure of many kinds of treatment, of rest cures, relaxation cures, hypnotism, faith cures, physical culture, and the ordinary medical prescriptions, and in the treatment of these cases, in my own observations, and in the appreciation of the patients themselves, I have had abundant opportunity to prove to my own satisfaction that in its application to present needs my theory has stood the test of practice in every circumstance and condition.

That the limits imposed by the present work render it woefully inadequate I am quite willing to admit, but the necessity for a certain urgency has been forced upon me, and I have deemed it wiser to outline my subject at once rather than wait for the time when I shall be ready to publish my larger work. Indeed, when I think of the material even now at my command, of the wonderful and ever-increasing list of illustrative cases that have passed and are still passing through my hands, it seems to me that this preliminary treatise might well grow, like Frazer's *Golden Bough*, from one volume to twelve. In the present volume, however, I must confine myself to the primary argument and to indicating the direction in which we may find physical completeness. In the work which will follow I shall deal with the detailed evidence of the application of my theory to life, of cases and cures, and all the substance of experience.

And there are many reasons why I should hesitate no longer in making my preliminary appeal, chief among them being the appalling physical deterioration that can be seen by any intelligent observer who will walk the streets of London or New York, for example, and note the form and aspect of the average individuals who make up the crowd. So much for the surface signs. What inferences can we not draw from the statistics? To take three instances only: What of the disproportionate and apparently undeniable increase in the cases of cancer, appendicitis and insanity? For that increase goes on despite the fact that we have taken the subject seriously to heart. Now I would not fall into the common fallacy of *post hoc ergo propter hoc,* and say that because the increase of these evils has gone hand-in-hand with our endeavours to raise the standard by physical-culture theories, relaxation exercises, rest cures, and *hoc genus omne*, therefore the one is the result of the other; but, lacking more definite proof on the first point, I do maintain that if physical-culture exercises, etc., had done all that was expected of them they must be considered a complete failure in the checking of the three evils I have instanced.

Are these troubles, then, still to increase? Are we to wait while the bacteriologist patiently investigates the nature of these diseases, until he triumphantly isolates some characteristic germ and announces that here, at last, is the dread bacillus of cancer?[1] Should we even then be any nearer a cure? Could we rely on inoculation, and even if we could, what is to be the end? Are we to be inoculated against every known disease till our bodies become depressed and enervated sterilities, incapable of action on their own account? I pray not, for such a physical condition would imply a mental condition even more pitiable. The science of bacteriology has its uses, but they are the uses of research rather than of application. Bacteriology reveals a few of the agents active in disease, but it says nothing about the conditions which permit these agents to become active. Therefore I look to that wonderful instrument, the human body, for the true solution of our difficulty, an instrument so inimitably adaptable, so full of marvellous potentialities of resistance and recuperation, that it is able, when properly used, to overcome all the forces of disease which may be arrayed against it.

In this thing I do not address myself to any one class or section of the community. I have tried in what follows to avoid, so far as may be, any terminology, any medical or scientific phrases and technicalities, and to speak to the entire intelligent public. I wish the scheme I have here adumbrated to be taken up universally, and not to be restricted to the advantage of any one body, medical or otherwise. I wish to do away with such teachers as I am myself. My place in the present economy is due to a misunderstanding of the causes of our present physical disability, and when this disability is finally eliminated the specialised practitioner will have no place, no uses. This may be a dream of the future,

---

[1] Modern investigators, however, almost unanimously incline now to the theory that the cause of cancer is a morbid proliferation of the cells not due to the primary influence or isolation of alien bacteria.

but in its beginnings it is now capable of realisation. Every man, woman, and child holds the possibility of physical perfection; it rests with each of us to attain it by personal understanding and effort.

F. MATTHIAS ALEXANDER.

16 Ashley Place,
Westminster,
London.

CONTENTS

PART III

THE THEORY AND PRACTICE OF A NEW METHOD OF RESPIRATORY RE-EDUCATION

INTRODUCTORY WORD

MANY persons have pointed out the strain which has come upon human nature in the change from a state of animal savagery to present civilisation. No one, it seems to me, has grasped the meaning, dangers and possibilities of this change more lucidly and completely than Mr. Alexander. His account of the crises which have ensued upon this evolution is a contribution to a better understanding of every phase of contemporary life. His interpretation centres primarily about the crisis in the physical and moral health of the individual produced by the conflict between the functions of the brain and the nervous system on one side and the functions of digestion, circulation, respiration and the muscular system on the other; but there is no aspect of the maladjustments of modern life which does not receive illumination.

Frank acknowledgment of this internecine warfare in the very heart of our civilisation is not agreeable. For this reason it is rarely faced in its entirety. We prefer to deal with its incidents and episodes as if they were isolated accidents and could be overcome one by one in isolation. Those who have seen the conflict have almost always proposed as a remedy either a return to nature, a relapse to the simple life, or else flight to some mystic obscurity. Mr. Alexander exposes the fundamental error in the empirical and palliative methods. When the organs through which any structure, be it physiological, mental or social, are out of balance, when they are unco-ordinated, specific and limited attempts at a cure only exercise the already disordered mechanism. In "improving" one organic structure, they produce a compensatory maladjustment, usually more subtle and more difficult to deal with, somewhere else. The ingeniously inclined will have little difficulty in paralleling Mr. Alexander's criticism of "physical culture methods" within any field of our economic and political life.

In his criticism of return or relapse to the simpler conditions from which civilised man has departed Mr. Alexander's philosophy appears in its essential features. All such attempts represent an attempt at solution through abdication of intelligence. They all argue, in effect, that since the varied evils have come through development of conscious intelligence, the remedy is to let intelligence sleep, while the pre-intelligent forces, out of which it developed, do their work. The pitfalls into which references to the unconscious and subconscious usually fall have no existence in Mr. Alexander's treatment. He gives these terms a definite and real meaning. They express reliance upon the primitive mind of sense, of unreflection, as against reliance upon *reflective* mind. Mr. Alexander sees the remedy not in a futile abdication of intelligence in order that lower forces may work, but in carrying the power of intelligence further, in making its function one of positive and constructive control. As a layman, I am incompetent to pass judgment upon the particular technique through which he would bring about a control of intelligence over the bodily organism so as not merely to cure but to prevent the present multitudinous maladies of adjustment. But he does not stop with a pious recommendation of such conscious control; he possesses and offers a definite method for its realisation, and even a layman can testify, as I am glad to do, to the efficacy of its working in concrete cases.

It did not remain for the author of these pages to eulogise self-mastery or self-control. But these eulogies have too frequently remained in the hortatory and moralistic state. Mr. Alexander has developed a definite procedure, based upon a scientific knowledge of the organism. Popular fear of anything sounding like materialism has put a heavy burden upon humanity. Men are afraid, without even being aware of their fear, to recognise the most wonderful of all the structures of the vast universe—the human body. They have been led to think that a serious notice and regard would somehow involve disloyalty to man's higher life. The discussions of Mr. Alexander breathe reverence for this wonderful instrument of our life, life mental and moral as well as that life which somewhat meaninglessly we call bodily. When such a religious attitude toward the body becomes more general, we shall have an atmosphere favourable to securing the conscious control which is urged.

In the larger sense of education, this whole book is concerned with education. But the writer of these lines was naturally especially attracted to the passages in which Mr. Alexander touches on the problems of education in the narrower sense. The meaning of his principles comes out nowhere better than in his criticisms of repressive schools on one hand and schools of "free expression" on the other. He is aware of the perversions and distortions that spring from that unnatural suppression of childhood which too frequently passes for school training. But he is equally aware that the remedy is not to be sought through a blind reaction in abolition of all control except such as the moment's whim or the accident of environment may provide. One gathers that in this country, Mr. Alexander has made the acquaintance of an extremely rare type of "self-expressive" school, but all interested in educational reform may well remember that freedom of physical action and free expression of emotion are means, not ends, and that as means they are justified only in so far as they are used as conditions for developing power of intelligence. The substitution of control by intelligence for control by external authority, not the negative principle of no control or the spasmodic principle of control by emotional gusts, is the only basis upon which reformed education can build. To come into possession of intelligence is the sole human title to freedom. The spontaneity of childhood is a delightful and precious thing, but in its original naïve form it is bound to disappear. Emotions become sophisticated unless they become enlightened, and the manifestation of sophisticated emotion is in no sense genuine self-expression. True spontaneity is henceforth not a birth-right but the last term, the consummated conquest, of an art—the art of conscious control to the mastery of which Mr. Alexander's book so convincingly invites us.

JOHN DEWEY.

PART I
MAN'S SUPREME INHERITANCE

CHAPTER I

FROM PRIMITIVE CONDITIONS TO PRESENT NEEDS

"Our contemporaries of this and the rising generation appear to be hardly aware that we are witnessing the last act of a long drama, a tragedy and a comedy in one, which is being silently played, with no fanfare of trumpets or roll of drums, before our eyes on the stage of history. Whatever becomes of the savages, the curtain must soon descend on savagery forever."

J. G. FRAZER.

THE long process of evolution still moves quietly to its unknown accomplishment. Struggle and starvation, the hard fight for existence working with fine impartiality, remorselessly eliminate the weak and defective. New variations are developed and old types no further adaptable become extinct, and thus life fighting for life improves towards a sublimation we cannot foresee. But at some period of the world's history an offshoot of a dominant type began to develop new powers that were destined to change the face of the world.

Speculations as to what first influenced that strange and wonderful development do not come within the province of this treatise, but I should like in passing to point out that the theory and practice of my system are influenced by no particular religion nor school of philosophy, but in one sense may be said to embrace them all. For whatever name we give to the Great Origin of the Universe, in the words of a friend of mine, "we can all of us agree . . . that we mean the same thing, namely, that high power within the soul of man which enables him to will or to act or to speak, not loosely or wildly, but in subjection to an all-wise and invisible Authority." The name that we give to that Authority will in no way affect the principles which I am about to state. In subscribing to them the mechanist may still retain his belief in a theory of chemical reactions no less than the Christian his faith in a Great Redeemer. But through whatever influence these new powers in man came into being I maintain that they held strange potentialities, and, among others, that which now immediately concerns us, the potentiality to counteract the force of evolution itself.

This is, indeed, at once the greatest triumph of our intellectual growth and also the self-constituted danger which threatens us from within. Man has arisen above nature, he has bent circumstance to his will, and striven against the mighty force of evolution. He has pried into the great workshop and interfered with the machinery, endeavouring to become master of its action and to control the workings of its component parts. But the machine has as yet proved too intricate for his complete comprehension. He has learned gradually the uses of a few parts which he is able to operate, but they are only a small fraction of the whole.

What then is man's position to-day, and what is his danger? His position is this. In emerging from the contest with nature he has ceased to be a natural animal. He has evolved curious powers of discrimination, of choice, and of construction. He has changed his environment, his food, and his whole manner of living. He has enquired into the laws which govern heredity and into the causes of disease. But his knowledge is still limited and his emergence incomplete. The power of the force we know as evolution still holds him in chains, though he has loosened his bonds and may at last free himself entirely. Thus we come to man's danger.

Evolution—a term we use here and elsewhere in this connexion as that which is best understood to indicate the whole operation of natural selection and all that it connotes—has two clearly defined functions; by one of these it develops, by the other destroys. By an infinitely slow action it has developed such wonders as the human eye or hand; by a process somewhat less tedious it allows any organ that has become useless to perish, such as the pineal eye or (in process) the vermiform appendix, and, if we can estimate the future course, the teeth and hair.

By the change he has effected in his mode of life, man is no longer necessarily dependent upon his physical organism for the means of his subsistence, and in cases where he is still so dependent, such as those of the agriculturist, the artisan, and others who earn a living by manual labour, he employs his muscles in new ways, in mechanical repetitions of the same act, or in modes of labour which are far removed from those called forth by primitive conditions. In some ways the physical type which represents the rural labouring population is, in my opinion, even more degenerate than the type we find in cities, and mentally there can be no comparison between the two. The truth is that man, whether living in town or country, has changed his habitat and with it his habits, and in so doing has involved himself in a new danger, for though evolution may be cruel in its methods, it is the cruelty of a discipline without which our bodies become relaxed, our muscles atrophied, and our functions put out of gear.

The antagonism of conscious as opposed to natural selection[2] has now been in existence for many thousands of years, but it is only within the last century or less that the effect upon man's constitution has become so marked that this danger of deterioration or decay has been thrust upon the attention, not only of scientific observers, but of the average, intelligent individual. No examination of history is necessary in this place to set out a reason for this comparatively sudden realisation of physical unfitness. Briefly, the civilisation of the past hundred years has been unlike the many that have preceded it, in that it has not been confined to any single nation or empire. In the past history of the world an intellectual civilisation such as that of Egypt, of Persia, of Greece, or of Rome, perished from internal causes, of which the chief was a certain moral and physical deterioration which rendered the nation unequal to a struggle with younger, more vigorous, and—this is important—wilder, more natural peoples. Thus we have good cause for believing that the danger we have indicated, though as yet incipient only, was a determining cause in the downfall of past civilisations. But we must not overlook the fact that destructive wars and devastating plagues held sway in the earlier history of mankind, and whilst the latter acted as an instrument of evolution in destroying the unfit, the former, by decreasing the population, threw a burden of initiative and energy on the remnant, necessitating the use of active, physical qualities in the business of all kinds of production.

Now the conditions have altered. Greater scientific attainments in every direction than have ever been known have combated, and will probably in the future overcome, the devastating diseases which have decimated the populations of cities, whilst a higher ethical ideal constantly tends to oppose the horrible and repugnant barbarism of war which, with the spread of civilisation even to the peoples of the Orient, becomes to our senses more and more fratricidal, a fight of brother against brother.

A hundred years ago Malthus, a prophet if not a seer, recognised our danger and within the past quarter of a century a dozen theorists have proposed remedies less stringent than those advocated by Malthus, but

[2]It should, however, be clearly understood in this connexion that certain laws of natural selection must, so far as we can see, always hold good; and it would not be advisable to alter them even if it were possible. For example, that curious law may be cited which ordains the attraction of opposites in mating and so maintains nature's average. The attraction which a certain type of woman has for a certain type of man, and vice versa is, in my opinion, a fundamental law, and any attempt to regulate it would be harmful to the race. This, however, is no argument against the regulation or prevention of marriages between the physically and mentally unfit.

almost equally futile. Among the theorists are those perhaps unconscious reactionaries who advocate the simple life, by a return to natural food and conditions, in endlessly varying ways. To them in their search for natural foods and conditions we would point out that countless generations separate us from primitive man, a lapse of time during which our functions have become gradually adapted to new habits and environment, and that if it were possible by universal agreement for the peoples of Europe to return instantly to primitive methods of living, the effect would be no less disastrous than the reversal of the process, the sudden thrusting of our civilisation upon savage tribes whereby, to quote one or two recent examples only, the aborigines of North America, New Zealand, and Japan (the Ainu tribes) have become, or are rapidly becoming, extinct.

When therefore we point out man's power of adaptability in this connexion, the emphasis is thrown on the slowness with which that adaptability is passed on to our descendants and on the relative permanence of the new powers acquired. For our purpose the argument remains good whether we admit or deny the inheritability of acquired characteristics, our point being that in either case the process is necessarily a slow one, though it is plainly more rapid if the hypothesis be true.[3]

From the savage to the civilised state, man passed, as I say, so slowly that the passing in the early stages caused neither difficulties nor changes sufficiently marked to force themselves on our recognition. In other words, the subject of these changes was unconscious of them, and the habit of depending upon these sensory appreciations ("feeling tones," or "sense of feeling"), dominant by right in the savage or subconsciously directed state, remained firmly established in the civilised experiences, so that to-day man walks, talks, sits, stands, performs in fact the innumerable mechanical acts of daily life without giving a thought to the psychical and physical processes involved.

It is not surprising that the results have proved unsatisfactory. The evils of a personal bad habit do not reveal themselves in a day or in a week, perhaps not in a year, a remark that is also true of the benefits of a good habit. The effects of the racial habits I am now describing have gone on unnoticed for untold centuries. But in the last hundred years the evil has become so marked that its effect has at last forced itself upon our attention. The failure of subconscious guidance in modern civilisation is now being widely admitted, and the consideration of this fact has led a few to the logical conclusion that conscious guidance and control is the one method of adapting ourselves not only to present con-

[3]For a further statement of one aspect of heredity, see Chapter VI of this book.

ditions, but to any possible conditions that may arise. We have passed beyond the animal stage in evolution and can never return to it.

For these reasons it becomes necessary, if we would be consistent, to reject at once all propositions for improving our future well-being which can by any possibility be described as reactionary. Even in this brief résumé of man's history one tendency stands out clearly enough, the tendency to advance. When that first offshoot from a dominant type began to develop new powers of intellect, a form was initiated which must either progress or perish. Atavism must be counteracted by the powers of the mind, and reaction is a form of atavism. No return to earlier conditions can increase our knowledge of the secret springs of life, or aid our formulation of world-laws by the understanding of which we may hope to control the future course of development.

The physical, mental, and spiritual potentialities of the human being are greater than we have ever realised, greater, perhaps, than the human mind in its present evolutionary stage is capable of realising. And the present world crisis surely furnishes us with sufficient evidence that the familiar processes we call civilisation and education are not, alone, such as will enable us to come into that supreme inheritance which is the complete control of our own potentialities. One of the most startling fallacies of human thought has been the attempt to inaugurate rapid and far-reaching reforms in the religious, moral, social, political, educational, and industrial spheres of human activity, whilst the individuals by whose aid these reforms can be made practical and effective, have remained dependent upon subconscious guidance with all that it connotes. Such attempts have always been made by men or women who were almost completely ignorant of the one fundamental principle which would so have raised the standard of evolution, that the people upon whom they sought to impose these reforms might have passed from one stage of development to another without risk of losing their mental, spiritual, or physical balance.

For in the mind of man lies the secret of his ability to resist, to conquer and finally to govern the circumstance of his life, and only by the discovery of that secret will he ever be able to realise completely the perfect condition of *mens sana in corpore sano*.

CHAPTER II

PRIMITIVE REMEDIES AND THEIR DEFECTS

> ". . . Having heard that Henry Taylor was ill, Carlyle rushed off from London to Sheen with a bottle of medicine, which had done Mrs. Carlyle good, without in the least knowing what was ailing Henry Taylor, or for what the medicine was useful."
>
> *LIFE OF* TENNYSON.

THE danger of mental, nervous, and muscular debility, which is the outcome of the conditions resulting from the trend of our development, has been widely recognised during the past fifty years, and we must turn aside for a moment to consider certain phases of its treatment as indicated by the well-known and widely applied terms "physical culture," "relaxation," and "deep-breathing."

With regard to "physical-culture," it must be clearly understood that I do not allude to any one system or practice, but speak in the widest terms; terms which are applicable alike to the most primitive forms of dumb-bell exercise, or to the most elaborate series of evolutions designed to counteract the effect of a particular malady. But lest my application of the term be misunderstood, I will explain that where I write "physical-culture" thus, between inverted commas and with a hyphen, I mean it to stand for "a series of *mechanical* exercises, simple or complicated, designed to strengthen a bodily function by the development of a set of muscles or of the complete system of muscles"; but where I use the words physical culture, currently and without a hyphen, I denote a general system for the improvement of the entire physical economy by a just co-ordination and control of all the parts of the system, particularly excluding any method which tends to the hypertrophy of any one energy without regard to the balance of the whole.

In the first place it will be recognised from what I have already said, that the whole theory upon which the present "physical-culture" school is based is but another aspect of the reversion to nature which we have stigmatised as a form of atavism. It is an attempt to stiffen the new garment of our intellectual development by lining it with the old fabric of so-called "natural exercise." "Physical-culture" as defined, is what one might term the obvious, uninspired method which naturally presents itself as a remedy for the ills arising from an artificial condition. The logic of it is of the simplest, and proceeds from the major premise that bodily defects arise from the disuse and misuse of muscles and energies in an artificial civilisation, which muscles and energies in a natural state would be continually called upon to provide the means of livelihood.

From this it seems obvious to argue that if we contrive an artificial mechanical means of exercising these muscles for, let us say, one, two, or three hours a day, they will resume their natural functions, and so—The lacuna cannot be satisfactorily filled. If we carry on the argument to its logical conclusion the fallacy is made evident. For the method arising from this argument creates civil war within the body. There is no co-ordination, and the outcome must be strife. This point will be at once made clear by an instance which must be taken to represent a broadly typical case, an allegory rather than a special example of particular application.

Let us take for example the case of John Doe, whose work keeps him indoors from 9 a.m. to 6 p.m., and makes a very urgent call upon his mental and nervous powers. By the time he is thirty-five, possibly five or ten years earlier, John Doe is suffering from anæmia, indigestion, nervous debility, lassitude, insomnia, heart weakness, and heaven only knows what other troubles. His bodily functions are irregular, his muscular system partly atrophied and unresponsive, his nerves irritated, and his general condition—there is really no better word—"jumpy."

Incidentally I must add that his mind is inoperative in many directions. He has a bad mental attitude towards the physical acts of everyday life. For him his body is a mechanism, the intricate workings of which he never pauses to examine, but which drives or forces through a certain series of evolutions similar in kind to those it has always performed within his experience. When this mechanism fails, it has to be forced on again by tonics and stimulants or given a "rest," which is followed by a return to the old methods of propulsion.

However, John Doe, who has already postponed far too long his search for a remedy, at last takes a course of "physical-culture," although his time is severely limited, and his exercises are confined to an hour or two morning and evening. At first he may say that he feels a wonderful benefit and probably advises every friend he meets in the city to follow his example. I am quite willing to grant that Doe may be benefited, I will even admit that if he continues his exercises it is possible he may not fall back into the same state of nervous prostration into which he fell originally, but the point I wish to make quite clear is that his cure did not in itself possess the elements of permanence. It was merely a tinkering or botching-up of the fabric of his body. For if we consider his case from a purely detached standpoint, we must see that Doe attempted to develop two systems or modes of life which could not in the nature of things work harmoniously together. On the one hand, for two, three or four hours a day, he was occupied in mechanically developing his muscular system without making any reference in the *manner* in which he drove his machine, and stimulating and accelerating the supply of blood which therefore required increased oxygenation or reinforced lung power; in brief, he was exercising those functions and energies which in a primitive state would have been called upon during the greater part of his waking life to supply him with food. On the other hand, for the remaining twelve hours or so during which he was engaged in his profession, in the eating of meals and in reading, in playing indoor games or in similar sedentary occupations, the newly developed powers were being neglected and a call was being made upon the old nervous energies and centres of control. John Doe's physical body thus had two existences, excluding the natural condition of sleep, one fiercely active, muscular, dynamic, the other sedentary, nervous, static.

These two existences are not correlated, they are antagonistic; they do not mutually support each other, they conflict. John Doe's body becomes the scene of a civil war, and the heart, lungs, and other semi-automatic organs are in a state of perpetual readjustment to opposing conditions, as they are called upon to support one side or the other in the perpetual combat. Such a condition cannot tend in the long run to the improvement of mankind as a whole.

For, as I shall show later,[4] in the case of John Doe and in all parallel cases, the consciousness of the person concerned is not changed in regard to the use of the muscular mechanism. Even if he exercises for six hours daily, on taking up his ordinary occupations once more he will immediately revert to the same muscular habits he has already acquired in connexion with such occupations. For it is clear that John Doe has a wrong mental attitude towards the uses of his muscular mechanism in the acts of everyday life. He has been using muscles to do work for which they were never intended, whilst others, which should have been continuously employed, have remained undeveloped, inert, imperfectly controlled. We may say in truth he is suffering from mental and physical delusions with regard to the uses of his body. To mention but one of many instances of his lack of recognition of the true uses and functions of his muscular system, we shall notice that whenever he thrusts his

[4]For a fuller analysis of this, see p. 61 et seq. of this volume.

head forward or throws it back his shoulders always accompany the movement in either direction, this movement of the shoulders being entirely unconscious and made without any recognition of the fact that they are being moved. Now in this condition of mental and physical delusion, the unfortunate man tries to do something with these mechanisms which he is unable to control, hoping that by the mere performance of certain physical exercises he can restore his body to a condition of perfect physical health.

It may be well at this point, seeing that I have admitted the possibility of some preliminary benefit to John Doe from his first experience of the "physical-culture" exercises, to show more in detail why that benefit was not maintained. The fact is that when this man realised the seriousness of his digestive troubles he was simply recognising a symptom and not a primary cause or causes of his increasing disorders. A proper psycho-physical examination would have revealed bad habits in his waking and sleeping moments which tended more or less to reduce his intra-thoracic capacity to a minimum; such a minimum is not only harmfully inadequate but also renders due functioning of the vital organs practically impossible.

Incidentally it may be of value to consider what this condition of minimum intra-thoracic capacity really means and to note some of the influences upon the whole organism. For as this thoracic cavity contains many of the vital organs, the whole abdominal viscera is directly or indirectly influenced by its capacity. Minimum thoracic capacity means that the organs within the thorax are harmfully compressed and that the heart and lungs do not get a proper chance to function adequately. A harmful strain is thrown upon the heart, the lungs are not adequately employed or sufficiently aerated, and the lung tissue deteriorates. The proper distribution of the blood is interfered with because of the undue accumulation in the splanchnic area, to the detriment of the lung supply. As the lungs are the chief distributors of blood it will be understood that this condition of minimum thoracic capacity interferes with the circulation and general nutrition. The respiratory processes are employed in sucking in air instead of creating a partial vacuum in the lungs by a co-ordinated thoracic expansion which will give atmospheric pressure its opportunity.[5] There is an undue intra-abdominal pressure and harmful flaccidity of the abdominal muscles, which means dropping of the viscera, imperfect functioning of the liver, kidneys, bladder, etc., stagnation in the bowels and irritation and distention of the colon, intestines, etc.; in other words, indigestion, constipation and all the con-

[5]For a fuller explanation, see Chapter VI, p. 89.

comitant disorders and general impairment of the vital functioning. Let us, for a moment, think of the thoracic and abdominal cavities as one fairly stiff oblong rubber bag filled with different parts of a working machine which are interrelated and interdependent, and which are held in position by their attachment to the different parts of the inner surface of this bag. We will then suppose, for the sake of our illustration, that the circumference of the inner upper half of this bag is three inches more than that of the lower half. As long as this general capacity of the bag is maintained the working standard of efficiency of the machinery is indicated as the maximum. Let us then, in our mind's eye, decrease the capacity of the upper part of the bag and increase that of the lower half until the inner circumference of the latter is three inches more than the former. We can at once picture the effect upon the whole of the vital organs therein contained, their general disorganisation, the harmful irritation caused by undue compression, the interference with the natural movement of the blood, of the lymph and of the fluids contained in the organs of digestion and elimination. In fact we find a condition of stagnation, fermentation, etc., causing the manufacture of poisons which more or less clog the mental and physical organism, and which constitutes a process of slow poisoning.

Now to revert to the experiences of John Doe. I have already stated that when he first tried physical exercises at home or in the gymnasium as a remedy for his digestive disorders, he experienced a sense of relief. This was only natural, seeing that he was leading a more or less sedentary life. Why, then, was the effect of these exercises gradually diminished until he considered the physical treatment a comparative failure? This brings us to the point of real interest. The fact is that any increased amount of exercise does give a sense of relief to those who lead sedentary lives, but unfortunately this sense of relief is too often a delusive mental exaggeration of the real changes in the right direction. It is not often a reliable register of benefits derived which make for permanent relief. Students of these questions know that the man whose conditions we are analysing has already developed debauched *kinæsthetic* systems which permit defective registrations of different sensations or feeling-tones, and hence it is very difficult for the person so constituted to arrive at a reliable estimate of the extent of his improvement through such faulty senses. We know, too, that, so far as he is concerned, the improvement is not permanent, a fact which he readily admits. There are scientific reasons for accepting the accuracy of this conclusion, and I will endeavour to explain the position. Let us admit, for the sake of our explanation, that benefits actually accrued in various directions in the early stages of his physical exercises. Whatever these benefits may have been, and however great they were, I contend that it was always certain that sooner or later if he persisted in the physical exercises, he would gradually develop defects which would counterbalance and finally outweigh the benefits we have admitted.

The following are some of the reasons which support these contentions. I shall deal more fully with them in later chapters.

(1) *A Defective Kinæsthetic System.* Experience has proved to us that the conditions present, when he took up the exercises, go hand in hand with an incorrect and defective kinæsthetic system.

The mere performance of physical exercises could not give him a new and correct kinæsthetic sense in connexion with the use of the mental and physical organism in his acts of everyday life.

(2) *Erroneous Preconceived Ideas.* It is impossible for me to set down the myriad dangers with which he is beset in consequence of erroneous preconceptions during his daily practice on "physical-culture" lines. The pages of a fairly large book will be necessary to do even meagre justice to this subject. But I can assure my readers that this is demonstrably true and I am daily convincing the most sceptical by practical procedures.

(3) *Defective Sense-Registration and Delusions.* This serious defect is in practice linked up with erroneous preconceptions resulting in mental and physical delusions which are far-reaching and dangerous.

An Example. Take a person who, prior to re-education, has the habit of putting the head back whenever an attempt is made to put the shoulders back. Ask this person to put the head forward and keep the shoulders still and it will be found that as a rule he fails to carry out the order, and moves his shoulders also. Ask him to put the head forward whilst the teacher holds the shoulders still, and the pupil will put the head back instead of forward.

(4) *Defective Mental and Physical Control.* The most common form of this defective control encountered in teaching work is when the teacher wishes to move the head, or hand, or arm, or leg for the pupil, in order to give the new and correct sensation in the proper use of the parts. Experience proves that the great majority are utterly wanting in the controls necessary to enable the person to gain this experience quickly.

The teacher asks the pupil to lift his arm. He does so but exercises an undue amount of tension. In order to give the pupil the new kinæsthetic register of the correct amount of tension necessary, the teacher asks to be permitted to lift the arm for him, but as a rule the pupil acts exactly as he did when he was requested to perform the act himself.

(5) *Defective Inhibition.* The practical teacher finds all pupils more or less hampered by lack of inhibitory control, the possession of which would make re-education and co-ordination from the pupil's standpoint comparatively easy. Consideration will show that our ordinary mode of life and the generally accepted teaching methods do not make for the development of the inhibitory powers. On the contrary, our powers in this direction rather tend to diminish, and the outward and visible signs of the serious results are everywhere for him who runs to read.

(6) *Self-Hypnotism.* This very serious and all too common evil has not been attacked on a practical basis. People have spoken of it and written about it in a general theoretical way, much as they have done about relaxation, but with no better results on the practical side, when applied to everyday life. The self-hypnotism I am referring to is a specific self-hypnotism indulged in at a given and particular time, and is cultivated unknowingly by teachers and pupils during lessons, and frequently by both in everyday life.

People will tell you they can think better by closing their eyes. This is a prevalent form of self-hypnotism, self-deception, and produces a state of dreaming which is particularly serious because it is a harmful condition assumed consciously. The ordinary dreamer falls into this condition unconsciously.

(7) *Cultivated Apprehension.* This is probably the most serious condition which we cultivate and which has been dealt with at length on pages 142-147.

(8) *Prejudiced Arguments and Attempted Self-Defence.* The real weakness and shallowness of human nature is shown in this connexion in a way which is uncomplimentary to our intellectual pride. The saddest fact is, that it is always intensified in the person who would be counted above the average in intellectuality by a consensus of opinion. We are all well aware that such an one to win an argument will strain his statement of his facts in the direction he desires them. His reason is so dominated by his emotions and his sense appreciation (feeling-tones) that an appeal to the former is at first in vain. The majority of mankind has over-compensated in these directions, and it is for this reason that in the education and development of the child of to-

day and the future, we must see to it that we relinquish all educational methods which tend to cultivate guidance and control through the emotions and the sensory appreciations (feeling-tones).

Some perception of the evils we have thus briefly summarised has been awakened in the minds of the more earnest thinkers during the last few years, and, as a result, the systems of exercises display a clearly marked tendency towards modification. They have lessened their muscle-tensing violence, and have become, and are becoming, ever less and less strenuous physical acts. Thus we find "physical-culture" advocates who a few years ago insisted upon the use of dumb-bells, and in some cases dumb-bells increasing in weight over a graduated series of exercises, now emphasising the necessity for *gentle* exercises without even mentioning the dumb-bell, which is perhaps as good a proof as any of the truth of my contentions.

My next instance, namely, "relaxation," is even less efficient. The usual procedure is to instruct the pupil, who is either sitting or lying on the floor, to relax, or to do what he or she understands by relaxing. The result is invariably collapse. For relaxation really is invariably collapse. For relaxation really means a due tension of the parts of the muscular system intended by nature to be constantly more or less tensed, together with a relaxation of those parts intended by nature to be more or less relaxed, a condition which is readily secured in practice by adopting what I have called in my other writings the position of mechanical advantage.[6] But apart from an incorrect understanding of the proper condition natural to the various muscles, the theory of relaxation, like that of the rest cure, makes a wrong assumption, and if either system is persisted in, there must inevitably follow a general lowering of vitality which will be felt the moment regular duties are taken up again, and which will soon bring about the return of the old troubles in an exaggerated form.

The last remedy mentioned at the opening of this chapter was "deep-breathing." This is a later form of "physical-culture" development, and is, in effect, a modification in the right direction. It is the logical outcome of the perception that strenuous, forcing, muscular exercises were resulting in new and possibly greater evils than those they professed to cure. "Deep-breathing" is indeed a step in the right direction, but only a step, because, while it does not always do serious harm and in some instances, perhaps, a certain amount of good, it does not go to the root of the matter, the eradication of defects, nor does it take cognisance of

[6] See Part II, p. 111.

the most important factor in the scheme of physical co-ordination. What the radical factor is I shall explain in detail in my next chapter, but I will first briefly review the chief points of the argument as far as it has been unfolded.

In imagination we have seen man through the darkness which covers his first appearance on the earth, the early Miocene man. As we have pictured him, he was a creature of simple needs and of a vigorous bodily habit, an animal in all save that spark of self-consciousness which burned feebly in his primitive, but increasing and differentiating brain. Again we have a somewhat clearer vision of him with wider powers of courage and cunning, adapting weapons to his use, and so specialising the functions of his mind through a long two million years, through palæolithic and neolithic periods into the age of bronze, where he has become a reasoning, designing creature, with powers of imagination and idealisation, powers still turned, however, to physical uses.

And at last we reach the differentiation of man from man and class from class which marks the historical period of civilisation, the period of dwelling in cities, of adaptability to new and specialized habits, of labour that makes little or no call upon the physical capacities, of food procured without energy, the period when the slow process of evolution, which has resulted in the product of a new and marvellous instrument of self-conscious, directive powers, was becoming gradually superseded by that which it had brought forth.

CHAPTER III

SUBCONSCIOUSNESS AND INHIBITION

> "You can have neither a greater nor a less dominion than that over yourself."
>
> LEONARDO DA VINCI.

WITHIN the last thirty years we have evolved a new science, the science of psychology. A generation ago psychology was subject-matter only for the philosopher, the metaphysician, the poet, or the ecclesiastic; now it is being investigated in the laboratory by tests of sensibility, reaction-times, and other responses to stimulation too technical to be explained here, tests carried out by means of elaborate and intricate instruments and machinery designed to weigh the *hidden springs of life* in the balance. The phrase I have italicised is purposely vague, for I have no wish to fall foul of a terminology or to make any *a priori* assumption which might involve me in controversial matters completely outside my province. At the same time I see clearly that some convenient phrase will become necessary, and I will therefore adopt one which is at least familiar and within certain limits descriptive enough, namely, the "subconscious self."

It may seem strange that one should look to any such formally organised science as modern psychology, to a science that is working in a laboratory with mechanical appliances, for any elucidation of a question which has for so long been regarded as strictly within the domain of the priest. But science, as Tyndall said, is only another name for common-sense, and a little consideration will show that the postulate I have insisted upon, namely, the growth and progress of intellectual control, demands that this admirable quality of common-sense or reason, should be applied to the elucidation of this all-important problem. Unhappily, psychology, from which we hope so much, is as yet in its infancy, and the few attempts that have been made, such as those of the late Professor Münsterberg, to apply the theories of the laboratory and the class room to practical work of the world, cannot be said to have produced any results worth considering. In any case I must transcend the present limits of academic psychology in this consideration of the subconscious.

The concepts which have grown up round this term, the "subconscious self," are in many cases curiously concrete in form. Much error has sprung from that earnest and well-intentioned work of the late F. W. H. Myers, *Human Personality and Its Survival After Bodily Death.* Mr. Myers pictured an entity within an entity, and his work, though inductive in form, was *a priori* in method, for he had formed the conception of a subjective personality taking shape within an objective, material shell, and had controlled his evidence to a definite, preconceived end.

The fallacies of Myers have been exposed again and again. His argument is intrinsically unsound, and when put to the test of newer knowledge his hypothesis fails to explain the fact. But because Myers' conception was so graphic and credible it took a strong hold upon the popular imagination, a hold which the eight years following the publication of *Human Personality* has not become weakened in the minds of a great number of people, full though these years have been of discovery and new knowledge. It is for this reason that I have reverted to Myers' conception of the subconscious, or as he called it, the "subliminal self," inasmuch as I wish it to be clearly understood from the outset that I use the term "subconscious self" to denote an entirely different concept. Indeed, anyone who has followed my argument to this point must have inferred the trend of my purpose, namely, that as the intellectual powers of man extend, we progress in the direction of *conscious control.* The gradual control of evolution by the child of its production has pointed always to this end, and by this means, and by this alone, can the human race continue in the full enjoyment of its physical powers without forfeiting a fraction of its progressive intellectual ideal.

It will inevitably be asked at this stage what I mean when I speak of the "subconscious self," and I must therefore answer that question to the best of my ability, even though I have to leave for a moment the limits of proved fact and tread on the wider ground of hypothesis. I do not propose, however, to overburden my theory with the detail of evidence, and what follows must therefore be taken as an inclusive statement, much of which I could prove conclusively in a larger work, whilst the unproved remnant must necessarily await confirmation from the researches of future investigators in the domains of psychology. In the first place then we must see not only that the subconscious self is not a possession peculiar to man, but that it is in fact more active, in many ways more finely developed, in the animal world. Among some animals the consciousness of danger is so keen that we have attributed it to prescience. The fear of fire in the prairies, of flood, or of the advance of some natural danger threatening the existence of the animal, is evidenced far ahead of any signs perceptible by human senses, and as we cannot, except sentimentally, attribute powers of conscious reasoning to the animal world, it is evident that this "fore-knowledge" is due to a delicate co-ordination of animal senses. Again, we see that animals which have not had their powers dulled by many generations of domestication make the majority of their movements, as we say, "instinctively." They can judge the length of a leap with astonishing accuracy, or take the one certain chance of escape among the many apparent possibilities open to them without an instant's hesitation, and as these powers are evidenced in some cases within a few hours or minutes after the birth of the animal, they are admittedly not the outcome of experience.

The whole argument for the evidence of the possession of a subconscious self by animals can be elaborated to any length, and depends upon facts of observation made over a long period of time. The few examples I have here cited merely illustrate that side of the question which throws into prominence the point of what we may call abnormal powers, or powers which seem to transcend those of human reason so far as it has been developed. It is this appearance of transcendent qualities in the human subconsciousness which misled Myers, who did not pause to apply his allegory of the subconscious entity to the animal world. Such an application would have tended to prove that the "soul" (for that is what Myers really intended, however carefully he may have avoided the actual word) of the animal was more highly developed than that of man.

In the second place, however, we are confronted with the unquestionable fact that the subconsciousness can be "educated" below the plane of reason. Acts very frequently performed become so mechanical that they can be repeated without any sense of conscious awareness by the operator. The pianist, after constant rehearsals, will perform the most intricate passage while his attention is engaged with an entirely unrelated subject,—although it is particularly worthy of remark in this connexion, that when such an art as the performance of music falls temporarily into such an automatic repetition, the connoisseur will instantly recognise the loss of some quality,—generally spoken of as "feeling,"—in the rendering. Again, it appears that in some cases a more or less permanent impression may be made upon the subconsciousness by casual suggestions, often related to fear, even though such suggestions be, in some cases, the result of a single experience. A nervous hysterical subject, already far too willing to submit to the guidance of emotion and what he or she fondly believes to be "instinct" or "intuition" may be so harmfully impressed in this way as to develop any of the many forms of "phobia," which are, as the suffix correctly implies, forms of morbid terror. These are but two instances of the "education" of the subconciousness below the reasoning plane, but a dozen others will suggest themselves to the reader out of his own experience. The important point is the fact that the phase of being with which we are dealing becomes, as we progress through life, a composite of animal instincts and habits acquired below the plane of reason either by repetition or by suggestion. But before I leave this general conception of the subconsciousness, I must emphasise the fact that up to this point we share the qualities of the subconscious mind with the animal kingdom. For in the lower organisms no less than in that of humanity, this subconsciousness can be educated. The observations of naturalists now confirm the belief that the young of certain birds—the swallow has been particularly instanced—are *taught* to fly by the parent birds; whilst any one who has trained a dog will know how such a trick as "begging" for food may become so habitual as to appear instinctive.

So much for general definition; I come now to the point which marks the differentiation of man from the animal world, and which is first clearly evidenced in the use of the reasoning, intellectual powers of inhibition.

Now it is evident that in the earlier stages of man's development, the inhibition of the subconscious animal powers was frequently a source of danger and of death. Reason, not as yet sufficiently instructed and far-seeing, was an inefficient pilot, and sometimes laid the ship aback when she would have kept before the wind if left to herself. To abandon the metaphor, the control was imperfect, it wavered between two alternatives, and by rejecting the guidance of instinct suffered, it may be, destruction. But the necessity for conscious control grew as the conditions of life came to differ ever more and more from those of the wild state. This, plainly, was due to many causes, but chiefly to the limitations enforced by the social habit which grew out of the need for co-operation.

This point must be briefly elaborated, for it marks the birth of inhibition in its application to everyday life, and in so doing it demonstrates the growth of the principle of conscious control which, after countless thousands of years, we are but now beginning to appreciate and understand.

It is true that we have evidence of conscious inhibition in a pure state of nature. The wild cat stalking its quarry inhibits the desire to spring prematurely, and controls to a deliberate end its eagerness for the instant gratification of a natural appetite. But in this, and in the many other similar instances, such instinctive acts of inhibition have been developed through long ages of necessity. The domestic kitten of a few weeks old, which has never been dependent on its own efforts for a single meal, will exhibit the same instinct. In animals the inherited power is there; in man also the power is there as a matter of physical inheritance, but with what added possibilities due to the accumulated experience gained from the conscious use of this wonderful force.

The first experience must have come to man very early in his development. As soon as any act was proscribed and punishment meted out for its performance, or as soon as a reward was consciously sought—though its attainment necessitated realised, personal danger—there must have been a deliberate, conscious inhibition of natural desires, which in its turn enforced a similar restraint of muscular, physical functioning. As the needs of society widened, this necessity for the daily, hourly inhibition of natural desires increased to a bewildering extent on the prohibitive side. There grew up first "taboos," and then the rough formulation of moral and social law, and on the other hand a desire for larger powers which encouraged qualities of emulation and ambition.

Among the infinite diversity of these influences, natural appetites and the modes of gratifying them were ever more and more held in subjection, and the subconscious self or instinct which initiated every action in the lower animal world fell under the subjection of the conscious, dominating intellect or will. And in this process we must not overlook one fact of supreme importance, viz., man still progressed physically and mentally. It is therefore clear that this control acquired by the conscious mind broke no great law of nature, known or unknown, for, if this acquired control had been in conflict with any of those great, and to us as yet incomprehensible forces which have ruled the evolution of species, the animal we call man would have become extinct, as did those early saurian types which failed to fulfil the purpose of development and perished before man's first appearance on this earth.

Before we attempt, then, any exact definition of the subconscious self we must have a clearer comprehension of the terms "will," "mind," and "matter," which may or may not be different aspects of one and the same force. More than two thousand years of philosophy have left the metaphysicians still vaguely speculating as to the relations of these three essentials, and personally, I am not very hopeful of any solution from this source. The investigation, though still in its infancy in this form, has taken the shape of an exact science, and it is to that science of psychology as now understood that I look to the elucidation of many difficult problems in the future. Without touching on the uncertain ground of speculative philosophy, I will try, however, to be as definite as may be with regard to my conception of the subconscious self.

In the first place, great prominence has been given to the conception of the subconscious self as an entity within an entity, by the claim made for it that it has absolute control of the bodily functions. This claim depends for its support upon the evidence of hypnotism and of the various forms of auto-suggestion and faith-healing. Under the first heading, we have been told that under the direction of the hypnotist the ordinary functions of the body may be controlled or superseded, as for instance, that a wound may be formed and bleed without mechanically breaking the skin,[7] or that a wound may be healed more rapidly than is consistent with the ordinary course of nature. Under the second heading, which includes all forms of self-suggestion, we have had examples of what is known as stigmatisation,[8] or the appearance on the bodies of hysterical and obsessed subjects of some imitation of the five sacred wounds. Indeed the instances of cures which seem to our uninstructed minds miraculous, and due by inference to the power of faith, are so numerous that no special example need be cited. These and many kindred phenomena have been explained on the hypothesis that the hidden entity when commanded by the will is able to exert an all-powerful influence either beneficent or malignant, the obscure means by which the command may be enforced being variously described. We see at once that the conception of a hidden entity is the primitive explanation which first occurs to the puzzled mind. We find the same tendency in the many curious superstitions of the savage who turns every bird, beast, stone, and tree into a Totem, and endows them with powers of evil or of good, and discovers a "hidden entity," all of a piece with this conception of the subconscious self, in a piece of wood that he has cut from a tree, or a lump of clay that he has modelled into the rude shape of man, bird, or beast.

My own conception is rather of the unity than the diversity of life. And since any attempt to define the term Life would be presumptuous, the definition being beyond the scope of man's present ability, I will merely say that life in this connexion must be read in the widest application conceivable. And it appears to me that all we know of the evolution or development of life goes to show that it has progressed, and will continue to progress, in the direction of self-con-

[7]Cf. *Hypnotism*, by Albert Moll. Good cases of suppuration, blistering, and bleeding, as the result of suggestion without any preliminary abrasion of the skin, are those supplied by the records of Professor Forel's experiments at the Zurich Lunatic Asylum. These experiments were conducted on the person of a nurse who is described as the daughter of healthy country people, and not a hysterical subject.

[8]There is much evidence on this point, some of it conflicting, but the main fact must be considered above question.

sciousness.[9] If we grant the unity of life and the tendency of its evolution, it follows that all the manifestations of what we have called the "subconscious self" are functions of the vital essence or life-force, and that functions are passing from automatic or unconscious to reasoning or conscious control. This conception does not necessarily imply any distinction between the thing controlled and the control itself. This may be inferred from the use of the word "self-conscious," but the further elucidation of this side of the theory is not germane to the present argument.

Now I am quite prepared to accept as facts phenomena of the kind I have instanced, such as unusual cures effected by hypnotism, and by the somewhat allied methods of the various forms of faith-healing, but I do deny, and most emphatically deny, that either procedure is in any way necessary to produce the same or even more unusual phenomena.[10] In other words, I maintain that man may in time obtain complete conscious control of every function of the body without, as is implied by the word "conscious," going into any trance induced by hypnotic means, and without any paraphernalia of making reiterated assertions or statements of belief.

Apart from my practical experience of the harm that so often results from hypnotic and suggestive treatment, an experience sufficient to demonstrate the dangers of applying these methods to a large majority of cases, I found my objection to these practices on a broad and, I believe, incontrovertible basis. This is that the obtaining of trance is a prostitution and degradation of the objective mind, that it ignores and debases the chief curative agent, the apprehension of the patient's conscious mind, and that it is in direct contradiction to the governing principle of evolution, the great law of self-preservation by which the instinct of animals has been trained, as it were, to meet and overcome the imminent dangers of everyday existence. In man this desire for life is an influence in therapeutics so strong that I can hardly exaggerate its potentiality, and it is, moreover, an influence that can be readily awakened and developed. The will to live has in one experience of mine lifted a woman almost from the grave, a woman who had been operated upon and practically abandoned as dead by her surgeons. A passing thought flashing across a brain that had all but abandoned the struggle for existence, a sudden consciousness that her children might not be well cared for if she died, was sufficient to reawaken the desire for life,

---

[9]Cf. Herbert Spencer, *Education*, Chapter XI, "Humanity has progressed solely by self-instruction."

[10]Moreover, I deny that hypnotism can possibly succeed except in comparatively rare instances. It is not universal in its applicability.

and to revivify a body which no medical skill could have saved.[11] But there is no need to quote instances. The fact is recognised, yet how small is the attempt made to use and control so potent a force! The same argument may be also applied to the prostration of the mind as a factor in the popular rest cures which really seek to put the mind, the great regenerating force, out of action.

Returning to my definition of the subconscious self, it will be seen that I regard it as a manifestation of the partly-conscious vital essence, functioning at times very vividly but on the whole incompletely, and from this it follows that our endeavours should be directed to perfecting the self-consciousness of this vital essence. The perfect attainment of this object in every individual would imply a mental and physical ability and a complete immunity from disease that is still a dream of the future. But once the road is pointed, we must forsake the many bypaths, however fascinating, bypaths which lead at last to an *impasse* and necessitate a return in our own footsteps. Instead of this, we must devote our energies along the indicated road, a road that presents, it is true, many difficulties, and is not straight and easy to traverse, but a road that nevertheless leads to an ideal of mental and physical completeness almost beyond our imaginings.

[11] Two years later this woman came to me in a state of collapse, the result of the after effects of a bad attack of pleurisy. She proved an admirable patient, and is now in perfect health. She was a magnificent instance of a case in which the power was there, finely developed, but not the knowledge which would enable her to make full use of that power.

CHAPTER IV

CONSCIOUS CONTROL

"Man one harmonious soul of many a soul
Whose nature is its own divine control."

SHELLEY.

ONE of the most recent phases of popular, as opposed to scientific, thought has been that which has endeavoured to teach the control of the mind. This teaching has been spoken of as the "New Thought" movement, though certain of its precepts may be found in Marcus Aurelius. This movement has had, and is still having, a considerable vogue in America, and the influence of it has been felt in England, many of the writings of its exponents having been published here within the last fifteen or twenty years. The object of the teaching is to promote the habit of "right thinking" which is to be obtained by the control of the mind. The "New Thought" teaches that certain ideas such as fear, worry, and anger, are to be rigidly excluded from the mind and the attention fixed upon their opposites, such as courage, complacency, calm. With certain of the tendencies expressed in this movement I am in sympathy, but following the usual course of such movements, the "New Thought" is losing sight of its principle, which was, indeed, never fully grasped, and is becoming involved in a species of dogma, the rigidity of which is in my opinion, directly opposed to its primary object. One of its earlier and most capable exponents, however, Ralph Waldo Trine, marked the principle with a phrase, and by naming one of his works *In Tune with the Infinite*, gave permanence to the central idea, though more recent writers in embroidering the theme have lost sight of the original thesis. Moreover, I have not found in the "New Thought" a proper consideration of cause and effect in treating the mental and physical in combination. These writings exhibit, and have always exhibited, the fallacy of considering the mental and physical as in some sense antitheses which are opposed to each other and make war, whereas in my opinion, the two must be considered entirely interdependent, and even more closely knit than is implied by such a phrase.

Again in all these writings we are confronted with one word which is dominant, and by its iteration must produce an effect on the mind of all readers. That word is "faith," and because it is so prominent and so little understood, I feel that it is essential I should give some explanation of it in the light of my own principles.

In the first place, it is perhaps hardly necessary for me to point out that faith in this connexion need not be allied with any conception of creed or religion. It is true that this is the form in which we are most familiar with it in mental healing, and the associations which are grouped round the word itself very commonly induce us to connect it with the conceptions that have had such a wide and general influence on the thoughts of mankind in all stages of civilisation. But we have abundant evidence now before us that in healing it is the patient's attitude of mind that is of the first importance, and that faith is every whit as effective when directed towards the person of the healer, a drug, or the medicinal qualities supposed to be possessed by a glass of pure water, as when it is directed to a belief in some supernal agency. This fact is indisputable, and it is only because the latter form of faith is so much more widespread, inasmuch as it lies at the very foundation of all religions, that this agency has effected a number of cures out of all proportion to those brought about by faith in some purely material object. What I here intend by faith, therefore, is its exercise in the widest sense and without any restriction of creed.

So far as we can analyse the effect of what we call an act of faith on the mental processes, it would seem that it is operative in two directions. The first is purely emotional. The patient having conceived a whole-hearted belief that he is going to be delivered from his pain or disease by the means of some agency supernal or material, experiences a sensation of profound relief and joy. He understands and believes that without effort on his part he is to be cured by an apparent miracle, and the effect upon him is to produce a strong, if evanescent, emotional happiness. In this we have an exact parallelism between the patient whose cure is physical and material, and the convert whose cure is spiritual. Now it is widely acknowledged by scientists and the medical profession generally that this condition of happiness is an ideal condition for the sufferer, that it is not only the most helpful condition of mind, but that it actually produces chemical changes in the physical constitution, changes which are the most salutary in producing a vital condition of the blood, and hence of the organisms.

The second way in which this act of faith operates is in the breaking down of a whole set of mental habits, and in the substitution for them of a new set. The new habits may or may not be beneficial from the outset apart from the effect produced by the emotional state which is hardly ever maintained for a long period, but even so the breaking down of the old habits of thought does produce such an effect as will in some cases influence the whole arrangement of the cells forming the tissues, and dissipate a morbid condition such as cancer.

Thus we see that this so-called act of faith is in reality purely material in its action, and there is no reason why we should have recourse to it to produce the same and greater effects. It may perhaps be asked by some objectors why we should seek to dismiss the act of faith, since it undoubtedly produces these ideal conditions in some cases. The answer is obvious. Faith-healing is dangerous in its practice and uncertain in its results. It is dangerous, because in the majority of cases its professors seek in the first place to alleviate pain. They may do this, leaving the disease itself untouched, but, as I shall point out later on, in such cases the disease will continue and eventually kill the patient, even though he may be able successfully to fight the pain. Faith-healing is also uncertain in its results, because, in addition to the danger I have mentioned, it merely substitutes one uncontrolled habit of thought for another. At first the new habit, because it is new, may bring about a change to a better condition, but if it remains, it will in its turn become stereotyped, and may very well lead at last to just as morbid a condition as was induced by the old mental habit it superseded. For these reasons, which are, I think, trenchant enough, I desire most earnestly to see all the present conceptions that surround this profession of faith-healing thrown aside in order that we may arrive at a sane and reasoned process of mental therapeutics. I have touched briefly on the movement here because it emphasises the fact that we are dimly grasping at a truth but paralysing our attempts to hold it by the premature assumption that we have it safe at last. At the same time I believe that underlying the teachings of these recent movements, "New Thought" and "Faith-healing" in general (and in these two closely allied influences I include all the offshoots and subdivisions), there is some apprehension of an essential, an apprehension which is liable to lose its grip by reason of the dogma and ritual that has grown up and tends to obscure the one fundamental.

All these sects, parties, societies, creeds—call them what you will—have a common inspiration; we need no further proof than this that no one of the many developments from the common source is in itself complete and perfect. There is good evidence that each new development as soon as it becomes specialised is separated from its true source, becomes overelaborated, and so works its own downfall, the principle becoming absorbed and dominated by the bias of some individual mind. This is my analysis of the phenomena. It follows that what we seek is the noumenon, the reality, the true idea that underlies all these various manifestations.

Before I attempt, however, to trace this common principle, I wish to make three statements.

> (1) I do not profess to offer a finally perfected theory, for by so doing I should lay myself open to the same arguments I have advanced against other theories of the same nature. I say frankly that we are only at the beginnings of understanding, and my own wish is to keep my theory as simple as possible, to avoid any dogma.
>
> (2) I do not propose for many reasons to consider in this place my own methods in any other connexion but that of their application to physical defects, to the eradication of diseases, distortions, and lack of control, and, progressively, to the science of race-culture and the improvement of the physique of the generations to come.
>
> (3) I wish it to be clearly understood that this treatise is not finally definitive. I hope in the future to have many opportunities of elaborating my general thesis, and of stating my experience of particular applications of my methods to peculiar cases, but I should not be true to my own principles if I were not willing to accept amendments, even perhaps to alter one or other of my premises, should new facts tend to show that I have made a false assumption in any particular.

Now that I have thus cleared the ground, I will examine what I believe to be the first and greatest stumbling block to conscious self-control, namely, "rigidity of mind." This rigidity results in the fixed habit of thought and its concomitant evils, among which is the subjection of functional and muscular habits to subconscious control.

In defining rigidity of mind, I must hark back for a moment to that suggestive phrase of Mr. Trine's, *In Tune with the Infinite*, although in the present application the rigidity I am concerned with is considered in a physical connexion and does not involve interference with any non-spatial conceptions. It is rather the first half of the phrase that is here of importance, for to be "In Tune" conveys to my mind, and I wish it to convey the same meaning to others, the idea of sensitiveness to impressions and responsiveness to the touch, when "all the functions of life are becoming an intelligent harmony." In a word, I want by this phrase to suggest the idea of being open-minded. For even in reading this, if the individual deliberately puts himself in opposition to my point of view, he can by no possibility hope to benefit. Wherefore I desire above all things that he or she will read at least with an open mind, and form no conclusion until I have finished, and will perhaps, more particularly, subdue the interference of that great and ruling predisposition which has in the past so long impeded the advance of science, and with which I will deal in my next chapter.

Let us consider for a moment the application of rigidity of mind to physical functions. A person comes to me with some crippling defect due to the improper use of some organ or set of muscles. When I have diagnosed the defect and shown the patient *how* to use the organ or muscles in the proper way, I am always met at once with the reply, "But I can't." Let me ask any one who is reading this and who suffers in any way, whether his or her attitude to the defect they suffer from is not precisely the same? This reply indicates directly that the control of the part affected is entirely subconscious; if it were not, we should merely have to substitute the hopeful "I can" for that despondent "I can't," to remove the trouble. By (a) hypnotic treatment, by (b) faith-healing, or by (c) the application of the principles of the "New Thought," the patient in such a case would have the subconscious control influenced, either (a) by the mechanical means of trance and suggestion by the hypnotist, which leaves the conscious mind in exactly the original condition and merely changes, and it may be only temporarily, the habit of the subconscious control, or (b) and (c) by reiterated commands of the objective mind. Even if these commands have been reinforced by the influencing suggestion of the healer, they either substitute by repetition one habit for another without any apprehension by the intelligence of the true method of the exchange, or, what is quite as frequent and far more harmful, they shut out the sensitiveness to pain from the cerebral centres, and so leave the radical evil, no longer labelled by nature's warning, to work the patient's destruction in secret. Briefly, all three methods seek to reach the subjective mind by deadening the objective or conscious mind, and the centre and backbone of my theory and practice, upon which I feel that I cannot insist upon too strongly, is that THE CONSCIOUS MIND MUST BE QUICKENED.

It will be seen from this statement that my theory is in some ways a revolutionary one, since all earlier methods have in some form or another sought to put the flexible working of the true consciousness out of action in order to reach the subconsciousness. The result of these methods is, logically and inevitably, an endeavour to alter a bad subjective habit whilst the objective habit of thought is left unchanged. The teachings of the "New Thought" and many sects of faith-healers set out clearly enough that the patient must think rightly before he can be cured, but they then set out, automatically, to carry out their teaching by prescribing "affirmatives" or some sort of "auto-suggestion" both of which are in effect no more than a kind of self-hypnotism, and, as such, are debasing to the primary functions of the intelligence.

I will take a simple instance from my own experience to illustrate a case in point. A patient, whom I will call X, came to me with an obstinate stammer arising from a congenital defect in the co-ordination of the face, tongue, and throat muscles. Whenever X attempted to speak he drew down his upper lip. This was the outward sign of a series of vicious acts connected with a train of muscular movements, a sign that the ideo-motor centres were working to convey a wrong guiding influence to the specific parts concerned in the act of speech. These guiding influences rendered X quite incapable of speech, and would, indeed, have had the same effect upon any other individual who produced the same working of the parts concerned. To insist in such a case that X should repeat "I can speak," or "I won't stutter," would be merely to endeavour to reach a supposed omniscient subconscious self which would counteract the evil by the exercise of some assumed and separate intelligence possessed by it. I undertook the case by appealing to X's intelligence.

Now, strange as it may seem (and I intend to treat this curious perversion in my next chapter), X's objective intelligence is not so easily reached and influenced as might appear. He has formed a muscular habit of drawing down his lip independently of his conscious control, and the line of suggestion set up by the wish to speak induces at once a reflex action of a complicated set of muscles. X has learned to do this automatically, and at first seems incapable of controlling those lip muscles when the wish to speak is initiated.

In this case my first endeavour must be directed to keeping in abeyance, by the power of inhibition, all the mental associations connected with the ideas of speaking, and to eradicating all erroneous, preconceived ideas concerning the things X imagines he can or cannot do, or what is or is not possible. My next effort must be to give X a correct and conscious guidance and control of all the parts concerned, including, of course, the lip and face muscles, and in order to obtain this control, he must have a complete and accurate apprehension of all the movements concerned. And in this apprehension must precede and be preparatory to any conception of "speaking," during the application of all the guiding orders involved. In originating some new idea which is to take the place of the old idea of drawing down the upper lip, it may be necessary at first to break the old association by means of some new order, such as deliberately to draw the lip up, to open the mouth, or to make some similar muscular act previously unfamiliar in its application to the act of speaking. This new order is then substituted for the command to speak. X is told not to speak but to draw up his lip, open his mouth, etc. It will be understood that I have omitted much detail touching the interdependence of the parts concerned, but I wish here to convey the essentials of method rather than the physiological explanation of their working. It must always be remembered that Nature works as a whole and not in parts, and once the true cause of the evil is discovered and eradicated all the affected mechanisms can soon be restored to their full capacity. I may note here that X was completely cured of his stammer, and that his was a particularly obstinate case, a fact chiefly due to the confirmation of a wrong habit in early childhood.

This is an example, chosen for its simplicity, to illustrate the prime essentials of my theory, but it is capable of a very wide application, so wide that it may be applied to the working not only of the ordinary controlled muscles, but of the semi-automatic muscles which actuate the vital organs. Not many years ago an Indian Yogi was examined by Professor Max Müller at Cambridge, and we have it on the authority of the latter that this Yogi was able to stop the beating of his own heart at will and suffer no harmful consequences.

Let it be clearly understood, however, that I have no sympathy with these abnormal manifestations which I regard as a dangerous trickery practised on the body, a trickery in no way admirable or to be sought after. The performances of the Yogis certainly do not command my admiration, and the well-known system of breathing practised and taught by them is, in my opinion, not only wrong and essentially crude, but I consider that it tends also to exaggerate those very defects from which we suffer in this twentieth century. I have merely quoted this case of the Yogi in support of my assertion that there is no function of the body that cannot be brought under the control of the conscious will.

That this is indeed a fact and not a theory, I do claim without hesitation, and I claim further that by the application of this principle of conscious control there may in time be evolved a complete mastery over the body, which will result in the elimination of all physical defects. Certain aspects of this control and the reasons why it has not been acquired I will treat under the next heading.

CHAPTER V

APPLIED CONSCIOUS CONTROL

A Conception of the Principles Involved

THE term "conscious control" is one which is employed by different people to convey different conceptions. The usual conception is one which indicates specific control, such as the moving of a muscle consciously, and is practised by athletes who give performances of physical feats in public. Again, there is the conscious movement of a finger, toe, ear, or some other specific muscle or limb.

The phrase "Conscious Control" when used in this work is intended to indicate the value and use of conscious guidance and control, primarily as a *universal*, and secondly as a *specific*, the latter always being dependent upon the former in practical procedure.

Furthermore, it is not used merely to indicate a guidance and control which we may apply in the activities of life with but doubtful precision in one or two directions only, but one which may be applied universally, and with precision in all directions, and in all spheres where the mental and physical manifestations of mankind are concerned.

Since the publication of my book, *Conscious Control*, I have received and continue to receive letters from interested readers concerning the practical application of conscious control, and also regarding my conception of the principles involved.

"It is all very well to talk of conscious control, but how are we to acquire it?" wrote one enquirer. "How far-reaching is its application?" wrote another, whilst a third remarked, "If your experience has proved that such far-reaching beneficial effects result from conscious guidance and control, your concept must be much more comprehensive than that usually accepted." "I have a friend who is cursed with a bad temper," wrote another enquirer, "and he realises the fact. He has applied to his medical and spiritual advisers for help. They have given him a certain amount of valuable advice, but the result is far from satisfactory."

We all know of cases of men and women who eat or drink more than is good for them, and we also know that only a small minority are able to master their unhealthy desires in these directions. Examination of the misguided majority would reveal the fact that they were badly co-ordinated, and that psycho-physical conditions were present which would lead an expert to expect an overbalanced state in one direction or another, a domination of conscious reasoned control by subconscious unreasoned desire.

Such cases may be readily and successfully dealt with on a basis of conscious guidance and control in the spheres of re-education, re-adjustment, and co-ordination.

To gain control where there is a tendency to overindulgence in alcohol or food is a very difficult problem for the ordinary human being while he remains in his badly co-ordinated condition. This is shown by the failure which succeeds failure until the unfortunate person arrives at the conclusion that it is impossible to break the habit.

He or she then drifts into the advanced stages of a condition which becomes as akin to disease as neuritis, neurasthenia, indigestion, or rheumatism. As a matter of fact these malconditions may be the immediate outcome of the indulgences before referred to.

The unfortunate fact which we must face is that such people are practically without control where these failings are concerned, and the general opinion is that these people lack will-power. In my opinion this is not really true.

Say that a man is a thief and is caught and punished. He tells his friends and relatives that he intends to reform. But does he really intend to do so? In the first instance does not the answer to this question depend upon the point of view of the person concerned? Let us take as an example two brothers. The one is a thief but the other is not, inasmuch as he has never stolen anything in his life. He would scorn such an act, but he has no hesitation in taking advantage of a friend with whom he makes an agreement. He may even fail to realise that he is acting unjustly towards his friend. The fact is, he is well acquainted with the details and possibilities of the business concern which this agreement represents. He is aware of his superior knowledge and he deliberately uses it in framing the clauses of the agreement so that he is certain to derive more benefit from the transaction than his less experienced friend, though at the same time he may thoroughly understand that the contract should be drawn upon lines which would ensure that equal benefits would be derived. This he calls business, not theft.

It is quite possible that the thief would scorn to take such advantage of a friend. I have known of such cases; hence the phrase, "Honour among thieves."

Now we do not speak of the other brother as lacking in will-power, but wherein lies the difference in this connexion between him and his thief brother?

In the case of the thief, the promise to reform was made. He steals again and again, so that people say in the ordinary way, "He is hopeless, he hasn't the will-power to enable him to reform." As I have before indicated, I fear this is not a correct solution.

For if we admit that in both instances all depends upon the point of view, we cannot be surprised that the mere promise to reform is usually futile, and we must furthermore realise that a changed point of view is the royal road to reformation. At the same time, experience of human idiosyncrasies has taught us that the most difficult thing to change is the point of view of subconsciously controlled mankind. The lack of power to reform is the result of the usually partial failure of the subconscious mental mechanisms in a sphere demanding reasoned judgment.

As a matter of fact this man possesses a great amount of will-power and energy in certain directions, just as he probably lacks it in others. This applies equally to his brother and, in a greater or less degree, to every human being. At the same time I think we are justified in concluding that the thief, as compared with his brother, exercises his energy, will-power and resourcefulness in but limited directions. This applies to all people cursed with what we call criminal tendencies in contrast to their more fortunate fellow beings. Here we arrive at the point where we are once more confronted with misdirected energies concentrated into narrow channels through abnormal tendencies; hence the overcompensation which inevitably follows.

A thief, unfortunately, too often confines his energies to what to his perverted outlook—the result of a wrong point of view—is a legitimate means of gaining the necessaries of life. From his perverted point of view he merely takes something from another person which he considers he has as much right to possess as any one else, if he is clever enough to get it by any means at his command. I have heard a certain type of Socialist express views which justify this mode of reasoning. His point of view is practically that of the thief, and he needs the same help if he is to come into communication with his reason. We know that men and women have continued to steal for years without being even suspected, and there cannot be any doubt that in thus escaping detection, they prove that they possess forms of exceptional will-power, energy, resourcefulness, courage, determination, and initiative, which, if directed into the right channels, would have made them highly successful and valuable members of society.

It must not be forgotten that if the thief is detected, his punishments are so formidable, not only because of the legal penalties he incurs, but also because of the scorn and derision with which he meets in the social sphere, even amongst his blood relations, that they would act as a deterrent upon the ordinary person.

Obviously, then, the problem to be solved in connexion with the thief or any other criminal, is concerned with the psycho-physical conditions influence him in the direction of crime, and also with the failure of punishment either to change his point of view or to direct his excellent mental and physical gifts into honest and valuable spheres of expression.

We are all aware that a conservative is rarely converted to the liberal viewpoint or vice versa in a day, or a month, or even a year. Such mental changes, in the subconsciously controlled person should, with rare exceptions, be made gradually and slowly; for the demands of re-adjustment in the psycho-physical self are great, and depend upon the conditions present in the particular person. It is conceivable that with certain conditions present, the process of re-adjustment may bring about such disorganisation as may cause a serious crisis. During an experience of this kind the person would for a period be in greater danger than ever,[12]and the length of this period would vary in different people. The process of re-adjustment in all spheres means immediate interference with the forces of strength and weakness, and in the case of the thief under consideration the force of strength was associated with mental and physical peculiarities in him as evil factors which had more or less controlled him; in fact, they constituted guidance and direction in his case. In all his physical and mental activities, which these evil factors stimulated, he experienced his maximum of confidence and directive power.

Now where his weaknesses were concerned, he had little to depend upon. His attempt to reform was a demand for re-adjustment, which, in turn, meant a period of comparative loss of confidence and directive power. His new efforts needed to be directed into channels where he not only lacked confidence, but where he suffered most from the overcompensation experienced in the past. In reality, his supports were suddenly wrenched from him, and replaced by those which his well-meaning friends and relatives considered infinitely superior and absolutely reli-

---

[12]In this connexion the following verses (24, 25, 26) from the Gospel according to St. Luke, Chapter XI, are interesting:

24. When the unclean spirit has gone out of a man, he walketh through dry places, seeking rest: and finding none, he saith, I will return unto my house whence I came out.

25. And when he cometh, he findeth it swept and garnished.

26. Then goeth he, and taketh *to him* seven other spirits more wicked than himself; and they enter in, and dwell there: and the last state of that man is worse than the first.

able. Their experiences of life had, to their satisfaction, proved them to be so; but their experiences were not his experiences, their strength was not his strength, their weaknesses were not his weaknesses; and it is in consequence of such facts as these that subconscious control fails, and reasoned conscious control is needed.

If I have succeeded in making my point clear to the reader he will recognise and admit this unfortunate thief's danger. He must, in a way, sympathise with this man who, through no fault of his own, is being directed during the period of comparative helplessness, in a round of unfamiliar and complex experiences by a delusive and debauched subconsciousness. If, on the other hand, conscious reasoned control had been substituted and employed in re-education and co-ordination, the process of readjustment would have presented the minimum of the difficulties and dangers we have enumerated.

In view of the foregoing, are we justified, except in rare instances, in expecting to change the thief any more than the liberal or conservative by ordinary methods on a subconscious basis? The evidence in the light of experience is against the proposition.

The conservative and the liberal of our example, no less than the thief, are equally dependent upon subconscious guidance and control, and are the victims of the particular tendencies, harmful and otherwise, which have developed and become established, as a rule, without recognition, and without any primary appeal to their reasoning faculties.

Therefore, we must turn our attention once more to that psychophysical process which we call habit, including developments which have their origin in consciousness as well as those which spring from the subconsciousness.

For instance, a man may be, as we say, born a thief. In other words, he is cursed with the subconscious abnormal craving or habit which makes a man a thief by nature.

On the other hand, he may be quite normal at birth, but in early life he may drift into simple and apparently harmless little ways which through carelessness and lack of sound training, develop very slowly and remain unobserved either by the person concerned or by his friends and relatives.

We all know of men and women who became drug fiends merely through wishing to experience the sensation or sensations produced by the drug. In the most unsuspecting way it is repeated at some future time. This innocent beginning has so often developed into the drug habit.

We know of apparently strong-minded scientific men who have taken drugs, in the first instance, from a purely scientific standpoint and so in a seemingly harmless way, but who, in spite of this, have rapidly fallen victims to the drug habit. Exactly the same process has served to create the majority of inebriates.

It is important to keep in mind that different men and different women fall victims to some particular stimulant or drug, whilst they are in absolute mastery of themselves where other seductive influences are concerned.

For instance, A became addicted to a certain drug habit, but although he had taken alcohol from an early age he never became an immoderate drinker. It was not until he came into contact with this particular drug that his latent abnormality or weakness or whatever one chooses to call it, became fully manifested. Again, B had lived in China, and had continually smoked opium with the Chinese. He did so for a year without the habit gaining any hold upon him, but the tea habit on the contrary became his danger. Despite the fact that his health was seriously affected by overindulgence in tea, and that according to his medical advisers' opinion he had, by its immoderate use, developed certain troubles which caused him considerable suffering, he continued his excesses in tea drinking, as others do who come under the influence of drugs, or of alcohol, in one or all of its forms.

When this point is reached these people are, in the words of Emerson, "out of communication with their reason"; a subconscious tendency. Herein lies the explanation of difficulties which they rarely surmount, difficulties which could not remain as such if subconscious control were supplanted by conscious guidance and control of the whole organism; for in practical procedures in life this conscious guidance and control connotes "bringing them once more into communication with their reason" and supplying the "means whereby" of successful readjustment.

That they were out of communication with reason is indicated by the fact that though they knew they were seriously ill, and were told by their doctors that in order to regain health they must abstain from certain foods and drinks, they did not so abstain. Their continuance in indulgence merely satisfied some inward craving which can only become a governing factor as against human reason, when men are controlled by the subconscious instead of by the conscious powers; for subconscious control (instinct) is the outcome of experiences in those spheres where the animal senses exercised the great controlling and directing influences in the early stages of man's evolution; whereas conscious control (reasoned experience) through re-education, co-ordination and readjustment is the result of the use of the reasoning powers in the conduct of life, by means of which man may fight his abnormal desires for harmful sensory experiences.

The fact that civilised human beings will take wine or sugar or drugs, when conscious that it is gradually undermining health and character, is proof positive of the domination of the physical over the mental self, exactly as in the Stone Age.

It shows that in the case of sugar, for instance, they have become victims to the sense of taste. In other words, the sensations produced by the sense of taste influence and finally govern their conduct in this connexion, whereas instead they should be governed by the faculties of reason. They have developed vicious complexes in which perverted physical sensations must be satisfied, even at the cost of mental and physical injury, and often of intense pain.

This psycho-physical state does not indicate satisfactory progress on the evolutionary plane up to the present time, and, furthermore, it does not give promise of greater progress in the future under this same subconscious direction. The domination of certain perverted sensations presents another interesting phase, inasmuch as these sensations are very often associated with comparatively superficial complexes.

For instance, take the case of a person who is suffering from the ill effects of taking sugar in harmful quantities. If he happens to decide to abstain from satisfying his taste desires in regard to sugar, and actually abstains, for, say, a week or ten days, it often happens that he loses the seductive pleasing sensation formerly derived from sugar, and frequently develops a positive dislike for it.

This also serves to reveal in the majority of people the unreliability of the different senses, such as taste, etc. Of course, in all these cases this unreliability is due to abnormality in one or more directions, usually more, and this fact emphasises the absolute necessity for the establishment of those normal conditions which demand conscious guidance and control, for their maintenance in civilisation; conditions which tend to eradicate and prevent abnormal cravings and desires in any direction.

When discussing the forgoing phenomena with friends and pupils, I am frequently asked questions like this: "To what are we to attribute the particular manifestations of strength or weakness in different people, where specific abnormal sensations are concerned?"

"Why is one person swayed unduly by some particular sensation which he knows is ruining his health and causing daily suffering, whilst another, equally abnormal and deluded though proof against this failing of his fellow being, succumbs to some other type of sensory influence?"

It is simply a matter of the psycho-physical make-up of the individual, of his inherent tendencies, and of his general experiences of life in different environments. All people whose kinæsthetic systems are debauched and delusive develop some form of perversion or abnormality in sensation. The point of real importance is to eradicate and prevent this kinæsthetic condition in order to make impossible in the human being such domination by sensation.

There is another point which exercises the layman's mind, and that is that great suffering, in consequence of abnormal indulgence in some direction, does not act as a deterrent.

Of course, if these unfortunates were in communication with their reason and were thus consciously guided and controlled, such suffering would serve to prevent them from repeating the experience which caused it.

To those who have studied this curious phase of mental and physical phenomena, it would almost seem that they derived a form of satisfaction or pleasure from such suffering; otherwise, one would conclude, they would not continue to repeat the acts, which, in their experience, have been followed by actual pain and discomfort.

And surely there is nothing very unreasonable in this suggestion, seeing that there is little doubt that *ill health* in some people is just as natural as *health* is in others.

It simply means an attempt on the part of nature to do her work where the conditions are *abnormal*, in accordance with the same process as where they are *normal*.

The person enjoying the latter condition abhors suffering and pain, and will act reasonably in order to prevent both, and it is quite consistent with our knowledge and experience of the abnormal in the human organism to incline to the idea that those who are afflicted with abnormal tendencies find a perverted form of pleasure in pain.

And all these suggestions serve to support the theory that the first principle in all training, from the earliest years of child life, must be on a conscious plane of co-ordination, re-education and re-adjustment, which will establish a normal kinæsthesia.

The abnormal condition referred to is more or less governed by the senses through the subconsciousness and we must remember that the great controlling forces in the animal kingdom are chiefly *physical*. It is also in keeping with the purely animal stage of evolution, and any advance from this stage demands that the balance of powers must gradually move in favour of the mental.

The controlling and guiding forces in savage four-footed animals and in the savage black races are practically the same; and this serves to show that from the evolutionary standpoint the mental progress of these races has not kept pace with their physical evolution from the plane of the savage animal to that of the savage human.

This brings us to the crux of my contentions regarding conscious guidance and control in its widest meaning, that is, as a universal.

Wherever we find the domination of subconscious (instinctive) control, it affords proof that in the lowly evolved states of life the physical is the great controlling force, and we are well aware that this condition does not ensure progress to those higher planes of evolution which should be the goal of civilised growth and development, the goal for which mankind was undoubtedly destined.

The inadequate relative progress of the mental evolution of the black races as compared with that of their physical evolution, when considered in relation to their approximation to the savage animals, cannot be considered other than a most disappointing result. It surely does not furnish any convincing evidence that mankind is likely to advance adequately on the evolutionary plane in civilisation by continuing to rely upon the original subconscious guidance and control.

CHAPTER VI

HABITS OF THOUGHT AND OF BODY

> "The man who has so far made up his mind about anything that he can no longer reckon freely with that thing, is mad where that thing is concerned."
>
> ALLEN UPWARD, *THE NEW WORD.*

WHEN speaking of the case of stammering, cited in my last chapter, I had occasion to note that it was not an easy task to influence X's conscious mind. The point is this: A patient who submits himself for treatment, whether to a medical man or to any other practitioner, may DO what he is told, but will not or cannot THINK as he is told. In ordinary practice the man who has taken a medical degree disregards this mental attitude in ninety-nine cases out of a hundred. Medicine, diet, or exercise is prescribed, and if the patient obediently follows the mechanical directions given with regard to the prescriptions, he is considered a good patient. The doctor does not trouble as to the patient's attitude of mind, except in that one case out of a hundred, possibly a case of flagrant hypochondria.

Indeed I am willing to maintain and prove in this connexion that a very large percentage of cases which are now being treated in our public and private lunatic asylums, have been allowed to develop insanity by reason of this disregard of the mental attitude. I cannot stop now to consider this interesting subject of insanity, but I must note in passing that the very large percentage of the cases I have mentioned should never have been allowed to arrive at the condition which made it necessary to send them to an asylum in the first instance. Very many of them, so far from lacking mental control, possess minds of quite exceptional ability. Some are instances of subjects who in the first place have assumed a deliberate attitude to subserve a private end, such as the avoidance of uncongenial work, or the overindulgence of some desire or perverted sense, the result being that the attitude which was first adopted deliberately, became afterwards a fixed habit, and so uncontrollable.

When therefore we are seeking to give a patient conscious control, *the consideration of mental attitude must precede the performance of the act prescribed.* The act performed is of less consequence than the manner of its performance. It is nevertheless a remarkable fact that although the patient or enquirer into the system may apprehend this truth, he often finds an enormous difficulty in altering some trifling habit of thought which stands between him and the benefit he clearly expects. And the simple explanation of this apparently strange enigma is that the majority of people fall into a mechanical habit of thought quite as easily as they fall into the mechanical habit of body which is the immediate consequence.

I will take an instance from a subject outside my own province in order to bring the matter home, but I will preface my illustration by pointing out that I personally am not in the least concerned to alter the habit of thought of either of the persons I bring forward as examples, and I only cite well-known political propaganda in order to give vividness to my picture.

Let us suppose then that A is a convinced Free-Trader, and that Z is no less certain of the glorious possibilities of Protection, and let us set A and Z to argue the matter. We notice at once that when A is speaking Z's endeavours are confined to catching him in a misstatement or in a fault of logic, and A's attitude is precisely the same when Z holds the stage. Neither partisan has the least intention from the outset of altering his creed, nor could either be convinced by the facts and arguments of the other, however sound. This is a fact within the experience of every intelligent person. The disputants have so influenced their own minds that they are incapable of receiving certain impressions; a part of their intelligence normally susceptible of receiving new ideas, even if such ideas are opposed to earlier conceptions, is in a state of anæsthesia; it is shut off, put out of action. The habit of mind which has been formed mechanically translates all the arguments of an opponent into misconceptions or fallacies. Neither disputant in our illustration has the least intention or desire to approach the subject with an open mind. Unfortunately, the rigid habit of mind does not only apply to political issues; it is evidenced in all the thoughts and acts of our daily life, and is the cause of many demonstrable evils.

And touching this question of mental rigidity, I may cite a very valuable criticism from Mr. William Archer, the well-known London dramatic critic, on the primary point of the "Desirability of the Open Mind." This criticism was published in *The Morning Leader* for 17th December, 1910. I replied in the same paper, and my answer was published on 23rd December, 1910.

As this brief discussion illustrates very clearly the misconception which most easily arises with regard to this question, I now reprint these two letters, precisely as they originally appeared.

THE OPEN MIND

By William Archer

"In the fifth chapter of an able and interesting book by Mr. F. Matthias Alexander, entitled *Man's Supreme Inheritance* (Methuen), there occurs a passage which I propose to take as the text of this week's discourse. Treating of 'mechanical habits of thought,' Mr. Alexander says:

> "'Let us suppose that A is a convinced Free Trader, and that Z is no less certain of the glorious possibilities of Protection, and let us set A and Z to argue the matter. We notice at once that when A is speaking, Z's endeavours are confined to catching him in a misstatement or in a fault of logic, and A's attitude is precisely the same when Z holds the stage. Neither partisan has the least intention from the outset of altering his creed, nor could either be convinced by the facts and arguments of the other, however sound. . . . The habit of mind which has been formed mechanically translates all the arguments of an opponent into misconceptions or fallacies. Neither disputant has the least desire to approach the subject with an open mind. Unfortunately this rigid habit of mind does not only apply to the issues of government; it is evidenced in all the thoughts and acts of our daily life, and is the cause of many demonstrable evils.'

"Very often, of course, the fact is as Mr. Alexander states it; but can we, I wonder, accept the ideal of the 'open mind' implied in his illustration? Is not a certain stability of conviction absolutely necessary to the efficient conduct of the business of life? And are we not almost as apt to err on the side of impressionability as on the side of rigidity? I seem to remember a warning in Scripture against being 'blown about by every wind of doctrine.'

"If we reflect for a moment, I think we shall see that the amount of open-mindedness which reason demands must vary according to the nature of the question at issue. On a question of fact, which is capable of absolute demonstration, it is, of course, folly to let prejudice or bias prevent us from perceiving the truth. But it is not on such questions that disputes commonly arise. Theology, I fancy, is, in the modern world, almost the only influence that frequently leads people to close their minds against demonstrable facts or overwhelming probabilities. But of the most important questions in life, many are not questions of fact at all, while as to others, the evidence is so complex or so inaccessible that demonstration is not, as the saying goes, humanly possible. It is proverbially futile to argue on questions of taste; for enjoyment consists in a relation of the perceiver to the thing perceived which cannot be produced by force of reason or of reasoning. No doubt, in going to "Salome" or to the Post-Impressionist Exhibition, we ought to take with us an open mind; that is to say, we ought not to go in a wilfully Philistine or frivolous mood. And in discussing them afterwards, we ought to preserve an open mind, in so far that we ought not to make a law of our own limitations, and accuse of folly or insincerity those people who see more in post-Wagnerism and post-Manetism than (perhaps) we do. Yet even here open-mindedness may be carried to excess; for undoubtedly there exists a great deal of affectation and charlatanism in matters of art, and it would be weak credulity to take every Maudle and Postlewaite at his own valuation. "A popgun remains a popgun," says Emerson, "though the ancient and honourable of this world affirm it to be the crack of doom"; and there are innumerable questions of quality and value on which no one who has any mind at all can possibly keep his mind open.

"Let us turn now to political questions of the order suggested by Mr. Alexander's illustration. They are not, as a rule, questions of ascertainable fact, but of speculation or conjecture as to the probable results of a given course of action. They are generally very complex questions; the present issue between the two Houses of Parliament is almost unique in its simplicity. And not only is each question complex in itself; it is inextricably interwoven with other questions of similar complexity. Can we reasonably expect or desire, then, that either A or Z, in a single discussion of such a topic and Tariff Reform, should have his whole system of thought revolutionised? When such a conversion occurs (and I suppose it does sometimes occur) ought we to praise the convert's open mind? Ought we not rather to pity his shallow mind, in which the new conviction can scarcely be deeper rooted than the old? A man's political opinions, I take it, if they have any substance and consistency, are, and ought to be, a sort of mosaic set in a cement of fundamental principle. You may alter the pattern by laborious picking and rearranging but not by a mere push at a single point. Does it follow from this that political discussion is an idle waste of time? Not at all. It forces us to rethink our thoughts, and to keep them consciously and clearly related to fundamental principles. Also it sifts our arguments; in looking out for our opponent's fallacies we not infrequently become aware of our own. Furthermore, a discussion may form part of the long course of thought, or evolution of feeling, whereby a really valid conversion may be ultimately brought about. Though we may think ourselves wholly unmoved by our opponent's reasoning, a subconscious effect may remain, and may in due time manifest itself. Without our realising it, one or two cubes in our mental mosaic may, in fact, have been loosened. A greater result than this, from any single discussion of a complex political question, is scarcely, I think, to be desired. No doubt it is highly desirable that we should at one time or another have brought a perfectly open mind to the study of such a question as Tariff Reform; and this many of us have done. For my own part, I can honestly say that when Mr. Chamberlain first threw the apple of discord into our midst, I so clearly realised the merely traditional and unreasoned character of my Free Trade ideas, that I was biased, if anything, against them, and fully prepared to find them fallacious. The fact that I have not done so may be due to insufficient or unintelligent study, but certainly not to any initial lack of openness of mind.

"Finally, I would note another limitation to the ideal of the open mind. There are certain questions on which we cannot safely keep our minds open, because we know that that way madness lies. I once spent a whole day at Concord, Mass., arguing with a friend who had become a convert to astrology, and was bent on drawing my horoscope. To that I had no objection; but I cannot pretend that my mind was for a moment open to his arguments. Somewhat more difficult is the case of the Bacon-Shakespeare theory: ought we to keep an open mind on that? I am inclined to answer, 'No'; for if we once lose grip of the fact that the whole thing is an insanity, we are in danger of being submerged in a swirling torrent of *'folie lucide.'* The origin and psychological conditions of the illusion are perfectly plain. It is, indeed, one of the oddest and most instructive incidents in the history of the human error, and in that sense worthy of study. Poor Bacon has been forced, by no fault of his own, into the position of the Tichborne Claimant of literature, and one cannot but wonder what he would think of the Onslows, Whalleys, and Kenealys, who are pleading what they believe to be his cause. But a really 'open mind' on the question is, I conceive, a symptom of an exorbitant love of the marvellous and an imperfect hold upon the reality of things. There are subjects on which no mind can remain open without in some degree losing its balance."

THE OPEN MIND

To the Editor of the "Morning Leader"

"Sir—Although Mr. William Archer has rather misapprehended my point of view in his very interesting article, I would not intrude a reply upon you did I not believe that this question is one that lies at the root of so many physical evils, and that it is a question, therefore, which must not be hastily put on one side—as, no doubt, many of your readers will be inclined to put it after their perusal of Mr. Archer's temperate and, apparently, logical reasoning. I say 'apparently,' because, though his syllogism is sound enough, it is based on a faulty premise due to his misapprehension of my statement; doubtless, I am to blame for not having made myself fully comprehensible.

"In the first place, let me admit at once that the whole question is relative. Mr. Archer's implied example of the man 'blown about by every wind of doctrine,' is an example, from my point of view, of rigidity rather than plasticity, inasmuch as he is necessarily a hysterical neurotic, and is almost entirely dependent on his subconscious processes. Now, it is these very subconscious processes which restrict the use of the conscious, reasoning centres; which form what we call habits of mind, that, becoming fixed, are almost beyond the control of reason; which, in extreme cases, take possession of what was once the intelligence, and are manifested as the *idée fixe*, the obsession, the monomaniacal tendency.

"But, disregarding these extremes, let me take an example from ordinary life, and, perhaps, no better one could be offered than Mr. Archer's own of the Bacon-Shakespeare controversy, a subject, among others, which Mr. Archer suggests is sufficient to upset our reason, should we attempt to maintain an open mind with regard to it.

"As a matter of fact, what he conceives as an open mind here is a mind with an inclination to be perverted (or converted) by specious reasoning. The right attitude of the open mind in this case is, 'I have weighed the arguments in favour of Bacon's authorship and have found them insufficient, and until such a time as new and better evidence is forthcoming, I shall continue to hold the view I have always held.'

"The rigid attitude which I condemn in this connexion is the one that says, 'You will never alter my opinion, whatever fresh evidence you may adduce.' In the first example we can come to a conclusion on the evidence; the conscious reason has been exercised and remains in command. It is not until the attitude becomes subconscious and fixed that any danger arises. When that comes about, the man who has decided for Shakespeare's authorship would remain unconvinced in face of any discovery of new evidence. Yet can any one doubt, any one who cares to walk through the world with open eyes as well as an open mind, that the vast majority of opinions given out by the average man and woman have become subconscious habits of thought?

"My professional experience has shown me how great an obstacle to the recovery of physical soundness this impeding habit of thought has become. The whole purpose of my book (*Man's Supreme Inheritance*), from which Mr. Archer quotes, is to submit that the course of evolution had tended in the direction of our obtaining conscious control of our own bodies, and argues that this is the only means by which we can rise above the artificial restrictions, often physically poisonous, imposed by civilisation. And I assure you, sir, that this ideal of conscious control is absolutely unrealisable by any person who is guided and restrained by these subconscious habits of thought, and who is, in consequence, quite unable to exercise the free use of his intelligence.

"So what I intend by the open mind, and in this, I think, Mr. Archer has not fully understood me, is the just use and exercise of conscious reason, a use which is the rare exception to a very delimiting rule.

Yours, etc.,

"F. Matthias Alexander."

To this letter Mr. Archer did not reply, but this brief correspondence covers very fairly, in my opinion, a statement of the popular objection to the "open mind," and my answer to that objection.

Returning now to my own province of therapeutics, I need hardly give any special instance to carry my point. Of late years much attention has been given to the consideration of mental attitude in relation to disease, and although no clearly defined remedy has been advanced, the condition has been diagnosed and defined. The "fixed idea," hallucination, obsession, are all terms used deliberately to denote a morbid condition, but we have to apply these terms much more widely and grasp the fact that they are applicable to small, disregarded mental habits as well as to the well-defined evils which marked their development. In the case of X, the mental habit which had grown up as the result of postulating, "I can't draw my lip up before speaking," was only another aspect of the attitude of A and Z towards the subject of their discussion, and it was precisely similar in kind. The aggregate of these habits is so characteristic in some cases that we see how easily the fallacy arose of assuming an entity for the subconscious self, a self which at the last analysis is made up of these acquired habits and of certain other habits, some of them labelled instincts, the predisposition to which is our birthright, a predisposition inherited from that long chain of ancestors whose origin goes back to the first dim emergence of active life. Fortunately for us there is not a single one of these habits of mind, with their resultant habits of body, which may not be altered by the inculcation of those principles concerning the true poise of the body which I have called the principles of mechanical advantage,[13] used in co-operation with an understanding of the inhibitory and volitional powers of the objective mind, by which means these deterrent habits can be raised to conscious control. The false pose and carriage of the

[13]Certain aspects of these principles will be found set out in detail in Part II of this volume.

body, the incorrect and laboured habits of breathing that are the cause of many troubles besides the obvious ill-effects on the lungs and heart, the degeneration of the muscular system, the partial failure of many vital organs, the morbid fatty conditions that destroy the semblance of men and women to human beings,—all these things and many more that combine to cause debility, disease, and death, are the result of incorrect habits of mind and body, all of which may be changed into correct and beneficial habits if once we can clear away that first impeding habit of thought which stands between us and conscious control.

I believe I have at last laid myself quite open to the attack of the habitual objector, a person I am really anxious to conciliate. I have given him the opportunity of pointing a finger at my last paragraph and saying, "But you only want to change one habit for another! If, as you have implied, the habit of mind is bad, why encourage habits at all, even if they are as you say, 'correct and beneficial'?"

Now this is a point of the first importance. But in the first place it is essential to understand the difference between the habit that is recognised and understood and the habit that is not. The difference in its application to the present case is that the first can be altered at will and the second cannot. For when real conscious control has been obtained a "habit" need never become fixed. It is not truly a habit at all, but an order or series of orders given to the subordinate controls of the body, which orders will be carried out until countermanded.

It will be understood, therefore, that the word "habit" as generally understood, does not apply to the new discipline which it is my aim to establish in the ordinary subconscious realms of our being. The reasons for this are two:

(1) The conscious, intelligently realised, guiding orders are such as may be continued for all time, becoming more effective year by year until they are established as the real and fundamental guidance and control necessary to that which we understand by the words growth and evolution.

(2) The stimuli to apprehension, or excitement of the fear reflexes, are eliminated by a procedure which teaches the pupil to take no thought of whether what he calls "practice," is *right or wrong*.

This second statement, however, requires further elucidation; and I feel that a lay description by a pupil of mine may present the case more clearly to the untrained reader than any technical account. The excerpt is from a letter written by the Rev. W. Pennyman, M.A.

"One great feature of Mr. Alexander's system as seen in practical use is that the individual loses every suggestion of *strain*. He becomes

> perfectly 'lissom' in body; all strains and tensions disappear, and his body works like an oiled machine. Moreover, his system has a reflex result upon the mind of the patient, and a general condition of buoyancy and freedom, and indeed of gaiety of spirit takes the place of the old jaded mental position. It is the pouring in of new wine, but the bottles must also be new or they will burst, and this is exactly what Mr. Alexander's treatment does. It creates the new bottles, and then the new wine can be poured in, freely and fully."

This quotation, however, describes a result, and the means to its achievement can only be attained under certain conditions. There must be, in the first place, a clear realisation by the pupil that he suffers from a defect or defects needing eradication. In the second place, the teacher must make a lucid diagnosis of such defects and decide upon the means of dealing with them. In the third place there must be a satisfactory understanding between teacher and pupil of the present conditions and the means proposed to remedy them.

These three preparatory realisations indicate the real psycho-physical significance of the pupil's mental position. He begins by a definite admission that the subconscious factors by which his psycho-physical organism is being guided are limited and unreliable. He acknowledges in fact that he suffers from mental delusions regarding his physical acts and that his sensory appreciation, or kinæsthesis, is defective and misleading; in other words, he realises that his sense register of the amount of muscular tension needed to accomplish even a simple act of everyday life is faulty and harmful, and his mental conception of such conditions as relaxation and concentration, impossible in practical application.

For there can be no doubt that man on the subconscious plane, now relies too much upon a debauched sense of feeling or of sense-appreciation for the guidance of his psycho-physical mechanism, and that he is gradually becoming more and more overbalanced emotionally with very harmful and far-reaching results.

The results indeed are all too obvious, and yet it must be presumed that the individual has endeavoured to do the *right* and not the *wrong* thing. Does any one set out to catch a train relying upon a watch which as he knows perfectly well is unreliable? Would any sane person place dependence on the reading of a thermometer that he knows to be defective? No, we must admit not only that there is a failure to register accurately in the sensory appreciation, but also that the fault is unrecorded in the conscious mind. And it is for this reason that the pupil must be given a new and correct guiding and controlling centre, before being asked to perform even the simplest acts in accordance with his own idea and judgment.

Some understanding of these slightly technical and practical details is necessary in order to form a clear idea of what is meant by the simple word "habit," which was the origin of this discussion; but I shall return to a fuller analysis of method in this relation in Part II of this work.[14] What I wish to emphasise in this place is that the evil, disturbing habit which it is necessary to eradicate is in the ordinary experience both permanent and unrecognised. It may in some cases have been originally incurred above the plane of reason, but this form of habit is invariably perpetuated in the subconsciousness. On the other hand, the mode of functioning which is substituted, but which may nevertheless be spoken of quite correctly by the same term of "habit," is as subject to control as the routine of a well-organised office. Certain rules are established for the ordinary conduct of business, but the controller of that business must be at liberty to break the rules or to modify them at his discretion. The man who allows an office to take precedence of any other consideration—and I have known instances of such a morbid concession to traditional procedure in business houses—is surely and steadily on the way to commercial failure.

I will now take an illustration of the principle from my own practice. Suppose a patient comes to me who has acquired incorrect respiratory habits, and suppose that he is plastic and ready to assimilate new methods, and that after receiving the new guiding orders from me, he soon learns consciously to make proper use of the muscular mechanism which governs the movements of the breathing apparatus, a word that fitly describes this particular mechanism of the body. Now it would be absurd to suppose that thereafter this person should in his waking moments deliberately apprehend each separate working of his lungs any more than we should expect the busy manager of affairs constantly to supervise the routine of his well-ordered staff. He has acquired conscious control of that working, it is true, but once that control has been mastered, the actual movements that follow are given in charge of the "subconscious self," although always on the understanding that a counter order may be given at any moment if necessary. Until, however, such counter order is given, if it ever need be given, the working of the lungs is for all intents and purposes subconscious, though it may be elevated to the level of the conscious at any moment. Thus it will be seen that the difference between the new habit and the old is that the old was our master and ruled us, while the new is our servant ready to carry out our lightest wish without question, though always working quietly and unobtrusively on our behalf in accordance with the most recent orders given.

---

[14]Certain aspects of these principles will be found set out in the two pamphlets which I have incorporated in this volume.

Briefly, as I see it, the subconsciousness in this application is only a synonym for that rigid routine we finally refer to as habit; this rigid routine being the stumbling block to rapid adaptability, to the assimilation of new ideas, to originality. On the other hand, the consciousness is the synonym for mobility of mind, that mobility which the subconscious control checks and impedes, mobility which will obtain for us physical regeneration and a mental outlook that will make possible for us a new and wider enjoyment of those powers which we all possess, but which are so often deliberately stunted or neglected.

Consider this point also in its application to the case of John Doe, cited in my second chapter. If the mental attitude of that individual had been changed, and he had learned to use his muscles consciously; if, instead of automatically performing a set of muscle tensing exercises, he had devoted himself to apprehending the control and co-ordination of his muscles, he could have carried his knowledge into every act of his life. In his most sedentary occupations he could have been using and exercising his muscular system without resort to any violent contortions, waving of the arms or kicking of the legs; and I cannot but think that he could better have employed the hours spent in this manner by taking a walk in the open air or by occupying himself with some other form of natural exercise. Still, if in his case certain mild forms of exercise at certain times were necessary, such exercises should have employed his mental and physical powers, and through these agencies should have used his muscular mechanism in such a way that its uses could have been applied to the simplest acts, such as sitting on a stool and writing at a desk. There would then have been no question of what we termed "civil war" within his body; the whole physical machinery would have been co-ordinated and adapted to his way of life.

In an earlier paragraph I pointed out that John Doe was suffering from certain mental and physical delusions, and I endeavored to show how these delusions militated against his recovery of health. Returning to this point now that the correct method has been indicated, I may use his case to give another example of this method. What John Doe lacked was a conscious and proper recognition of the right uses of the parts of his muscular mechanism, since while he still uses such parts wrongly, the performance of physical exercises will only increase the defects. He will, in fact, merely copy some other person in the performance of a particular exercise, copy him in the outward act, while his own consciousness of the act performed and the means and uses of his muscular mechanism will remain unaltered. Therefore before he attempts any form of physical development, he must discover, or find some one who can discover for him, what his defects are in the uses indicated. When this has been done he must proceed to inhibit the guiding sensations which cause him to use the mechanism imperfectly; he must apprehend the position of mechanical advantage, and then by using the new, correct guiding sensations or orders, he will be able to bring about the proper use of his muscular mechanism with perfect ease. If the mechanical principle employed is a correct one, every movement will be made with a minimum of effort, and he will not be conscious of the slightest tension. In time a recognition will follow of the new and correct use of the mechanism, which use will then become provisionally established and be employed in the acts of everyday life.

For instance, if we decide that a defect must be got rid of or a mode of action changed, and if we proceed in the ordinary way to eradicate it by any direct means, we shall fail invariably, and with reason. For when defects in the poise of the body, in the use of the muscular mechanisms, and in the equilibrium are present in the human being, the condition thus evidenced is the result of an *undue rigidity* of parts of the muscular mechanisms associated with *undue flaccidity* of others. This undue rigidity is always found in those parts of the muscular mechanisms which are forced to perform duties other than those intended by nature, and are consequently ill-adapted for their function.

As Herbert Spencer writes:

> "Each faculty acquires fitness for its function by performing its function; and if its function is performed for it by a substituted agency, none of the required adjustment of nature takes place, but the nature becomes deformed to fit the artificial arrangements instead of the natural arrangements."

Unfortunately, all conscious effort exerted in attempts at physical action causes in the great majority of the people of to-day such tension of the muscular system concerned as to lead to exaggeration rather than eradication of the defects already present. Therefore it is essential at the outset of re-education to bring about the relaxation of the unduly rigid parts of the muscular mechanisms in order to secure the correct use of the inadequately employed and wrongly co-ordinated parts.

Let us take for example the case of a man who habitually stiffens his neck in walking, sitting, or other ordinary acts of life. This is a sign that he is endeavouring to do with the muscles of his neck the work which should be performed by certain other muscles of his body, notably those of the back. Now if he is told to relax those stiffened muscles of the neck and obeys the order, this mere act of relaxation deals only with an effect and does not quicken his consciousness of the use of the right mechanism which he should use in place of those relaxed. The desire to stiffen the neck muscles should be inhibited as a preliminary (which is not the same thing at all as a direct order to relax the muscles themselves), and then the true uses of the muscular mechanism, i.e., the means of placing the body in a position of mechanical advantage, must be studied, when the work will naturally devolve on those muscles intended to carry it out, and the neck will be relaxed unconsciously. In this case the conscious orders, by which I mean the orders given to the right muscles, are preventive orders, and the due sequence of cause and effect is maintained.

I will, here, only note one more point in concluding my reference to the hypothetical John Doe, who, nevertheless, stands as the representative of a very large body of people. This point is the question of the storing and reserving of energy, and to use a phrase which has a mechanical equivalent, the registration of tension. If you ask a man to lift a *papier-mâché* imitation of an enormous dumb-bell, leading him to believe that it is almost beyond his capacity to raise it from the floor, he will exert his full power in the effort to do that which he could perform with the greatest ease. In a lesser degree the same expenditure of unnecessary force is exerted by the vast majority of "physical-culture" students, and by practically every person in the ordinary duties of daily life. The kinæsthetic system has not been taught to register correctly the tension or, in other words, to gauge accurately the amount of muscular effort required to perform certain acts, the expenditure of effort always being in excess of what is required, an excellent instance of the lack of harmony in the untutored organism. This fact may be easily tested by any interested person who will take the trouble to try its application. Ask a friend to lift a chair or any other object of such weight that, while it may be lifted without great difficulty, will in the process make an undoubted call on the muscular energies. You will see at once that your friend will approach the task with a definite preconception as to the amount of physical tension necessary. His mind is exclusively occupied with the question of his own muscular effort, instead of with the purpose in front of him and the best means to undertake it. Before he has even approached it, he will brace or tense the muscles of his arms, back, neck, etc., and when about to perform the act he will place himself in a position which is actually one of mechanical disadvantage as far as he is concerned. Not only are all these preparations of course quite unnecessary, but the whole attitude of mind towards the task is wrong. In such instances as this, any preconception as to the degree of tension required is out of place. If we desire to lift a weight with the least possible waste of energy, we should approach it and grasp it with relaxed muscles, assuming the position of greatest possible mechanical advantage, and then gradually exert our muscular energies until sufficient power is attained to overcome the resistance.

Returning now to the consideration of that bias or predisposing habit of mind which so often balks us at the outset, we may see at once that this predisposition takes many curious forms. Sometimes it is frankly objective, and is outlined in the statement, "Well, I don't believe in all this, but I may as well try it." In this form a single unlooked-for result is generally enough to change disbelief into credulity. I write the word "credulity" with intention, for I mean to imply that the reaction in a certain type of mind is little, if any, better than the profession of disbelief. What is required is not prejudice in either direction, but a calm, clear, open-eyed intelligence, a ready, adaptive outlook, an outlook, believe me, which does not connote indefiniteness of purpose or uncertainty of initiative.

Another form of predisposition arises from lack of purpose, and the mental habits that go with this condition are hard to eradicate, more particularly when the original feebleness has led to some form of hypochondria or nervous disease which has been treated with the usual disregard of the radical evil. It is not difficult for the most superficial enquirer to understand that in treating cases like these any method which relieves the subject still further of the exercise of initiative—such a method as the rest cure, for instance, though I could quote many others—only increases the original evil. The lack of purpose is pandered to and cultivated, and after the six weeks or so of treatment, the patient returns to his or her duties in ordinary life, even more unfitted than before to perform them. As I have said before, no account is taken of the instinct for self-preservation or the will to live. This is the very mainspring of human life, yet in the routine of our protected civilisation even its power tends at times to become relaxed, and the machinery runs down. The machinery should then be wound up again, instead of being allowed to become still further relaxed by resting. This lack of purpose, the immediate effect of our educational methods, is unhappily very common in all classes, but especially among those who have no occupation, or those whose employment is a mechanical routine which does not exercise the powers of initiative. The curious thing about this very large class is that they do not really want to be cured. They may be suffering from many physical disabilities or from actual physical pain, and they may and will protest most earnestly that they want to be free from their pains and disabilities, but in face of the evidence we must admit that if the objective wish is really there, it is so feeble as to be non-existent for all practical purposes. In many cases this attitude of submission to illness is the outcome of a strong subjective habit. The trouble, whatever it is, is endured in the first instance; it is looked upon as a nuisance, perhaps, but not as an intolerable nuisance; no steps are taken to get rid of it, and the trouble grows until, by degrees, it is looked upon as a necessity. Then at last, when the trouble has increased until it threatens the interruption of all ordinary occupations, the sufferer seeks a remedy. But the habit of submission has grown too strong, and as long as the disease can be kept within certain bounds, no effort is made to fight it. This is of course one of the commonest experiences in the healing profession. A patient is treated and benefited and seems on the high road to perfect health. Then follows a relapse. The first question is, "Have you been following the treatment?" and the answer, if the patient is truthful, is "I forgot," or "I didn't bother any more about it." In a recent experience of a medical friend of mine, a patient confessed to having stayed in the house for a week after a certain relapse occurred, although the very essence of the prescription by which he had previously benefited was to be in the fresh air as much as possible. This simply means that the subjective habit of submission has grown so strong that the objective mind, weakened in its turn by the neglect of its guiding functions, is unable to conquer it. No prescription or course of treatment can have any effect upon such a patient as this, unless the subjective habit can be brought within the sphere of conscious control. In other cases this apparent lack of desire for health is due to an attachment to some dearly loved habit, which must be given up if the proper functions of the body are to be resumed. It may be a habit of petty self-indulgence or one that is imminently threatening the collapse of the vital processes, but the attachment to it is so strong that the enfeebled objective mind prefers to hold to the habit and risk death sooner than make the effort of opposing it. Even in cases where no harm can be traced directly to a markedly influencing habit, the general all-pervading habit of lassitude or inertia is so strong that any régime which may be prescribed is distasteful if it involves, as it must, the exercise of those powers which have been allowed to fall more or less into disuse.

Space will not permit of my giving further instances of the predisposing habit, but very little introspection on the part of my readers should enable them to diagnose their own peculiar mental habits, the first step towards being rid of them. We must always remember that the vast majority of human beings live very narrow lives, doing the same thing and thinking the same thoughts day by day, and it is this very fact that makes it so necessary that we should acquire conscious control of the mental and physical powers as a whole, for we otherwise run the risk of losing that versatility which is such an essential factor in their development.

If, at this point, the reader feels inclined to analyse these habits and to set about a control of them, I will give him one word of preliminary advice, "Beware of so-called concentration."

This advice is so pertinent to the whole principle that it is worth while to elaborate it. Ask any one you know to concentrate his mind on a subject—anything will do—a place, a person, or a thing. If your friend is willing to play the game and earnestly endeavours to concentrate his mind, he will probably knit his forehead, tense his muscles, clench his hands, and either close his eyes or stare fixedly at some point in the room. As a result his mind is very fully occupied with this unusual condition of the body which can only be maintained by repeated orders from the objective mind. In short, your friend, though he may not know it, is not using his mind for the consideration of the subject you have given him to concentrate upon, but for the consideration of an unusual bodily condition which he calls "concentration." This is true also of the attitude of *attention* required for children in schools; it dissociates the brain instead of compacting it. Personally, I do not believe in any concentration that calls for effort. It is the wish, the conscious desire to do a thing or think a thing, which results in adequate performance. Could Spencer have written his *First Principles*, or Darwin his *Descent of Man*: if either had been forced to any rigid narrowing effort in order to keep his mind on the subject in hand? I do not deny that some work can be done under conditions which necessitate such an artificially arduous effort, but I do deny that it is ever the best work. Nor will I admit that such a case as that of Sir Walter Scott can logically be argued against this view. For the real earnest wish to write the Waverley novels was there, even if it originated in the desire to pay the debts he took upon himself, and not in the desire to write the novels because he took a pleasure in the actual performance. Briefly, our application of the word "concentration" denotes a conflict which is a morbid condition and a form of illness; singleness of purpose is quite another thing. If you try to straighten your arm and bend it at the same moment, you may exercise considerable muscular effort, but you will achieve no result, and the analogy applies to the endeavour to delimit the powers of the brain by concentration, and at the same time to exercise them to the full extent. The endeavour represents the conflict of the two postulates "I must" and "I can't"; the fight continues indefinitely, with a constant waste of misapplied effort. Once eradicate the mental habit of thinking that this effort is necessary, once postulate and apprehend the meaning of "I wish" instead of those former contradictions, and what was difficult will become easy, and pleasure will be substituted for pain. We must cultivate, in brief, the deliberate habit of taking up every occupation with the whole mind, with a living desire to carry each action through to a successful accomplishment, a desire which necessitates bringing into play every faculty of the attention. By use this power develops, and it soon becomes as simple to alter a morbid taste which may have been a lifelong tendency as to alter the smallest of recently acquired bad habits.

The following is an interesting experience with a pupil who was strongly inclined to a belief in the value and power of concentration. This pupil contested vigorously my attacks on the object of her faith, as practised in accordance with the orthodox conception. She put forward the usual arguments, of course, and I quite failed to make any impression on her mental attitude towards the vexed question under discussion. But at last, some days after our first encounter, my opportunity came. We were not at the time directly discussing concentration, but we were dealing with kindred subjects, and presently my pupil began to speak of the attitudes adopted by people towards the things in life that they like or dislike to do. Her own plan, she said, with a touch of pride, had been to develop the habit of keeping her mind on other and more pleasant subjects whenever she had been engaged in a task that was unsympathetic to her, and she had so far succeeded in the cultivation of this habit that the disagreeable sensations of any unpleasant duty were no longer experienced by her. I then put one or two questions to her and elucidated among other facts that for years she had been unable "to concentrate" when reading and that this difficulty was becoming constantly more pronounced. Fortunately this instance opened those locked places of her intelligence that I had been unable to reach by argument. I showed her how she had been cultivating a most harmful mental condition, which made concentration on those duties of life which pleased her appear as a necessity. She had been constructing a secret chamber in her mind, as harmful to her general well-being as an undiagnosed tumour might have been to her physical welfare. I am glad to say that she came to admit the truth of my original position and has since begun her efforts to carry out the suggestions I offered for the correction of her bad habit.

And in all such efforts to apprehend and control mental habits, the first and only real difficulty is to overcome the preliminary inertia of mind in order to combat the subjective habit. The brain becomes used to thinking in a certain way, it works in a groove, and when sent in action, slides along the familiar, well-worn path; but when once it is lifted out of the groove, it is astonishing how easily it may be directed. At first it will have a tendency to return to the old manner of working by means of one mechanical unintelligent operation, but the groove soon fills, and although thereafter we may be able to use the old path if we choose, we are no longer bound to it.

In concluding this brief note on mental habits I turn my attention particularly to the many who say, "I am quite content as I am." To them I say, firstly, if you are content to be the slave of habits instead of master of your own mind and body, you can never have realised the wonderful inheritance which is yours by right of the fact that you were born a reasoning, intelligent man or woman. But, I say, secondly, and this is of importance to the larger world and is not confined to your intimate circle, "What of the children?" Are you content to rob them of their inheritance, as perhaps you were robbed of yours by your parents? Are you willing to send them out into the world ill-equipped, dependent on precepts and incipient habits, unable to control their own desires, and already well on the way to physical degeneration? Happily, I believe that the means of stirring the inert is being provided. The question of Eugenics, or the science of race culture, is being debated by earnest men and women, and the whole problem of contemporary physical degeneration is one which looms ever larger in the public mind. It is the problem which has exercised me for many years, and which is mainly responsible for the issue of this book, and in my next chapter I shall treat it in connexion with the theory of progressive conscious control which I have outlined in the foregoing pages.

CHAPTER VII

RACE CULTURE AND THE TRAINING OF THE CHILDREN

> "In what way to treat the body; in what way to treat the mind; in what way to manage our affairs; in what way to bring up a family; in what way to behave as a citizen; in what way to utilise those sources of happiness which nature supplies,—how to use all our faculties to the greatest advantage; how to live completely? And this being the great thing needful for us to learn, is, by consequence, the great thing which education has to teach. To prepare us for complete living is the function which education has to discharge."
>
> HERBERT SPENCER, *EDUCATION.*

EVERY child is born into the world with a predisposition to certain habits, and furthermore, the child of to-day is not born with the same development of instinct that was the congenital heritage of its ancestors a hundred or even fifty years ago. Many modern children, for example, are born with recognisable physical disadvantages that are the direct result of the gradually deteriorating respiratory and vital functioning of their forbears.

For many months, the period varying with the sex and ability of the individual, the vital processes and movements are for all practical purposes independent of any conscious control, and the human infant remains in this helpless, dependent condition much longer than any other animal. The habits which the child evidences during this protracted period are those hereditary predispositions which are early developed by circumstance and environment, habits of muscular uses, of vital functioning, and of adaptability. If it were possible to analyse the tendencies of a child when it is, say, twelve months old, we could soon master the science of heredity which is at present so tentative and uncertain in its deductions, but the child's potentialities lie hidden in the mysterious groupings and arrangement of its cells and tissues, hidden beyond the reach of any analysis. The child is our material; within certain wide limits we may mould it to the shape we desire. But even at birth it is differentiated from other children; our limits may be wide but they are fixed. Within those limits, however, our capacity for good and evil is very great.

There are two methods by which a child learns. The first and, in earlier years, the predominant method is by imitation, the second is by precept or directly administered instruction, positive or negative.

With regard to the first method, parents of every class will admit the fact not only that children imitate those who are with them during those early plastic years, but that the child's first efforts to adapt itself to the conditions surrounding it are based almost exclusively on imitation. For despite the many thousand years during which some form of civilisation has been in existence, no child has yet been born into the world with hereditary instincts tending to fit it for any particular society. Its language and manners, for instance, are modelled entirely on the speech and habits of those who have charge of it. The child descended from a hundred kings will speak the language and adopt the manners of the East End should it be reared among these associations; and the son of an Australian aboriginal would speak the English tongue and with certain limitations behave as a civilised child if brought up with English people.

No one denies this fact; it has been proved and accepted, yet how often do we seek to make a practical application of our knowledge? Although science of heredity is still tentative and indeterminate, no reasoning person can doubt from this and other instances that in the vast majority of cases at least, the influence of heredity can be practically eradicated. Personally, I see very clearly from facts of my own observation that when the characteristics of the father and mother are analysed, and their faults and virtues understood, a proper training of the children will prevent the same faults and encourage the same virtues in their children.

To appreciate to the utmost the effect of training upon the children, we must remember that the first tastes, likes, or dislikes of the infant begin to be developed during the first two or three days after birth. Long before the infant is a month old, habits, tending to become fixed habits, have been developed, and if these habits are not harmful, well and good. The first sense developed is the sense of taste, a sense that develops very quickly and needs the most careful attention. Artificial feeding is in itself a very serious danger, but when this feeding is in the hands of careless or ignorant persons the danger becomes increased a hundredfold. An instance of this is the common idea that considerable quantities of sugar should be added to the milk. This is done very often to induce the child to take food against its natural desire. It may be that the child has been suffering from some slight internal derangement, and Nature's remedy has been to affect the child with a distaste for food in order to give the stomach a rest. Then the unthinking mother tempts the child with sugar, and all sorts of internal trouble may follow. But in such a case as this the taste for a particular thing, such as sugar, is encouraged, and apart from the direct harm which may result, the habit becomes the master of the child, and may rule it through life; the child, in fact, is sent out into the world the slave of the sense of taste.

Unfortunately, in ninety cases out of a hundred, children up to the age of six or seven years are allowed to acquire very decided tastes for things which are harmful. Women are not trained for the sphere of motherhood, they do not give these matters the thought and attention they deserve, and hence they do not understand the most elementary principles concerning the future welfare of their offspring in such matters as feeding and sense guidance. Children are not taught to cultivate a taste for wholesome, nourishing foods, but are tempted, and their incipient habits pandered to, by such additions as the sugar I have more particularly cited.

At the present time I know a child of five years old whose taste is already perverted by the method, or lack of method, I have indicated. This child dislikes milk unless undue quantities of sugar are added, will not eat such food as milk puddings or brown bread, and has a strong distaste for cream. It is almost impossible to make the child eat vegetables of any kind, but he is always ready to take large quantities of meat and sweets. The child is already suffering from malnutrition and serious internal derangement. The latter would be greatly improved by small quantities of olive oil taken daily, but it is only with the greatest difficulty that the child can be induced to take it. If he lives with his parents for the next ten years, he will grow into a weak and ailing boy, and will suffer from the worst forms of digestive trouble and imperfect functioning of the internal organs.

Apropos of this point, I remember hearing a question put to my friend, Dr. Clubbe of Sydney, by a London specialist, who asked what, in Dr. Clubbe's opinion, was the primary cause of the derangement of the natural working of a child's muscular mechanism and respiratory system. The answer was given without hesitation, "Toxic poisoning as a result of artificial feeding." The logic of this answer will be readily apprehended by the layman, when he considers the interdependence of every part of the system, for in this case the nerve centres connected with the sensory apparatus of the digestive organs and the urea control also the respiratory processes. As a consequence, when these centres are dulled in their action as a result of toxic poisoning, there is a loss of activity in the processes of respiration, with consequent maladjustments of those parts of the muscular mechanism more nearly concerned, and so the whole machine is thrown out of gear.

Thus we see that in such instances the mischief begins very early in the life of the child, and it is carried on and exaggerated with every step in its development. Even in babyhood precept and coercion should come into play. Usually when the child cries, little effort is made to discover the cause. Often the child is soothed by being carried up and down the room. It is wonderful how soon the infant begins to associate some rudiments of cause and effect. The child who is unduly pandered to will soon learn to cry whenever it desires to be rocked or dandled, and thus the foundations of pandering to sensation are quickly laid.

But as the child comes to the observant age its habits begin to grow more quickly. We have admitted that a child imitates its parents or nurses in tricks of manner and speech, yet we do not stop to consider that it will also imitate our carriage of the body, our performance of muscular acts, even our very manner of breathing. This faculty for imitation and adaptation is a wonderful force, and one which we have at our command if we would only pause to consider how we may use it in the right way. The vast majority of wrong habits acquired by children result from their imitation of the imperfect models confronting them. But how many parents attempt to put a right model before their children? How many learn to eradicate their own defects of pose and carriage so that they may be better examples to the child? How many in choosing a nurse will take the trouble to select a girl whom they would like their children to imitate? Very, very few, and the reason is simple. In the first place they do not realise the harmful effect of bad example, and, in the second, the great majority of parents have so little perception of truth in this matter that they are incapable of choosing a girl who is a good specimen of humanity, and are sublimely unconscious of their own crookedness and defects.

Children too accept their parents' defects as normal and admirable. The boy of 12 or 14 never dreams for instance that his father's protruding stomach is anything but the condition proper to middle-age, and often, doubtless, figures to himself the time when he will arrive at the same condition. The time will come when such things as these—I refer to the abnormality of the father—will be considered a disgrace. What then can we hope from these parents who are at the present time so unfit, so incapable of teaching their own children the primer of physical life? And I may note here that this principle has a wider application than that of the nursery; it holds, also, in connexion with the model of physical well-being set by the teachers in all primary and secondary schools. There is no need for me to elaborate this theme. The iniquity of allowing children to be trained in physical exercises, in our Board Schools for instance, by a teacher who is obviously physically unfit, is sufficiently glaring.

The crux of the whole question is that we are progressing towards conscious control, and have not yet realised all that this progress connotes. Children, as civilisation becomes continually more the natural condition, evidence fewer and fewer of their original savage instincts. In early life they are faced by two evils, if they are developed on the subconscious plane. If they are trained under the older methods of education they become more and more dependent upon their instructors; if under the more recent methods of *"free expression"* (to which I shall presently refer at some length) they are left with the vagaries of the imperfect and inadequate directions of subconscious mechanisms that are the inheritance of a gradually deteriorated psycho-physical functioning of the whole organism.

In such conditions it is not possible for the child to command the kinæsthetic guidance and power essential to satisfactory free expression, or indeed to any other satisfactory form of expression for its latent potentialities. As well expect an automobile, if I may use the simile, to express its capacity when its essential parts have been interfered with in such a way as to misdirect or diminish the right impulses of the machinery.

The child of the present day, once it has emerged from its first state of absolute helplessness, and before it has been trained and coerced into certain mental and physical habits, is the most plastic and adaptable of living things. At this stage the complete potentiality of conscious control is present but can only be developed by the eradication of certain hereditary tendencies or predispositions. Unfortunately, the usual procedure is to thrust certain habits upon it without the least consideration of cause and effect, and to insist upon these habits until they have become subconscious and have passed from the region of intellectual guidance.

I will take one instance as an example of this, the point of right-and-left-handedness. We assume from the outset, and the superstition is so old that its source is untraceable, that a child must learn to depend upon its right hand, to the neglect of its left. This superstition has so sunk into our minds by repetition that it has become incorporated in our language. "Dexterous" stands for an admirable, and "sinister" for an inauspicious quality, and we may even find ignorant people at the present day who say that they would never trust a left-handed person. As a result of this attitude and of the absolute rule laid down that a child must learn to write and use its knife with the right hand only, the number of ambidextrous people is limited to the few who, by some initial accident, used their left hand by preference and were afterwards taught to use their right. In a fairly wide experience I do not remember having heard of a father or mother who has said: "This child may become an artist or a pianist," for example, "and may therefore need to develop the sensitiveness and powers of manipulation of the left hand as well as the right," although I have known many cases where much time and trouble had to be expended in acquiring the uses of the left hand later in life; such cases as those of persons suffering from writers' cramp and dependent for their living on their ability to use a pen.

I have cited this example of right-handedness because it exhibits the pliability of the physical mechanism in early life and the manner in which we thoughtlessly bind it to some method of working, without ever stopping to think whether that method is good in itself, or whether it is the one best adapted for the conditions of life into which the child will grow. We thrust a rigid rule of physical life and mental outlook upon the children. We are not convinced that the rule is the best, or even that it is a good rule. Often we know, or would know if we gave the matter a moment's consideration, that in our own bodies the rule has not worked particularly well, but it is the rule which was taught to us, and we pass it on either by precept, or by holding up our imperfections for imitation and then we wonder what is the cause of the prevailing physical degeneration!

What is intended by these methods of education is to inculcate the accumulated and inferentially correct lessons derived from past experience. It is true that the lesson varies according to the religious, political, and social colour of the parent and teacher, but speaking generally, the intention would be logical enough, if we could make the primary assumption that each generation starts from the same point,—the assumption, in other words, that a baby is born with the same potentialities, the same mental abilities and assuredly the same physical organism whether he be born in the 16th or the 20th century.

And even as recently as a hundred years ago, that assumption might have been made with some show of reason. For the changes were so slight and have evolved so slowly as to attract little attention. Granted similar conditions of parentage and upbringing, the differences between the child of 1800 A.D. and that of 1700 A.D. were hardly noticeable.

That statement, however, does not apply to the child of 1917. For many years past there has been unrest and dissatisfaction in the world of education. New methods have been tried, superimposed for the most part on the top of the older ones, and even more daring experiments have been made, experiments which sought to throw over the old traditions, bag and baggage. All these trials have so far failed, in my opinion; and one reason for the failure has been due to the fact that educationalists as a body have been unable to recognise the obvious truth that the child of the twentieth century cannot be judged by the old standards.

This truth is so evident to me that I hesitate at the necessity to prove it. It seems incredible to me that any one of my generation could fail to realise the extraordinary differences between the contemporaries of his own growth and the children of our present civilisation. I could produce a dozen instances of this difference, but one must suffice in this place. It is, however, an example that is peculiarly typical. For I remember, and my experience has not been in any way an abnormal one, the facility with which the children of my generation learnt the uses of common tools. In a sense they may be said to have inherited a certain dexterity in the handling of such things as a hammer, knife, or saw. To-day many parents are greatly impressed if a child of from $2^{1}/_{2}$ to 6 years old can use one of these implements with a reasonable show of efficiency. I have known fathers and mothers representative of the average parent of to-day who find any instance of this efficiency in their own children an almost startling thing and certainly matter for boast to their relations and friends.

Unhappily the real difference goes far deeper than this superficial effect would at first seem to indicate. The early attempts of the modern child to employ his physical endowment in such common and necessary acts as walking, running, sitting or speaking, are far below the standard of ability that I remember a generation ago. The standard of kinæsthetic potentiality has been lowered. Elements that I will not attempt to trace, lest I be tempted on to the fascinating ground of evolutionary theory, have intervened most amazingly in the past thirty years, and the most evident result of this intervention has been the marked change in the subconscious efficiency of the modern child.

Thus, even from the birth of the infant, our problem is not precisely that of the old educationalists; and this primary congenital difference between the children of two generations has been, and is being, exaggerated in the nurseries of the independent classes both in England and America. (Doubtless in other countries of Europe the same effects are being produced, but I prefer to speak only of that which I have observed and closely studied for myself.) There is still a tendency to take all responsibility and initiative away from the child of wealthy parents. Nurses first and governesses later perform every possible act of service that shall relieve the child of trouble. It is not even allowed to invent its own games. Toys are supplied in endless quantities, expensive, ingenious toys, that need no imaginative act to transform them into reduced models of the motors, trains, or animals they are manufactured to represent, and some one, some adult, is always at hand to amuse the child and *teach him how to play*. I must italicise the absurdity of that last sentence. For what does this teaching mean, if it does not mean that it is seeking to substitute the adult idea of play for the childish one? In my day, any old brick played the part of a train or a horse, and in the mental act required to see the reality under so uncompromising a guise my imagination was exercised. Then I, and the other children of my time, grew dissatisfied with so poor a substitute, and as we progressed in experience, the stimulated imaginations found expression in *inventing* and in *making* better replicas of the realities of our childish experience. And we grew with the exercise. We had our little responsibilities and we taught ourselves not only how to play but how presently to adapt our play to the great business of social life. But what equipment is furnished to the child who never has an independent moment throughout its nursery career? How can such a child hope to succeed in life, should the fortune it hopes to inherit from its parents be suddenly lost or diverted? Every one knows the answer. We can see the results in any great city of modern civilisation, in London slums and in the Bowery of New York. A few generations of such teaching as this and we should have had a differentiated race as helpless as the slave-keeping ants.

But although this petrifying method of teaching and supervision is still practised, the reaction against it has already set in both in England and America. Unhappily that reaction has been too violent as such reactions commonly are. From one extreme of permitting the child no opportunity of the exercise of independent thought and action, we have flown to the other in adopting the principle which is now known as "Free Expression"—a principle which I can show to be no less harmful than over-supervision. In fact so far as the physical expression of a child is concerned, the methods of Free Expression are even more dangerous than those of the opposite school.

In England, this movement towards "Free Expression" has not so far been crystallised into a definite propaganda, nevertheless a number of thoughtful but unhappily inexpert parents are trying to adopt the principle in their own homes. Mr. Shaw's Preface to his *Misalliance* puts the theory of the method in a very clear and convincing argument. His main assumption is as follows: "What is a child? An experiment. A fresh attempt to produce the first man made perfect; that is, to make humanity divine. And you will vitiate the experiment if you make the slightest attempt to abort it into some fancy figure of our own. . . ." That represents, of course, an idealist attitude, and every idealistically minded parent in Great Britain who reads that Preface of Mr. Shaw's on "Parents and Children" at once attempts to put the theory into practice. The results, if the theory is persisted in, will be disastrous; and although in many cases the parents realise their error by practical experience before the child reaches the age of seven or so, certain cases I have seen demonstrate all too clearly that much mischief is being done even at the age of seven; faults and bad habits have become so far established that it is sometimes very hard to eradicate them.

And in America the mischief is going further still. So called "free" schools have been instituted which, although they may differ in the detail of their methods, are based on the same underlying principles. As far as I have examined the theory and practice of these schools their purposes are:

(1) To free the child as far as possible from outside interference and restraint.

(2) To place him in the right environment and then to give him materials and allow him activities through which he may "freely express himself."

Now this presupposes, firstly, that the child if left to himself has the power of expressing himself adequately and freely; secondly, that through this expression, he can educate himself. How far both these suppositions are fallacies will be understood by any one who has followed my argument and my citations of actual cases even up to this point; but the matter is so important that I do not hesitate to bring forward further evidence to establish my objection to this new and dangerous method.

I will begin by drawing attention to the practical side of two of the channels for self-expression, which are specially insisted upon in schools where the new mode is being practised, namely, dancing and drawing. A friend of mine always refers to them as the two D's, a phrase that refers very explicitly to these two forms of damnation when employed as fundamentals in education.

The method of the "Free Expressionists" is to associate music with the first of these arts. Now music and dancing are, as every one knows, excitements which make a stronger emotional appeal to the primitive than to the more highly evolved races. No drunken man in our civilisation ever reaches the stage of anæsthesia and complete loss of self-control attained by the savage under the influence of these two stimuli. But in the schools where I have witnessed children's performances, I have seen the first beginnings of the madness which is the savage's ecstasy. Music in this connexion is an artificial stimulus and very potent one.

And though artificial stimuli may be permissible in certain forms of pleasure sought by the reasoning, trained adult, they are uncommonly dangerous incitements to use in the education of a child of six.

Need I defend still further my description of music as an artificial and powerful stimulus? During the present war it has been reported that the influence of alcohol and drugs has been resorted to by the Germans to drive their men to the attack. But we know that in earlier wars, the greatest effects could be attained by music, effects that drive the fighters into the most delirious excesses of savagery. And, doubtless, if the sound of music could have made itself heard above the awful din of guns that precede a modern advance, the old stimulus would have been preferred by the Germans to the administration of drugs. As it is, I have heard that bands are used whenever possible. Full-grown men and women will admit that they can become "drunk" with music and by "drunk" I mean that the motions of the subconsciousness are excited to such a pitch that they take control, until they completely dominate the reasoning faculties. Alcohol produces this result by partial paralysis of the peripheral cilia, music and dancing by over-exaltation of the whole kinæsthetic system. In the latter case, however, no evil effects can be produced in the first instance, without the reasoning consent or submission of the subject. Savages and *young children have not yet learnt to withhold that consent.*

And altogether apart from this question of intoxication—to which by the way every individual is not susceptible—these unrestrained, unguided efforts of the children to dance are likely to prove extremely harmful. I have watched while first one air and then another has been played on the piano, the intention of these changes being to convey a different form of stimulus with each air, and I admit that the children responded in accordance with the more or less limited kinæsthetic powers at their command. But it was very obvious to me that all these little dancers were more or less imperfectly co-ordinated; that the idea projected from the ideomotor centre constantly missed its proper direction; that subconscious efforts were being made that caused little necks to take up the work that should have been done by little backs; that the larynx was being harmfully depressed in the efforts to breathe adequately causing both inspiration and expiration to be made through the open mouth instead of through the nostrils; and that the young and still pliable spines were being gradually curved backwards and the stature shortened when the very opposite condition was essential even to a satisfying aesthetic result.

And when we realise that the teachers who witness these lessons are entirely ignorant of the ideal physical conditions that are proper to children, and so are woefully unaware of the dangerous defects that are being initiated by these efforts to dance, we must admit that, as practised, this particular form of free expression is being encouraged at a cost that far outweighs any imagined advantage.

Here, for instance, is an example that came directly under my notice. A little girl six years old was brought to me for kinæsthetic examination and I found her to be in really excellent physical condition. She was then sent to school where she became interested in dancing. The dancing at this school was considered a form of free expression, and the children were encouraged to make their own movements, undirected. Different airs were played to which the child was expected to react, and the little girl of my example found great pleasure in this part of her school work and gave much of her time to it, until she was considered to express herself more freely than any of the other children in the form of art she had chosen. I may point out that one of the essential principles of these free-expression schools is to permit a child to choose its own activity and to pursue it for practically as long as it desires.

Her mother, however, became dissatisfied after a time with her child's general condition. Curious and somewhat alarming physical distortions were beginning to manifest themselves, most noticeably a tendency to carry her head on one side, a tendency she was unable to rectify. At last the mother brought back the child to me for re-examination.

Now less than a year before I had passed this child as an unusually fine example of correct physical co-ordination. When she came back to me she was in little better condition than a congenital degenerate. All that fluent co-ordination of her muscular mechanisms had disappeared, and in place of it I found rigid tendons, stiffened muscles, and, worst of all, faulty habits of guidance and control, among them a habit of governing the muscles of her body and legs by stiffening the unrelated muscles of her neck. (Incidentally I may note in passing that in the human being the neck is very often the indicator of inadequate and false controls. There are good reasons why this should be the case, *a priori*, but they are too technical for this book.) A further particular defect was due to a tensing and shortening of the upper muscles of the thighs where they are attached to the torso, a defect that was tending to warp and shorten the child's stature. Lastly, the most significant change of all, the child who a year before had been outspoken and fearless, and clear of speech, was now timid and shy, and mumbled her words so badly that I could with difficulty understand her.

Here then is a case of a child, starting in the best physical condition, who was placed in what was considered the right environment and permitted the exercise of free activity. And I claim that the harmful result was so inevitable that any one of real experience might have anticipated it with almost absolute certainty.

The second ominous "D" is drawing, and this comes into another category of damnation, since mental rather than physical effects are concerned, although the latter are involved both in the harmful, uncorrected poses adopted by the children when seated at the table, and in the false directions of the ideo-motor centres of which only a few reach the essential fingers that are holding or more often grotesquely clutching the pencil. It may seem a small thing to the layman that a child should try to guide a pencil by movements of its tongue, but to the expert that confusion of functions is indicative of endless subconscious troubles.

Let me describe the practical procedure of a certain type of "free-drawing" lesson. Pencils, paper, and the usual paraphernalia are placed on tables or desks in different parts of the school-room, in the hope that the child may be tempted to use them in drawing. Then, one day, a pupil takes up a pencil and makes an attempt to draw, another follows his example and so on, until all the pupils have made some kind of effort in this direction.

Now the act of drawing is in the last analysis a mechanical process that concerns the management of the fingers, and the co-ordination of the muscles of the hand and forearm in response to certain visual images conceived in the brain and imaginatively projected on to the paper. And the standard of functioning of the human fingers and hand in this connexion depends entirely upon the degree of kinæsthetic development of the arm, torso, and joints; in fact upon the standard of co-ordination of the whole organism. It is not surprising, therefore, that hardly one of these more or less defectively co-ordinated children should have any idea of how to hold a pencil in such a way as will command the freedom, power, and control that will enable him to do himself justice as a draughtsman.

Any attentive and thoughtful observer who will watch the movement and position of these children's fingers, hand, wrist, arm, neck and body generally, during the varying attempts to draw straight or crooked lines, cannot fail to note the lack of co-ordination between these parts. The fingers are probably attempting to perform the duties of the arm, the shoulders are humped, the head twisted on one side. In short, energies are being projected to parts of the bodily mechanism which have little or no influence on the performance of the desired act of drawing, and the mere waste projection of such energies alone is almost sufficient to nullify the purpose in view.

But I have already said enough to prove that no free expression can come by this means. The right impulse may be in the child's mind, but he has not the physical ability to express it. Not one modern child in ten thousand is born with the gift to draw as we say "by the light of Nature," and that one exceptional child will have his task made easier if he is wisely guided in his first attempts.

But my chief objection to this teaching of drawing is the encouragement it gives to profitless dreaming. Drawing is an art, and we know some of the characteristics that are commonly imputed to the artist,—though many of the greatest artists have been exemplarily free from them. These characteristics are eccentricity, lack of balance, power of self-hypnotism, and a general irrationality. Yet surely it cannot be emphasised too strongly that the artist succeeds in spite of these impediments to expression, and not because of them. These characteristics that I have instanced are by-products of the artistic genius. They are developed through erroneous conceptions and overconcentration on a particular creative activity, and time and again in the history of the world these by-products have ruined, incapacitated, and disgraced men of real genius.

Nevertheless, if I can judge by my experience of this form of free expression, the child is encouraged to practise the eccentricity as a means to obtain the gift of drawing, which as a principle is about the same as trying to breed race horses with weak lungs because it has been noted that certain very fast horses have been rather deficient in this respect. To encourage eccentricity is not to breed genius, and genius itself is more free and more creative when it is not hampered by eccentricity. Let us, at least, have some appreciation of rational cause and effect.

So much for my two "D's," but my general criticism of the "free expression" experiment does not end there. For I must confess that I have been shocked to witness the work that has been going on in these schools. I have seen children of various ages amusing themselves—somewhat inadequately in quite a number of cases—by drawing, dancing, carpentering, and so on, but in hardly a single instance have I seen an example of one of these children employing his physical mechanisms in a correct or *natural* way. I insist upon the use of the word *natural* even though it be applied to such relatively artificial activities as drawing and carpentering. For there is a right, that is to say a most effective, way of holding and using a pencil or a carpenter's tool. But the children I saw commonly sat or stood in positions of the worst mechanical advantage, and the manner in which they held their pencils or their tools demonstrated very clearly that until their management of such instruments was corrected, they could never hope to produce anything but the most clumsy results. Worse still, these children were forming physical habits which would develop in a large majority of cases into positive physical ills. A child who tries to guide its pencil by futile movements of its head, tongue, and shoulders may be preparing the way to ills so far-reaching that their origin is often lost sight of.

As an instance of this, I recently had a case of a boy of 3 1/2 years who suffered from fear reflexes. If a stranger entered a room when the child was present, he would cry and cling to his mother or nurse. At the seaside after asking to be allowed to bathe with other children, he was subsequently afraid to go near the water. And in many other ways he exhibited unreasoning terrors which, according to the general diagnosis common in such cases, were presumed to be the cause of his general backwardness, a symptom particularly marked in his speech, for he was only able to articulate a few words and those very imperfectly.

My first examination of him revealed the fact that he lacked proper control of his lips and tongue, and of one internal physical function, the latter chiefly at night. And that the lack of control in these particulars was the direct cause of his psycho-physical condition was very conclusively proved by my treatment of him. Treated on a basis of conscious guidance and control, re-educated and co-ordinated, the child made rapid advancement, and he progressed towards a condition approximating more closely to what one might call normal, than he had experienced since birth. The fear reflexes became less and less subject to excitement, he grew less irritable, his temper was more controlled, and his outbursts of crying were exhibited far less often.

I have cited this instance to show what strange psychic effects may spring from apparently purely physical causes,—though, indeed, the complement of psycho-physical is so unified that it is impossible to divide the components and place them on one plane or the other. In this boy's case, the primary cause of the trouble was probably congenital, but equal and greater troubles may arise from much smaller original defects if the initial habit is confirmed and crystallised by use, as I fear will be the case, if the child is left to develop itself on the lines of the free expression advocates. It is quite certain, for example, in the case just referred to, that no amount of "free" activity could have released the child from his constrictions whilst the influence caused by his malcoordinations still existed.

But surely I have given enough to prove my case against this last development in education. In an ideal world into which children were born with ideal capacities, Mr. Shaw's thesis might have some weight. In this rapidly changing world of the 20th century we require, more than ever before, a system that shall guide and direct the child during his earlier years. This implies no contradiction of what I have said earlier anent the method of constant supervision. The necessary correction of physical and mental faults that I am advocating is a very different thing from the attempt to mould a child into one particular preconceived form. I would only insist that the children of to-day, born as they are with very feeble powers of instinctive control, absolutely require certain definite instructions by which to guide themselves before they can be left to free activity. And these directions must be based on a principle that will help the child to employ his various mechanisms to the best advantage in his daily activities. These directions involve no interference with what the child has to express; they represent merely a cultivation and development of the *means* whereby he may find adequate and satisfying release for his potentialities.

It is true that the foregoing principles must and will involve certain necessary prohibitions, but if we select those essentials that deal with the root cause of the evil instead of with the effects, we render unnecessary the continual admonitions and "naggings" which represented one of the vices of the old system, a vice from which it has been the object of the new education to free the child.

To sum up this aspect of child-training, I find that on the whole the methods of the older educationalists, with their definite prohibitions and their exact instructions, were less harmful than the extremes of the modern school that would base their scheme of education upon a child's instinctive reactions. The older methods failed, I admit, for one reason, because the system was carried too far; for another, because the injunctions and prohibitions were based on tradition, prejudice, and ignorance, instead of upon a scientific principle dictated by reason. But the new methods fail because they are founded on an entirely erroneous assumption which is demonstrably fallacious. Can any method be defended that is open to such a charge?

Give a child conscious control and you give him poise, the essential starting point for education. Without that poise, which is a result aimed at by neither the old nor the new methods of education, he will presently be cramped and distorted by his environment. For although you may choose the environment of a nursery or a school, there are few, indeed, who can choose their desired environment in the world at large. But give the child poise and the reasoned control of his physical being and you fit him for any and every mode of life; he will have wonderful powers of adapting himself to any and every environment that may surround him. And if he be one of those exceptional individuals that, by some rare gift of nature or by some force of personality, are able to bend life to their own needs, be very sure that so far from having suppressed his power of free expression, you will have strengthened and perfected just those abilities which will enable the genius to put forth all that is best and greatest in him.

My last charge against the advocates of free expression is that they themselves are not free. So many propagandists and teachers show an unwarranted intolerance towards the exponents of the old systems. They are, in fact, too constricted in their mental attitude to give play to their imagination. From one extreme they have flown to the other, and so have missed the way of the great middle course which is wide enough to accommodate all shades of opinion.

For let me state clearly in concluding this comment on a new method, that I am, myself, as strong an advocate for free expression, rightly understood, as any propagandist in the United States of America. But I am convinced by long observation and experiment that the untrained child has not the adequate power of free expression. There are certain mechanical and other laws, deduced from untold centuries of human experience, laws that are only in the rarest cases unconsciously followed by the natural child of to-day. (One of these rare cases that has recently come under my notice has been the billiard playing of Mr. George Gray. I am of the opinion that the mechanical principle of the position adopted by him could be scientifically demonstrated as being as nearly perfect for its particular purpose as any position could be. And according to my observation of him, Mr. Gray manifests in his play the most remarkable and controlled kinæsthetic development I have yet witnessed. But how many George Grays has the world so far produced?)

Over twenty-two years ago in Australia, I was teaching what I still believe to be the true meaning of free expression. My pupils in this case came to me for lessons in vocal and dramatic expression. Now by the old methods these pupils would have been taught to imitate their master very accurately in vocal and facial expression, in gesture, in the manner of voice production; and it would have been at once apparent to any one acquainted with the manner and methods of the teachers, where each pupil had received his training. Furthermore, pupils educated by those methods were taught to interpret each poem, scene, or passage on the exact lines that were considered correct by their respective teachers.

My own method, which at that time was regarded as very radical and subversive, was to give my pupils certain lessons in re-education and co-ordination on a basis of conscious guidance and control, and in this way I gave the reciter, actor, or potential artist the means of employing to the best advantage his powers of vocal, facial, and dramatic expression, gesture, etc. He could then safely be permitted to develop his own characteristics. A few suggestions might be necessary as to interpretation, but the individual manner was his own. No pupil of mine could be pointed to as representing some narrow school of expression, although most of them could be recognised by the confidence and freedom of their performances.

And in this connexion it may be of interest to my readers to know that in 1902-3 I decided to test the principles I advocated, and to this end I organised performances of "Hamlet" and "The Merchant of Venice" for which I gave special training on the lines I have just indicated to young men and women, none of whom had previously appeared in a public performance of any kind whatsoever. I trained all these young people on the principles of conscious guidance and control, principles that I had then developed and practised. My friends and critics naturally anticipated a wonderful exhibition of "stage fright" on the evening of the first performance, but as a matter of fact not one of my young students had the least apprehension of that terror. By the time they were ready to appear the idea of "stage fright" was one that seemed to them the merest absurdity. It may be said that they did not understand what was meant by such a condition. And this, although I would not allow a prompter on the nights of the public performance! I regard this as one of the most convincing public demonstrations I have yet made of the wonderful command and self-possession that may be attained by the inculcation of these principles.

For it must be observed that I sent these tyros to the performance capable of expressing their own individualities. If they had been hedged about or boxed in by an endless series of "Dont's" confining their performances by a rigid set of rules, the majority of them would almost certainly have broken down within the first two minutes. On the other hand, it is hardly necessary to picture the chaos that would have ensued, had I sent them on the stage without training of any kind, poor, helpless, ignorant examples of what they supposed to be free expression.

The foregoing is an example of education in only one sphere of art, but it serves as an excellent indication of the essential needs of education, in general, where the child is concerned. We must give the child of to-day and of the future as a fundamental of education as complete a command of his or her kinæsthetic systems as is possible, so that the highest possible standard of "free expression" may be given in every sphere of life and in all forms of human activity. We must build up, co-ordinate, and re-adjust the human machine so that it may be *in tune*. We are all acquainted with the expression *"tune up"* where the automobile is concerned, and when we wish to command the best expression of this machine we avail ourselves of the *"tuning up"* process of the mechanical expert. And as the human organism is, as Huxley says, a machine, we must remember that if we wish it to express its potentialities adequately it must be *"in tune."* This will represent what we consider to be that satisfactory condition of the child's kinæsthetic systems which will enable him to express himself freely and adequately. It constitutes the "means whereby" of free and full expression, of adaptability to the ever changing environment of civilised life, and to all that these two essentials connote.

In this note on race culture and the training of children, I have thus far dwelt almost exclusively on the earlier years of childhood. But I have much to say at some future time on the questions of primary and secondary education, that is, of the boy and girl at school between the ages of, say, seven and eighteen. No one who has read so far with attention and has earnestly attempted to comprehend my point of view, will now be able to urge that the question of education, secular or religious, is outside my province, for the mental and physical are so inextricably combined that we cannot consider the one without the other, but, at the risk of being accused of repetition, I will briefly state my case in this connexion once again, as follows:

I wish to postulate:

That conscious guidance and control, as a universal, must be the fundamental of future education.

That civilisation and education, as manifested up to the present, cannot be said to have compelled man to advance adequately from the lower to those higher planes of satisfactory evolution, where his savage animal instincts will not under any circumstances, or in response to any stimuli, dominate his transcendent tendencies, or put him out of communication with his reason.

That mankind should progress by slow continuous processes from one stage of evolution to another. This will be particularly the case when he is passing from his animal subconscious stage to the higher, reasoned conscious stages, during which process he will develop a new subconsciousness (cultivated, not inherited) under the guidance of consciousness, likewise an increasing control which holds his animal proclivities in check.

That the evolutionary progress from childhood to adolescence, and so through the vicissitudes of life which follow, is determined by the process adopted, the ratio of progress being in accordance with the standard of efficacy of this process, and that this principle of evolution applies equally to a nation.

That subconsciously developed mechanisms (subconscious guidance and control) function satisfactorily during those stages of our evolution which approximate to the more or less animal plane.

That the old moderate methods of education are not incompatible with cultivation and development on the animal subconscious plane.

That "free expression" principles cannot bring satisfactory results while the subject's mechanisms are operated by inherited subconscious guidance and control.

For this very reason, all aid to progressive development must conform to the principle to the projection of guiding orders and controls in the right direction or directions with the simultaneous employment of positions of mechanical advantage, irrespective of the correctness or otherwise of the immediate result. The result may be unsatisfactory to-day and to-morrow, or during the next week, but if the position of mechanical advantage is employed and orders and controls in the right direction are held in mind and projected again and again, a new and correct complex sooner or later supersedes the old vicious one, and becomes permanently established.

That consciously controlled mechanisms (conscious guidance and control) are essential to man's satisfactory development and progress to the higher stages of his evolution; and to that continued adequate vital functioning of his physical or mental organism necessary in these advanced stages, where more rapid adaptability to the swiftly and ever-changing environment, and the power to *see*, and *comprehend new ideas*, are the urgent demands of an advancing civilisation.

That consciously controlled mechanisms are essential to the successful inculcation of the principle of "free expression" and all that it connotes in Education.

Conscious guidance and control, as the fundamental in education, commands the fundamentals of "free expression." The words free or freedom are herein used in their true meaning, not in the ordinary acceptation. I refer to the point of view which causes one to ask, "Is there such a thing as real freedom?" For we know that we cannot have freedom without restraint, any more than we can have psycho-physical harmony without antagonism.

It is said that the dividing line between tragedy and comedy is not one that the majority of people readily recognise, and this is also the case in regard to what is called freedom and licence. This is the danger which the new democracies of the world are facing at this very moment, and their dangers will be increased a thousandfold in the near future, when they will be called upon to pass through that critical period of re-adjustment which must follow the present world crisis.

In this matter of education I am, admittedly, an iconoclast. I would fain break down the idols of tradition and set up new concepts. In no matters do we see more plainly the harmful effect of the rigid convention than in this matter of teaching. We speak commonly of training the minds of children. It is a happy expression in its origin, and we still retain its proper intention when we apply the word to its uses in horticulture.

The gardener does, indeed, train the young growth. He draws it out to the light and warmth and leads it into the conditions most helpful for its development.

And so, in teaching, the first essential should be to cultivate the uses of the mind and body, and not, as is so often the case, to neglect the instrument of thought and reason by the inculcation of fixed rules which have never been examined. Again, where ideas that are patently erroneous have already been formed in the child's mind, the teacher should take pains to apprehend these preconceptions, and in dealing with them he should not attempt to overlay them, but should eradicate them as far as possible before teaching or submitting the new and correct idea. I say "teaching or submitting" and perhaps the latter word better expresses my meaning, for by teaching I understand the placing of facts, for and against, before the child, in such a way as to appeal to his reasoning faculties, and to his latent powers of originality. He should be allowed to think for himself, and should not be crammed with other people's ideas, or one side only of a controversial subject. Why should not the child's powers of intelligence be trained? Why should they be stunted by our forcing him to accept the preconceived ideas and traditions which have been handed down from generation to generation, without examination, without reason, *without enquiry as to their truth or origin*? The human mind of to-day is suffering from partial paralysis by this method of forcing these unreasoned and antiquated principles upon the young and plastic intelligence.

The educational system itself is grievously inadequate and detrimental, as all thinking educationalists are aware, but the decision regarding the necessity for physical exercise and "deep-breathing" in our schools has added another evil. I wish to say here deliberately that the many systems of physical training generally adopted show an almost criminal neglect of rational method, and of the test which can demonstrably prove the practice to be unsound and hurtful.

Some years ago I wrote in the *Pall Mall Gazette*:

> "I will merely point out that in our schools and in the Army human beings are actually being developed into deformities by breathing and physical exercises. I have before me a book on the breathing exercises which are used in the Army, and any person reasonably versed in physiology and psychology, and knowing they are inseparable in practice, will at once understand why so much harm results from them. Take either the officers or the men. In a greater or less degree the unduly protruded upper chests (development of emphysema), unduly hollowed backs (lordosis), stiff necks, rigid thorax, and other physical

> eccentricities have been cultivated. It is for these reasons that heart troubles, varicose veins, emphysema, and mouth breathing (in exercise) are so much in evidence in the Army. As this is a matter of *national importance, I am prepared to give the time necessary to prove to the authorities (medical or official) connected with the Army, the schools, or the sanatoria, that the 'deep breathing' and physical exercises in vogue are doing far more harm than good,* and are laying the foundations of much graver trouble in the future. The truth is that all exercises involving 'deep breathing' cause an exaggeration of the defective muscular co-ordination already present, so that even if one bad habit is eradicated many others—often more harmful—are cultivated."

And again in my pamphlet *"Why We Breathe Incorrectly"* (Nov., 1909) I wrote:

> "Let me make myself clear by explaining that the man who breathes incorrectly and inadequately, does so as an immediate and inevitable consequence of abnormal and harmful conditions of certain parts of his body. The man who breathes correctly and adequately does so as an immediate and inevitable consequence of normal and salubrious conditions of the same parts. It therefore follows that if the conditions present in the second man can be induced in the first, he will then, but not otherwise, be a correct and adequate breather. And the process by which this is achieved is simply a readjustment of the parts of the body by a new and correct use of the muscular mechanisms through the directive agent of the sphere of consciousness. This change brings about a proper mechanical advantage of all the parts concerned, and causes, thanks to the right employment of the relative machinery, such expansion and contraction of the thoracic cavity as to give atmospheric pressure its opportunity. Now here we have (a) the directive agent of the sphere of consciousness, and (b) the use of the muscular mechanisms—the combination causing certain expansions and contractions, and *the result being what is known as breathing.* It will at once be seen, therefore, that the act of breathing is not a primary, or even a secondary, part of the process, which is really *re-education of the kinæsthetic systems associated with correct bodily postures and respiration,* and will be referred to universally as such in the near future. As a matter of fact, given the perfect co-ordination of parts as acquired by my system, breathing is a subordinate operation which will perform itself."

I stand by every word of this to-day. Hundreds of soldiers every year have to leave the British Army on account of heart trouble directly brought about by the "drill-sergeant's chest" and its concomitant strains and rigidities. Not long ago, Mr. Punch had a picture of a young boy riding in the Row with his groom and answering that worthy's question as to how he would salute a Royal Personage—"Same as the soldiers do; hold my hand up to my hat and look as if I was going to burst!" Certainly a straw showing which way the wind blows.

These same soldiers will start on a long route march with chest "well set" and stiff. The strain of marching inevitably brings them later into an easier slouching position, which makes continuance possible and at its worst is not so positively harmful as is the tension of the other posture.

Compare the free, loose but more healthy physical attitude of the sailor ashore with that of the "smart" soldier strutting in town like a pouter pigeon for the honour of the regiment. It is your team of sailors that is the readier and the more effective for hard work.

And but a few weeks (now years) ago, I saw with dismay in a popular illustrated daily paper a truly pathetic picture of a class of schoolboys with hollowed backs and protruding chests looking like nothing so much as very ruffled pouter pigeons. And the master was commended for his zeal in producing such results by "deep breathing." (See photographs facing this page.)

Is it, I would ask, likely on the face of it that the right position in which a man or woman should stand for health's sake should be one needing positive strain to preserve? The thing is preposterous, and I am convinced that nothing can result from the application of such principles but complete chaos, physical and mental.

To return to my general theory of training, I fear I must not particularise too definitely in some directions, but my instance of right-handedness has its application. On the one hand we are willing to sacrifice reason for such a tradition and convention as this; on the other for an untried and possibly illogical idea. The defence for the latter sacrifice is generally based either on the need for enthusiasm or the necessity for proceeding by a system of trial and error. Well, as to enthusiasm, I will claim that no one is a greater enthusiast than I am myself, but I will not permit my enthusiasm to dominate my reason. One day I hope to write an account of how I arrived at the practical elucidation of my principles of conscious control, and when I do, I shall show very plainly how one of the greatest, if not *the* greatest danger against which I had to fight was my own enthusiasm. It is as vivid and keen to-day as it was over twenty years ago, but I should never have worked out my principles, if I had allowed it to dominate my reason. Again, as to the argument pleading the necessity for empiricism, I admit also that my own methods have been and still are, in some directions, experimental. But with regard to the "free expression" movement, I claim that the error in practice has been sufficiently demonstrated, and further than that, I must insist that we are not justified in experimenting on children. I have

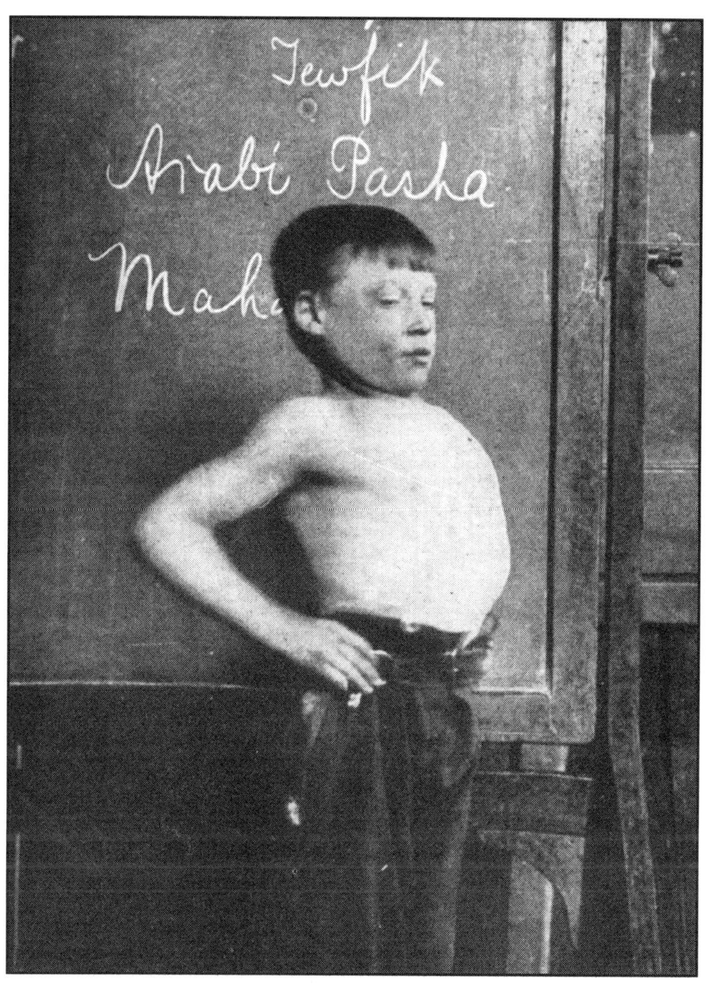

This photograph, published a few years ago in an English daily paper, represents a member of a class in a London country council school performing deep breathing exercises. On the back of this page this lad may be seen at work in the class. These unfortunate boys as here shown are simply being developed into deformities. Luckily of late a change for the better has taken place in school calisthenics.

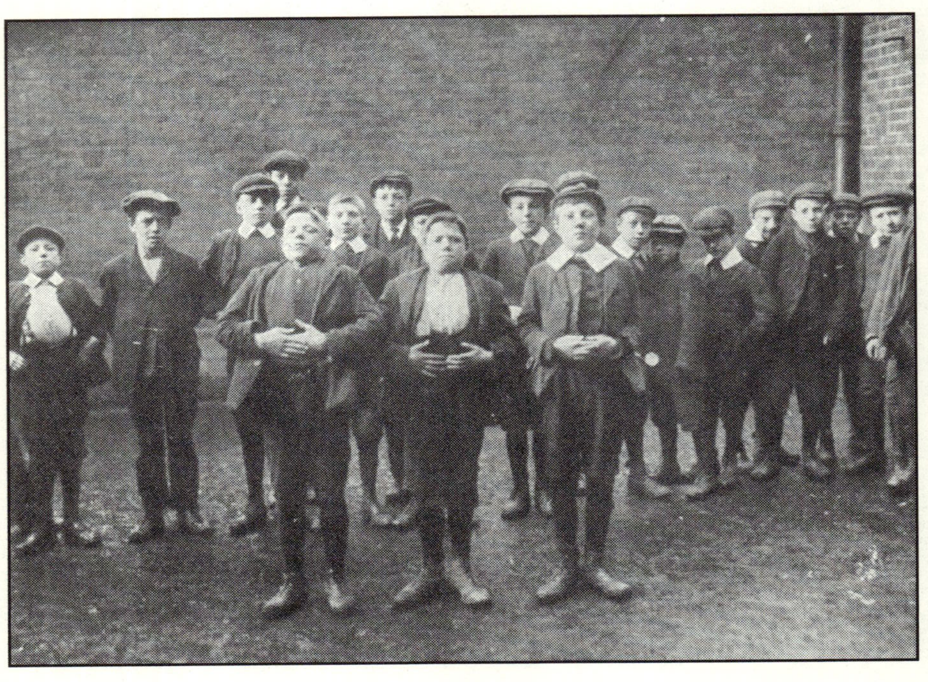

See note on front of page.

never done that inasmuch as I have realised that the error may be irreparable. Could any fault weigh heavier on a human conscience than that by which, however unwittingly, another human life had been distorted?

Wherefore, pleading on behalf of my most important client, the child of this younger generation, I demand that we shall proceed to neither of the dangerous extremes that threaten his physical and mental well-being. On the one hand we must avoid the thrusting upon him of fixed ideas, by which you may narrow his mind, for I know that when you limit him, imparting to him deliberately your own mental habits, the effects go far beyond what we are pleased to call the "formation of character." On the other hand we are not justified in leaving him entirely to himself. Whilst he has the right of choice within certain limits, he has not, unhappily, the ability to choose in his earlier years. We need not bind him to choose this or that, but we must educate him in such a way as to give him the power of choice. In Mr. Allen Upward's delightful work, *The New Word*, which I have already quoted, he says: "Give the child leave to grow. Give the child leave to live. Give the child leave to hope and to hope truly. . . . He is the plaintiff in this case. I say that he is mankind . . . and his birthright is the truth." And to that I would add, "Give the child leave, also, to learn. Give him opportunity to profit by all the knowledge we can give him out of our experience. His birthright, indeed, is the truth, but we must aid him in making the discovery."

It is full time that we gave more earnest thought to this matter. I cannot in this brief outline dwell on the many phases of proper food, clothing, and physical training, and all those other points which we must consider. The Kinæsthetic Systems concerned with correct and healthy bodily movements and postures have become demoralised by the habits engendered in the schoolroom through the restraint enforced at a time when natural activity should have been encouraged and scientifically directed, and in the crouching positions caused by useless and irrational deskwork.

And I may note in this connexion that I am continually being asked, both by friends and unknown correspondents, for my opinion concerning the correct type of chair, stool, desk or table to be used in order to prevent the bad habits which these pieces of furniture are supposed to have caused in schools. In my replies I have tried to demonstrate that the problem is being attacked from the wrong standpoint.

Let us consider the problem in the light of common sense. Suppose, for example, that there is an ideal chair, some wonderful arrangement of perfect angles, hollows, and supports that will almost magically rectify or prevent every fault in the child's physical mechanism. Suppose further that the child finds great ease and repose when seated in this ideal chair. How then can he avoid suffering the tortures of all that is uncomfortable, when he rides in the cars, or sits down in his own home, or visits a friend, or goes for a picnic on the river or in the woods? I see nothing else for it; when that ideal chair has been found, our child will have to carry it about with him wherever he goes.

In the second place, how is it possible for this ideal chair to be miraculously adaptable to every age and type of child? Are we to treat children as plastic lumps of clay to be fitted to the model insisted upon by the lines of our ideal chair; or are we to study and measure each individual and have a chair built to his measure, once a year, say, until he is adult?

No, what we need to do is not to educate our school furniture, but to educated our children. Give a child the ability to adapt himself within reasonable limits to his environment, and he will not suffer discomfort, nor develop bad physical habits, whatever chair or form you give him to sit upon. I say, "within reasonable limits," for it is obviously absurd to expect a Brobdingnagian child to use a Lilliputian chair. But let us waste no valuable time, thought, or invention in designing furniture, when by a smaller expenditure of those three gifts we may train the child to win its own conscious control, and rise superior to any probable limitations imposed by ordinary school fittings.

For the problem to be solved in education is that same problem which needs solution in the social, political, religious, industrial, economic, ethical, æsthetic and other spheres of progressive human activity. In every sphere of life we have for years given "effects" the significance of "causes" and have made worthy attempts to put matters right on this unsound basis. In the case of education certain symptoms have been recognised as more or less harmful, and the whole blame has been placed upon the method or methods of education involved.

For at least half a century, the method of the social worker was conceived on the lines of giving money, food, and clothing to the poor, in an attempt to ameliorate their condition. The evils of this false policy came home to them in a practical way, and nowadays, the object of the social worker is to give the poor the "means whereby" of general advancement and of getting money, clothes, and food by their own efforts.

The same principle holds good in the treatment of the children. Hitherto educationalists have given them what they considered they needed. What we must do in the future is to give them the "means whereby" they may themselves satisfy their needs and command their own advancement.

The adoption of new methods is a procedure which always demands a due and proper consideration of the thing, person, or persons to which they are to be applied. Investigation along these lines would probably have revealed the real *cause* of the difficulties to be faced in the education of the child of to-day, which is that the process of civilised life has gradually changed the child's psycho-physical condition at birth. In this process much has been gained and much lost. From the educator's point of view the losses have been stupendous as compared with the gains, for the all-important kinæsthetic systems have been deteriorated by man's attempt to pass from the lower (animal) to the higher stages of the evolutionary plane while depending upon a subconsciously controlled organism.

I have still very much more to say on this subject of education, and I hope to have an opportunity in the near future of elaborating my methods and of setting them out so that they may be practically and universally applied. But if by these few remarks I can arouse some interest in this world problem, I shall have done something towards its solution. It is a problem which is very urgent at the present time, and is growing more urgent every day. All that we have done up to the present time is to enforce one rule or another upon the children as an experiment, for all the rules have been rigid in their enforcement, however unscientific in their conception. In place of these rules I look for an ideal which I believe to be comparatively easy of realisation. I look for, and already see, a method of training our children which shall make them masters of their own bodies; I look for a time when the child shall be so taught and trained that whatever the circumstance which shall later surround it, it will without effort be able to adapt itself to its environment, and be enabled to live its life in the enjoyment of perfect health, physical and mental. For, as I have already pointed out, man has progressed towards the higher and more complex stages of civilisation. He has continued to change his habits of life and being still far from the highest state attainable he will continue to change. The farther he becomes removed from the primitive uncivilised stage of his evolution the less likely is he to have the opportunity in the daily routine of his life so to exercise the physical machinery that it will be prevented from working imperfectly by the controls of instinct. "Conscious control" will enable man to adapt himself more readily to changing conditions of life. No one who looks out upon this latter day world with discerning eyes can fail to see that the changes tend to become more rapid and more radical than ever before in the history of the world's progress.

We look towards the goal, and it is best to seek the highest and be content with no less, but at the same time it is necessary that we should consider the practical detail of our journey. What follows in Parts II and III may seem trivial by comparison with the high endeavour I have outlined, but it is the triviality of the essential detail.

I wish to point the road still more clearly, and to show how every man and woman may learn to walk upon it.

CHAPTER VIII

EVOLUTIONARY STANDARDS AND THEIR INFLUENCE ON THE CRISIS OF 1914

In the previous chapters I have dealt briefly with the fundamentals upon which our whole structure of education and civilisation is based, and have attempted to point to the different tendencies developed by the individual in the struggle to progress upon this basis. At the same time I have indicated that which I am confident is the only true fundamental upon which mankind in a state of civilisation may progress and evolve to a condition commanding freedom for all time from those limiting, narrowing, and debasing qualities which belong to the animal spheres of existence.

It seems to me that the present world crisis indicates that this is the psychological moment to make a wide application of my principles, though my reader may consider that I should not enter the debatable ground of hypothesis in a work which has been devoted, up to this point, to arguments almost entirely drawn from personal experiences and observation.

I have dealt with the fundamentals employed in the development of the child and the adult, and I have postulated that the evolutionary progress from childhood to adolescence, and on through the vicissitudes of life which follow, is determined by the process adopted, the ratio of progress being in accordance with the standard of efficacy of this process, and that this principle of evolution applies equally to a nation.

It then devolves upon us to consider the different processes adopted by different nations, in order to gauge accurately their different stages of evolution and their possibilities of growth and development towards real individual and national progress.

After centuries of endeavour in the direction of progress in accordance with well-defined processes, founded upon approved educational, religious, economic, political, industrial, ethical and æsthetic principles, and after a century of unprecedented progress in the realm of Arts and Sciences, we are faced with the spectacle, in a supposedly civilised nation, of a debauched kinæsthesia which has manifested itself in such a display of savage instincts as will present us in the eyes of a more highly evolved universe as plunged in the depths of barbarism.

During the past three years the people of the world have been shocked and stirred by events which even four years ago were considered impossible in the stage of civilisation then reached. In consequence, we find that a special and earnest endeavour is being made to solve problems of vital importance which have a bearing upon the future development and cultivation of the potentialities of mankind.

It is, therefore, essential to recognise that we have reached a point in the process called civilisation which will be recorded as one of the most critical and vital in the world's history.

At this moment the great nations of Europe are engaged in the most terrific conflict of force ever recorded, whilst in America, a land of peace, there is being witnessed what is probably the most bitterly contested conflict of opinion ever experienced regarding the conduct, policy, and duty of the American nation where the old world is concerned.

(This was penned prior to American intervention in the war.)

The happenings of the past three years must influence our present and future opinion of the value of our educational, political, moral, social, industrial, religious and other principles where the progress of man is concerned, as he passes from the animal plane of his evolution to those higher planes for which he is undoubtedly destined.

The conclusions thus reached will so influence the future welfare of mankind that the facts from which these conclusions are deduced demand the most serious attention and study of every human being.

It is therefore essential that we make an earnest endeavour to discover fundamentals. In this connexion we must consider the available evidence concerning the cause or causes of this conflict in Europe which has shaken our boasted advancement in civilisation to its very roots. What does this recrudescence of barbarity mean when viewed with an open and unprejudiced mind in its relation to the future of those principles which alone make for the real mental, physical, and spiritual growth of mankind in progressive civilisation?

It signifies a tremendous clash of opposing forces, a desperate conflict between the lowly-evolved peoples of the world as against the more highly evolved races, the struggle of an open-minded, mobile idealism for the supremacy of the individual against a narrow-minded, rigid, material automatism which entails the suppression of the individual and the obliteration of his reason in the supposed interests of the State.

Let us take, then, a general comparative view of the compelling psycho-physical forces in the life of primitive and civilised nations up to the crisis. America in this stands apart and must be considered separately.

In Primitive Nations. The compelling forces were chiefly physical and subconscious. The very essentials of life depended almost entirely upon brute force. Daily experiences gave a keen edge to savage instincts and unbridled passions, to an automatic development which opposed the cultivation of the faculty of adaptability to new environments. Even the spheres of courage were limited, and when confronted with the unusual these peoples quaked like cowards, and fled panic-stricken from the unaccustomed, as in the case of the negroes in the Southern States of America when the men of the Ku-Klux Klan pursued them on horseback dressed in white.

In Civilised Nations. The compelling forces have become less and less physical and less subconscious than in the case of primitive nations, but the advance from the physical to the mental and from the subconscious to the conscious has not been adequate or sufficiently comprehensive to establish the mental and conscious principles as the chief compelling forces in the progress of the nation or even of the individual. The essentials of life do not depend upon brute force, and daily experiences become less and less associated with factors which make for the development of savage instincts and unbridled passion, or automatic development. But experience has proved that civilised nations have failed to come through the ordeal of adaptation to the ever-changing environment of civilisation with satisfactory results. The spheres of courage are still more or less limited, and when brought suddenly face to face with the unusual and unexpected people still exhibit a tendency to panic and loss of control. The progress made by civilised nations from the primitive state to the present has not been upon comprehensive lines. The result has been that the majority of the activities of the nation have been limited, and in those few activities where the widening influence held sway, the freedom became licence and led to overcompensation. This condition was sufficiently harmful as long as it applied to the individual and to individual effort, the individual being more or less held in check by collective opinion; but when it applied to the nation and to national effort, that nation which ignored the opinion of other nations developed unchecked, and the national decision to stifle the individual, body and soul, if it seemed to be for the welfare of the State, constituted the most powerful force in the prevention of progress on the evolutionary plane.

For this decision, once it became the result of national conception, carried with it the most damaging and impossible of all mental processes in the sphere of true evolutionary advancement. In the first place the national decision was the result of an erroneous national conception, the outcome of what I have called, for the want of a better name, "manufactured premises."

Manufactured premises are the forerunners of unsound and delusive deductions—a stultification of reason—and demand the cultivation of a form of self-hypnotism which is fatal to national or individual progress.

A few observant people noted this dangerous habit even in the early literature of the German nation, and watched with keen interest its cultivation in all spheres of activity in recent years. This explains the stupendous failure of German judgment in all matters of national and international importance, of the impossibility of the peoples of that nation to see anything from any other point of view but their own, of their crass stupidity in gauging the psychology of other nations, and particularly that of the American nation.

In the foregoing we have fundamentals worthy of consideration. They must occupy the attention of all thinking people who wish to make a contribution towards the uplifting of mankind and the establishment of a standard of reasoned guidance and control which should make another barbarous conflict unthinkable and therefore impossible.

Naturally, every nation is ready enough with a more or less humane reason for its madness. Self-protection, an altruistic regard for the rights of smaller nations, a sense of high duty towards mankind at large, all these pleas have been urged as explaining the single principle which has drawn this or that nation into the whirlpool. And each and every nation must surely have pleaded liberty as their excuse at some time or another, liberty being one of those adaptable terms that may be used to mean almost anything. Before the war Germany was maintaining a right for "liberty" of expansion, a defensive use of the word that has hardly anything in common with the American use at the present time.

On the other hand philosophers, economists, psychologists, commercial experts, and the public at large have been busy with a dozen other theories of the primary causes of the war. We have heard much talk of race hatred, of business rivalry, of high commercial and political intrigues, and a dozen other influences, and all of them have been put forward at one time or another as the sole reason for the present welter of blood and fury. We have, in fine, so many reasons from which to choose that we may be quite sure no single one of them can possibly afford us an inclusive and adequate explanation.

But I will go still further than that. For I maintain on grounds which I find logically unshakeable, that if we admit, as seems the only sensible course, that something of all these reasons and excuses has entered into the conditions producing such awful results, we must still seek some explanation of the preceding state that made these conditions possible. All our reasons, in fact, are mere effects, and we are groping for our primary cause among resultant phenomena. We can never solve our problem by such a method as this. We might as well hope to find the origin of a child by dissecting its limbs and intestines. Our only hope is to shift our viewpoint, to cease our muddled examination of the details just in front of us, and try to see our problem in the broad terms of one who can stand back and see life moving through the centuries.

With all people, in all spheres of life, we know only too well that certain mental and physical manifestations give an absolute clue to their character, to their aims in life, their ideals, and, what is more to the point, to the stage they have reached in the process called evolution.

Incidentally, I would point out that education as generally understood, even when it implies the most up-to-date methods, does not necessarily mean progress on the evolutionary plane any more than ability as a linguist need denote a high standard of mentality.

This applies also to most arts and particularly to those where music and dancing are concerned. The lower the stage of evolution, within certain limits, the greater the appeal of music and dancing.

When we review the history and general progress of humanity we find the instincts and traits of the animal—the brute force principle—predominating at certain stages. If we go back far enough we find that there was a stage when it was always predominant.

Therefore, a test as to the ratio of progress of nations on the evolutionary plane is to be found in their tendency and desire to advance beyond that stage where the mental and physical forces, which should only belong as inherited instincts to the brute animals and savages, hold sway; and with this in view, if we take a survey of the history, ideals, habits of life, mental outlook, and general tendencies of the German nation, it will show conclusively that these self-hypnotised people approximated too closely to the lower animals and savages in their mode and chief aims of life.

The great and noble ideals and aims of mankind making for progress towards the more highly evolved states were cast aside for the unreasoning, brutal, and ignoble principles which make for the debasement of man's elevating potentialities, and hold him a slave to the cruel and lowly-evolved state of the primitive creatures. That any nation or nations should deliberately adopt, as their highest ideals and aims, brute force in all its hideous aspects, desecration of mind, body, and soul for the State, justification of criminal instincts and acts if employed on behalf of the State, destruction, rape and plunder, murder and torture to terrify innocent civilians; that they should adopt, in short, the brutal principle that "Might is Right" in that special national form in which it has been manifested in the last half century and directed towards what is now known as "Militarism,"—all this is surely proof positive that they have progressed but little on the upward evolutionary stage from the state occupied by the brute beast and the savage. The criminal aspect of the outrage of all that right-thinking human beings hold dear is intensified by the fact that the nations which perpetrated the deed were among the most prosperous of the world, and enjoyed, as aliens, the same privileges as the subjects of those nations whose hospitality and confidence they abused.

The nations bearing the brunt of the struggle against this outburst of primitive brutal instincts and desires have long since reached a stage in their evolution which made the methods of Attila unthinkable. If forced into war they conducted it on the evolved plane of the human, and not that of the animal. They treated their captives as honourable men and extended to them every conceivable consideration within their power. Prior to this war the ideals and aims of these nations were the antithesis of those of their lowly-evolved enemies, and they were ideals and aims which made for the right to live in peace with all other nations. They aimed at the reduction of armaments, and gave practical proof of their aims. They opened their ports and their markets to their present enemies and gave them a free hand in every respect in all spheres of activity. They had no desire to beat down the ideals and principles which make for the ennoblement of mankind, they had no wish to dominate the world by brute force and to establish a system of living and a form of conduct which grinds the individual into a mere heartless unreasoning automaton, rigid-brained, driven like an animal, and not daring to claim even his soul as his own.

For many years prior to the crisis of 1914 we listened to the blatant outbursts of German professors and other educated authorities of that nation concerning its superiority to other nations. We were asked to believe that certain individuals of that nationality had reached the stage of the superman. These unfortunate and deluded people have for some time been cursed with this obsession.

Thinking men and women of other nations listened and wondered when these claims were made concerning these supermen, and after examining the evidence advanced to support these claims became convinced that they were not justified. The stupendous failure of the supposed supermen in every sphere of mental and physical activity in the present war proves the correctness of these convictions.

It seems inconceivable that supermen could so have guided and directed the whole national energy of Germany that it became more and more narrowed,—like the German mind,—until it concentrated almost solely upon the stupid conception of the domination of the world by Germany. To this end, the national energy was diverted chiefly into two channels:

COMMERCIAL INDUSTRY AND MILITARISM

One of the great features connected with the former was the extraordinary development of machinery, which demanded for its successful pursuance that the individual should be subjected to the most harmful systems of automatic training.

The standardised parts of the machine made demands which tended to stereotype the human machine. The limitations of human activity, mental and physical, reached the maximum. The power to continue work under such conditions depended upon a process of deterioration in the individual. He was slowly but surely being robbed of the possibility of development. The very soul of man was crushed to foster an industrial process which was to provide the sinews of the war machine, to support that curse called militarism, and the demoralisation of Germany came chiefly through that nation's conceptions of militarism which, in the first and last analysis, stands for the worst manifestation of those savage instincts and unbridled passions associated with the lowest stages of primitive race development.

The horrible results of the sum total of the national madness which the foregoing represents are now revealed before us, for to Germany this militarism constituted a rigid plan, a system, and a world-philosophy.

She is convinced, against all the evidence, that her plan, system, or philosophy, is so undeniably right as to constitute an absolute. As a nation she has no mobility, no poise. She is influenced by a stultifying idea, the perfection of her own "Kultur" (a word more properly translated as a civilisation than by the word "culture" as used in the English or American sense). She is, in fact, just as badly co-ordinated, as unable to follow the true mandate of reason, as any individual who is dominated by a fixed idea.

For the trouble is that when reason is so far held in check that is loses its power of denial, it must have lost its power of control. The original "idea" formulated in the conscious mind has sunk so deep into the subconscious that it cannot be changed except under the influence of some stronger outside power. For nearly fifty years Germany, in her schools, her gymnasiums, her universities, her civic and her political life, has been inculcating a rigid and mentally demoralising system, and she is suffering now—as the monomaniac in private life must suffer—for her particular form of insanity.

Even in the conduct of her great campaign, this weakness of hers has begun to defeat her. She has lost the power of adaptability in military matters. She repeats the faults of her original plan, despite the endless illustrations that have been afforded by her Western antagonists that that plan can be very considerably bettered. No doubt the Higher Command may realise in some instances the weakness of the old method in conditions that have been immensely modified since August, 1914, but they are impotent to change, in a year or in a decade, the effect of their own teaching on the millions of Germany's army. The massed attack, for example, has been demonstrated to be a disastrous failure—a single well-placed machine-gun can defeat it—but Germany's soldiers will not advance in a scattered attack. They have learnt to depend upon the nearness of their comrades. Separate a German battalion and it has neither confidence nor courage.

Again, can one reasonably doubt that the German nation suffers from some form of self-hypnotism when one sees evidence of the almost pathetic belief apparently still placed in the campaign of "frightfulness"? The German people themselves are afraid—an inevitable symptom of certain forms of monomania—of the horrible devices they themselves are using, and no evidence can bring home to them the fact, that the plan of terrorising their enemies not only fails but recoils even upon their own heads. London—I speak from experience—is not intimidated by Zeppelin raids by night, nor by seaplane raids by day. The inhabitants of London do not cower under these terrible afflictions and beg for peace; on the contrary each horrible incident arouses afresh their determination to prevent, if possible, a recurrence of such savagery in the world's history. Any sane nation must have realised this fact eighteen months ago; Germany, blind and rigid in the trance of her self-hypnosis, still staggers on to her own destruction.

In the opposite direction it is interesting to note the methods of the British. In their case, we can trace no such clear effort for narrowness and organisation. The general policy of the nation, whether internal or international, had that haphazard air which is so commonly cited as being a characteristic of the English method as a whole. We saw an almost complete inability to govern or even to manage that still largely subconsciously ruled country of Ireland. We witnessed the most astounding blunders of policy with regard to foreign countries (witness Lord Salisbury's cession of Heligoland to Germany in 1890, Gladstone's handling of the first Boer War, and a dozen other instances), and even with regard to the treatment of Britain's own colonies, whilst internally her educational and administrative systems were the result of a method of trial and error which was sometimes well-nigh disastrous.

The British have in them a peculiar kind of empiricism. They are ready to laugh at and to criticise their own defects. They admit quite freely, for example, that they "blundered through somehow" in the Boer War, and that they have blundered again and again (most destructively in Gallipoli) in the present campaign. Their criticism of the rigidity of their own military methods is a proof that if the criticism is sometimes justified, the people at home—aye! and the New Army abroad—have never been infected with that rigidity themselves. But, in truth, that rigidity of discipline is now little in evidence in the field. And how little it has affected the British and French plan of campaign may be judged by the fact that every new device of any importance during the war, whether a device of method or of mechanical invention, has been originated by France and Great Britain. Now, from the German point of view, this adaptability to circumstances would be pronounced, *a priori*, as certain to lead to disaster. I put it to America, on the evidence afforded by the battle-fields of France, which method is the more likely to achieve ultimate success?

Returning now to my single reason for the cause of the present war, I feel that the explanation has already been given. Granted a nation educated and trained as Germany has been, some explosion was inevitable sooner or later. If we have in our midst an individual suffering from a fixed idea, he must in time become intolerable to us. Never in the history of the world have thought and the tendency to organisation been more fluid than they were in the first years of the 20th century. Yet one great and powerful nation interfered with us at every turn, impeding the flow of liberal thought by her obsession with the ideas of her own greatness and the omnipotence of her military machine. Nevertheless the other nations of Europe adapted themselves within limits to the demands of this rigid mechanism in their midst. And it may be that these very powers of endurance and adaptability hastened the crisis. They were regarded by the monomaniacs of Germany as signs of weakness, and just as their own philosopher Nietzsche went mad by concentration on his own invariable theme, so at last Germany crossed the bounds of sanity, imbued with a crazy belief in her own omnipotence. She ran amuck in the wide streets of Europe, and even yet she has not realised her own madness. I seriously question whether she will come to anything like a proper realisation of that madness in the present generation. She has allowed a habit of mind to become fixed; and it has fallen into the realms of her subconsciousness. We must treat her as mad, but she is nevertheless to be pitied.

Earlier in this chapter, I separated America from the rest of the world. And my reason for this is that I regard this great nation of the United

States as still in its early childhood from one point of view. I have an immense confidence in the future of America. I see that she has potentialities and opportunities such as no other nation has ever had. For her the possibilities of control by reason are illimitable. But at the same time I must issue a very serious warning to every American reader of this book. For already I have seen the imitation of certain habits of thought, habits which, if they are persisted in, will sink deep into the national subconsciousness and prove a source of danger to the body politic.

My wish for America is that she should preserve as far as possible an open mind. She has recently entered the Great War for reasons that every right-minded man and woman must applaud and respect. I trust that she will come out of it with the same balance and power of choice, so that when she has to turn again to her own affairs, to matters of education, of government, and of her commercial interests, she will be able to form a national mind, sane enough and strong enough to control the great national body.

No finer ambition is possible than this. The old ambition of dominance, whether commercial or military, defeats itself by its very exaggeration. Such ambitions mount up until they become topheavy, and, even if they could be achieved, the result would be nothing but a decadence such as that which followed the Empire of Rome.

But given such a power of co-ordination and of self-control in the race, as a unit, as could be compared with the balance of a wise and healthy man, that nation would be free, with a greater liberty than history can record, and to such a nation little would be impossible. She would become the teacher of the world by the force of her reason and example. She would inaugurate the coming of a greater and wiser humanity.

END OF PART I

PART II
CONSCIOUS GUIDANCE AND CONTROL

EDUCATION

"It is because the body is a machine that education is possible. Education is the formation of habits, a superinducing of an artificial organisation upon the natural organisation of the body; so that acts, which at first require a conscious effort, eventually become unconscious and mechanical."

HUXLEY.

RE-EDUCATION

"It is because the body is a machinc that (RE) education is possible. (RE) education is the formation of (NEW AND CORRECT) habits, a (RE-INSTATING OF THE CORRECT) artificial organisation upon the natural organisation of the body; so that acts, which at first require conscious effort, eventually become unconscious and mechanical."

INTRODUCTION TO PART II

IN the first part of this volume I have endeavoured to explain the general principle which underlies my work. I will now present my proposition from a slightly different angle, as it were, to ensure a clearer view of it, that is, I shall deal with it in the light of its practical application to the acts of everyday life.

I trust I may do something to convince thinking men and women that conscious control is essential to man's satisfactory progress in civilisation, and that the properly directed use of such control will enable the individual to stand, sit, walk, breathe, digest, and in fact live with the least possible expenditure of vital energy. This will ensure the highest standard of resistance to disease. When this desirable stage of our evolution is reached the cry of physical deterioration may no longer be heard.

I will write out as concisely, as definitely, and as boldly as possible, my claims and my main argument. In a second part I have added some more discursive notes and comments, which I trust will meet the many requests I have received for further light on certain points in my former book.

With the records of my casebooks for over twenty years before me I feel it right to set down my convictions in terms that do not admit of any doubt or uncertainty. My conclusions upon the urgent question of physical decadence have not been formulated in haste. They are deductions from a long series of striking results and observed facts, and, frankly, I consider them so important that I cannot hesitate to deliver my message in a tone which may appear to some to savour of over-confidence. So be it!

CHAPTER I

SYNOPSIS OF CLAIM

1. My first claim is that psycho-physical guidance by conscious control, when applied as a universal principle to "living," constitutes an unfailing preventive for diseases mental or physical, malformations, and loss of general efficiency. It is commonly considered that these conditions are brought about by such evils of civilisation as the limitation of energy, and by that loss of so-called "natural conditions" which civilisation entails.

It is my earnest belief that the intelligent recognition of the principles essential to guidance by conscious control are essential to the full mental and physical development of the human race. Due consideration will convince even the sceptical that if mankind is to evolve to the higher stages of mental and physical perfection, he must be guided by these principles. They alone will bring men and women of to-day to the highest state of well-being, enabling them to grapple effectively with the problems of the day in the world of thought and action, gradually widening the dividing line which separates civilised mankind from the animal kingdom.

There is no sphere of human activity, of human feeling or philosophy where the adoption of the principles of conscious guidance and control would not bring invaluable benefits.

At present man is held in bondage by many subconscious instincts which enslave the animal kingdom, the savage, and the semi-savage. Let me illustrate this. Animals and savages become immediately unbalanced when they experience the unusual, as for instance, when they see an express train dash along for the first time. Such a new experience would cause the bravest animal to become overwhelmed with that degree of fear which momentarily suspends his normal guidance by instinct. So also with the savage, who would be equally unbalanced by an experience of this kind. In most spheres of normal life, he, like the animal, depends on instinctive guiding principles which act with perfect balance under accustomed circumstances. In the face of the unusual, however, he is unable to meet suddenly the requirements of a new environment. To meet these he needs reasoned, conscious guidance which is the outcome of the habit of conscious control, and marks the dividing line between the animal kingdom, where instinct is the guide, and the human kingdom where its members are in communication with reason.

The mental and physical limitations and imperfections of men and women of the present day make it impossible for them to meet satisfactorily the great majority of the requirements of their present environment, and render them quite incapable of making the best of their capabilities in any new environment. These instinctive guiding principles, not even perfectly balanced as in the case of the savage and the animal, are miserably insufficient to meet the conditions of the modern world with its ever changing environment. Yet it is upon these instincts that men and women rely, to the detriment of their mental and physical attainments.

2. My next claim is that all such diseases as those referred to above (e.g., cancer, appendicitis, bronchitis, tuberculosis, etc.) are too often permitted to remain uneradicated and frequently undetected, and so to develop in consequence of the failure to recognise that the real cause of the development of such diseases is to be found in the erroneous preconceived ideas of the persons immediately concerned, ideas which affect the organism in the manner described in Part I of this book.

The only experience which the average man or woman has in the use of the different parts of the human organism is through his or her subconsciousness. The result is a subconscious direction which in the imperfectly co-ordinated person is based on bad experiences and on the erroneous preconceived ideas before mentioned. Small wonder, then, that such direction is faulty and leads to the development of serious defects and imperfections. With this erroneous direction even the attempt to carry out a simple action in accordance with subconscious habit is fraught with danger, for it invariably affects in a detrimental manner other parts of the subject's organism which have nothing to do with the particular act or acts attempted. For instance, in the subconsciously controlled person the attempt to lengthen the neck is invariably preceded by a movement of the eyes in an upward or downward direction. Wrong use of the eyes in this or some similar manner too frequently is the forerunner of what eventually develops into an established habit, often causing an unnecessary and undue strain of the eyes which seriously impairs their efficiency, and which in the ordinary way of life leads to the specific treatment of these organs. It is obvious, however, that what is needed in such a case is the eradication of the erroneous preconceived idea and harmful habits, thereby removing gradually the undue and unnecessary strain upon the organs of sight. This will enable them to regain their lost efficiency and it is almost certain that specific treatment of any kind on orthodox lines will be unnecessary. In consequence of faulty guidance misdirected energies are not confined to one part of the organism. They affect the hands, arms, shoulders, legs, thorax, hips, knees, ankles and other parts of the organism, frequently causing strain and interference with the functioning of the different organs and finally seriously injuring them. To support this second claim I bring forward the following arguments:

(a) Till now little or no attention on a practical psycho-physical basis has been given to the vital and harmful influence of this faulty direction (of subconscious origin) and of the erroneous preconceived ideas and faulty posture associated therewith. Under such influences the subject can hardly fail to cultivate a wrong mental attitude towards life in general and towards the art of living (evolving satisfactorily), especially in regard to the primary causation of the defects which may be present or which may develop eventually, but also in regard to the essential laws connected with the eradication of these defects.

(b) Owing to the lack of distinction between reasoned (conscious) and unreasoned (subconscious or partly conscious) actions, the subject suffers from various forms of mental and physical delusions, notably with regard to the physical acts he performs. Incidentally it should be pointed out that if this is true of the ordinary acts of everyday life how much more so of those physical acts which may be necessary to meet the demands of some new environment! As a striking instance of delusion in physical acts let us take the case of a man *who believes himself to be merely overcoming what he regards as essential inertia, when he is really fighting the resistance of undue antagonistic muscular action exerted by himself*, a resistance of which he is not consciously aware. In all such cases there is a constant conflict between two great forces, the one (subconscious) destined to exercise supreme directive powers during the early stages of human evolution, the other (conscious) to supersede this limited direction and finally to prove the reliable guide through the higher and highest stages of the great evolutionary scheme which leads to the full enjoyment of his potentialities. It must be remembered that the former became firmly established during centuries of subconscious direction, holding undisputed sway until the first glimmering of reasoned conscious guidance came in its crudest form to disturb its power, a power which it is destined one day to overthrow. In the present stage of our mental and physical progress the conflict continues with gradually increasing energy, and while the conflict is being waged the subject is influenced first in one direction by the dictates of his subconsciousness (called by some "instinct," by others "intuition"), and then in another by his awakened conscious powers which he is gradually but slowly developing. Of the real significance of this conflict he has, unfortunately, no true realisation. At the same time he undoubtedly feels the force of these two influences as conflicting energies, but only in a dim, mysterious way. He is swayed first by one force and then by the other as happens when we hear a man or woman say, "Well, that seems the thing to do, but I feel that I shouldn't do it."

Very often he does what he feels instead of what seems to be the correct thing, and, moreover, the former is very frequently right. This is not surprising, seeing that the subconscious instinct in us is much more developed than the conscious faculty. But granting the subconscious its fullest degree of merit, we are forced to recognise its serious limitations in the mode of life (civilisation) with its ever changing environment which human progress demands. We must have a guiding principle without these limitations, to enable us to adapt ourselves much more quickly to the new environments which are inevitable in the progress of civilisation towards its legitimate goal.

We must have something more reasoned and definite than that which subconscious direction offers, and so we come to the need of reasoned guidance. Up to the present neither of these forms of direction really reaches the mind as a definite tangible idea consciously conceived. This is because of the fundamental principles upon which subconscious direction has been built up, and in consequence of the undeveloped condition of conscious guidance. Furthermore, the subject has not yet made any serious attempt to analyse these two forces, of whose particular workings he is but dimly aware. The fundamental principle which we call evolution demands that every human being shall be enabled to make this analysis, so that he may differentiate between the impulses springing from his subconsciousness (instinct-inhibition) and the conceptions created in his reasoning conscious mind.

The subject will thus cultivate the habit of distinguishing between reasoned and unreasoned actions and this will at once tend to the prevention of mental and physical delusions in all directions, notably in regard to his physical acts in old or new environments.

(c) Whilst these delusions remain, the subject will continue to perform wrong or detrimental actions, for as long as his settled mental attitude towards such actions remains unchanged, he will believe that he is performing them in a correct manner. It is owing to this involuntary, and on his part unrecognised, misapprehension, that many malformations and inefficiencies become established, which sooner or later may lead to definite disease. The popular misconception of the subject's responsibility in the matter leads him to be commonly pitied as for unavoidable defects, whereas it is of the first importance that he should realise the responsibility is his and his alone. He must be made aware that such defects arise from his own fault, and are the outcome of his ignorance or wilful neglect.

Once this new mental attitude is firmly established there is hope for the afflicted person and he will have the satisfaction of knowing that he is, as it were, working out his own salvation on common-sense practical lines, devoid of pernicious sympathy, face to face with real facts, and stimulated by a principle which cannot fail to secure the very best efforts in the right direction of which any ordinary person is capable.

(d) It is essential in the necessary re-education of the subject through conscious guidance and control that in every case the "means whereby" rather than the "end," must be held in mind. As long as the "end" is held in mind instead of the "means," the muscular act, or series of acts, will always be performed in accordance with the mode established by old habits. When each stage of the series essential to the "means whereby" is correctly apprehended by the conscious mind of the subject, the old habits can be broken up, and every muscular action can be consciously directed until the new and correct guiding sensations have established the new proper habits which in their turn become subconscious, but on a more highly evolved plane.

In effect these new habits ensure conditions which give new life to, and maintain in a high state of efficiency, every organ of the body, the automatic functions being reacted upon by the consciously controlled energies. By my system of obtaining the position of "*mechanical advantage*,"[15] a perfect system of natural internal massage is rendered possible, such as never before has been attained by orthodox methods, a system which is extraordinarily beneficial in breaking up toxic accumulation; thus avoiding evils which arise from auto-intoxication.

The position of mechanical advantage, which may or may not be a

[15]A simple, practical example of what is meant by obtaining the position of mechanical advantage may be given. Let the subject sit as far back in a chair as possible. The teacher, having decided upon the orders necessary for the elongation of the spine, the freedom of the neck (i.e., requisite natural laxness), and other conditions desirable for the particular case in hand, will then ask the pupil to rehearse those orders mentally, at the same time that he himself renders assistance by the skilful use of his hands. Then holding with one hand one or two books against the inner back of the chair, he will rely upon the pupil mentally rehearsing the orders necessary to maintain and improve the conditions present, while he, with the other hand placed upon the pupil's shoulder, causes the body gradually to incline backwards until its weight is taken by the back of the chair. The shoulder blades will, of course, be resting against the books. The position thus secured is one of a number which I employ and which for want of a better name I refer to as a position of "mechanical advantage."

normal position, is the position which gives the teacher the opportunity to bring about quickly with his own hands a co-ordinated condition in the subject. Such co-ordination gives to the pupil an experience of the proper use of a part or parts, in the imperfect use of which may be found the primary cause of the defects present. It is by the repetition of such experiences of the proper use of his organism that the pupil is enabled to reproduce the sensation and to employ the same guiding principles in everyday life. The placing of the pupil in what would ordinarily be considered an abnormal position (of mechanical advantage) affords the teacher an opportunity to establish the mental and physical guiding principles which enable the pupil after a short time to repeat the co-ordination with the same perfection in a normal position.

I maintain in this connexion, that any case of incipient appendicitis may be treated successfully by these methods. Further, when this position of mechanical advantage has been attained through the employment of the first principles of conscious guidance and control, a rigid thorax may regain mobility, no matter what the age of the subject, and full thoracic expansion and contraction may be acquired and, with the minimum of effort, maintained. During the practical process by which this thoracic elasticity and maximum intra-thoracic capacity is gradually established, the body of the subject is at the same time readjusted and mental principles are inculcated which will enable him to maintain the improved conditions in posture and co-ordination which are being set up, and which will secure the normal and necessary abdominal pressure in the right direction, thus constituting a natural form of massage of the digestive organs which is maintained during the ordinary actions of everyday life.

3. I am able to re-adjust and to teach others to re-adjust the human machine with the hands; to mould the body, as it were, into its proper shape, and with an open-minded pupil it is possible to remove many defects in a few minutes, as, for example, to change entirely the production of a voice, its quality and power.

4. In prescribing the principles of conscious guidance and control, we are dealing not with an epidemic of physical or mental degeneracy, but with a stage in the progress of the human race from the subconscious and instinctive to the conscious and reasoned command of the whole human mechanism. In other words, we have reached a stage in the process of civilisation where demands are being made which we are unable to meet satisfactorily, and with the serious results which may be seen on every hand, results from which we can escape only by passing from those primitive modes of guidance which approximate too closely to those of the animal kingdom where the greater potentialities of the

human being remain latent.

The suggested adoption of conscious guidance and control as a universal principle on the lines heretofore outlined will enable us to move slowly but with gradually increasing speed towards those higher psychophysical spheres which will separate the animal and human kingdoms by a deep gulf, and mankind will then enjoy the blessings which will be the natural result of capacities fully developed.

CHAPTER II

THE ARGUMENT

THE marked tendency toward physical degeneracy among the men and women of all civilised races has been the constant theme of physiologists, therapeutists and other specialists; endless explanations have been put forward to account for it, and countless remedies suggested to counteract it. In this question, as in the details of medicine and surgery, the general inclination of the human mind is always towards a treatment of epidemic symptoms, towards vague generalisations in the diagnosis and treatment of individual symptoms, whether the word "individual" in this case refers to a specific sufferer or a correlated class of diseases, towards a regard of effects rather than of causes.

As a reaction against this long-accepted method of dealing with individual symptoms by differentiated treatment, there has arisen a great diversity of so-called "mind-healers," whose *a priori* methods and lack of any clearly conceived system have brought their efforts into disrepute. Such were the conditions which over twenty years ago I sought to understand, believing—as I still do—that the whole human race was at some great psycho-physical turning point in its history, and that if the true nature of this evolutionary stage could be understood, it might and should be possible to direct man's physical and mental progression and so combat, and in time eliminate, a thousand evils which seem to have no counterpart in the world of the lower animals, save in very exceptional cases.

In embarking upon this enquiry I realised from the outset that I was dealing not with a world-wide epidemic but with a stage of progress, and that it was essential therefore that I should at once discard all theories which advocated, implicitly or explicitly, a return to similar conditions. Evolution knows no such return to extinction. The species must go forward to a triumphant perfection, or give place to a more dominant, more complete, self-controlled type.

Now if man as an animal, with an animal body differing little in anatomical structure from other families of the order of Primates, is yet differentiated physically by a susceptibility to disease and bodily degeneration, which, save in very exceptional cases, finds little or no parallel in the lower animals, we must determine the prime cause of such differentiation. The solution of the problem which is commonly put forward, and which has found support in the body calling themselves in England and in the United States "Eugenists," I cannot accept as universal. This theory rests mainly on the contention that in the human body polity the physical struggle for existence has ceased to have effect, that the unfit are permitted to produce offspring equally with the fit, and that for the natural selection imposed by circumstances which are fatal to the weak we must substitute an arbitrary selection in order to maintain the high efficiency of the natural type. Though I am in sympathy with many principles of Eugenics I reject this theory as a universal one. It is inconsistent with the great and inspiring ideal of the progress of the human race toward a mental and bodily perfection. If we believe in the idea of a Purpose running through life, unfolding itself to each successive generation and expressing itself in the terms of human experience; if, in other words, we believe in any scientific theory of development, in any large scheme of progress, it is impossible to accept a theory which assumes the lack of adaptability in man's physical body to thrive in the conditions which have grown up around him, or to enter its true and natural kingdom of perfect soundness. If we postulate that a third of civilised humanity is unfit to continue the race, we can only conclude that man's physical evolution has proved a failure, and that the race is doomed ultimately to extinction. And, in the last analysis, it is inconceivable that the prime instinct and desire for reproduction can be overruled at the dictates of any small body of men, or even that such a method, if possible, could be productive of any highly desirable results.

Wherefore I take my stand firmly on the ground that the body of civilised man is capable not only of continuing the struggle for existence but of rising to a higher potentiality. So, returning to the point of differentiation between man and the lower animals, I am now convinced that we must seek for the cause of this physical degeneration not in the pressure of new circumstances of life, but in the progress from one state of being to the next. I maintain that in order to discover the solution of this twofold problem of universal disease and its universal remedy, we must look to this enormous growth of reasoning power, and to the consciousness and realisation of the means whereby the desired effect can be obtained. For the animal and the lower races of mankind do not perform physical acts by any process of reason. They are the servants of that strange directing law which governs the flower in its curiously ingenius devices to ensure cross-fertilisation, no less than the higher mammalia in the rules of their gregarious societies, the law for which we have found no better term than Instinct. It is this "instinct" which guides all the nervous muscular mechanisms of the animal's anatomical structure, and is traceable as the motive in all functional processes. But in the physical economy of mankind this instinct is actually at war with, and is ever being controlled and superseded by conscious, directive reason.

The number of man's instinctive actions grows ever more limited, (1) as the result of a complete change of habit, and (2) more noticeably, as the outcome of a mental evolution which prompts him continually to seek a cause for every action, to analyse and endeavour to comprehend the secret springs of his being. Moreover civilisation, with its multitudinous problems of life and its perpetual interplay of personalities, demands even in the minutiæ of physical action a constant reasoning, a deliberate and comparatively rapid adaptation to surroundings such as instinct is quite unable to provide. Thus man's whole body is a polity ruled by two governors whose dictates are not invariably consistent one with the other; and one governor is frequently disobeyed at the expense of the other. This fact, indeed, is obvious when it is thus considered, but we have to determine the possible outcome. There are three alternatives. The first, a return to the sole guidance of instinct, is unthinkable. The second, the continuance of this dual government, is the very condition which has led to the evils we seek to remedy. There remains the third, namely, that man's physical evolution points to progress along the road of reasoned, conscious guidance and control. It was this last conclusion which over twenty years ago led me to investigate and to practise the means by which this conscious guidance and control could be obtained, so as to apply it to the eradication and prevention of human ills, and to the maintenance of the body in a high degree of physical perfection.

CHAPTER III

THE PROCESSES OF CONSCIOUS GUIDANCE AND CONTROL

THE formulation of the method of conscious guidance and control arises in practice from a close study of the imperfect uses of the mental and physical mechanisms of the human organism. Since, as has been shown, conscious guidance and control is necessary and is being practised to some extent, inefficiently, by every civilised man and woman, it is essential that its principles should be thoroughly understood. The method is based firstly on the understanding of the co-ordinated uses of the muscular mechanisms, and secondly, on the complete acceptance of the hypothesis that each and every movement can be consciously directed and controlled.

In re-educating the individual, therefore, the first effort must be directed to the education of the conscious mind. The words "re-educating" and "re-education" have a specific meaning. In the individual the normal processes of education in the use of the anatomical structure is conducted subconsciously, certain instincts commanding certain functions, whilst other functions are conducted deliberately. The effects of this haphazard process have either to be elaborated or broken down, according to the defects established by misuse of the mechanisms, and the first step in re-education is that of establishing in the pupil's mind the connexion which exists between cause and effect in every function of the human body.

In the performance of any muscular action by conscious guidance and control there are four essential stages:

(1) The conception of the movement required;

(2) The inhibition of erroneous preconceived ideas which subconsciously suggest the manner in which the movement or series of movements should be performed;

(3) The new and conscious mental orders which will set in motion the muscular mechanism essential to the correct per-

formance of the action;

(4) The movements (contractions and expansions) of the muscles which carry out the mental orders.

The process of re-education concerns itself with establishing these principles, and for the purpose of illustration we may take a typical example of a patient who has had no experience of them.

A well-built, muscular man in the prime of life, conducting during business hours a sedentary occupation and taking more or less violent exercise during his leisure, becomes a chronic sufferer from indigestion with all its concomitant troubles. He complains that physical exercises of the gymnasium no longer do him any good, but appears to think that if he gave up his office work altogether, an economic impossibility for him, he might recover.

Suppose he is asked to stand upright and take a "deep breath." It will be found that he immediately makes movements which tend to retard the proper action of the respiratory processes rather than to promote such action. For instance, it is almost certain that in the attempt to make the movement referred to he will stiffen the muscles of his neck, throw back the head, hollow the back, protrude the stomach, and take breath by audibly *sucking* air into the lungs. The muscles over the entire surface of the bony thorax will be unduly tensed, tending to more or less harmful thoracic rigidity at the very moment when the maximum of mobility is needed. How could the result be otherwise? For, in telling the pupil to take a "deep breath," the teacher starts out with the assumption that the pupil can do so. But why such an assumption? What guide in carrying out the order has the pupil except his own admittedly erroneous guidance? I say "admittedly" erroneous, for I contend that the pupil's condition, together with the fact that he and the teacher deem it necessary to remedy it, is tantamount to this admission. So common, so almost universal is such a response as the above to these orders that the truth of the statement may be tested on any average individual. Now the mistakes of this response need not be dwelt upon here. They have proved in every case in my experience sufficient explanation for the trouble of the digestive organs. Examination of the subject will reveal the hollowing of the back with the accompanying protrusion of the abdominal wall, whilst the abdominal muscles will be deficient in the energy and tone necessary to the maintenance of efficiency in the digestive organs. Now in dealing with this case, many parts of the organism will require readjustment. The spine must be straightened and lengthened, the mean thoracic capacity permanently increased in order to give free play to the internal organs, and the firmly established habit of drawing breath by *sucking* air into the lungs must be broken.

It is essential in this place to point out that no system of physical exercises will alter the present condition of the subject in respect to these faults, since all exercises will be conducted under a primary misconception with regard to the use of the muscles involved in the re-adjustment and co-ordination of the organism.

We may now follow the individual through the four stages in the inculcation of the principles of conscious control. In the first place it is necessary that he should have a clear understanding of the faults we seek to remedy. No tacit compliance on his part to a treatment, the processes of which he does not understand, will be of the slightest value. He must accept completely the principle in detail. In the second place he must be taught to realise his erroneous conceptions which result in erroneous movements, and this, whether the conceptions be conscious or subconscious. He must also be taught to inhibit, and, finally, to eradicate these preconceived ideas and the mental order or series of orders which follow from them. Only then can he give correct guiding orders as next described.

In the third place, then, he must learn to give the correct mental orders to the mechanisms involved, and *there must be a clear differentiation in his mind between the giving of the order and the performance of the act ordered and carried out through the medium of the muscles.* The whole principles of volition and inhibition are implicit in the recognition of this differentiation. Thus, to return to the example under consideration, we will suppose that I have requested the pupil *to order* the spine to lengthen and the neck to relax. If, instead of merely framing and holding this desire in his mind, he attempts the physical performance of these acts, he will invariably stiffen the muscles of his neck and shorten the spine, since these are the movements habitually associated *in his mind* with lengthening his spine, and the muscles will contract in accordance with the old associations. In effect it will be seen that in this, as in all other cases, stress must be laid on the point that it is *the means* and not the *end* which must be considered. When the end is held in the mind, instinct or long habit will always seek to attain the end by habitual methods. The action is performed below the level of consciousness in its various stages, and only rises to the level of consciousness when the end is being attained by the correct "means whereby."

In the fourth place, when the correct guiding orders have been practised and given by the mind, a result attained by attention and the instruction of the teacher, the muscles involved will come into play in different combinations under the control of conscious guidance, and a reasoned act will take the place of the series of habitual, unconsidered movements which have resulted in the deformation of the body. And it must be kept clearly in mind that the whole of the old series of movements has been correlated and compacted into one indivisible and rigid sequence which has invariably followed the one mental order that started the train; such an order, for instance, as "Stand upright."

Leaving this specific example, I come now to a consideration of the general principles involved. Firstly, as to the teaching method.

Every one who has had experience, personally or vicariously, of the many "methods" and "systems" of teaching breathing, speaking, singing, physical culture, golf, fencing, etc., must have noticed that whilst the failures of these "methods" are many, the successes are comparatively few.

The few successes are of course set down to exceptional natural aptitude, whilst the teacher has an explanation of those cases more flattering to himself and prefers not to consider too closely the average of his failures. The truth is that all these systems break down because the pupil, in the attempt to adopt them, is guided always by his subconscious direction and is forced to depend too much on what is called natural aptitude. When guidance by conscious control and reason supersedes guidance by instinct, we shall be able to develop our potentialities to the full.

My own analysis of the matter is that the teaching method is, as a rule, entirely wrong, and wrong because of a fundamental misconception and an entirely inaccurate analysis resulting in a false premise. The pupil's defects are dealt with commonly through their effects and not their causes. It is not recognised that every defective action is the result of the erroneous preconception of the doer, whether consciously or subconsciously exercised, and the orders which directly or indirectly follow. Nor is it understood that a pupil under the influence of such erroneous preconceptions can make no real progress till he is made to realise that it is he himself who is actually bringing about the defective action. The teacher does not attach sufficient importance to the fact that the pupil is often under a complete misapprehension as to his own actions, being under the delusion that he is doing one thing when he is often doing the exact opposite.

No real progress in the overcoming of faults can be made until the pupil consciously ceases to will or to do those things which he has been willing and doing in the past, and which have led him to commit the faults that are to be eradicated. "Don't do this, but this," says the teacher, dealing with *effects*. In other words, it is assumed that the defective action on the part of the pupil can be put right by "doing something else." The teacher accepts and preaches this doctrine without ever analysing the defect to its root cause in the human will, the motor of the whole mechanism. He forgets that in "doing something else" the pupil must use the same use the same machinery which, *ex hypothesi*, is working imperfectly, and that he must be guided in his action by the same erroneous conceptions regarding right or wrong doing. Neither teacher nor pupil seems to remember that to know whether practice is *right* or *wrong* demands judgment. Judgment is the result of experience. Faulty or wrong experience means faulty or bad judgment, whereas correct experience means good judgment.

The very fact that the pupil was beset with defects and needed help proves that his *kinæsthetic* experiences were incorrect and even harmful, and as his judgment on the kinæsthetic basis has been built upon such faulty experience, the judgment will prove most misleading and unsound.

Therefore we are forced to dispense, for the time being, with the sense of feeling as a guide in its old sphere of associations. We cannot deny that we are beset with defects, that even when the way is made clear for their eradication we cannot follow that way on our old mode of procedure, because our guides in the form of sensory appreciation (feeling-tones), general experience, and judgment are unworthy of our confidence, and will guide us in such a way that, even if we succeed in eradicating some specific defect, it will be found that in the process we have cultivated a number of others which are as bad or even worse than the original.

It seems also to me that practice so-called is so rarely directed by a reasoned analysis on a reasoned plan. Nor does the teacher analyse and instruct with accuracy. He demands from the pupil merely imitative not reasoned acts. This makes practice so often futile for the imperfectly co-ordinated person, and teaching both halting and inadequate.

With regard to this question of the imitative method I have frequently had to point out to vocal pupils that certain effects and capacities, which they hoped to acquire in a few lessons, were a result of a proper conscious knowledge on my part of the "means whereby" the voice is produced. To achieve these results they must study and master the same principles, but they could never reproduce them by a series of imitative acts divorced from knowledge of the processes involved and skill in using these processes. There is no royal road to anything worth having, and the imitative method of teaching seems to me pure charlatanry.

The position of the teacher and pupil is a very hopeless one as long as their standpoint is still on the subconscious plane, and the physical and mental conditions of our time, when considered in the light of the teaching methods adopted in the past, afford abundant proof of this.

My reader can rejoice that the foregoing is a faithful representation of our position to-day. He can rejoice because these tremendous forces demand that if he wishes to progress he must leave the subconscious plane of animal growth and development, and adopt the reasoned conscious plane of guidance and control by means of which mankind may rise to those high evolutionary planes for which his latent and undeveloped potentialities fit him.

I will now endeavour to outline the teaching method which should be adopted if we are to pass successfully from subconscious to conscious guidance and control, in the endeavour to remove defects and delusions and to develop and establish correct guiding centres and senses.

The conscious guidance and control advocated here is on a wide and general, and not on a specific basis. Conscious control applied in a specific way in unthinkable, except as a result of the principle primarily applied as a universal. For instance, the conscious controlling of the movements of a particular muscle or limb, as practised by athletes and others, is of little practical value in the science of living. The specific control of a finger, of the neck, or of the legs should primarily be the result of the conscious guidance and control of the mechanism of the torso, particularly of the antagonistic muscular actions which bring about those correct and greater co-ordinations intended to control the movements of the limbs, neck, respiratory mechanism and the general activity of the internal organs.

In order to describe the teaching method necessary in this connexion, I will indicate the procedure which should be adopted in the attempt to help a pupil in whom undue tension of the muscles of one side of the neck causes the head to be pulled down on that side. In the ordinary way, the pupil is told to relax and straighten the neck and he and his teacher devote themselves to this end. This attempt may be attended with more or less success, chiefly less. If they do succeed in removing the specific trouble it is almost certain that new defects will have been cultivated during the process. In any case the teacher's order to relax and straighten the neck is incorrect and primarily the result of a wrong assumption. It started from a false premise which led to false deductions. The pupil and his teacher decided that something was wrong and that therefore something specific had to be done to put it right. The "end" was held in mind primarily and not the "means whereby."

The correct point of view is: Something is wrong in the use of the psycho-physical mechanism of the person concerned. Is this imperfection or defect a direct or indirect result of this person's own direction and action, or is it the result of some influence outside of himself and beyond his power to control? It can be proved conclusively that his imperfections or defects are due entirely to causes springing directly or indirectly from his own ideas and acts.

It is therefore obvious that the correct order of procedure for teacher and pupil is first for the pupil to learn to prevent himself from doing the wrong things which cause the imperfections or defects, and then, as a *secondary* consideration in procedure, to learn the correct way to use the mental and physical mechanisms concerned.

If there is any undue muscular pull in any part of the neck, it is almost certain to be due to the defective co-ordination in the use of the muscles of the spine, back, and torso generally, the correction of which means the eradication of the real cause of the trouble.

This principle applies to the attempted eradication of all defects or imperfect uses of the mental and physical mechanisms in all the acts of daily life and in such games as cricket, football, billiards, baseball, golf, etc., and the physical manipulation of the piano, violin, harp and all such instruments.

My reader must not fail to remember that mental conceptions are the stimuli to the ideo-motor centre which passes on the subconscious or conscious guiding orders to the mechanism. In dealing with human defects or imperfections we must consider the inherited subconscious conceptions associated with the mechanisms involved, and also the conceptions which are to be the forerunners of the ideo-motor guiding orders connected with the new and correct use of the different mechanisms.

In order to establish successfully the latter (correct conception), we must first inhibit the former (incorrect conception), and from the ideo-motor centre project the new and different directing orders which are to influence the complexes involved, gradually eradicating the tendency to employ the incorrect ones, and steadily building up those which are correct and reliable.

It will therefore be understood that if we eliminate the conception established and associated with our defects or imperfections, it means that we are really eliminating our inherited subconsciousness, and all the defective uses of the psycho-physical mechanism connected therewith.

In our attempts on these lines we are, at the outset, confronted with the difficulty of mental rigidity. The preconceptions and habits of thought with regard to the uses of the muscular mechanisms are the first if not the only stumbling-blocks to the teaching of conscious control. Many of these preconceptions are the legacy of instinct, others arise from habitual practices started by a faulty comprehension of the uses of the mechanism, others again by conscious or unconscious imitation of faults in others. In this last case it may be noted that although we are always deploring the degeneracy of civilised man the exemplars held up for the child's conscious and unconscious imitation are nearly always faulty specimens. These preconceptions and habits of thought, therefore, must be broken down, and since the reactions of mind on body and body on mind are so intimate, it is often necessary to break down these preconceptions of mind by performing muscular acts for the subject vicariously; that is to say, the instructor must move the parts in question while the subject attends to the inhibition of all muscular movements. It would be impossible, however, to describe the method in full detail in this place, owing to the extraordinary variability of the cases presented, no two of which exhibit precisely the same defects. On broad lines it is evident that the misuses must be diagnosed by the instructor who may be called upon to use considerable ingenuity and patience in correcting the faults, and substituting correct mental orders for the one general order which starts the old train of vicious habitual movements. The mental habit must be first attacked and this mental habit usually lies below the level of consciousness; but it may be reached by introspection and analysis, and by the performance of the habitual acts by other than the habitual methods, that is by physical acts performed consciously as an effect of the conscious conception and the conscious direction of the mind.

Speaking generally, it will be found that the pupil is quite unable to analyse his own actions. Tell a young golfer that he has taken his eye off the ball or swayed his body, and he feels sure, in his heart, that you are mistaken. The imperfectly poised person has not a correct apprehension of what he is really doing. In this apparently simple matter of the carriage or poise of the body I find in quite nine-tenths of my cases a harmful rigidity[16] which is quite unconsciously assumed. When it is pointed out to them, and physically demonstrated, they almost invariably deny it indignantly. I ask a new pupil to put his shoulders back and his head forward, and he will consistently put both back or forward. I tell a new pupil he is shortening his spine, and in attempting to lengthen it he invariably shortens it still more. The action is one over which he has neither learnt not practised any control whatever. He is simply deluded regarding his sensations and unable to direct his actions. I do not therefore in teaching him actually order him to lengthen his spine by performing any explicit action, but I cause him to rehearse the correct guiding orders, and after placing him in a position of mechanical advantage I am able by my manipulation to bring about, directly or indirectly as the case may be, the desired flexibility and extension.

[16]A very notable though trivial instance of mental "rigidity" was brought to me by a pupil while writing these pages. A fireman on duty at a theatre had neglected to unbolt the escape doors. When severely reprimanded he pleaded that he had been instructed by an assistant manager to do duty in another part of the theatre at the time he usually opened the escapes. The following night the assistant manager instructed him to make the same change in his routine on which the man pleaded, "Don't ask me to do that, sir. I forgot the escapes last night and I am sure to forget 'em again if you make me go that way round. You see, sir, I've gone round the other way so long that if I make a change I seem to lose my memory."

The process is of course repeated until the pupil gains a new kinæsthetic sense of the new and correct use of the parts, which become properly co-ordinated, and the correct habit is established. He will then no longer find it easy to cause his physical machinery to work as it did before the fault was thus effectively eradicated.

I frequently have to treat cases of congenital or acquired crippling and distortion. I protest against the mental attitude which looks upon such ailments as incurable and beyond the control of the patient—the mental attitude of the person who says "Poor fellow," to the sufferer, and induces him to repeat and be dominated by this paralysing formula. As a matter of plain fact the condition is maintained by the pupil's erroneous ideas concerning "cause" and "effect," and the working of his own mechanism, and so, subconsciously but quite effectively, he is really causing and maintaining the trouble. My method is to make an examination and then to apply tests to discover the real cause or causes, namely, erroneous preconceived ideas, and to find out what minimum of control is left, and therefrom to develop a healthy condition of the whole organism by a simple and practical procedure which step by step effects the desired physical and mental changes. Like the faith-healer, then, I lay much stress on the mental attitude of the patient; unlike him, instead of denying the existence of the evil I make the pupil search out with me its cause. I then explain to him that his own will (not mine or some higher will) is to effect the desired change, but that it must first be directed in a rational way to bring about a physical manifestation, and must be aided by a simple mechanical principle and a proper manipulation. In this way a reasoned and permanent confidence is built up in the pupil instead of a spurious hysterical one which is apt to fail as suddenly as it arose. I will not, for instance, allow my pupils to close their eyes during their work, in spite of a constant plea that they can "think better" or "concentrate" better with their eyes shut, for, as a rule, I find that this resolves itself into an attempt at self-hypnotism. I make them endeavour to exercise their conscious minds all the while. As I have already said, I maintain further and I am prepared to prove that the majority of physical defects have come about by the action of the patient's own will operating under the influence of erroneous preconceived ideas and consequent delusions, exercised consciously or more often subconsciously, and that these conditions can be changed by that same will directed by a right conception implanted by the teacher.

In this connexion I am able to give particulars of an interesting case.

A well-known actor fell during rehearsal and injured his arm so severely that he was unable to raise it more than five or six inches from his side without intense pain. He consulted many medical men without relief, and had been disabled for six weeks when he was sent to see me.

I diagnosed the case as a subjective subconsciously willed disablement. Of course, the last thing I mean is that it was "affected" in the usual sense; all the patient's interests and character made this impossible.

I asked him to lift his arm. "I can't." "But please try." He did so and the cause of his trouble was immediately apparent to me. He was using the muscular mechanisms of the arm and neck in such a way as to place a severe strain on the injured muscle, such a strain indeed as would have been harmful to a normal arm and which caused him intense pain. For instance, he was exerting force sufficient to lift a sack of flour and he *looked* as if he had been called upon for such an exertion! He was stiffening all the muscles which he should have relaxed, and was altogether acting as the subconsciously controlled person of to-day does habitually act when something unusual occurs. To put the matter in the terms of my thesis, he acted in accordance with a subconscious guiding influence which had long since lost the standard of accuracy of instinct possessed by his early ancestors, whilst nothing had been given to or cultivated by him in his civilised state to compensate for its loss. The "cure" was so simple as to appear ludicrous. I had diagnosed that the subconsciously stiffened muscles were the cause of the trouble. My efforts were devoted to obtaining the correct action of the arm with the minimum of tension. This was done by manipulation and by giving him guiding orders which brought about the correct use of the parts concerned. Within ten minutes he was able to lift his arm with very little pain and resumed his professional work at once and without relapse. Note that the relaxing was not brought about by a preliminary order to relax, an action which entailed processes of which he had no true consciousness and over which therefore he had no control. Note also that this demonstration is much more effective for the treatment of similar later accidents and for general self-development and control, than any hypnotic "suggestion" that there was no pain.[17]

[17] "This experimental observation is so far to our interest that it has proved that hypnotic suggestion is by far surpassed in the duration of its effects by suggestion in the waking state, and this again by regular teaching and practice. But this is physiologically explicable: Hypnotic suggestion obtains its results solely through the intensity of the isolated stimulus and through the brain-track it leaves behind, which has an abnormally slight connexion with the whole associative mechanism of the brain. Regular instruction, on the contrary, is based on the strong associative implanting of the stimulus and the brain-track it leaves behind, with the normal activity of the brain, i.e., on the many-sidedness of the nervous connexions and their reproductive effect; whilst, in the first case, the trace is more or less easily effaced, in the second the accompanying reproductive, sympathetic stimulus increases and preserves the result obtained, as well as effecting the other bodily functions dependent on it."—*The Psychic Treatment of Disease,* Berthold Kern.

I do not deny, for it would be against the evidence, that the healers do contrive to remove pain; but apart from the danger of removing mere symptoms (that is, removing nature's danger signals and leaving the danger untouched), their methods have the obvious limitation of being repugnant to many, and have fallen into some discredit amongst those who are by no means amongst the least capable, accomplished, and thoughtful human types.

Another very interesting case was that of a man who stuttered and came to me for help. All stutterers have their particular and peculiar little accompaniments to the main defect. His was a harmful habit of moving his arm up and down from the elbow as he attempted to speak. I asked him why he did this, and he replied that he *felt* it assisted him in speaking. I explained and demonstrated to him that this was a delusion, that this movement of the limb was really a hindrance and not an assistance. He saw that a considerable amount of valuable mental and physical energy, which should have been conveyed to the mechanisms and organs of speech, was being diverted to a limb which might have been amputated without interfering in any way with those mental and mechanical processes upon which his powers of speech entirely depended. He became convinced on these points and intimated his willingness to endeavour to carry out my instructions. I assisted him to establish a working conscious control basis and improved his co-ordination generally.

Then I made the following request:

"I wish you to project orders to these newly developed co-ordinators. You will then be prevented from employing your arms as an aid in speaking, and in your general attempts at conscious guidance in private. In public I which you to adopt the following mode of procedure:

> "Whenever a person speaks to you, asking a question or in any way trying to open up a conversation, you must as a primary principle refuse to answer by mentally saying *No.* (This will hold in check the old subconscious orders—the bad habit of moving the arm. It constitutes the inhibition of the old errors before attempting to speak.)
>
> "Then give the new and correct orders to your general co-ordinations and command the 'means whereby' of the act of correct and controlled speaking.
>
> "Make this a principle of life."

Perhaps I should add here that I convinced this pupil by practical demonstrations that the energy directed to his arm was wasted and misdirected; that, if this energy were correctly directed to the proper co-ordinations concerned with the mechanism of breathing and speaking, the process would represent the difference between correct and incorrect attempts in the direction of ultimate satisfactory breath and speech control. In this particular case the desired end was gained in a few weeks.

The observant person must have noted the singularly small range of physical control exercised by the average adult outside the narrow sphere of his daily routine actions. In the realm of sport, for instance, take the golf swing. A novice, or for that matter a player of some experience carefully "addresses" the ball and is instructed *to swing up and down again in the same orbit,* without moving the head or swaying the body. The professional has arranged the stance; the drive seems the simplest of actions; yet, more often than not, it fails lamentably. And the player, nine times out of ten, *has no sort of consciousness* of what has interfered with his stroke.

This is a very common instance of the failure to achieve the desired end in those who depend solely upon subconscious direction. Even the accomplished and practised golfer has periods when he acknowledges that he is "off his game" or "out of form," times when his skill leaves him altogether *because he cannot register consciously* the method which, when he uses it instinctively, enables him to play well.

Where the novice is concerned, however, the stubborn fact to be faced is that it is practically impossible for the ordinary person to carry out such instructions as *swing up and down again in the same orbit, etc.*, with precision and accuracy. At the first attempt the pupil may, by mere chance, succeed. He may even make a second successful attempt, and a third, and so on. But such instances are very rare. On the other hand, he may begin badly and after a few days record a series of successes. Incidentally, I will point out that this applies more or less to the majority of experienced golf players. We all know that to vary is to be human. But there should not be such an alarming gulf between our best and our worst. It is very serious from the mental point of view. It shakes our confidence in ourselves to the very roots of our mental and physical foundations. Such experiences have a bad effect even upon the emotions generally, and the person concerned develops irritation, bad temper, and other undesirable traits at a time (a time of recreation and pleasure) when there should be an absolute absence of these harmful conditions.

It will readily be conceded that during our attempts at this or any other game the mental condition of the performer should be in keeping with a pleasurable and health-giving form of outdoor exercise.

But to return to the stumbling-blocks in the way of the correct performance of an act which requires one "to swing up and down in the same orbit." These arise mainly from the tendency of the great majority to curve and shorten the spine unduly and otherwise to interfere with the correct conditions of the muscular system of the back, the spine, and the thorax in the performance of certain physical acts.[18] These tendencies are particularly marked when the arms are employed in such a movement as the "swing down" to make the stroke following the preparatory "swing up." Consequently not one person in a thousand is capable of maintaining during the *down* stroke those conditions of the back and spine present during the *up* stroke. Consideration of these points will indicate that in order "to swing up and down in the same orbit," it is essential that the position of the spine—particularly as regards its length and relative poise during the up and down movement—must be maintained. Other conditions are of course necessary but I cannot deal with more than one or two of the chief factors.

In order to secure the proper use of the arms and legs correct mental guidance and control are necessary. Such guidance and control should, of course, be conscious. Furthermore, this mental guidance and control must co-ordinate with a proper position and length of the spine and the accompanying correct muscular uses of the torso, if these limbs are to be controlled by that guidance and co-ordination which will command their accurate employment at all times within reasonable limits.

The foregoing are a few of the fundamental difficulties with which the golf teacher and pupil are beset. Those who have taken lessons will at once admit that the ordinary teaching methods fail to reach these difficulties satisfactorily. As a matter of fact they are not even taken into consideration. The orthodox teaching method holds the "end" in view and not the "means whereby." It depends upon the giving of orders on the "end-gaining" principle, such an order, for instance, as "Swing up and down again in the same orbit," without consideration of the "means whereby"; that is, without making certain that the pupil has the power to maintain a proper position of his spine and back and to use the limbs correctly during the performance of such physical acts. In other words, the teacher should first discover if his pupil is reasonably correctly co-ordinated in those muscular uses of his organism which are essential to the proper carrying out of instructions necessary to the performance of definite physical acts demanding co-ordination in the use of the human body and limbs.

If these tests are not made the beginner will waste much valuable

[18]A simple experiment will serve to prove this shortening by the increase of, say, the lumbar curve. Take a piece of cardboard of six inches in length and place it flat on a table or against the wall. With a pencil draw lines on the table or wall as close to the upper and lower ends of the cardboard as possible. Remove the cardboard and curve it slightly across the lower portion about an inch from the end which touched the lowest line. Replace it on the lower line without interfering with the curve and you will find that it does not reach the upper line any longer. A similar condition occurring in the human being means a shortening of the stature.

time, dissipate his energies, suffer needless worry and suspense, and become unduly apprehensive in his attempt to gain even a very moderate standard of dependable excellence in playing golf or other games to which he may devote himself.

If we employ as the fundamental in teaching the principles of conscious guidance and control on a basis of re-education and general coordination the following advantages should accrue:

(1) The pupil will be made aware of his specific defects in the employment of his mental and physical organism in physical performances.

(2) When he has been made aware of these defects, he can be taught to inhibit the faulty movements, and his teacher can assist him to gain slowly but correctly the necessary experiences in the correct use of those muscular mechanisms which will enable him sooner or later to govern them properly without the aid of the teacher, and to employ them with accuracy and precision in his game of golf and other physical performances.

(3) In the golf act under consideration he must first be given the correct experiences in the use of the muscular mechanisms of the torso and legs with the arms falling naturally at his side.

(4) The correct experiences should then be given with the use of the arms in making the "up stroke." When this act can be performed without interference with the satisfactory conditions of the torso and legs, the correct experiences should be given in making the "down stroke" but without attempting to *drive* the ball. This latter portion of the whole act should not be attempted until the pupil is familiar with the different movements described in 1, 2, 3 and 4.

(5) When the attempt to drive is finally made, the idea to be held in mind is that of *repeating the experiences as a whole* (in other words, the "means whereby"), not the idea of making a drive. If the pupil holds the "end" (i.e., making a drive) in mind he will at once revert to all his old subconscious habits in the use of his mental and physical organism, whereas, on the other hand, if he holds in mind the "means whereby" (his new correct experiences) he will sooner or later put them correctly into practice and make his drives with an accuracy and precision which will give the maximum of satisfaction and pleasure.

I have personal knowledge of a person who, by employing the principles of conscious control which I advocate, mounted and rode a bicycle down-hill without mishap on the first attempt, and on the second day rode 30 miles out and 30 miles back through normal traffic. This same person was also able to fence passably on first taking the foil into his hands. In each case the principles involved were explained to him and he carefully watched an exhibition, first analysing the actions and the "means whereby," then reproducing them on a clearly apprehended plan. This, it seems to me, should be a normal, not an abnormal human accomplishment. Just as a cat by sheer instinct, the first time she essays to jump, gauges her powers and the distances with accuracy, so, with more reason and with greater ease, the human subject, by employing consciously controlled intellect and kindred experience in place of instinct, should be able to direct his powers to a definite ordained end with less physical strain and less frequent physical repetition, i.e., "Practice."

In this connexion I have been often asked the difference between instinct and intuition. I define instinct as the result of the accumulated subconscious psycho-physical experiences of man at all stages of his development, which continue with us until, singly or collectively, we reach the stage of conscious control: whilst intuition is the result of the *conscious reasoned* psycho-physical experiences during the process of our evolution.

The word "subconsciousness" is but a formula for our habits of life. I hold strongly that when we shall have reached the state of conscious control in civilisation, and have established thereby new and correct habits, a new and correct subconsciousness will become established.

I might here with advantage re-emphasise my view regarding the supreme importance of conscious control.

Conscious control is imperative, as I have pointed out, because instinct in our advancing civilisation largely fails to meet the needs of our complex environment. Without conscious control the subject or patient may know he has defects, may know further what those defects are, may even know at what explicit improvement he is to aim, and yet may be quite unable by means of imitation or the orthodox and traditional methods of instruction to effect the desired end.

With conscious control, on the other hand, true development (unfolding), education (drawing out), and evolution are possible along intellectual as against the old orthodox and fallacious lines, by means of reasoned processes, analysed, understood, and explicitly directed. Conscious control enables the subject, once a fault be recognised, to find and readily apply the remedial process.

It is my belief, confirmed by the research and practice of nearly twenty years, that man's supreme inheritance of conscious guidance and control is within the grasp of any one who will take the trouble to cultivate it. That it is no esoteric doctrine or mystical cult, but a synthesis of entirely reasonable propositions that can be demonstrated in pure theory and substantiated in common practice.

I will now consider at greater length a characteristic case for the elucidation of these various points of theory and practice.

M. H., a youth fourteen years old, was sent to me by a well-known throat specialist. He had removed two nodules from the boy's vocal chords, and had given him special treatment in a nursing home for a month, but without any satisfactory improvement. The mother came to me with the boy and was present during my treatment. I found that his attempts to speak resulted in a hoarse whisper accompanied by spasmodic twitchings of various parts of the body and by facial contortions, all this being brought about by erroneous conceptions, left untouched by the former teacher, as to the amount of effort needed in order to speak. In his former lessons he had been told to try and improve the utterance of simple sounds and words, without any analysis or pointing out of the wrong means which he had previously employed to this end. All his efforts to carry out his teacher's directions were made in accordance with his original preconceptions and former experience. His muscular mechanisms were employed in the same (wrong) way and his whole consciousness and explicit and implicit self-directions were exactly the same as they had been previously.

He had opened his mouth imperfectly and had been ordered by his teacher to open his mouth wider. But there had been no recognition by the pupil that he had not opened his mouth sufficiently, neither had there been any analysis by the teacher of the pupil's failure to open the mouth (a seemingly simple thing but *ex hypothesi* not simple to the patient), or of the concomitant contortions and automatic reaction. As well say "You have been speaking improperly, now speak properly," and call that a lesson, as indeed it would have been called in the early Victorian era, as, "Open your mouth wide, speak up, and don't make nervous movements." It is not the "end" that the teacher and pupil must work for, but the "means whereby." And this discovery of the "means whereby," differing in different subjects and not to be stated in a general formula, can only be the result of trained observation and careful, patient investigation and experience. In practice, the anxiety of this particular pupil to *speak* along the lines of his old preconceived ideas, which nothing had been done to remove, had made his many lessons fruitless, and had set in motion the old habitual train of irrelevant and hampering actions.

My own treatment then is: First to observe and analyse and bring about a proper working of the machinery in general (nature does not work in parts but as a whole): then to point out the first guiding order or orders to be brought into play by the pupil, namely, the inhibiting of the tension of the muscles working the lower jaw. The pupil must be made to realise clearly that this involves no action whatever on his part, but that he need only remember the correct inhibiting orders and employ them in accordance with definite instructions. When he does this it at once results in the freeing of his jaw, enabling me to move it for him with my hand. This gives him for the first time the correct kinæsthetic sense in connexion with the action of his jaw and makes it clear once and for all to him that the desired action is perfectly and easily possible. The subconscious jerkings and contortions pointed out one by one are patiently inhibited by the pupil, sometimes directly but more often by the explicit use, under my direction, of guiding orders which gradually co-ordinate and remedy the whole faulty system of the pupil's muscular action. One by one the wrong actions and reactions are inhibited, the tightening of the neck, the throwing back of the head, the tension of the lower jaw, the deep "sucking" breath, the jerks of the limbs, the grimaces; and then, on the positive side, the right actions are gradually built up, such as the free controlled opening of the mouth, the even "pneumatic" breath, the upright balanced poise, the clear enunciation and correct vocalisation.[19]

The brain of both pupil and teacher are at work the whole time. No use is made of "hypnotism" or of auto-suggestion, but the confident, skilful, patient and explicit directions of the teacher should tend to remove flurry and vagueness and consequent waste of mental and physical effort.

The analysis of even the simplest processes is apt to appear unduly complex. This case can be stated briefly on the practical side. It took twenty lessons to break down the bad habits and another twelve to effect a complete and permanent cure.

With regard to such a simple act as opening the mouth two or three factors should be emphasised: firstly, the tendency to yield to erroneous preconceived ideas, secondly, the delusions of the pupil in regard to thought and action, thirdly, a pernicious dependence on sensation which has been based soley upon experience of defective action.

There are very few men, for instance, who when told to open the mouth, will not throw the head back with the idea, as it were, of lifting the upper jaw away from the lower. They do not observe or reflect that an inhibition of the subconscious orders which cause the mechanisms to keep the mouth closed will bring about such a relaxation of that mus-

[19]As I have already explained in Part I, inspiration is not a sucking of air into the lungs but an inevitable instantaneous rush of air into the partial vacuum caused by the automatic expansion of the thorax.

cular tension as will allow the jaw to drop. It does in fact commonly drop in the case of that type of idiot who is most often open-mouthed; whilst it is common knowledge that in boxing a blow on the head, heavy enough to throw out the controlling gear, causes the jaw of the injured boxer to drop of itself and to remain dropped for a considerable time.

When I ask a pupil to let me move his lower jaw away from his upper he usually increases instinctively the tension that keeps the lower jaw in place. As I have frequently pointed out, an enormous aggregate waste of energy is involved in these constant and irrational tensions.

But the matter becomes seriously harmful in, let us say, such actions as singing and speaking, for when the mouth is opened with this unconscious and absurd expenditure of force, the neck is unduly stiffened, the head is thrown backwards, the larynx unduly and harmfully depressed, and thereby in a position most unfavorable to good vocalisation. As I have for years pointed out and demonstrated in my own practice, from these ill-considered tensions spring the different forms of throat and ear trouble which are so common and which so frequently defy ordinary or for that matter extraordinary and highly specialised medical treatment. By inducing a proper conception of the right method of opening the mouth, I can command in the patient, and what is more important, teach him to command in himself, a free condition in which the larynx tends to be slightly raised and relaxed instead of tightened and depressed; whilst there will surely follow and that with a minimum of effort, a greater mobility of the facial muscles and those of the lips and tongue so essential to good and clear enunciation and vocalisation.

This, in the briefest summary, is the method of teaching the process of conscious control of the muscular mechanisms. I come now to an equally brief consideration of the effects of this method. Speaking generally, I have found that the first immediate effects are a general stimulation and increased efficiency of the whole organism. Nor is this difficult to understand. For it would seem that in the life led by civilised man so little demand is made upon any but the commonly exercised muscles, and these are called upon for comparatively so little effort, that a general sluggishness supervenes, with consequent stagnation resulting in the commonly observed effects of auto-intoxication. With the breaking up of the old motor habits, the muscular mechanisms are brought into full play, the toxins which have accumulated are broken up and disturbed, and increased vitality, a sense of power, and enormously improved efficiency follow as a matter of course. Beyond this, and still speaking generally, I find that there are increased powers of resistance against the attacks of infectious diseases, and—possibly the greatest effect since it guarantees the lasting qualities of the change which is brought about—an ability to check the formation of any bad, incipient muscular or mental habit. This last is, in my opinion, of the very first importance, for it demonstrates the power of the individual, once these principles of conscious guidance and control are mastered, to be the lord of his own body.

Of the specific effects procured by the inculcation of these methods I cannot speak at length, but I am able to produce a list of cases which have been treated by me, in some of which I can only say that I have been astonished at the results. These include cases diagnosed by prominent physicians in England, Australia, and the United States of America as paralysis, varicosity, tuberculosis, asthma, adhesions of the lungs, hæmorrhage, congenital and other malformations, effects of infantile paralysis, many varieties of throat, nose and ear trouble, hayfever, chronic constipation, incipient appendicitis and colitis; and in no case that has come under my personal supervision have I discovered any relapse that was not curable by a few further instructions in the principles enunciated. Looking to the future and to the development and elaboration of this method, I foresee that a race which has been educated on the lines of what I have called "conscious guidance and control" will be eminently well fitted to meet any circumstance which the civilizations of the future may impose. The minds and bodies alike of such a race will be adaptable to any occupation that may be their lot. To those who have been educated in these principles no severe physical exercise is a necessity, since there are no stagnant eddies in the system in which the toxins can accumulate, and to them will belong a full and complete command of their physical organisms. That this practical and by no means visionary or untried psycho-therapy will in time supersede the tentative and restricted methods of somato-therapy, I am confident, and I sincerely hope that the great benefits which these principles confer will not be confined to any one race or people. The wonderful improvements in physical health—often deemed "miraculous" by the uninitiated—which have been effected in adults, adumbrate the potentialities for efficiency which may be developed in the children of the new race.

It is essential that the peoples of civilisation should comprehend the value of their inheritance, that outcome of the long process of evolution which will enable them to govern the uses of their own physical mechanisms. By and through consciousness and the application of a reasoning intelligence, man may rise above the powers of all disease and physical disabilities. This triumph is not to be won in sleep, in trance, in submission, in paralysis, or in anæsthesia, but in a clear, open-eyed, reasoning, deliberate consciousness and apprehension of the wonderful potentialities possessed by mankind, the transcendent inheritance of a conscious mind.

CHAPTER IV

CONSCIOUS GUIDANCE AND CONTROL IN PRACTICE

WHILST under the guidance of the subconscious mind, mankind cannot readily adapt itself to the rapidly and everchanging conditions imposed by civilisation. A proper standard of mental and physical perfection implies an adaptability which makes it easy for a man to turn from one occupation in which a certain set of muscles are employed, to another involving totally different muscular actions. Under the present subconscious guidance such an easy transference is, to say the least of it, likely to be a very rare occurrence.

For the purpose of demonstration we may assume that a man who has been engaged in clerical work all his life is suddenly called upon to become a ploughman and to make a success, within a reasonable time, of his new occupation. This is an extreme instance, but the argument will apply equally well in a less extreme case. As he is subconsciously controlled he will attack the problem through his sense of feeling—through his feeling-tones—and strive directly for the desired "end." He will make no reasoned estimate of the "means whereby" he may make a success. He will not, as a preliminary to the act of ploughing, consider the particular demands which will be made on different parts of his organism, nor will he take into account the elemental laws which are essential to a satisfactory use of the plough as an instrument to be controlled in its legitimate sphere. His mind is fixed from the start on the achievement,—on the act of ploughing. He looks only to the end he desires to attain.

So he will grip the handles of his plough, set the horses in motion, and will be pleased to find that the plough moves more or less through the earth, chiefly less, for he finds it difficult to keep the share embedded and to keep the furrow straight. When he succeeds, he is almost certain to be thrown from side to side by the movements of the plough, which are affected by the hard or soft ground it meets in its progress. He holds no conscious reasoned guiding principles in his mind. His efforts are simply subconscious, in a chance endeavour to gain the end in view.

In order to maintain his own equilibrium and the efficient working of the plough, it is highly probable that he will unduly tense muscles which are precisely those which should not be tensed, and relax those which should do the most work. The tension of the muscles of the arm will almost certainly be unnecessarily high, and the general use of the wrong muscles will tend to destroy the proper equilibrium rather than to maintain it. We thus see that the moment he steps into his new occupation (which he no doubt had congratulated himself would bring perfect health in its train), he immediately begins to cultivate new and harmful habits during his daily round.[20] He becomes a badly co-ordinated, imperfectly guided ploughman precisely as he was a badly co-ordinated and imperfectly guided clerk. When the principles of reasoned conscious control are adopted, the man leading a sedentary life will be able to take up the occupation of ploughman without any fear of cultivating harmful habits. Moreover, he will attain proficiency in ploughing in one-tenth part of the time that the subconsciously controlled man took to obtain a half-mastery of it.

Let us see how he would set about it from the point of view of reasoned conscious guidance and control. Acting under the guiding principles of reasoned and conscious control he will consider first the "means whereby" he may achieve his object, rather than that object itself. He will take time to consider well the factors to be overcome. It will be obvious to any one who will take the trouble to watch another man at the plough, that a great deal of proper manipulation is necessary to keep the share embedded and a straight furrow. The manipulation requires firstly the maintenance of the ploughman's equilibrium under very difficult circumstances. This consideration will make it clear to him that his body must remain comparatively steady and support the arms and legs as the trunk of a tree does its limbs, following as nearly perpendicularly as possible the line the furrow should take. It will be evident to him that the "give and take" of the joints of the arms and legs are the chief moving factors which should meet the different movements of the handles of the plough. His highly trained guiding sensations will not permit him to make more physical tension with any part of the muscular system than is absolutely necessary, and only the particular muscles best adapted for the control of his equilibrium and his plough will be called into special use. For instance, when the left handle of the plough is forced upwards and the right downwards by the plough being thrown into a position leaning towards the right, the ploughman's

[20]It is worthy of note in this connexion that during the past two years the English hospitals have been crowded with cases of men who, formerly accustomed to sedentary occupations, have "broken down" with army training.

left arm will bend at the wrist, elbow, and shoulder, and the right straighten in order to maintain his equilibrium and general control without undue strain and interference with the proper position of the torso. Of course the left arm should exercise a downward pressure on the left handle, and the right should tend to pull the right handle upwards in order to straighten the plough again in its most effective position in the furrow. The left leg should be slightly bent at the knee, and the right leg should be kept straight and firm. The ploughman would thereby exercise his maximum of control in the right direction with the minimum of effort, and freedom from harmful strain. It will be clear from this example that in the consciously controlled stage of psycho-physical development men and women will be able, without fear of mental or physical harm, to adapt themselves at once to any strange or unusual circumstances in which they are placed. They will act in the face of the unaccustomed or the unsuspected at the direction of their conscious reasoning minds, before any promptings springing from the subconscious mind can take possession of them. Just as they will be able by conscious reasoning to change their habits at will, to be to-day a clerk, to-morrow a reasoning ploughman, so they will meet sudden surprise by that same conscious reasoning and accurate judgment which follows it. I have already drawn attention to the conduct of animals and of men and women in the lower stages of evolution when they are confronted with any phenomena to which they are unaccustomed; how that they stand terror-struck and immovable, and betray themselves. Such a condition of mind contains no element of control or reasoning, and the high importance of re-educating civilised men and women to a condition in which their control and reason are the main factors, need scarcely be emphasised at this point. On all sides is seen the destruction, the waste, the loss in human lives and human energy which are the direct outcome of a civilisation based on subconscious action.

It is our duty now to superimpose a new civilisation founded on reason rather than on feeling-tones and debauched emotions, on conscious guidance and control rather than upon instinct. The savage is terror-struck when an eclipse passes over the sun; he bows to wood and stone, quivering with fear at any desecration of any of his puppet gods. Anything which has no place in his limited range of experience he approaches through instinct which may preserve but is more likely to betray him. To-day the greater part of mankind carries out the normal responsibilities of a lifetime guided by the same imperfect forces. Men have learnt the meaning of many things which to the savage were inscrutable, but when faced with the unknown they betray the same lack of control. Suddenly-angered men will make a retort which in the light of reflection appears to them foolish and inadequate. It is an everyday experience. In the calmer moments that follow, they think of the "things they might have said," the things they might have done, which is a simple indication of the fact that in the heated moment their emotions held sway over them, whilst their reason and control were in abeyance. The subconsciously controlled person is immediately thrown into a state of panic when faced by any emergency which presents an element of danger.

Under such circumstances many become self-hypnotic and in this state will be found absolutely out of communication with their reason. As an instance of this, one may quote the behaviour of unbalanced people in a fire. In trying to save some of their possessions before making their escape they will throw from the windows as likely as not articles which will certainly be broken to atoms in their fall. The man who threw the drawing-room clock through the window and carried the hearth-rug downstairs is no fictional figure. His action represents the kind of behaviour that may be expected from the uncontrolled person in such an emergency. The following instance from my own experience may prove interesting in this connexion.

I arrived late one evening at a large hotel in a well-known mining town in one of the Colonies. I was told that there was not a room available, but that if I cared to share a room with two beds in it, with the two little sons of the proprietor, I might have a night's rest. Those who have any experience of a mining town where there is a "gold rush" on will appreciate my good fortune. Eight weary souls that night slept on the billiard-table and I do not remember how many found a bed on the hard, draughty floor of that same room. A great friend of mine was living at the hotel. He was a man of considerable learning and accounted by all who knew him as a fine scholar and the possessor of a fine intellect. The last injunction we received from the proprietor before he retired was, "Be sure to lock your door." After a long chat with my friend we went very late to bed. Remembering the request of my host I bolted the door, extinguished the light and almost immediately fell into a sound sleep. Within an hour I was awakened by the crackling sound of burning wood and the roar of flames. I realised at once that the hotel was on fire and almost immediately the tongues of flame found their way into my room through the top of the wooden walls and began to lick the ceiling of the bedroom.

My first thought was for the little lads who were sleeping in the room. I unbolted the door, and taking one under my left arm began to search for the other. By this time the room was filled with smoke, so I took the one boy out and returned to the search in the dense smoke. He had evidently jumped out of his bed half awake, for I found him under the bed. Taking both under my arms I rushed down the stairs and ran with them to their father's bedroom. He dashed out and calling his men-servants at once proceeded to take measures to extinguish the fire. I, of course, rushed to my friend's room, awakened him, and after lighting his candle and seeing him jump to the floor I left him, and proceeded to give the general alarm. I then joined those who were fighting the flames, which after a while were successfully extinguished. My readers will be able from this account to judge of the time which elapsed between the visit to my friend's room and the complete extinguishing of the fire. When all was over I looked round to exchange a word with my friend and was surprised to find that he was not of the number by whom we were surrounded. I walked back to his room and was amazed to find him absolutely dressed. When I entered the room he was calmly buttoning up his waistcoat as on any other morning when he had nothing to fear. He was self-hypnotised as regarded his chances of being burned alive, and had even shaved.

Thousands of instances of similar behaviour in unusual circumstances might be given, and the list might well be completed with the now famous story concerning Carlyle's failure to keep in "communication with his reason," on the occasion that Henry Taylor was ill. He heard the news, and became overanxious to help his friend. We can only conclude that he was under the domination of his subconsciousness, when he rushed off to Sheen with the remaining portion of a bottle of medicine which had helped Mrs. Carlyle, without knowing the particular uses of the medicine or the cause of his friend's illness.

The managing director of one of the largest business houses operating in Great Britain and America had been sent to me for treatment by his medical adviser. We had frequently discussed the psychological tendencies and characteristics of young men likely to make their way in the business world. One day, after a chat on this subject in which we were both interested, he informed me that there was always room in his firm for the right kind of young man, and intimated that if I knew one he would be glad if I would send him along. For some weeks prior to this time I had been asked to interest myself in a young man I had never met. I mentioned this to my pupil, and he said, "Ask the young man to write to me and I will fix an appointment." This was done, and the following is the young man's account of the interview: "I called on Mr. ——— and he positively insulted me. When I entered his office he asked me to sit down while he finished a letter. After about five minutes he jumped suddenly from his chair, walked towards me, and banging his fist with great vigour on a table near me, shouted, 'What the devil do you know about business?' Of course," the young man continued, "I was so unnerved that I could not even collect my thoughts and I was so flurried that I could not answer his further questions. He told me he hadn't any position to suit me." "My dear young man," I remarked, "why did you allow Mr. ——— to insult you? Why did you not remonstrate with him and assure him that you could not permit him to speak to you in such a way?" "I was so upset by his sudden attack, and I didn't expect to be treated in such a way." "Just so," I replied, "you were nonplussed by the unexpected. But I hope this will be a lesson to you. Mr. ——— was only testing you, and he wants men who are capable of dealing with unexpected events and situations in his business. If you had made an instant protest against his manner, you would now be in a position in his firm because you would have come successfully through his test."

In that stage of evolution which may be defined as purely animal, the powers of instinct in accustomed circumstances are quite remarkable, and it is due to this fact that the animal, in certain conditions of danger, will do the one right thing to escape. On the other hand, in proof of the limitations of instinct, we have only to name the noble and subconsciously controlled ostrich, so wily in its movements, and so clever in many directions, which when confronted with more than an ordinary danger, presses its head into the sand and allows its pursuer to kill it. The powers of instinct are undoubtedly limited in the animal kingdom, in uncivilised mankind, and in all stages of evolution where subconscious control is the guiding principle. This fact perhaps accounts more than anything else for the rise and fall of nations and of races, for no community as yet has cultivated and developed a national consciousness in communication with reason. The psychology of nations is too large a subject to deal with here, but, logically, if the principles of conscious guidance and control, as I have outlined them in application to the individual, were further adopted by the rising nation, it is unthinkable that it should ever suffer from deterioration.

It would act in all crises strictly in accordance with the dictates of reason, and, guided by a judgment born of tested experiences, it would be supreme.

CHAPTER V

CONSCIOUS GUIDANCE AND CONTROL

APPREHENSION AND RE-EDUCATION

THE average person may exhibit complete nerve control and balance during accustomed experiences and accomplishment of the different mental and physical demands made during the ordinary round of life, but, when suddenly confronted with the unexpected or unknown, he betrays undue apprehension and loss of control, even when the new experience may not hold any real terrors for him. The fact is, he becomes panic-stricken by the effects of the new experience. He is mentally incapable of considering the "facts of the case," for his reasoning power is thrown completely out of use by the unusual, and he is reduced to the level of the terrified animal or savage. This shows that we have not reached the stage of evolution where, by employing the reasoning faculties, we should be able to meet any emergency with control and calmness and do the right thing at the psychological moment. The really clever barrister takes advantage of this human weakness, and when cross-examining proceeds to unbalance the witness by an unexpected attack on a new line. If the barrister is successful in his choice in this connexion he will assuredly gain his end with the witness who has not learnt to meet the unusual with reasoned judgment. He will become unnerved, and the barrister can hardly fail to succeed in disconcerting him.

Let me point out, however, that the barrister himself can be caught in the same trap if the witness adopts a mode of procedure which will be new to his rival. It will be merely a matter of which gets his blow in first. As an instance, in a case of special interest at which I was present, the following took place. Incidentally I should mention that the barrister and witness had a mutual friend by whom they had sent uncomplimentary messages to one another before the meeting in court. Naturally both were on guard. The barrister opened by, "Now, Mr. ———, might I *suggest* ———" and made the unfortunate mistake of repeating this the second time, whereupon the witness calmly remarked, "May

I remind you that you are here to *ask questions, not to suggest.*" The barrister was quite nonplussed for the moment. This disturbed his usual control and allowed his feeling to dominate his judgment, and during the remainder of the case he failed to regain his balance and gave so much attention to trying to get even with the witness that he missed many points of the greatest value to his case and the verdict was gained by his opponents.

The removal of the Hunt Club Cup from its stand at Ascot Race Course is a trenchant example of the practical application of the knowledge of the weakness of men and women in the direction indicated. Constables and employees of the makers of the cup were on duty to ensure its safety, and moreover, there were always crowds of people round it. To any ordinary person it would have seemed absolutely impossible to remove such a large article without being detected. Despite this fact it was taken from its stand and removed from the Ascot grounds. One of those who successfully carried out this scheme must have been a highly developed psychologist, a man who knew only too well the weaknesses of his fellow-men. Presumably he knew that something unexpected must be done suddenly in order to attract and divert for a considerable length of time the constables guarding the Cup, during which time the thief would be enabled to get some distance away with his prize before its removal would be noticed. We are told that a group of men caused a disturbance, that heated words were exchanged and blows followed, no doubt at a prearranged signal. The thief counted on the psychological fact that the constables were unlikely to use their reason and so preserve their self-control by continuing to watch the Cup in the face of this unexpected occurrence, and during the distraction therefore the theft was accomplished.

It must be obvious that there is going on a wicked waste of this wonderful power of reasoning, where reliance is placed on an automatic subconsciousness which permits the suspension of our common-sense and upsets our balance, thus narrowing our sphere of usefulness. Therefore if we are really to progress in the future, subconscious guidance must be superseded by a reasoned and conscious guidance which can safeguard us in unusual circumstances and at critical moments. For with real progress on a sound basis we must expect a great increase in "critical moments" and "unusual circumstances," and our development must be on those lines which will enable us to meet them with calmness and common-sense, doing the one right thing the latter will suggest. This failing in reasoned action is as common amongst the educated as amongst the uneducated, and it is a most serious indictment of our present educational system that it should be so, and that as it is at present constituted it does not offer any real solution of the problem to be applied by the men and women of the future.

Take as an example a very prevalent form of human weakness, namely, our attitude of mind in regard to simple worries, whether real or imaginary. It is an interesting psychological fact that there are millions of highly educated people who have cultivated unwillingly what may be called the "worry habit." This worry habit is directly the outcome of the lack of use of our reasoning faculties, as is conclusively proved to me in my long professional experience by the fact that people suffering in this way worry exactly in the same degree when the cause has been removed as when it was actually a reality. I can hear my readers say, "But the person is not convinced that the cause has been removed." In the experience I refer to they were absolutely convinced, and in my next book there will be a fitting opportunity, I hope, to explain at considerable length this mental condition which seems so extraordinary and unreasonable.

This is one of the most difficult mental defects a teacher can be called upon to eradicate, because it shows that the person so afflicted is dominated by a subconsciousness built up of delusion and undue apprehension without any relation to common sense or fact. Another instance of the disregard of reasoned judgment is demonstrated to me constantly in the mental attitude of my pupils when they first come to me for lessons. In the endeavour to perform some particular act, however simple, many pupils exhibit a degree of apprehension out of all proportion to the point at issue. This makes progress almost impossible and causes considerable distress. It is not my intention to deal with any of the complex examples which come to my notice in my daily experience with intelligent and educated pupils, but merely to set down some of the very simple examples of difficulties which seriously retard the progress of well-meaning people while undergoing any training.

Naturally a teacher is forced to point out at the beginning that this or that is wrong. All too frequently the pupil at once shows distinct signs of unnecessary apprehension. As this condition is the most retarding feature in any teaching work, I have for years in my own work devoted special attention to it and at once make an attempt to prevent it by endeavouring to put the pupil into "communication with his reason." There are numerous and widely differing means to this end in the early stages of re-education to the description of which a whole book might easily be devoted, but it is sufficient here to mention it in a general way. I begin by pointing out that we expect these different things to be wrong, that their being so is not a case for worry or apprehension, seeing that they assuredly can be corrected. I draw attention to the obvious fact that a pupil comes to a teacher because there is something wrong. That must be the primary idea, otherwise the teacher's help is superfluous. Then, why worry when the defects or failings are discovered and made known to one? Surely it is something that should evoke pleasure rather than worry. In other words, if we have imperfections and defects, we seek help because we are conscious of their existence, because we wish to know definitely what they are, so that we may have an opportunity to eradicate them. Common-sense dictates that we should find a teacher who can detect these defects and diagnose their cause, and when this is done the pupil has much to ease his mind, much to bring him real satisfaction when the teacher can assure him of their eradication, and a changed mental attitude should immediately follow. But many people are so out of communication with their reason that it needs days of re-education to establish a satisfactory working basis.

Now, to bring about the correct performance of any act by the principles of my system of teaching it is not necessary at the beginning to call upon the pupil for any specific physical efforts. This very fact should remove immediately any cause for worry or apprehension, but in many cases it does not. When this is the case the teacher must explain that the reason that the pupil is unable to perform the act correctly is that he believes that there is something for him to do physically, when as a matter of fact the very opposite is necessary. He *is doing* what is wrong. Obviously he should begin then by ceasing to do what is wrong, not by endeavouring blindly to do what is right. The process is this: Apprehensively he tries to do what he thinks his teacher desires him to do. The old wrong subconscious orders follow in their usual channels, and before he realises the fact he is performing the act in the old wrong manner. Therefore he must learn to inhibit these incorrect subconscious orders, which result in undue physical tension and the imperfect use of his muscles. But instead of employing inhibition he adds to his difficulties by renewing his efforts on the old basis to put right what he is told is wrong, and he actually employs increased force in accordance with his own estimate of the amount needed to perform the act. And why so? Chiefly because the ordinary human being has lost the habit of inhibition, and because he is guided here by his sense of feeling, in this connexion the most unreliable guide.

When it is explained to such a pupil that inhibition is the first step in his re-education, that his apprehensive fear that he may be doing wrong and his intense desire to do right are the secrets of his failure, he will invariably endeavour to prevent himself from doing anything, by exerting force usually in the opposite direction. And so he creates a second harmful force which, in conjunction with the first, serves only to increase the undue physical tension and to intensify the already exaggerated apprehensive condition. The fundamental principle in the re-education of such a subject is the prevention of this undue and unnecessary apprehension. He must not attempt to remedy any defect by "doing something" physically in accordance with his sensory appreciation, which is the outcome of his erroneous preconceived ideas and incorrect psycho-physical experience. His reasoning power is dominated by his sense of feeling where his psycho-physical self is concerned, so that he cannot even attempt to carry out any physical act excepting the one he *feels* to be right, despite the fact that by his reasoning faculties and practical proof, he knows that his sense of feeling is misleading and is the outcome of erroneous preconceived ideas. We must therefore make him understand that so very frequently in re-education the correct way to perform an act *feels* the impossible way. There is only one way out of the difficulty. He must recognise that guidance by his old sensory appreciation (feeling) is dangerously faulty and he must be taught to regain his lost power of inhibition and to develop conscious guidance. The teacher must with his hands move the pupil's body for him in the particular act required, thereby giving him the correct kinæsthetic experience of the performance of the act.

To the uninitiated this may seem a simple matter, but if my reader will put it to the test, it will not be necessary for me to convince him that it is quite otherwise in the majority of cases. This is not surprising when it is realised that as soon as the teacher places his hands on the pupil and attempts to move him, he is at once in contact with his faulty and deceptive sense of feeling, the dominating sense in the subconsciously controlled person under such circumstances. My experience has proved that the pupil at first will act in precisely the same way if I attempt to perform the act for him as if I had asked him to do it without my assistance. He is just as apprehensive as a result of one request as of the other, and in this state of apprehensiveness he is, mentally and physically, impossible to deal with from the standpoint of re-education. He conjures up in his mind all kinds of fears that he will do this or that incorrectly. If you mention that he did a certain thing when you placed your hands on him, he will make an endeavour physically to prevent himself the next time. This, of course, is one of the worst errors a pupil can make. It is usually attended by far more tension and apprehension than when he performed the act which you pointed out was incorrect. The re-education work really begins here and it takes weeks, nay, sometimes months to bring the pupil to a stage in his co-ordination when he will be really once more in communication with his reason. With these facts before us I feel that my reader will advocate with me the necessity of adopting principles which will create new and correct habits, and eradicate needless apprehension and fear from the souls of human beings. To this end we must break the chains which have so long held them to that directive mental plane which belongs to the early stages of his evolution. The adoption of conscious guidance and control (man's supreme inheritance) must follow, and the outcome will be a race of men and women who will outstrip their ancestors in every known sphere, and enter new spheres as yet undreamt of by the great majority of the civilised peoples of our time. The world will then make in one century greater progress in evolution towards a real civilisation than it has made in the past three.

CHAPTER VI

INDIVIDUAL ERRORS AND DELUSIONS

FREQUENT reference has already been made to individual delusions, errors, and misconceptions of a more or less harmful nature associated with our mental and physical efforts in the different rounds of daily life. I wish now to draw special attention to those which may be said to have a more strictly personal bearing than those referred to heretofore, and which have not been fully recognised despite the fact that they are forerunners of unusually harmful and persistent bad habits. The individual misconceptions, errors, and delusions to which I refer are indicated in the cases which follow. They are the direct result of most laudable attempts to accomplish something considered necessary to the welfare of life, something which seemed essential to success in life, something which was felt to be a worthy achievement in life. Among these I would instance:

The attempt to bring about some change considered necessary in the shape or use of a part or parts of the physical organism, and to conceal or change some supposed or real psycho-physical peculiarity, weakness, or defect.

The clinging to erroneous reasoning, in the face of undoubted evidence which revealed the errors in such reasoning, regarding the mode of procedure adopted in the attempt to prevent or "cure" attacks of illness and painful or disagreeable experiences.

The decision that a certain condition is present, and the definite conclusion as to its degree of harmfulness or the extent of its general effect upon the organism, or its influence upon the daily conduct of life.

The attempt to remedy what the subject considers a lack of concentration.

The attempt to gain benefit by relaxation in consequence of the recognition of undue tension of the muscular mechanisms, not only in physical acts, but also during the attempt to rest by sitting in a chair, lying on a bed or couch, etc.

The detection by the subject of symptoms which are always considered serious and call for immediate eradication and future prevention. The original conception in this connexion is influenced by warped and incorrect subconscious experiences, and consequently a narrow and perverted view is taken of the conditions present.

The "one-brain-track" method is in operation and the *modus operandi* adopted by the subject is therefore deduced from false premises. Symptoms are considered causes and furthermore the chief aim of the subject in practical procedure is the attainment of the "end" desired, not the due and proper considered analysis of the "means whereby" which will secure that "end."

Perusal of the following history of cases will serve to draw attention to the little-recognised but all-important fact that mankind's attempts at self-help on a subconscious basis in the spheres indicated cause him to live in a self-created danger zone. Moreover, the area of this zone is being gradually but surely extended by each and every new experience in those psycho-physical activities where attempts are being made in what may be termed preventive and curative spheres.

The foregoing applies to a very wide range of bad habits over the whole organism, such as:

(1) The cultivation of harmful habits in consequence of misdirected energy and mental delusions which cause disorders and defects of the eyes, ears, nose and throat, etc.

(2) The development of the dangerous habit of not hearing any instructions, opinions, advice or argument which if put into practical procedures would be contrary to the psycho-physical subconscious habit associated with some defect, peculiarity or other abnormal condition.

(3) The development of overcompensation in some direction. "Running an idea to death," as we say.

(4) The harmful domination by a "fixed idea," on account of which the subject struggles to gain an "end" without adequate and sound consideration of the correct "means whereby," or of possible consequences to him in the cultivation of defects during this process.

CASE I

An attempt to hide a thin neck.

The subject's wife intimated that the thinness of his neck made him look many years older than his real age. This occupied his mind for some time and he was increasingly worried by his wife's statement. He felt that he must find a practical remedy, but in the plan which he conceived he only thought of the "end" he had in view which was to hide what he believed to be an unsightly and unsatisfactory part of his anatomy. He conceived the idea of wearing as high a collar as possible and, not being satisfied with the result, he took a second and very harmful step in the hiding plan. This was a deliberately cultivated habit of shortening his neck until the under part of the jaw rested on the top of the collar, while the head was pulled back until the lower part of the back of the head pressed on the back of the collar. From his point of view a satisfactory remedy had been found and the denounced neck was at last concealed from view.

In the standing, sitting, and walking positions these uses, or rather misuses, of the muscles of the neck soon grew into a very firmly established habit which became associated with a general tendency towards the shortening of the neck and spine, whilst the muscular co-ordinations of the whole organism were gradually and harmfully interfered with.

Some of my impressions at the first interview were:

> (1) The exaggerated rolling movement of his body when walking.
>
> (2) The pressure of the under part of the jaw and the lower part of the back of the head or upper part of the neck on the collar.
>
> (3) The marked lumbar curve of the spine with the usual shortening of stature and protruding abdominal wall. Harmful flaccidity of the abdominal muscles and general stagnation of the abdominal viscera.
>
> (4) The fallen arches of the feet—one foot caused very considerable pain at times when standing or walking.
>
> (5) That colour of the skin and condition of the eyes which indicates serious internal disorder.
>
> (6) The upper part of the front of the chest was held unusually high (pouter-pigeon style). The thorax was harmfully rigid.
>
> (7) The apprehensive mental condition in his own personal affairs and also in his contact with the practical affairs of life.

His medical advisers were unanimous in declaring that he was suffering from nerve and digestive disorders and he failed to make any improvement during many years of treatment. In his own words he "had year by year gone from bad to worse" until he was often too nervous to cross a street with ordinary traffic, and his fears in this connexion were increased by frequent attacks of giddiness when he almost lost his sense of equilibrium. He complained of painful distention after meals and suffered much from insomnia.

CASE II

An attempt to conceal his height when interviewing actor-managers of shorter stature.

It is well known in professional circles that there is a prevailing idea in the mind of the actor-manager that he should be taller than the actors who support him. The actor to whom I refer in this instance discovered that he had missed several lucrative engagements by being taller than the actor-manager with whom he had arranged personal interviews. Incidentally I may mention that he possessed a fine physique and enjoyed at this time good health. It is obvious that an actor must endeavour to prevent the loss of good engagements in his profession, and as his height was the only stumbling-block to his desires and necessities he considered his problem from this point of view only. Never for a moment did it occur to him that any mental or physical harm could result. With this *"one idea"* view he sought his remedy and soon decided that he must train himself to use his mechanisms in such a way that he could shorten his stature during interviews when seeking professional engagements. He succeeded in this direction, but unfortunately subconscious guidance and control takes no heed of the "means whereby" to be employed. His idea was merely to make an effort to gain the "end" he desired, and he was never really conscious of the actual means he ultimately employed. He merely conceived the idea of standing in a way which made him appear as short or even shorter than the person he was interviewing. Of the real mechanical happenings he was quite ignorant, and he had never thought it necessary to improve his knowledge in these all-important processes. This man came to me for help some four or five years after beginning to adopt this way of standing during the interviews. He had then been suffering for a considerable time from loss of voice, general exhaustion, and nerve and digestive disorders. On one occasion he experienced a mental and physical crisis which his medical advisers called "a nervous breakdown."

Some of my impressions at the first and subsequent interviews were:

(1) The undue and harmful lumbar curve of the spine with the corresponding intra-abdominal pressure.

(2) The harmful and undue depression of the larynx and its accessories.

(3) The exaggerated "gasping" in breathing in vocal and dramatic efforts.

(4) The undue rigidity of the thorax and a minimum intra-thoracic capacity.

(5) The lack of mental control in any attempts in psycho-

physical re-education and co-ordination.

(6) A pessimistic mental outlook with recurring fits of depression.

(7) In the standing and walking positions the hips were held too far forward, the knee joints were pressed too far back and the angle of the torso from the hips was harmfully inclined backwards, with a general tendency, as we say, to narrow the back.

CASE III

A fixed idea regarding a definite mode of procedure adopted after experiencing a week's illness in bed.

This lady developed certain symptoms for the first time. She then decided upon a practical common-sense method of dealing with them which would undoubtedly have been the correct one in the long run. The day following her first efforts in this direction her feeling-tones registered that she was much worse, in fact that she was very ill indeed and that the latest symptoms were worse than those she had hoped to remove and ultimately prevent. She decided that her attempted remedy had actually been the cause of additional trouble without in the least relieving the original symptoms. The remedy referred to was one of activity, mental and physical. She therefore came to the conclusion that this new phase of her illness had been actually brought about by the attempt she had made to fight her symptoms by simple but active methods. This conclusion became with her an *idée fixe.*

In discussing the matter the foregoing facts were vouchsafed to me. She said that she had given due consideration to them and had concluded in consequence of her experiences that the real remedy must be to go to bed and to allow the disorder to take its own course. This unfortunate experience caused her to continue to hold the idea that as soon as she felt any of the symptoms which preceded the first attack she should at once go to bed, to "prevent," as she put it, "the possibility of increasing the severity of the attack." She was absolutely convinced that she must not make any effort, mental or physical, in the way of removing or resisting the disorder as she had done on the first occasion of the attack. She decided upon the easy way of inactivity and non-resistance. Once the conscience seized upon an excuse for what the mental and physical "make-up" really craved she was doomed, and her conclusions were really influenced by this subconscious tendency. It is not surprising that after pursuing such a mistaken course for six months the attacks became more frequent and severe despite medical help, and the periods during which she was confined to her bed, and which she considered necessary to her recovery, became longer and longer. But the worst feature in her case was her increasing inability to make a real effort in the direction of health. She was actually developing her tendency to allow things to take their course, she was cultivating the serious habit of being guided and controlled by what she "felt" rather than by her reason. Her relatives at last came to the conclusion that her psycho-physical condition was serious and I was asked to express an opinion from this point of view.

At the outset one suspected some incorrect and harmful mental outlook and after a few lessons succeeded in securing the pupil's admission of the fact. A review of this mental conception may prove interesting and perhaps of great value to my readers, as it shows that as long as it existed her chances of permanently eradicating these symptoms were nil. The whole procedure constituted a prostitution of those physical, mental, and spiritual forces which are inseparable from and absolutely essential to that condition of the human organism which we call good health. This lady was suffering from the inadequate functioning of the vital organs associated with and responsible for good digestion and adequate elimination. This was proved conclusively by the results which accrued from a method of psycho-physical treatment which restored the adequate functioning after the eradication of the mental conception referred to above.

The position then was as follows:

> Certain symptoms were recognised which were the result of the stagnation of organs which needed increased activity in functioning. As a matter of fact they happened to be such as would have yielded more or less to a steady walk of a mile or so daily. The effect, therefore, of lying in bed for days was only a palliative measure. But in consequence of her first impressions through her debauched sense of feeling when she adopted active measures as a remedy, she made a definite decision against their adoption in the future; in fact, she absolutely objected to a second trial of the active method. In the intervals of freedom from these attacks the one idea was rigidly held in mind that on the recognition of the slightest symptom she must go to bed and remain there. She even considered any other mode of procedure harmful. These ideas became an obsession. She became less and less in communication with her reason and the fact that she admitted that the attacks became more frequent and the symptoms more serious did not cause her to relinquish her bed treatment in favour of some other. The fact is that her debauched emotions and feeling-tones had taken control instead of remaining secondary factors to reason.

It is possible to give hundreds of such cases, and attention is specially drawn to the fact that the *one idea* principle of meeting life's difficulties is the real cause of these serious results. If Case I, for instance, had held in his mind the "means whereby" for the concealment of his neck and had watched carefully the effect of his attempts in this particular upon his whole organism, he would assuredly have come to the conclusion that the thin neck, natural in his case, was to be preferred to the positive evils he was unconsciously cultivating. Neither he nor his wife detected any of the numerous defects as they developed during the neck-concealing process. On the other hand, they were both aware that he was gradually failing in health and had reached a stage which his medical advisers considered serious. Of course, never for a moment was the influence of the process of shortening the neck connected with his increasing troubles and disorders. His mental training had been solely on the lines of working for an "end" ("one brain track method") instead of holding in his mind the "means whereby."

He had never doubted for a moment the fallibility of the sensory appreciation of his organism. He firmly believed that immediately he decided to effect a change in his physical self he could command it by the employment of his subconscious guiding principles. He was unaware that these instinctive factors were delusive and unreliable as his directive agents.

If the reader's interest can be aroused in this connexion, all-important benefits must accrue in even the simplest spheres of daily life. Furthermore, the more difficult problems of living will be sensibly considered without fear of the disastrous results which are now so common.

CHAPTER VII

NOTES AND INSTANCES

SINCE this book was published in England, I have received a steady flow of letters from interested readers, lay and professional, which have been of great value to me. Among this correspondence, three pertinent questions occur again and again, and I am forced to infer (1) that these points are of peculiar interest to my readers and (2) that no satisfactory explanation of them is suggested by the application of the broad principles I have laid down. I feel, therefore, that in this, the American edition of my work, it may be well to treat these questions and various other matters which arise out of them for the benefit of future readers.

The three main questions—two of which occur in about eighty per cent. of the letters I have received—are these:

> (1) What is the correct standing position, and the position of mechanical advantage?
>
> (2) How is the reader to apply the principles of conscious control as here laid down, to specific bad habits such as overindulgence, whether in tobacco, alcohol, particular foods, etc., or to the cure of such diseases as asthma, tuberculosis, constipation, spinal curvature, appendicitis?
>
> (3) What are the outward signs of improvement to be noted during treatment, and are there scientific reasons for these results? In this connexion I have several times been asked to give particulars of some of my more striking and representative cases.

I will take these three questions *seriatim*, and devote as much space as possible to each of them.

I. "*What is the correct standing position, and the position of mechanical advantage?*"

I think the average man is very apt to forget that he cannot assume a position of stable equilibrium and a position which ensures a perfect mobility, unless his feet are so placed as to furnish at once a stable pose and a ready pivot and fulcrum. The most perfect base is obtained by setting the feet at an angle of about forty-five degrees to one another. In all other erect positions (the defects becoming exaggerated as this angle is decreased), it will be found that there is a tendency to hollow and shorten the back and to protrude the stomach, and if any effort is made to avoid these serious faults in posture, such effort will only result—unless the feet are moved to the correct position—in a stiffened, uneasy, and unstable attitude. It is not possible, however, to set out in written language the correct pose of the feet and legs in the ideal standing position, and I therefore subjoin four photographs which have been specially taken for this purpose (first published on 22nd October, 1910), and which show quite clearly not only the correct position of the feet, the fundamental problem, but also how the whole body of the person is thereby thrown into gear.

But when this ideal position is realised, the task of obtaining it by each individual has still to be undertaken. With reference to this task, I cannot do better than quote my pamphlet of July, 1908, entitled *Why "Deep Breathing" and Physical Culture Exercises Do More Harm than Good*, from which it will be clearly seen that the ideal position varies slightly according to the idiosyncrasies of the person concerned. The passage in question is as follows:

> "In the first place, to allow a pupil to assume, of himself, a certain standing position, means that his own perceptions and sensations are given the sole onus of bringing about the co-ordination upon which such standing position depends, an onus which they are quite unable to bear.
>
> "The perceptions and sensations of all who need respiratory and physical re-education are absolutely unreliable. It is the teacher who should have the responsibility of certain detailed orders, the literal carrying out of which will ensure for the pupil *what is then the correct standing position for him.* I emphasise this last, because no one stereotyped position can be correct for each and every pupil. When the person so employs the different parts of his body that one can speak of his 'harmful position in standing or walking,' it is only by causing the physical machinery gradually to resume correct and harmonious working, thus changing the position from time to time, that serious harm can be averted and satisfactory results secured. I may point out, moreover, that in trying to assume the 'proper standing position' at the outset, the pupil unavoidably puts severe strain upon the throat, thereby paving the way for throat, ear, and eye disorders."

Take the case, for example, of a boy who stoops very much, and combines a sinking above and below the clavicles with abnormal protrusion of the shoulder-blades. If he is told to "stand up straight" he will at once make undue physical effort to carry out the order thus crudely given, with the result that the shoulders will be thrown backward and upward, the shoulder-blades still further protruded, and the front and upper parts of the chest unduly elevated and expanded. There will also be a narrowing, a sinking, and a flabbiness of the lower dorsal and posterior thoracic region, with corresponding fixed protrusion and rigidity of the front chest wall, undue arching of the lumbar spine, shortening of the body and harmful stiffening of the arms and neck, instead of a fulness, broadness, and firmness of the back, with free mobility of the chest walls, resulting in normal curve of the lumbar region and comparative lengthening of the spine. With the arms hanging vertically, the relative position of that part of the thorax where the lungs are situated will be seen to be in front of the arms, instead of being, as it should be, behind them. In such a position, the boy feels helpless and tires rapidly, owing to the imperfect co-ordination, and any attempt to accustom him to this erect posture will ultimately result in deterioration rather than improvement.

Now the narrowing and arching of the back already referred to is exactly opposite to what is required by nature, and to that which is obtained in re-education, co-ordination, and re-adjustment, viz., *widening of the back and a more normal and extended position of the spine.* Moreover, if these conditions of the back be first secured, the neck and arms will no longer be stiffened, and the other faults will be eradicated.

In order to obviate the evils enunciated in the last two postulates the teacher must himself place the pupil in a position of mechanical advantage,[21] from which the pupil, by the mere mental rehearsal of orders which the teacher will dictate, can *ensure the posture specifically correct for himself,* although he is not, as yet, conscious of what that posture is.

I further elaborated the same point in *Why We Breathe Incorrectly* (November, 1909), and from this pamphlet I will now quote another passage which bears directly on some important points involved, viz.:

> "There can be no such thing as a 'correct standing position' for each and every person. The question is not one of correct position, but of correct co-ordination (i.e., of the muscular mechanisms concerned). Moreover, any one who has acquired the power of co-ordinating correctly, can readjust the parts of his body to meet the requirements of almost any position, while always commanding adequate and correct movements of the respiratory apparatus and perfect vocal control—a fact which I demonstrate daily to my pupils. Continual re-adjustment of the parts of the body without undue physical tension is most beneficial, as is proved by the high standard of health and long life of acrobats. It is a significant fact that the very reverse is the case with athletes, showing that undue muscular tension does not conduce to health and longevity."

[21]See also note, Part I, p. 57.

From what I have now said, it will be quite evident that the primary principle involved in attaining a correct standing position is the placing of the feet in that position which will ensure their greatest effect as base, pivot, and fulcrum, and thereby throw the limbs and trunk into that pose in which they may be correctly influenced and *aided* by the force of gravity. The weight of the body, it should be noted (see diagram AA), rests chiefly upon the rear foot, and the hips should be allowed to go back as far as is possible without altering the balance effected by the position of the feet, and without deliberately throwing the body forward. This movement starts at the ankle, and affects particularly the joints of the ankles and the hips. When inclining the body forward, there must be no bending of the spine or neck; from the hips upwards the relative positions of all parts of the torso must remain unchanged. When the position is assumed, it is further necessary for each person to bring about the proper lengthening of the spine and the adequate widening of the back. The latter needs due psycho-physical training such as is referred to in the two extracts quoted above.

This standing position as now explained is physiologically correct as a primary factor in the act of walking. The weight is thrown largely upon the rear foot, and thus enables the other knee to be bent and the forward foot to be lifted; at the same time the ankle of the rear foot should be bent so that the whole body is inclined slightly forward, thus allowing the propelling force of gravitation to be brought into play.

The whole physiology of walking is, indeed, perfectly simple when once these fundamental principles are understood. It is really resolved into the primary movements of allowing the body to incline forward from the ankle on which the weight is supported and then preventing oneself from falling by allowing the weight to be taken in turn by the foot which has been advanced. This method, simple as it may appear, is not, however, the one usually adopted. The mechanical disadvantage displayed in what is known as a "rolling gait," for instance, a gait which is common enough, is absolutely impossible when the instructions given are carefully followed. And the effect upon the whole mechanical mechanism of the person concerned is shown by the fact that when the co-ordinating principles brought about by this method are established, there is a constant tendency for the torso to lengthen, whereas the usual tendency—due to faulty standing position and the incorrect co-ordinations which follow—is for the torso to shorten.

Nearly every one I examine or observe in the act of walking, employs unnecessary physical tension in the process in such a way that there is a tendency to shorten the spine and legs, by pressing—if I may so put it

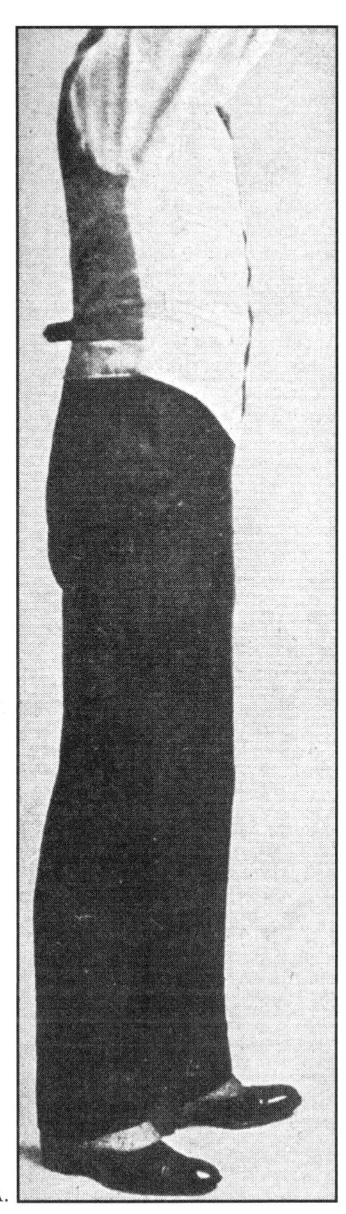

A.

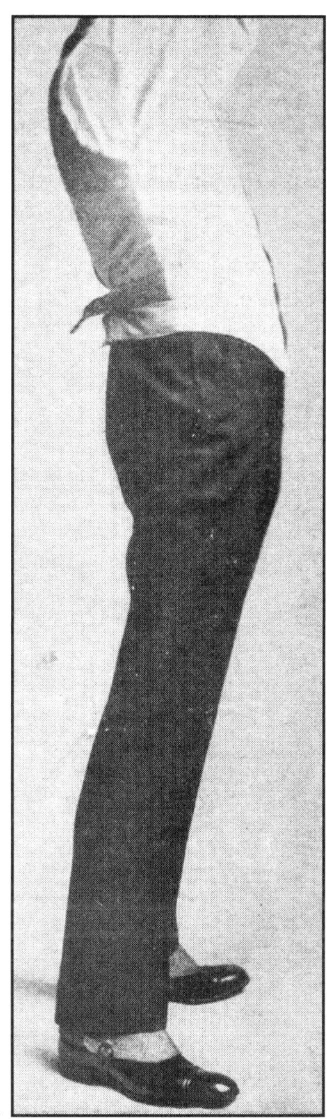

B.

A.A. THE FEET ARE HERE PLACED IN THE IDEAL POSITION FOR OBTAINING PERFECT EQUILIBRIUM OF THE HUMAN MACHINE, AND FOR PERMITTING THE MAXIMUM ACTIVITY OF THE FUNCTIONING OF THE WHOLE ORGANISM. NOTE.—IT IS EVIDENT THAT EITHER THE RIGHT OR LEFT FOOT MAY BE IN ADVANCE WITHOUT AFFECTING THE CORRECTNESS OF THE POSE.

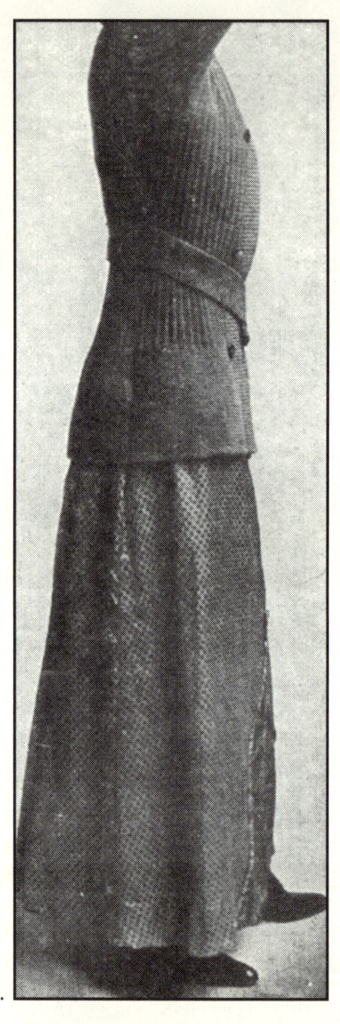

A.

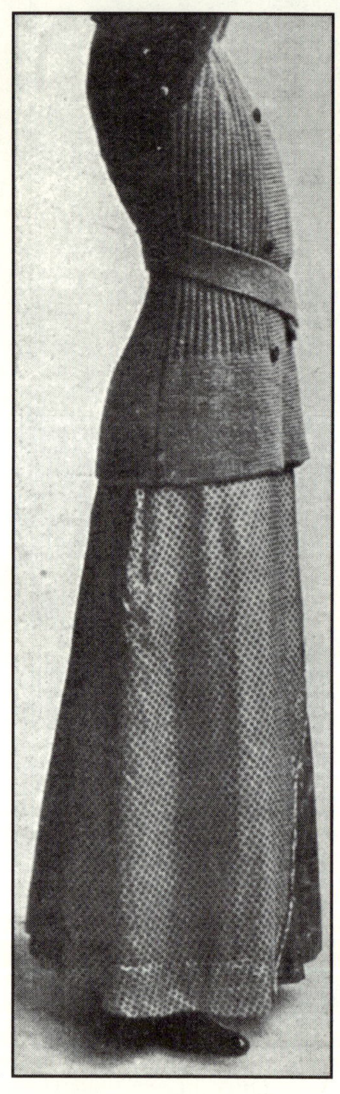

B.

B.B. The feet are here placed in a position which compels an imperfect adjustment of the whole organism in order to secure even an imperfect equilibrium. This position results in the minimum activity of the vital functioning

familiarly—down through the floor instead of, as it were, lightening that pressure by lengthening the body and throwing the weight forward and moving lightly and freely. In consequence of the "shortening" and "pressing down" just referred to, the civilised peoples are becoming more and more flat-footed. The properly co-ordinated person employs a due amount of tension in such a way that the tendency of the spine and legs is to lengthen, and the equilibrium is such that the undue pressure through the floor is absent and there is a lightness and freedom in the movements of such a person that is most noticeable. The person who is flat-footed has only to establish these conditions to restore the natural arch of the flatfoot.

We can find, perhaps, no better instance of the necessity for the application of the principles of conscious control to these fundamental and essential propositions of standing, walking, and running, than in the photographs taken of Dorando as he appeared when he was making his last terrible efforts to reach the tape at the conclusion of the Marathon race in London in 1908. One sees that he was desperately wearied, and that whatever conscious control of his muscular mechanisms he may ever have obtained, he was at this moment completely under the domination of subconscious (or subjective) control, that he was out of "communication with his reason." His body, as we see him in these photographs, is thrown back from the hips, his arms are outstretched behind him, and his legs are bent forward at the knee. As a consequence, he is compelled to use almost all his physical force in order to save himself from falling backwards. He is struggling against a tremendous gravitational pull which is dragging him away from his goal. If Dorando, magnificent athlete as he undoubtedly is, had been trained in the principles of conscious control, such an attitude would have been impossible for him, tired and exhausted even as he was. For if he had not been subconsciously controlled, he would have employed his common-sense at this moment and would have acted according to the guidance of its mandate. It is at such critical moments that we have urgent need for the control of reason, for it is then that we suffer most from the loss of the animal equivalent—instinct.

Dorando's muscles may have been taxed to their utmost capacity, but if he had been consciously controlled he would have leaned forward, not back, and while he had the strength necessary (but a very small part of the strength he was actually expending) to prevent himself from falling on his face, that gravitational force would have dragged him on instead of dragging him back from the object of his achievement, as was actually the case. He would, in short, have been able to make the *best* instead of the *worst* use of his powers.

Faults such as we see exaggerated in this instance are to be found in the carriage of many people to-day, and the fact is one of great importance to medical men. Patients are constantly advised to take walking exercise, although in many cases that exercise undoubtedly does more harm than good. In my opinion it is very essential that all doctors should devote more attention to this subject than they are devoting at the present time, in order that they may be in a position to advise which of their patients will be benefited by taking walking exercise, and which of them by so doing will aggravate the troubles from which they are suffering. For it should be evident, I think, that the good effects of fresh air and gentle exercise will be practically nullified, if the patient can only obtain them by exaggerating and perpetuating the defects which have led him to the prescription.

These same rules are equally applicable in principle to the acts of sitting and of rising from a sitting position. Very few people have the right mental conception of the "means whereby" of these acts or of the correct use of the parts which should be employed in their performance, and this despite the fact that we are performing these acts continually, and with such apparent ease from our own point of view. If you ask any of your friends to sit down you will notice, if you observe their actions closely, that in nearly all cases there is undue increase of muscular tension in the body and lower limbs; in many cases the arms are actually employed. As a rule, however, the most striking action is the alteration in the position of the head which is thrown back, whilst the neck is stiffened and shortened. Now I will describe the correct method, but it must be borne in mind that it is useless to give what I here call "orders" to the muscular mechanism, until the original habit and the principle of mental conception connected with this action have been eradicated. If, for instance, before giving any of the "orders" which follow, the experimenter has already fixed in his mind that he is to go through the performance of sitting down, *as that performance is known to him*, this suggestion will at once call into play all the old vicious co-ordinations, and the new orders will never influence the mechanisms to which they are directed, because those mechanisms will already be imperfectly employed, and will be held in their old routine by the force of the familiar suggestion. Firstly, then, rid the mind of the idea of sitting down, and consider the exercise and each order independently of the final consequence they entail. In other words, study the "means," not the "end." Secondly, stand in the position already described as the correct standing position, with the back of the legs almost touching the seat of the chair. Thirdly, order the neck to relax, and at the same time order the head *forward* and up. (Note that to "order" the muscles of the neck to relax does not mean "allow the head to fall forward on the chest." The order suggested is merely a mental preventive to the erroneous preconceived idea.) Fourthly, keep clearly in the mind the general idea of the lengthening of the body which is a direct consequence of the third series of orders. And fifthly, order simultaneously the hips to move backwards and the knees to bend, the knees and hip-joints acting as hinges. During this act a mental order must be given to widen the back. When this order is fulfilled, the experimenter will find himself sitting in the chair. But he is not yet upright, for the body will be inclined forward, unless he frustrates the whole performance at this point by giving his old orders to come to an upright position. Sixthly, then, and this is of great importance, pause for an instant in the position in which you will fall into the chair if the earlier instructions have been correctly followed, and then after ordering the neck to relax and the head *forward* and up, the spine to lengthen and the back to widen, come back into the chair and to an upright position by using the hips as a hinge, and without shortening the back, stiffening the neck, or throwing up the head.

The act of rising is merely a reversal of the foregoing. Draw the feet back so that one is slightly under the seat of the chair, allow the body to move forward from the hips, always keeping in mind the freedom of the neck, and the idea of lengthening the spine. Let the whole body come forward until the centre of gravity falls over the feet, that is to say, until the poise is such that if the chair were removed at this point, you would be left balanced in the position of a person performing the "frog dance," then by the exercise of the muscles of the legs and back, straighten the legs at the hips, knees, and ankles, until the erect position is perfectly attained.

If you care to experiment on a friend in this act of rising, you will observe that in the movement as performed by an imperfectly co-ordinated person, the same bad movements occur, tending to stiffen the neck, to arch the spine unduly, to shorten the body, and to protrude the abdominal wall.

This completes the co-ordinating idea with regard to standing, walking, and sitting, and the exercises indicated in the explanations I have made will be found exceedingly helpful as a first step towards a proper and healthful use of the muscular mechanisms in these simple acts of everyday life.

II. *"How are the principles of Conscious Control to be applied to the cure of specific bad habits, or to the cure of specific diseases?"*

The following letter is typical of many:

> "Dear Sir,—I have read your book, *Man's Supreme Inheritance*, with much interest, and I hope you will forgive me if I venture to point out

> a difficulty which presents itself to my mind, and probably to the mind of the ordinary reader.
>
> "It is this: In what way is it proposed to *apply* the principle of 'conscious control' in a given case—say in the overcoming of a habit, such as smoking, to take a common example—or in the case of functional disorders, as constipation? It seems to me that the great attraction to most people of the popular books on so-called 'New Thought' is that they lay down clear and precise rules which can be put into practice, so that the reader knows what he must do to be saved. But I confess I am unable to gather how you would recommend setting about the attainment of your principles. It would be a great help to me, and no doubt to others, if this could be explained, and probably in the larger work which you contemplate this will be more fully done.
>
> "In the meantime, however, if it is not asking too much, I should be extremely grateful to you if you could very kindly indicate the method you propose by which the principles could be applied in such cases as I have suggested. . . ."

Now, I may be doing the writer of this letter an injustice, but I am inclined to class him among the many enquirers who seem confidently to anticipate a miracle. In my introduction I have said, "In this brochure will be found no mention of royal roads, panaceas, or grand specifics," yet I feel sure that some of my readers have, nevertheless, imagined that by some marvellous means they may be cured by taking thought, despite all that I have written with regard to that procedure. We see in one paragraph of the letter quoted above a nice example of the desire to lean towards any mechanical method. "The great attraction . . . of the popular books on so-called 'New Thought,'" we read, "is that they lay down clear and precise rules which can be put into practice." It is true that I have not laid down any "clear and precise rules" which may cover every conceivable form of physical and mental trouble, as do the exponents of "New Thought" and "faith healing," and I think that my reason should be plain enough, for in my experience I have never found two cases exactly alike, and the detailed instructions which I might lay down for A might be extremely detrimental to B or C.

Nevertheless, since I see that some further explanation is needed, I will adumbrate the general principles which embrace the rule of application, however diverse the method may be in practice.

In the first place, all specific bad habits such as overindulgence in food, drink, tobacco, etc., evidence a lack of "control" in a certain direction, and the greater number of specific disorders such as asthma, tuberculosis, cancer, nervous complaints, etc., indicate interference with the normal conditions of the body, lack of control, and imperfect working of the human mechanisms, with displacement of the different parts of that mechanism, loss of vitality and its inevitable concomitant, lower activity of functioning in all the vital organs. When the subject has arrived at this condition, harmful habits become established and the standard of resistance to disease is seriously lowered.

To regain normal health and power in such cases, what I have called "re-education" is absolutely imperative. This treatment begins, in practically all cases, by instructions in the primary factors connected with the eradication of erroneous preconceived ideas connected with bad habits, and the simplest correct mental and physical co-ordination. The displaced parts of the body must be restored to their proper positions by re-education in a correct and controlled use of the muscular mechanisms. In this process the blood is purified, the circulation is gradually improved, and all the injurious accumulations are removed by the internal massage which is part and parcel of the increased vital activity from such re-education.

Thus the first stage in the eradication of bad habits and disorders is reached when improved conditions of health are established. Nor must it be forgotten that in this process of re-education a great object lesson is given to the controlling mind. In the very breaking up of maleficent co-ordinations or vicious circles which have become established, a new impulse is given to certain intellectual functions which have been thrown out of play. The reflex action which is setting up morbid conditions can only be controlled and altered by a deliberate realisation of the guiding process which is to be substituted, and these new impulses to the conscious mind have, analogically, very much the same effect as is produced on the body by the internal massage referred to above. The old accumulations of subconscious thought are dispersed, and room is made for new conceptions and realisations.

When the first stage is passed, it is just as easy at almost any time of life to establish "good" habits ("good" that is, by the test of all our experience and knowledge) as "bad" ones. Bad habits mean, in ninety-nine per cent. of cases, that the person concerned has, often through ignorance, pandered to and wilfully indulged certain sensations, probably with little or no thought as to what evil results may accrue from his concessions to the dominance of small pleasures. This careless relaxation of reason, in the first instance, makes it doubly difficult to assert command when the indulgence has become a habit. Sensation has usurped the throne so feebly defended by reason, and sense, once it has obtained power, is the most pitiless of autocrats. If we are to maintain the succession that is our supreme inheritance, we must first break the power of the usurper, and then reestablish our sovereign, no longer dull and indifferent to the welfare of his kingdom, but active, vigilant, and open-eyed to the evils which result from his old policy of *laissez-faire*.

So many people, I find, seem to regard the principles of conscious control as a kind of magic which may be worked by some suitable incantation. They appear to think that we may obtain conscious control of, say, the secretive glands, that we may be able to give an order to secrete more or less bile or gastric juice by a command of the objective mind. If such a thing were possible, and if I could endow any person with such power to-morrow, I should know perfectly well that I should, by so doing, be signing that person's death warrant; I might equally well give him a dose of poison. To refer to my metaphor of the sovereign ruler, you might as well expect a king to order and superintend the detail of his subjects' private life as expect the conscious mind directly to order and superintend every function of the body. If the king will ordain good and just laws, his policy will prosper; the detail of organisation must be left to inferior officers. In the care of the body the organisation is there, aptly and perfectly adjusted to its functions, and when the ruling power of conscious control has ordained the sane laws which shall establish peace and prosperity within the assembly, the organisation already in force will work in harmony to its fit and proper ends. On the other hand, there is great danger in underrating the power of conscious control which, if it must not be prematurely forced and made to intrude on automatic functions, must in no way be undervalued or delimited.

For instance, though it may not be possible to control directly each separate part of the abdominal viscera, we can control directly the muscles of the abdominal wall which encloses the viscera, and in reducing a protruding abdomen we can control many other muscles, notably those of the back, which when they are properly employed and co-ordinated will, by widening and altering the shape of the back, make place for the protruded stomach, allow it to occupy the natural position from which it has been ousted, and so give free play once more to the natural functions of the viscera that have been distorted and pinched by the forced positions they have had to assume. Here we see that though conscious control does not affect by a process of direct command, as it were, the lower automatic functions, there is great danger in assuming that such functions are beyond the reach of my methods.

This danger was brought before me when I read, in the *British Medical Journal* for December, 1909, an article on one side of my teaching contributed by Dr. S———, an old pupil of mine.

In this article Dr. S——— says:

> "Man's education does not always demand conscious instruction; in the absence of unfavourable circumstances he can learn by unconscious imitation of good models."

Now this is not demonstrably untrue, but at the same time it is, as I shall show, extraordinarily misleading, and is, in effect, just as valuable as the prescription of champagne and hothouse grapes for a pauper patient.

In the first place, we must remember, and Dr. S——— has himself admitted the fact, that the normal is the rarest of all states. Medical experts find that their most constant source of error in diagnosis arises from the overreadiness to assume normal conditions in patients whose internal economies and muscular co-ordination are, in fact, far from the ideal standard of proportion and interdependence. Yet if the expert trained in physiology fails to note the distortions which are upsetting the whole economy, what body is to be named the supreme authority that shall select the "good models" for unconscious imitation?

In the second place, we have to reckon with a psychological factor which at once determines the question of the validity of unconscious imitation. This factor is the demonstrable truth that unconscious imitation does in nine hundred and ninety-nine cases out of a thousand lay hold of the faults of the imitated and pass over the virtues. In a long experience of re-educating many professional men and women for the stage in this country, I have had abundant opportunity to observe the methods of the "understudy" set to "imitate" his or her principal, and my invariable experience has been that subconscious imitation has always been shown by a reproduction of the actor's or actress's most prominent failings. The intellectual reading of the part, the subtler inflexions of voice and the finer details of gesture are passed by, and the "understudy" reproduces the "mannerisms," all those obvious tricks of speech, manner, and gesture which are the least essential factors in the true reading of the part. Again, my experience in cases of stammering has shown me very clearly that especially among boys and young men, the stutter has in a very large majority of cases come about by the imitation of some other boy. We do not find boys so apt to imitate one of their fellows who speaks particularly well.

Now this imitation of a fault in speech is subconscious and will not always right itself naturally, and the reason for this will become clear with a little consideration. Set a man to work on an elaborate and intricate piece of machinery. Tell him that if he moves a switch here and a lever there, certain effects will be produced and certain desired results obtained. The movements are simple ones, and the man left to himself will be able to control the working of the machine with ease and certainty. But let us suppose that some essential part of the machine is put out of gear, and that the machine instead of running smoothly and easily begins to jerk and hiccough. Our assumed operator is immediately at a loss. He sees that there is something wrong, and that there is obvious friction where there was ease before; noise has taken the place of silence; but he knows nothing of the working of the machine save the elementary movements of the switch and lever, in the uses of which he has had instruction. Now, he may perform these movements again and again; but the machine still stutters, and our operator, quite at a loss, can do nothing to obviate these faults. He must allow the machine to continue working badly if it works at all.

The boy we have adduced as an example of a stammerer, who has copied some fault of another boy and found that fault become permanent, is in exactly the same position as the unskilled operator of our illustration. This boy knows the ordinary uses of his vocal machine which have heretofore produced normal results, but he does not know enough of the machine to repair it when it is put out of gear; he cannot control the machinery so that it may at once be restored to its previous efficiency. But just as the unskilled operator may be instructed in the complete mechanism he is set to supervise, and may then stop the machine when any fault becomes evident, discover the source of the defect and set it right; so will any person who has been instructed in the principles of conscious control be able to detect and obliterate any fault in his vocal or any other bodily mechanism, even if that fault was originated below the level of consciousness.

These marked examples furnish a sound and unfailing analogy to the principles of unconscious imitation in their application to physiology. The perfectly co-ordinated man or woman does, as a matter of fact, offer less mark for imitation to the ordinary observer than the man or woman who displays an obvious defect, just as the perfectly dressed man or woman passes with less remark than those people who affect some exaggeration of costume in order to attract attention. Were we able at this time to set the Greek model before our children, we should be able to display it only on occasion, and the unconscious imitative powers of the child would seize hold far more readily of the marked defects with which it would be forced into contact during the greater part of its waking life. In a perfect world, unconscious imitation would not be able to exert a perverting influence, and to the conception of such a world we may well turn our attention, but we shall never attain it by any means other than these principles of conscious, reasoning, deliberate construction, or reconstruction, upon which I have based the whole of my theory and practice.

And, finally, there is still a serious danger to be reckoned with, even should we find sufficient methods in our present civilisation from which we might learn by unconscious imitation. We must remember that during the advance of civilisation mankind has lost the faculty we call instinct, the faculty which guided mankind in a state of nature as it still guides the lower animal world. During our advance from this primitive condition, the one great defect in our mental, physical, and educational training has been the failure to recognise that civilised life is the death-bed of instinct, and that in civilised life man's education must always demand conscious instruction. For we see that it is at the critical moments that men fail to rise to the occasion. In such a case as that of Dorando, already cited, we see that a perfectly trained athlete, a man capable of the magnificent effort he made in the great Marathon race, was robbed of his victory by his dependence at the critical moment upon unconscious control as opposed to the conscious control which is the thesis of *Man's Supreme Inheritance.* And every day we are told that at critical moments, at the crisis of a debate, when suddenly called upon to decide a question of moment, or when faced with terrifying physical danger, men "lose their heads"— and fail. It is more especially at these times, at the crises of life, that the men who had been *educated* in the principles of conscious control would be capable of acting with the same reason and common-sense that characterised their mental and physical acts on the ordinary occasions of life. If they had relied upon *unconscious* imitation they would still be dependent, to a certain degree, upon instinct.

Before leaving Question II, however, I will deal specifically with two of the prevailing maladies of our time, viz., spinal curvature and appendicitis, and show how the principles I have enunciated have a particular bearing on the prevention and cure of these two serious ailments.

1. *Spinal Curvature.* A perfect spine is an all-important factor in preserving those conditions and uses of the human machine which work together for perfect health, yet there are comparatively few people who do not in some form or degree suffer, perhaps quite unconsciously, from spinal curvature.

The present attitude towards this very serious mark of physical degeneration would be ludicrous were it not that the matter is one of almost tragic importance, and I may quote in this connexion a letter of mine which appeared in *The Pall Mall Gazette* for 14th March, 1908. After dealing with certain other matters which need not be reproduced here, I cited the following instances of the results of our present attitude:

> "In our schools and in the army, human beings are actually being developed into deformities by breathing and physical exercises. I have before me a book on the breathing exercises which are used in the army, and any person reasonably versed in physiology and psychology, and knowing they are inseparable in practice, will at once under-

stand why so much harm results from them. Take either the officers or the soldiers. In a greater or less degree the unduly protruded upper chests (development of emphysema), unduly hollowed backs (lordosis), stiff necks, rigid thorax, and other physical eccentricities have been cultivated. It is for these reasons that heart troubles, varicose veins, emphysema, and mouth breathing (in exercise) are so much in evidence in the army. As this is a matter of national importance, I am prepared to give the time necessary to prove to the authorities (medical or official) connected with the army, the schools, or the sanatoria that the 'deep breathing' and physical exercises in vogue are doing far more harm than good, and are laying the foundation of much graver trouble in the future. The truth is that all exercises involving 'deep breathing' cause an exaggeration of the defective muscular co-ordination already present, so that even if one bad habit is eradicated, many others, often more harmful, are cultivated.

"In this connexion it is only necessary to point to the serious effects of 'deep breathing' and physical culture exercises in the causation of throat and ear disorders, following upon the undue and harmful depression of the larynx—the crowding down of the structures of the throat—such depression occurring with every inspiration, and as a rule with every expiration. This disorganisation and consequent strain in the region of the throat is always found exaggerated, and tends gradually to increase in people who are subject to asthma, bronchitis, and hay fever, and the removal of the factors causing such strain and disorganisation means great relief and gradual progress towards the eradication of these disorders; but, of course, all organic troubles should be removed in such cases."

Now I may say further that I have not, up to now, examined any method of physical culture or respiration which has not tended to bring about in time some form of directly harmful lumbar spinal curvature. And I have never examined a case of the (alleged) cure of spinal curvature in which the front of the chest has not been harmfully altered, and very often seriously deformed. The original idea in diagnosis of spinal curvature which has led to the methods producing these results is "that the activity of muscles is necessary to the retention of the spine in an erect position, in consequence of which, therefore, the primary cause for the scoliosis must be sought in an abnormal function of the muscles influencing the spine." This is the myopathic theory of Eulenburg, an authority whose dicta have had an important influence in medical practice.

The error of advocating physical exercises, as generally understood, of any kind in the treatment of spinal curvature is even greater than in the case of John Doe, whom I cited in the earlier part of this work and whose case should be again referred to in this connexion. The question here also is one of correct conscious recognition, and it is much more marked in the case of spinal curvature than in the case of my earlier illustration, a case in which there was no special deformity, and in which the muscle-tensing exercises I deprecated did not work to emphasise a marked structural malformation.

The important factors in relation to spinal curvature are these:

(a) The bent or curved and therefore shortened spine.
(b) The decreased internal capacity of the thoracic cavity.

Plainly, attention must first be given to straightening and lengthening the curved and shortened spine. This can be done by an expert manipulator who is able to diagnose the erroneous preconceived ideas of the person concerned, and cause the pupil to inhibit them while employing the position of mechanical advantage. And it can be done without asking the pupil to perform what he understands as a single physical act. Moreover, if the correct guiding orders are given to the pupil by the teacher, and the pupil makes no attempt to hold him or herself in the lengthened position, such use of the muscular mechanism will, nevertheless, be brought about as will ensure that the torso is held in a correct position. Formerly, the consciousness in regard to the correct action has been erroneous, a mere delusion, and the muscular mechanisms have worked to pull the body down. The truth of the matter is that in the old morbid conditions which have brought about the curvature the muscles intended by Nature for the correct working of the parts concerned had been put out of action, and the whole purpose of the re-educatory method I advocate is to bring back these muscles into play, not by physical exercises, but by the employment of a position of mechanical advantage and the repetition of the correct inhibiting and guiding mental orders by the pupil, and the correct manipulation and direction by the teacher, until the two psycho-physical factors become an established psycho-physical habit.

During this process of re-education, factor (b) has not been forgotten. A little consideration will show that any alteration in the spine must necessarily affect the position and working of the ribs. (The analogy of the keel of a boat and the ribs which spring from it may well be held in mind to make clear the following explanation.) It will be seen that as the ribs are held apart by muscular tissues (analogous to the boards of a boat), a bending of the spine will not buckle the ribs unless great force is applied, force sufficient to rupture the muscular tissue. But it is equally evident that there must be some play in the ribs in order that they may adjust themselves to the new position. This play is effected in the human body (and would be effected mechanically in the ribs of a boat, if they possessed sufficient elasticity) by the coming together of the ends of the "false" and "flying" ribs, that is, those lower ribs which are not attached to the bony sternum. This flattening of the curve of the ribs, and the approach of their free ends towards each other, reduces the thoracic cavity, just as in our illustration of the boat its capacity would be reduced if we forcibly narrowed the distance between the thwarts. On the other hand, we see that by increasing the thoracic capacity and so increasing the distance between the ends of these ribs, we are applying a mechanical principle which by a reverse action tends to straighten the spine.

These two actions, the re-education of the "Kinæsthetic Systems"and the increasing of the thoracic capacity which applies a mechanical power by means of the muscles and ribs to the straightening of the spine, are both aspects of the one central idea, and are not separate and divisible acts.

2. *Appendicitis.* The prevalence of appendicitis has always seemed to me one of the most striking proofs of the inefficiency of present-day methods in regard to health. At times I am filled with wonder that we permit such bad conditions to become established as may necessitate the removal of the appendix. It is, of course, well known that the operation is frequently performed when the conditions do not warrant such extreme measures, but cases have come under my notice, nevertheless, and those not among the uneducated classes, in which the symptoms had become so aggravated by years of harmful habits of life as to necessitate the major operation. Fortunately there is a section of the medical profession which objects, on scientific grounds, to the removal of the appendix in all but extreme cases, and this opposition and the evidence adducible as to the comparative ease with which the exaggerated condition may be avoided and the trouble completely cured by natural means, is doing much to limit the sphere of those champions of the knife who are never content unless they can be dissecting the living body.

There can be no question or shadow of doubt that when the whole frame is properly co-ordinated and the adjustment of the body is correct and controlled according to the principles I have enunciated, it is a practical impossibility to get appendicitis. The cause of the trouble is due to imperfect adjustment of the body which allows or forces the abdominal viscera to become displaced and to fall. The first consequence of this is a change of pressures and the loss of the natural internal massage, present in normal conditions. This leads to constipation among other symptoms, and permits the gradual accumulation of toxic poisons.

When the trouble has already shown itself and there is some positive inflammation of the appendix and tenderness in that region, it is by no means too late to apply my methods. The new co-ordinations which may in such cases be brought about very quickly, and established later, at once relieve false internal pressures and permit a natural readjustment of the viscera, and the furtherance of a rapid return to a healthy and normal condition is greatly accelerated by the internal massage.

With regard to this latter treatment to which I have already referred in this chapter, I may mention that many pupils have asked me if I use internal massage in my system of re-education. In my brochure on the *Theory and Practice of Respiratory Re-education*, included in Part III, it will be found that I used this description, as I said, for lack of one that was sufficiently comprehensive, but the principle itself is one of the first importance.

When a patient or pupil is placed in the position of mechanical advantage I have so often had occasion to refer to, the manipulator can secure the maximum movement of the abdominal viscera in strict accordance with the laws of nature and will obtain at the same time a maximum functioning of all the internal organs. In this way foreign accumulations are dissipated, constipation is relieved, and the more or less collapsed viscera—the cause of all the trouble—are restored to their proper places and resume their natural functions.

All these things, it will be seen, are essential factors in the prevention and cure of appendicitis, and I may add that the application of these principles in a very large number of cases in which an operation has been medically advised has conclusively demonstrated their value to the individual and to the race.

Appendicitis, like influenza, is probably almost an impossibility in the natural state; it is one of the results of civilisation and subconsciously controlled mechanisms, and is possible only through the conditions we have developed; and these adventitious troubles and ailments will continue to appear and to do their work of destruction until some general recognition is made of the necessity for substituting conscious control for the partly superseded forces which in a wild state render these ailments impossible.

III. "*What are the outward signs of improvement to be noted during treatment?*"

The signs of improvement are manifold and they necessarily vary according to the nature of the original defect, but I will set out here some of the more characteristic, such as occur in generally typical cases.

We see, in the first place, that the characteristic defects of the body, whether displacements of some part or parts of the muscular mechanism (in some cases even displacement of the bones), or defects of pose which throw some unusual strain upon a muscle, or, more commonly, a group of muscles not intended to take such strain, all have some correlated defects, which may be observed by the instructed as certain visible peculiarities and abnormalities. And we must draw particular attention in this connexion to the fact that these outer signs are *correlated* with the inner defects. Neither outer sign nor inner defect is from one point of view the *result* one of the other. The original cause is some faulty or imperfect co-ordination or conception of function; the inner defect and outer sign-mark are equally a consequence as they are to us an index.

As we should naturally expect, the chief sign-manual is to be found in the face. To me, that is a most valuable document upon which is written many curious, intricate, sometimes alarming confessions. The expression of the eyes, the set of the lips, the drawing of the forehead, and the more pronounced dragging of the flexible face muscles, are all marks which may be read by the expert, and, to answer the question directly, one of the earlier outward signs of improvement is to be found in a relaxation of the forced and unnatural expression which results from these contortions. It must be obvious that I cannot here set out in detail the symptomatic distortions which accompany the various internal defects, but one may be noted as an exemplar for the others however diverse.

The case in question was one of dilation of the heart and as such was brought to me by a medical friend, and, as a matter of fact, though this was the most alarming symptom, it was but one of many springing from deep-seated causes. Incidentally I may note that the spine was arched inwards, the legs were unduly and most abnormally stiffened when the patient was in a standing position, and the upper part of the chest was held most harmfully high—this last symptom being the influence which produced what was really a tertiary effect, though in this case the most threatening one, viz., the dilation of the heart. Now this patient carried certain very curious marks in the face: first a general expression of strain in the eyes and cheek muscles, and secondly four very marked indents or pits in the forehead. Here, indeed, were marks which the expert might read, and it was extremely interesting to note, as my treatment progressed and the patient recovered the proper use of the body and a consequent return to perfect health, first, the disappearance of the strained expression of eyes and face muscles, and secondly, the gradual filling up of the four curious indentations in the forehead. In this case the original symptoms were so marked that the patient's friends all commented on the change of expression during the progress of the treatment.

The face, however, is by no means the only index. Many defects lead, by way of stiffened neck and throat muscles, to an alteration in the quality and power of the voice. There too the mode of movement and the failure to express purpose in muscular action, the fumbling, indirect attempt to perform a simple act, are aids to diagnosis, either of the original defect, or, by their reversion to natural, easy functioning, of the progress of the cure.

Generally, also, we observe a clearing of the skin and eyes as the defects are eradicated, improvements which are due to better circulation and the improved quality of the blood, factors which bring about a continually increasing power in the organism to purge itself not only through the bowels and kidneys, but also through the skin.

Lastly, we may note a general improvement in physique, in the carriage of the body, in the whole appearance of co-ordinated, reasoned control.

Another curious and interesting test of the co-ordinated person who is attaining conscious control of the uses of his body is obtained by observing his hands when they fall to his sides in the position which comes naturally to him. One may say that there are three main stages to be observed in man's development in this particular, though the gradations are many and not, perhaps, always strictly progressive. The first stage may be observed in the lowest savages, the Hottentot, the Australian aboriginal, and many races at an early stage of development. Such examples stand with body thrown back from the hips, stomach protruded, and—here is the test—*with the palms of the hands forward*, the elbows bent into the sides, the thumbs sticking out away from the body. The second stage is evidenced in the averaged civilised man of to-day who stands as a rule with the palms of his hands towards his body, his elbows to the back, his thumbs forward. In the third stage, the properly co-ordinated person stands with the back of his hands forward, the thumbs inwards, and the elbows slightly bent outwards. This is a curious but little known test, which, in my experience, has never failed as an index to imperfect muscular co-ordination.

I believe I have now answered in sufficient detail the somewhat wide intention of these three main questions, but in conclusion I will note one further point that has been raised.

This is the question as to why the great majority of men and women breathe from their stomach or the upper chest and so allow, among other evils, the costal arch to be narrowed and the flying ribs to become constricted and stiffened. In the case of many women there can be no doubt that this is due to the use of tight corsets which confine these ribs, and do great general harm in constricting the natural play of the vital functions. But another and, in my opinion, the primary cause is the common practice of swathing a child in bands almost immediately after birth, and keeping him so fettered during many months of infancy. The idea of this practice is to prevent rupture in male children should they be subject to violent fits of crying or coughing, but the question of the relative tightness or looseness of these swathings is left in the hands of a nurse, who, in the great majority of cases, thinks it well to be on the "safe side" by winding the child unnecessarily tightly. Obviously the early habit is retained through life unless it is broken by some outside influence. The pliancy of the young organisms is such that the functioning of the breathing apparatus is quickly readjusted, but the evils which gradually accumulate, from this and similar causes, do not show themselves as a rule till much later in life.

Another cause is any imperfect adjustment of the muscular mechanism, a failure which may be due to incorrect training, to unconscious imitation, or to any of the chances which are always being presented to the child in the haphazard system of physical education which obtains in our nurseries and schools.

And on this note I may well conclude my chapter, for no argument I can advance in favour of a careful consideration of the principles I have laid down can have such cogency and force as the most superficial examination of the physique of the children in our schools and the adults in our streets. We are indeed suffering, not only in Great Britain but on the continents of Europe and America, from a failure to recognise that man is no longer a natural animal, whose life-habits were dependent upon the development of the faculty of instinct, and that all systems of physical culture (and how diverse they are!) must necessarily fail unless they take into account that first and last essential, the free use and consciousness of the reasoning, controlling mind.

PART III
THE THEORY AND PRACTICE OF A NEW METHOD OF RESPIRATORY RE-EDUCATION

First published 1907.

"Whoever hesitates to utter that which he thinks the highest truth, lest it should be too much in advance of the time, may reassure himself by looking at his acts from an impersonal point of view. . . . It is not for nothing that he has in him these sympathies with some principles and repugnance to others. He, with all his capacities, and aspirations, and beliefs, is not an accident, but a product of the time. He must remember that while he is a descendant of the past he is a parent of the future; and that his thoughts are as children born to him, which he may not carelessly let die."

HERBERT SPENCER.

INTRODUCTORY

It may be of interest to my readers to know that the method I have founded is the result of a practical and unique experience, for my knowledge was gained—

(1) While vainly attempting to eradicate personal, vocal, and respiratory defects by recognised systems.
(2) While afterwards putting into practice certain original principles, which enabled me to eradicate these defects.
(3) While giving personal demonstrations of the application of these principles from a respiratory, vocal, and health-giving point of view.

I first imparted the method thus evolved to patients recommended by medical men over ten years prior to June, 1904. At that date I introduced it to leading London medical men, who, after investigation, decided that the method was, as one doctor put it, "the most efficient known to (him)."

The method makes for—

In *Education*:

(1) Prevention of certain defects hereinafter referred to.
(2) Adequate and correct use of the muscular mechanisms

concerned with respiration.

In *Re-education*:

(1) Eradication of certain defects hereinafter referred to.

(2) Co-ordination in the use of the muscular mechanisms concerned with respiration.

The result of (2) is not only to make that function efficient, but also to ensure that normal activity and natural massage of the *internal organs* so necessary to the adequate performance of the vital functions and the preservation of a proper condition of health.

F. MATTHIAS ALEXANDER.

CHAPTER I

THE THEORY OF RESPIRATORY RE-EDUCATION

THE artificial conditions of modern civilised life, among which is comparative lack of free exercise in the open air, are conducive to the *in*adequate use of breathing power. Indulgence in harmful habits of feeding and posture have caused these same habits, through heredity and unconscious imitation, to become "second nature" in the great majority of adults to-day and frequently in children, even at an early age.

The normal condition of vigour in the action of the component parts of the respiratory mechanisms is greatly interfered with; general nervous relaxation is brought about, and a feeble, flabby action becomes permanent.

Certain muscles of the thoracic mechanisms which should take the lead in the performance of the breathing movements remain entirely inert for the greater part of life, whilst others, which were never intended by nature to monopolise this particular act but only to serve as a relief or change, are used solely for the act of breathing.

Hence arises a condition in which the posture, the symmetry of the body, the graceful normal curves of the whole frame, suffer alteration and change.

The capacity and mobility of the thorax (chest) are decreased, its shape (particularly in the lumbar region, clavicles, and lower sides of the chest) is changed in a harmful way, and the abdominal viscera displaced, whilst the heart, lungs, and other vital organs are allowed to drop below their normal position. Inadequate holding-space of the thorax—which means a distinct lessening of the "vital capacity"—and displacement of the vital organs within it, are great factors in retarding the natural activity of the parts concerned, which are therefore unable fully and naturally to perform their functions. Under these circumstances the natural chemical changes in the human organism cannot be adequate.

The serious interference with the circulatory processes and the inadequate oxygenation of the blood prevent the system from being properly nourished and cleansed of impurities, for the action of the excretory processes will be impeded and the whole organism slowly but surely charged with foreign matter, which, sooner or later, will cause acute symptoms of disease.

It will at once be understood that the defects enumerated produce distinct deterioration in the condition of the different organs of the body, and it is well known that an organ's power of resistance to disease depends upon the adequacy of its functioning power, which in turn depends upon adequate activity.

Records exist which prove that Chinese physicians as early as 2000 B.C. employed breathing exercises in the treatment of certain diseases. It is therefore obvious that the people concerned had reached:

(1) A stage in their evolution which corresponds with that of our time, i.e., demanding re-education.

(2) A stage of observation of cause and effect similar to that of to-day, which led them to see the need of re-education. Such re-education is essential to the restoration of the natural conditions present at the birth in every normal babe, though gradually deteriorated under conditions of modern life.

In recent years the following members of the medical profession have urged the inestimable value of the cultivation and development of the respiratory mechanism, and their conclusions have been borne out by the practical results secured by respiratory re-education combined with proper medical treatment.

MEDICAL OPINIONS CONCERNING THE EVIL EFFECT OF INTERFERENCE WITH AND INADEQUATE USE OF THE RESPIRATORY PROCESSES

Mr. W. Arbuthnot Lane, surgeon to Guy's Hospital, in his lecture published in the *Lancet*, December 17, 1904, p. 1697, urges that reduction in the respiratory capacity is a very great factor in lowering the activity of all the vital processes of the body, and that in the first instance inadequate aeration and oxygenation is the result of a serious alteration in the abdominal mechanisms, and afterwards this insufficient aeration impairs the digestive processes.

Dr. Hugh A. McCallum, in his clinical lecture on "Visceroptosis" (dropping of the viscera), as published in the *British Medical Journal*, February 18, 1905, p. 345, points out that over ninety per cent. of the females suffering from neurasthenia (exhaustion of nerve force) are victims of visceroptosis, and that the conditions present are bad standing posture, imperfect use of the lower zone of the thorax, and the lack of tone in the abdominal muscular system which leads to defective intra-abdominal pressure. He also mentions that Drs. John Madison Taylor of Philadelphia and Keith of England were the two first to point out that the origin of this disease begins in a faulty position and use of the thorax.

In a leading article in the *Lancet*, December 24, 1904, p. 1796, this passage occurs:

> "Whatever may be the causes, it is certain that an increasing number of town-dwellers suffer from constipation and atony of the colon, and that purgatives, enemata, and massage are powerless to prevent their progress from constipation to coprostasis."

CONVALESCENTS

The value of respiratory re-education in the treatment of convalescents was pointed out recently (1905) by M. Siredey and M. Rosenthal in a paper read at a meeting of the Société Medicale des Hôpitaux.

An excerpt from the *Lancet*, February 18, 1905, p. 463 reads as follows:

> "They said that respiratory insufficiency was one of the causes of the general debility which showed itself after an acute illness. It was easily recognised by the following symptoms, which the patient presented, namely, thoracic insufficiency, shown by absence or impairment of the movement of the thorax; and diaphragmatic insufficiency, shown by immobility or recession of the abdomen during inspiration—a condition met with in pseudo-pleurisy of the bases of the lungs.
>
> "Respiratory re-education was, in their opinion, the specific treatment for respiratory insufficiency. In the case of convalescents it constantly produced a progressive threefold effect, namely, expansion of the thorax, diuresis, and increase of weight. It promoted in a marked degree the recuperation of the vital functions which followed acute illness, and the general health of the patients improved rapidly. It ought to be combined with other forms of treatment, and the action of the latter was enhanced by it."

The matter of preventing defective and restoring proper action clearly calls for attention. The foregoing will enable the reader definitely to understand what is necessary, viz.,

(1) In *Prevention.* The inculcation of a proper mental attitude towards the act of breathing in children, to be followed by those detailed instructions necessary to the correct practice of such respiratory exercises as will maintain adequate and proper use of the breathing organs.

(2) In *Restoration.* A body possessing one or other or all of the defects previously named will need re-education in order to

eradicate the defects brought about by bad habits, etc., and to restore a proper condition. As the breathing mechanism is ordinarily *unconsciously* controlled, it is necessary, in order to regain full efficiency in the use of it, to proceed by way of *conscious* control until the normal conditions return. Afterwards, when perfected, unconscious control—as it originally existed prior to respiratory and physical deterioration—will supervene.

CHAPTER II

ERRORS TO BE AVOIDED AND FACTS TO BE REMEMBERED IN THE THEORY AND PRACTICE OF RESPIRATORY RE-EDUCATION

> "Each faculty acquires fitness for its function by performing its function; and if its function is performed for it by a substituted agency, none of the required adjustment of nature takes place; but the nature becomes deformed to fit the artificial arrangements instead of the natural arrangements."
>
> HERBERT SPENCER.

ANYTHING that makes for good may be rendered harmful in its effect by injudicious application or improper use, and many authorities have referred to this fact in connexion with breathing exercises. For the guidance of my readers I will detail some of the harmful results which accrue from the attempt to take what are known as "deep breaths" during the practice of breathing and physical exercises, in accordance with instructions set down and principle advocated in recognised breathing systems.

At the outset, let me point out that respiratory education or respiratory re-education will not prove successful unless the mind of the pupil is thoroughly imbued with the true principles which apply to atmospheric pressure, the equilibrium of the body, the centre of gravity, and to positions of mechanical advantage where the alternate expansions and contractions of the thorax are concerned. In other words, *it is essential to have a proper mental attitude towards respiratory education or re-education, and the specific acts which constitute the exercises embodied* in it, together with a proper knowledge and practical employment of the *true primary movement* in each and every act.

I may remark that I recognised this factor and put it to practical use over twelve years ago, but it has been quite overlooked or neglected in the other systems formulated before and since that time. In fact, when I introduced my method to leading London medical men they quickly admitted the value of this important factor, and expressed their surprise that on account of its importance it had not been previously advocated, seeing that from a practical point of view it is so essential, not only in the eradication of respiratory faults or defects (re-education), but also in preventing them (education).

A proper mental attitude, let me repeat then, is all-important. From its neglect arise many of the serious defects ordinarily met with in the respiratory mechanism of civilised people, all of which are exaggerated in the practice of customary "breathing exercises."

1. *"Sniffing"* or *"Gasping."* If the "deep breath" be taken through the nasal passages there will be a loud "sniffing" sound and collapse of the alæ nasi, and if through the mouth, a "gasping" sound. The pupil has not been told that if the thorax is expanded correctly the lungs will at once be filled with air by atmospheric pressure, exactly as a pair of bellows is filled when the handles are pulled apart.

It is a well-known fact, but one greatly to be regretted, that many teachers of breathing and physical exercises actually tell the pupils that, in order to get the increased air-supply, they *must* "sniff."

Worse than this, many medical men are guilty of similar instruction to their patients, and when giving a personal demonstration of how a "deep breath" should be taken, they "sniff" loudly and bring about a collapse of the alæ nasi, throw back the head, and interfere with the centre of gravity. Of course, it is only necessary to remind them of the law of atmospheric pressure as it applies to breathing, and they at once recognise their error.

Such a state of affairs serves to show that lamentable ignorance prevails even in the twentieth century in connexion with so essential a function as breathing, and on reflection we must realise the seriousness of a situation which, from some points of view, is really pathetic.

Most people, if asked to take a "deep breath," will proceed to—I use the phrase spoken by thousands of people I have experimented upon—"suck air into the lungs to expand the chest," whereas, of course, the proper expansion of the chest, as a primary movement, causes the alæ nasi to be dilated and the lungs to be instantly filled with air by atmospheric pressure, without any harmful lowering of the pressure.

2. During this harmful "sniffing" act it will be seen that—

(a) The larynx is unduly depressed; likewise the diaphragm.

The undue strain, caused by this unnatural crowding down of the larynx and its accessories, is undoubtedly the greatest factor in the causation of throat troubles, especially where professional voice-users are concerned. This has been abundantly proved by the practical tests I have made during the past twelve years.

My success in London with eminent members of the dramatic and vocal profession, sent to me by their medical advisers, might be mentioned in this connexion.

(b) The upper chest is unduly raised, and in most cases the shoulders also.

(c) The back is unduly hollowed in the lumbar region.

(d) The abdomen is generally protruded, and there is an abnormally deranged intra-abdominal pressure.

(e) The head is thrown too far back, and the neck unduly tensed and shortened at a time when it should be perfectly free from strain.

(f) Parts of the chest are unduly expanded, while others that should share in the expansion are contracted, particularly the back in the lumbar region.

(g) During the expiration there is an undue falling of the upper chest, which harmfully increases the intra-thoracic pressure and so dams back the blood in the thin-walled veins and auricles and hampers the heart's action.

(h) Undue larynx depression prevents the proper placing and natural movements of the tongue, the adequate and correct opening of the mouth for the formation of the resonance cavity necessary to the vocalisation of a true "Ah."

It is well known that the tongue is attached to the larynx, and therefore any undue depression of the latter must of necessity interfere with the free and correct movements of the former.

(i) The head is thrown back to open the mouth.

This is a common fault, even with professional singers, but a moment's consideration of the movements of the jaw—from an anatomical point of view—will show that it should move downwards without effort, and that it is not necessary to move the head backwards in order to effect the opening of the mouth by the lowering of the jaw, since, as a matter of fact, the latter movement will be more readily and perfectly performed if the head remains erect without any deviatory posture.

Every voice-user should learn to open the mouth without throwing back the head. Very distinct benefits will accrue to those who succeed in establishing this habit.

It is well known that the practice of "physical-culture" exercises has caused emphysema, and it has been suggested that unnatural breathing exercises have also been responsible for the condition. I refer to this because I wish to show that it would not be possible to cause emphysema by the method of respiratory education and re-education I have formulated.

Emphysema may be caused by:

(1) The reduction of the elasticity of the lung cells and tissue resulting from undue expansion of the lungs and from their being held too long in this expanded position.

(2) The undue intra-thoracic pressure, during an attempt at expiration or some physical act, upon the air cells, which remain filled with air in consequence of the means of egress from the lungs being temporarily closed by the approximation of vocal reeds and ventricular bands.

If the fundamental principles of my method are observed, these conditions cannot be present during the practice of the exercises, and emphysema therefore not only cannot be produced but is likely to be even remedied where previously existing.

In the first place, the tendency unduly to expand any part or parts of the thorax in particular, to the exclusion of other parts, is prevented by the detailed personal instruction given in connexion with each exercise in its application to individual defects or peculiarities of the pupil. Moreover, the mechanical advantages in the body-pose and chest-poise assumed in these exercises cause them to be performed with the minimum of effort, and lead to an even and controlled expansion of the whole thorax. There is not, as is too often the case, an undue expansion of one part of the chest, while other parts, which should share in such expansion, are being contracted—a condition that obtains, for instance, when the diaphragm is unduly depressed in inspiration. In this latter case there is a sinking above and below the clavicles, a hollowing in the lumbar region of the back, undue protrusion of the abdomen, displacement of the abdominal viscera, reduction in height, undue depression of the larynx, and the centre of gravity is thrown too far back.

The *striking feature* in those who have *practised customary breathing exercises* is an *undue lateral expansion* of the lower ribs, when several or all of the above defects are present. This excessive expansion gives an undue width to the lower part of the chest, and there are thousands of young girls who present quite a matronly appearance in consequence. The breathing exercises imparted by teachers of singing are particularly effective in bringing about this undesirable and harmful condition.

The guiding principle that should be invariably kept in mind by both teacher and pupil is to secure, with the minimum of effort, perfect use of the component parts of the mechanisms concerned in respiration and vocalisation. Then, sooner or later, adequate mobility, power, speed, absolute control, and artistic manipulation must follow.

Most people—teachers as well as pupils—when thinking of or practicing breathing exercises, have one fixed idea, viz., that of causing a *great expansion* of the chest, whereas its proper and adequate *contraction* is equally important. There are, indeed, many cases in which the expiratory movement calls for more attention than the inspiratory.

Careful observation will show that those who take breath by the "sniffing" or "gasping" mode of breathing always experience great difficulty with breath-control in speech and song, or during the performance of breathing exercises. This remains true whether the air is expelled through the mouth or nasal passages, and is due to the imperfect use of the thoracic mechanism, and the consequent loss of mechanical advantage already referred to at the end of the inspiration.

The natural and powerful air-controlling power is therefore absent, and its absence causes undue approximation of the vocal reeds, and probably of the ventricular bands in the endeavour to prevent the escape of air, which air, when once released under these conditions, is thereafter inadequately and imperfectly controlled.

In vocal use there is considerable increase in this lack of breath-control, the upper chest being more rapidly and forcibly depressed during the vocalisation.

This is not a matter for surprise, for if a mechanical advantage is essential to the proper expansion of the thorax for the intake of air, it is equally essential to the controlling power during the expiration, and if during the expiration the upper chest is falling, it clearly proves that the advantage indicated is not present.

CHAPTER III

THE PRACTICE OF RESPIRATORY RE-EDUCATION

HABIT IN RELATION TO PECULIARITIES AND DEFECTS

> "If we contemplate the method of Nature, we see that everywhere vast results are brought about by accumulating minute actions."
>
> HERBERT SPENCER.

THE mental and physical peculiarities or defects of men and women are the result of heredity or acquired habit, and the most casual observer has noticed that certain peculiarities or defects are characteristic of the members of particular families, as, for instance, in connexion with the standing and sitting postures, the style of walking, the position of the shoulders and shoulder-blades, the use of the arm, and the use of the vocal organs in speech, etc.

Such family peculiarities or defects are unconsciously acquired by the children, often becoming more pronounced in the second generation such acquirements making for good or ill, as the case may be. I will, however, confine myself to an enumeration of those with a harmful tendency, as an understanding of bad habits is essential to consideration of the teaching principles adopted in my method of respiratory-physical re-education.

The chief peculiarities or defects may be broadly indicated as:—

(1) An incorrect mental attitude towards the respiratory act.

(2) Lack of control over, and improper and inadequate use of, the component parts of the different mechanisms of the body, limbs, and nervous system.

(3) Incorrect pose of the body and chest poise, and therefrom consequent defects in the standing and sitting postures, the interference with the normal position and shape of the spine, as well as the ribs, the costal arch, the vital organs, and the abdominal viscera.

Re-education, when one or other or all of these peculiarities or defects are present, means eradication of existing bad habits, and the following will indicate some of the chief principles upon which the teaching method of this re-education is based:—

That where the human machinery is concerned Nature does not work in parts, but treats everything as a whole.

That a proper mental attitude towards respiration is at once inculcated, and each and every respiratory act in the practice of the exercises is the direct result of volition, the primary, secondary, and other movements necessary to the proper performance of such act having first been definitely indicated to the pupil.

It may prove of interest to mention that W. Marcet, M.D., F.R.S., and Harry Campbell, M.D., B.S., London, are of the opinion that volition as such makes a direct demand upon the breathing powers quite apart from all physical effort, and with these great advantages, that, unlike the latter, it neither increases the production of waste products nor tends to cause thoracic rigidity, thus more or less retarding the movements of the chest. The experiments made by Dr. Marcet show that the duration of a man's power to sustain the muscle contraction necessary to raise a weight a given number of times depends upon the endurance of the brain-centres causing the act of volition rather than upon the muscular power. An instance is quoted of a man who lifted a weight of 4 pounds 203 times, and who, after resting and performing forced breathing movements, raised the same weight the same height 700 times.

Regarding muscle development and chest expansion, Dr. Harry Campbell has in his book on breathing taken the case of Sandow. His conclusion will prove of interest. He pointed out that Sandow claimed to be able to increase the size of the chest 14 inches—that is, from 48 to 62 inches in circumference. Dr. Campbell then expressed the opinion that this increase is almost entirely the result of the swelling up of the large muscles surrounding the chest, and that most probably the increase in his bony chest (thorax) is not more than 2 to 3 inches, seeing that his "vital capacity" is only 275 cubic inches.

(For ten years past I have drawn the attention of medical men to the deception of ordinary chest measurements and to the evils wrought by the physical training and the "stand-at-attention" attitude in vogue in the army, and also to the harmful effects of the drill in our schools, where the unfortunate children are made to assume a posture which is exactly that of the soldier, whose striking characteristic is the undue and harmful hollow in the lumbar spine and the numerous defects that are inseparable from this unnatural posture.)

There is such immediate improvement in the pose of the body and poise of the chest whatever the conditions (excepting, of course, organised structural defects), that a valuable mechanical advantage is secured in the respiratory movements, and this is gradually improved by the practice until the habit becomes established, and the law of gravity appertaining to the human body is duly obeyed.

The mechanical advantage referred to is of particular value, for it means prevention of undue and harmful falling of the upper chest at the end of the expiration, which is always present in those who practise the customary breathing exercises, the pupil being then deprived of the mechanical advantage so essential to the proper performance of the next inspiratory act.

Then follows due increase in the movements of expansion and contraction of the thorax until such movements are adequate and perfectly controlled.

Further, these expansions are primary movements in securing that increase in the capacity of the chest necessary to afford the normal oscillations of atmospheric pressure, without unduly lowering that pressure—or, in other words, they give opportunity to fill the lungs with air, while the contractions overcome the air pressure and force the air out of the lungs, and at the same time constitute the controlling power of the speed and length of the expiration.

The excessive and harmful lowering of the air pressure in the respiratory tract, and the consequent collapse of the alæ nasi, is prevented by so regulating the respiratory speed that the lungs are filled by atmospheric pressure.

The value of this will be readily understood when it is remembered that such lowering, which is always present in the "sniffing" mode of breathing, causes collapse of the alæ nasi. It also tends to cause congestion of the mucous membrane of the respiratory tract on the sucker system, setting up catarrh and its attendant evils, such as throat disorders, loss of voice, bronchitis, asthma, and other pulmonary troubles.

From the first lesson the effect upon the splanchnic area is such that the blood is more or less drawn away from it to the lungs, and is then evenly distributed to other parts of the body. The intra-abdominal pressure is more or less raised, and there is a gradual tendency to the permanent establishment of normal conditions.

The use of bandages or corsets is to be condemned as treatment in protruding abdomen instead of the adoption of practical means to remove the cause. Such support to the abdominal wall is artificial and harmful, since it tends to make the muscles more flaccid. The respiratory mechanism should be re-educated, for this would mean a re-education or strengthening of the supports Nature has supplied. In other words, the sinking above and below the clavicles and the undue hollowing of the lumbar spine—the great factors in the direct causation of the protrusion of the abdomen—are removed, and a normal condition of the abdominal muscles established. This means a very decided improvement in the figure and general health.

The improvement in the abdominal conditions (the improved position of the abdominal viscera and the development of the abdominal muscles) is proportionate to that of the respiratory movements—a fact that can be readily understood when I point out that the movements of the parts are interdependent. When the faulty distension of the splanchnic area is present it will be found that the diaphragm is unduly low in breathing; and when there is excessive depression of the diaphragm in respiration there is interference with the centre of gravity by displacement forward, and the compensatory arching backward in the lumbar region.

After a time there is such improvement in the use of the component parts of the mechanism that an inspiration may, if desired, be secured by a depression of the diaphragm, while at the same moment the condition in the splanchnic area is actually improved.

Improvement in respiratory exchange is secured by gradual increase in the expansions and contractions of the thorax, which increases the aeration of lungs, the supply of oxygen, and the elimination of CO_2.

The quantity of residual air in the lungs is greatly increased, and if the expired air is always converted into a controlled whispered vowel during the practice of the breathing exercises very great benefits accrue, notably those derived from the prolonged duration of air in the lungs, and the proper inter-thoracic pressure necessary to force the adequate supply of oxygen into the blood and eliminate the due quantity of CO_2.

The employment of these whispered tones means the proper use of the vocal organs in a form of vocalisation little associated with ordinary bad habits, and that perfect co-ordination of the parts concerned which is inseparable from adequately controlled whisper vocalisation.

There is a rapid clearing of the skin, the white face becoming a natural colour, and a reduction of fat in the obese by its being burnt off with the extra oxygen supply.

This reduction in the weight and size is often quite remarkable, as also the development of the flaccid muscles of the abdominal wall and the consequent improvement in the activity of the parts concerned.

CONCLUDING REMARKS

THE foregoing will serve to draw attention to the far-reaching and beneficial effects of what, for the lack of a more satisfactory and comprehensive name, I refer to as respiratory re-education.

It is a method that makes for the maintenance and restoration of those physical conditions possessed by every normal child at birth, the presence of which ensures a proper standard of health, adequate resistance to disease, and a reserve power which, if a serious illness should occur, will serve to turn the tide at the critical moment towards recovery. The insurance of such a condition for a generation would mean the regeneration of the human race as constituted to-day; and I have no hesitation in stating that the results secured during the past twenty years, and particularly during the past thirteen years in London in co-operation with leading medical men, justify me in asserting that the practical application of the principles of this new method in education and re-education will be invaluable in overcoming the disadvantages and bad habits of our artificial civilised life, and that they will prove the great factor in successfully checking the physical degeneration of mankind.

INDEX

CONSTRUCTIVE CONSCIOUS CONTROL OF THE INDIVIDUAL

WITH AN INTRODUCTION BY

PROFESSOR JOHN DEWEY

DEDICATED TO THE MEMORY OF

MY MOTHER

PREFACE

THE demand for this book has been an insistent one for some time past, particularly from the American readers of *Man's Supreme Inheritance*, and, out of gratitude, I have a keen desire to make a contribution to our knowledge worthy of the written encouragement I have received from a large circle of readers, from the Press, and from scientific men in Australia, England and America.

This mass of correspondence is of the greatest interest and value to me, for every letter contains a request for further enlightenment on some particular point, or points, of special interest to the writer of the letter. Of course, it is quite impossible to answer all these queries in this volume, but, whenever possible, I shall give practical illustrations to shew, in a general way, the fundamental principle or principles which are involved in these queries, in the hope that these illustrations will help my correspondents to a better understanding of the practical side of their problems. I have sufficient matter for several volumes, and in making my selections I have been influenced by the relative importance of this matter to each portion of my subject. It may, therefore, be a source of satisfaction to any reader who may be disappointed in this respect to know that I have given due consideration to this essential part of my work.

In *Man's Supreme Inheritance* I have set down my thesis, together with practical procedures and illustrations, and, if I may judge from the correspondence received from readers, the way has thus been cleared to a new outlook and to the desire for a better understanding of the *means whereby* life may be lived sanely in the environment of twentieth-century experiences and rapid changes. In this book I am most anxious to answer such oft-repeated questions as, "Why are our instincts less reliable than those of our early ancestors?" "At what stage of man's evolution did this deterioration begin?" "What is the cause of our present-day individual and national unrest?" "Can you set down principles which will enable us to decide as to the best methods of educating our children?" "Evidently your conception of conscious control, co-ordination and re-education differs from the usual conception; if so, will you explain the difference in your next book?" I am of opinion that if I succeed in answering these questions, I shall have made a distinct step forward in helping to clear away, once and for all, the doubts of any person who, in the midst of worldwide unrest and dissatisfaction, is seeking honestly for truth amidst the mass of methods, systems, "cures" and treatments in what are called "physical," "mental" and "spiritual" spheres. In this connexion, it is important to note that the enthusiasts for these different methods point to excellent *specific* results (that is, according to their idea or conception of results) in support of their contentions and beliefs, but the fact remains that in spite of these results, associated with human effort during the past five hundred years in all spheres of remedial and curative activity, the standard of sensory appreciation, of general co-ordination and of reliable use of the mechanisms of the organism has been and still is being gradually lowered, with the associated serious conditions which are apparent to-day on every hand.

I intend to deal with a wide range of more or less generally accepted statements and principles laid down by experts in these spheres, in an attempt to shew my readers how they may arrive at a definite and reliable decision as to which method, system or "cure" may prove satisfactory.

To a certain point I am in sympathy with all workers in either "physical," "mental," or "spiritual" spheres, for I believe that "there are more things in heaven and earth than are dreamt of in our philosophy," but it has always seemed to me that the first duty of man was and is to understand and develop those potentialities which are well within the sphere of his activities here on this earth. For this reason I intend, in this volume, to adhere to my earlier scheme of practical illustration, endeavouring, as far as possible, to give a demonstrable illustration in connexion with statements and arguments. This formula, I venture to predict, will prove to be more and more the rule and not the exception as we progress towards a plane of constructive, conscious guidance and control. It has two advantages over other formulas. In the first place, it forces the philosopher or teacher to give to the world practical procedures, which may be applied to the actual activities of life, instead of theoretical conclusions which too often have no practical bearing upon life. In the second place—and this is all-important—it transfers his work from the doubtful field of individual or collective opinion to the more reliable field of demonstrable conclusion, inasmuch as he is in duty bound to devote years of labour and investigation to the valuable but difficult process of converting to practical use each and every original idea (opinion). This is a process of years, but if at the end of each experiment he gives to the world only those ideas which he has succeeded in reducing to practical procedures, rejecting all others, he will be making a great contribution to humanity: he will be offering practical experiences in a field where for centuries we have too often been offered little but personal opinions. As the thesis of *Man's Supreme Inheritance* is unfolded, volume by volume, it will be found that it covers ground that has been smoothed or roughened, as the case may be, by numberless combats among adherents of the various theories which tend in practical application towards the separation instead of the unity of human potentialities; and that, on the constructive side, it provides principles which are fundamental to that condition of unity which we all agree should be inseparable from the processes of living. The subject matter of this book represents an endeavour to shew that the great problems involved in the present condition of individual and national unrest demand for their solution a recognition, not only of their unity, but also of the unity of their underlying causes.

This reference to my thesis gives me an appropriate opening to lay before my readers the difficulty I have encountered in my attempts to set down, in a sufficiently clear and direct way, the results of my experiences in unfamiliar fields. This difficulty lies in the fact that the adequate description of these experiences, for purposes of practical application, calls for new and more comprehensive words than we have at our command. It is obvious that the most appropriate word (or words) chosen in order to convey an idea, will prove inadequate to express the aggregate, after an element that is new has been added to the idea. In such a case, we are forced either to use a word (or words) which is inadequate, or to coin one in an attempt to express adequately the expanded idea.

Expanding ideas are the fore-runners of human advancement. The conveyance of the knowledge concerned with expanding ideas, whether by the written or spoken word, calls urgently for the recognition of the fact that expanding ideas demand new words which will adequately express the original as well as the new thought or thoughts involved.

This book is really the second volume of *Man's Supreme Inheritance* and I have named it *Constructive Conscious Control of the Individual.* I am offering constructive arguments and a constructive plan, and the fact that I have indulged freely in destructive criticism does not affect this statement, for a consideration of the needs and aims of such a book reveals at once that this is a necessity. It will be found that my criticism is directed solely towards what I believe to be the impeding factors in our progress towards a constructive plan of life and education.

The preparation of the subject matter of this book has proved a very difficult task, in which I have needed considerable assistance, and I take this opportunity to express my gratitude to Professor John Dewey for the invaluable suggestions he made after reading the manuscript; to my assistants, Miss Ethel Webb and Miss Irene Tasker, for their valuable help in and their untiring devotion to the work of revising and preparing the subject matter for publication; to Dr. Peter Macdonald and to the Rev. W. G. Pennyman for assisting me by reading the manuscript and offering criticism; to Miss Mary Olcott for undertaking the responsibility connected with the correction of the proofs; and to Miss Edith Lawson and Miss Carla Atkinson for their help in connexion with proofs and typescripts. To each and all of these I owe a deep debt of gratitude.

F. MATTHIAS ALEXANDER.

16 Ashley Place,
Westminster, London.

PREFACE TO NEW EDITION

MANKIND today stands at bay. In the world outside himself his plans and schemes have not worked out as he expected. Theories and beliefs faithfully held have failed when brought to the test of actual practice. Hence it is not unreasonable to conclude that even if the bases of these theories and beliefs were sound, man's reaction in translating them into practice has led him into error and consequent failure.

One thing is certain. The bridging of the gap between theory, with its associated beliefs, and practice, depends at every step upon the human element, for it is the nature of the reaction of the individual engaged in the task of this bridging—the carrying-out of the plan or theory—that will determine the measure of success or failure. The all-important consideration, therefore, in bridging the gap between theory and practice is the make-up of the individual, particularly the sensory make-up. The manner of the use and functioning of the psycho-physical mechanisms responsible for his reactions in carrying out the activities required for this bridging (as for all his activities), depends upon the nature of the registering of sensations and experiences, and where this registering is trustworthy, the beliefs and judgments which result may be correspondingly trustworthy, but not otherwise.

The high estimate I hold of the part played by the human sensorium in the use and functioning of the self will be clear from this book, for its four parts are devoted to Sensory Appreciation in its Relation to Man's Evolutionary Development, Learning to Do, Man's Needs, and Happiness. In an interesting passage quoted in my book *The Use of the Self* (p. 474), Sir Arthur Eddington points out that religious belief is based upon experience, but goes on to admit that "there is such a thing as illusion," and that not "every experience is to be taken at face value." Hence it may be of interest and value to give consideration to the use and functioning of the human self that makes possible the registering of experience upon which religious and other belief is based. Certain it is that without the functioning of the human sensorium this registration would not be possible, and hence it will be seen how all-essential it is that the human sensorium should function as a reliable register in order to minimize the effect of sensory illusion in the forming and assessing the validity of the beliefs upon which our judgment of reality depends.

For the nature of this functioning determines the nature of this registration, and this in turn determines the nature of the experience upon which belief is based, and is, therefore, the forerunner of all we finally accept in arriving at our judgment in the matter of reality. If the Leaders in the religious life of the past and the Prophets had given due recognition to this in assessing the nature and value of the experiences upon which they believed religious and other beliefs should be based, their followers would not have been so frequently led into error by mistaking illusion for reality. Instead, they might have been led to unknown experiences far beyond the present limit of human conception of experience, as they passed from the instinctive to the conscious in changing and improving the use and functioning of the human self.

In this connexion I think it may be of general interest to quote the following passage from *The Thought and Character of William James*[1] by Ralph Barton Perry which shows the attitude of William James towards sensory experience. Professor Perry writes:

> "In speaking, first, of James's sensibility, I do not mean his susceptibility to feeling or emotion, but the acuity of his *senses*—the voluminousness and richness of the experience which he received through them, and the prominence of that experience and of its underlying motive in his life as a whole. . . . His psychological writings testify to his discrimination of organic sensations.
>
> "Having a high sensuous endowment and being avid of sensory experience, it is not surprising that he should have felt such experience to convey the authentic revelation of reality. It is the unsaid but fundamental premise of his whole metaphysics that only he can speak authoritatively of the universe who is most sensitively attuned to it. Metaphysics is an apprehending of reality in its most immediate and lifelike aspect, or a listening to hear 'the pulse of Being beat.' When he said that he found 'no good warrant for even suspecting the existence of any reality of a higher denomination than that distributed and strung-along and flowing sort of reality which we finite beings swim in,' he was placing his ultimate reliance on the human sensorium."

This is of particular interest to me because a member of the medical profession, a close friend of William James, had interested him enough in my work to persuade him to come to me in London for a course of lessons. Unfortunately, unforeseen circumstances interfered with this plan, so I did not have the pleasure and honour of numbering him among my pupils. For me this has been a lifelong regret, because from

[1]Vol. II, pp. 682-3. Quoted by the courtesy of Little, Brown & Co. Boston. (1935.)

what this friend told me, there can be little doubt that much could have been done to help him to enlarge his experience by means which would tend to restore trustworthiness to the sensory processes which were more or less untrustworthy, and bring the psycho-physical processes which activated his "high sensuous endowment" under conscious control, thus enabling him to bridge the gap between the instinctive and the conscious way of living.

I am emboldened to make this claim because of the knowledge I have gained through the evolution of my technique, first in teaching myself and then in my long experience of teaching others. As my technique evolved it became increasingly clear that by its procedures, provision is made for coming into contact with the unknown, because the improved condition of psycho-physical functioning brought about is not the result of working for a previously conceived and directed end (the known), but emerges as the indirect result of the employment of reasoned means whereby improved conditions in the use of the self are brought about (the unknown). This result does not come about by inducing self-hypnotism, or because of some chance happening, as for instance, the coming into contact with an outside influence, personal or otherwise, or the possession of some natural aptitude (habitual reaction) which is fitted to produce a certain desired result. In all these cases, instinct rather than the thinking and reasoning processes are relied upon, whereas "reasoning from the known to the unknown," as in my technique, depends upon the conscious employment of means that conform to biological, physiological and other laws known to us; in which, also, the observation of phenomena in cause and effect can be tested according to strict scientific method, so that as Dr. Dewey writes in his Introduction, "the causes that are used to explain the consequences, or effects, can be concretely followed up to show that they actually produce these consequences and not others."

Today I do not know of any person who doubts that if man is to evolve in the right direction, the gap between instinctive and conscious control of the self must be bridged, in order to bridge "the gap between idealistic theory and actual practice." During the past fifty years I have had a unique experience in helping men and women in many walks of life to do this, by employing their conscious reasoning processes in changing and improving their human sensorium as they pass from known (wrong) to unknown (right) experiences of their use of themselves. Moreover and all-important, the prerequisite to each step in this process was the restoration of trustworthiness to the human sensorium without which a human being could not register experience so as to be able to test its validity.

The untrustworthiness of the sensory appreciation of the people of this age is demonstrable, and will be found to be extreme in the rapidly increasing number of people afflicted with so-called "mental" and criminal tendencies. Few people would accept as trustworthy the experiences related to them by any person who was a so-called "mental" case, and by the same token we should be wise not to accept "at face value" the experiences of anyone else, or place implicit confidence in the judgment and conclusions based on these experiences, unless we have good reason for believing that the sensorium of that person is a trustworthy guide in functioning and in registering impressions.

Summed up, the foregoing meets the wellknown point at issue between the adherents of science and of religion, the scientist finding fault because of the want of what he calls "operational verification" of the experiences of the unknown upon which religious faith is based, and the adherents of religion claiming that many of their experiences, although not verifiable objectively, should not on that account be rejected by the scientist, for they are none the less real.

My earnest plea is for the unprejudiced consideration of the education that I have advocated for the gaining of unknown experiences in the improvement in the use of self. This is an education equally for the adult as for the child and involves improvement of the nature of their sensory appreciation as an essential training for a more trustworthy registration of any other experiences which may come to them, so minimizing their present liability to fall into error even if they inherit a "high sensuous endowment" such as Professor Perry tells us that William James possessed.

It is true that dependence upon instinctive reaction meets the needs of the animal kingdom, but the world crisis of our day serves to show that such dependence no longer meets man's needs when he tries to translate into practice his idealistic theories with regard to self-improvement, growth and progress.

F. MATTHIAS ALEXANDER.

Hotel Braemore
Commonwealth Avenue
Boston, Mass.

CONTENTS

CONCLUSIONS

INTRODUCTION

THE principle and procedure set forth by Mr. Alexander are crucially needed at present. Strangely, this is the very reason why they are hard to understand and accept. For although there is nothing esoteric in his teaching, and although his exposition is made in the simplest English, free from technical words, it is difficult for anyone to grasp its full force without having actual demonstration of the principle in operation. And even then, as I know from personal experience, its full meaning dawns upon one only slowly and with new meanings continually opening up. Since I can add nothing to the clear and full exposition that Mr. Alexander has himself given, it has occurred to me that the most useful form this introductory word can take is an attempt to explain wherein lies the difficulty in grasping his principle.

The chief difficulty, as I have said, lies in the fact that it is so badly needed. The seeming contradiction in this statement is just one instance of the vicious circle which is frequently pointed out and fully dealt with in the pages of the text. The principle is badly needed, because in all matters that concern the individual self and the conduct of its life, there is a defective and lowered sensory appreciation and judgment, both of ourselves and of our acts, which accompanies our wrongly-adjusted psycho-physical mechanisms. It is precisely this perverted consciousness which we bring with us to the reading and comprehension of Mr. Alexander's pages, and which makes it hard for us to realize his statements as to its existence, causes and effects. We have become so used to it that we take it for granted. It forms, as he has so clearly shewn, our standard of rightness. It influences our every observation, interpretation and judgment. It is the one factor which enters into our every act and thought.

Consequently, only when the results of Mr. Alexander's lessons have changed one's sensory appreciation and supplied a new standard, so that the old and the new condition can be compared with each other, does the concrete force of his teaching come home to one. In spite of the whole tenour of Mr. Alexander's teaching, it is this which makes it practically impossible for anyone to go to him with any other idea at the outset beyond that of gaining some specific relief and remedy. Even after a considerable degree of experience with his lessons, it is quite possible for one to prize his method merely on account of specific benefits received, even though one recognizes that these benefits include a changed emotional condition and a different outlook on life. Only when a pupil reaches the point of giving his full attention to the *method* of Mr. Alexander instead of its results, does he realize the constant influence of his sensory appreciation.

The perversion of our sensory consciousness of ourselves has gone so far that we lack criteria for judging the doctrines and methods that profess to deal with the individual human being. We oscillate between reliance upon plausible general theories and reliance upon testimonies to specific benefits obtained. We oscillate between extreme credulity and complete scepticism. On the one hand, there is the readiest acceptance of all claims made in behalf of panaceas when these are accompanied by testimonies of personal benefits and cures. On the other hand, the public has seen so many of these panaceas come and go, that it has, quite properly, become sceptical about the reality of any new and different principle for developing human well-being. The world is flooded at present with various systems for relieving the ills that human flesh is heir to, such as, systems of exercise for rectifying posture, methods of mental, psychological and spiritual healing, so that, except when there happens to be an emotional wave sweeping the country, the very suggestion that there is fundamental truth in an unfamiliar principle is likely to call out the feeling that one more person, reasonably sensible about most things, has fallen for another one of the "cure-alls" that abound. "How," it will be asked, "can the teaching of Mr. Alexander be differentiated from these other systems?" "What assurance is there that it is anything more than one of them, working better perhaps for some persons and worse for others?" If, in reply, specific beneficial results of Mr. Alexander's teaching are pointed out, one is reminded of the fact that imposing testimonials of this kind can be produced in favour of all the other systems. The point, then, to be decided is: What is the worth of these results and how is their worth to be judged? Or, again, if it is a question of the theories behind the results, most of the systems are elaborately reasoned out and claim scientific or spiritual backing. In what fundamental respect, then, do the principles and consequences of Mr. Alexander's teaching differ from these?

These are fair questions, and it seems to me that probably the best thing that this introduction can do is to suggest some simple criteria by which any plan can be judged. Certain other questions may suggest the path by which these criteria may be found. Is a system primarily remedial, curative, aiming at relief of sufferings that already exist; or is it fundamentally preventive in nature? And if preventive rather than merely corrective, is it specific or general in scope? Does it deal with the "mind" and the "body" as things separated from each other, or does it deal with the unity of man's individuality? Does it deal with some portion or aspect of "mind" and "body," or with the re-education of the whole being? Does it aim at securing results directly, by treatment of symptoms, or does it deal with the *causes* of malconditions present in such a way that any beneficial results secured come as a natural consequence, almost, it might be said, as by-products of a fundamental change in such conditioning causes? Is the scheme educational or non-educational in character? If the principle underlying it claims to be preventive and constructive, does it operate from without by setting up some automatic safety-device, or does it operate from within? Is it cheap and easy, or does it make demands on the intellectual and moral energies of the individuals concerned? Unless it does the latter, what is it, after all, but a scheme depending ultimately upon some trick or magic, which, in curing one trouble, is sure to leave behind it other troubles (including fixations, inhibitions, laxities, lessening of power of steady and intelligent control), since it does not deal with causes, but only directs their operation into different channels, and changes symptoms from such as are perceptible into more subtle ones that are not perceived? Anyone who bears such questions as the above in mind whilst reading Mr. Alexander's book will have little difficulty in discriminating between the principle underlying his educational method and those of the systems with which it might be compared and confused.

Any sound plan must prove its soundness in reference both to concrete consequences and to general principles. What we too often forget is that these principles and facts must not be judged separately, but in connexion with each other. Further, whilst any theory or principle must ultimately be judged by its consequences in operation, whilst it must be verified experimentally by observation of how it works, yet in order to justify a claim to be scientific, it must provide a method for making evident and observable what the consequences are; and this method must be such as to afford a guarantee that the observed consequences actually flow from the principle. And I unhesitatingly assert that, when judged by this standard, that is, of a principle at work in effecting definite and verifiable consequences, Mr. Alexander's teaching is scientific in the strictest sense of the word. It meets both of these requirements. In other words, the plan of Mr. Alexander satisfies the most exacting demands of scientific method.

The principle or theory of Mr. Alexander and the observed consequences of its operation have developed at the same time and in the closest connexion with each other. Both have evolved out of an experimental method of procedure. At no time has he elaborated a theory for its own sake. This fact has occasionally been a disappointment to "intellectual" persons who have subconsciously got into the habit of depending upon a certain paraphernalia of technical terminology. But the theory has never been carried beyond the needs of the procedure employed, nor beyond experimentally verified results. Employing a remarkably sensitive power of observation, he has noted the actual changes brought about in individuals in response to the means which he has employed, and has followed up these changes in their connexions with the individual's habitual reflexes, noting the reactions due to the calling into play of established bad habits, with even greater care than the more obvious beneficial consequences obtained. Every such undesirable response has been treated as setting a problem, namely, that of discovering some method by which the evocation of these instinctive reactions, and the feelings associated with them, can be inhibited, and, in their stead, such acts called into play as will give a basis for correct sensory appreciations. Every step in the process has been analysed and formulated, and every changing condition and consequence, positive or negative, favourable or unfavourable, which is employed as a means for developing the experimental procedure, has been still further developed. The use of this developed method has, of course, continuously afforded new material for observation and thorough analysis. To this process of simultaneous development of principles and consequences, used as means for testing each other, there is literally no end. As long as Mr. Alexander uses the method, it will be a process tending continually towards perfection. It will no more arrive at a stage of finished perfection than does any genuine experimental scientific procedure, with its theory and supporting facts. The most striking fact of Mr. Alexander's teaching is the sincerity and reserve with which he has never carried his formulation beyond the point of demonstrated facts.

It is obvious, accordingly, that the results obtained by Mr. Alexander's teaching stand on a totally different plane from those obtained under the various systems which have had great vogue until they have been displaced by some other tide of fashion and publicity. Most of those who urge the claims of these systems point to "cures" and other specific phenomena as evidence that they are built upon correct principles. Even for patent medicines an abundance of testimonials can be adduced. But the theories and the concrete facts in these cases have no genuine connexion with each other. Certain consequences, the "good" ones, are selected and held up for notice, whilst no attempt is made to find out what other consequences are taking place. The "good" ones are swallowed whole. There is no method by which it can be shewn what consequences, if any, result from the principle invoked, or whether they are due to quite other causes.

But the essence of scientific method does not consist in taking consequences in gross; it consists precisely in the means by which consequences are followed up in detail. It consists in the processes by which the causes that are used to explain the consequences, or effects, can be concretely followed up to shew that they actually produce these consequences and no others. If, for instance, a chemist pointed, on the one hand, to a lot of concrete phenomena which had occurred after he had tried an experiment and, on the other hand, to a lot of general principles and theories elaborately reasoned out, and then proceeded to assert that the two things were connected so that the theoretical principles accounted for the phenomena, he would meet only with ridicule. It would be clear that scientific method had not even been started; it would be clear that he was offering nothing but assertion.

Mr. Alexander has persistently discouraged the appeal to "cures" or to any other form of remarkable phenomena. He has even discouraged keeping records of these cases. Yet, if he had not been so whole-heartedly devoted to working out a demonstration of a principle—a demonstration in the scientific sense of the word—he would readily have had his day of vogue as one among the miracle-mongers. He has also persistently held aloof from building up an imposing show of technical scientific terminology of physiology, anatomy and psychology. Yet that course also would have been easy in itself, and a sure method of attracting a following. As a consequence of this sincerity and thoroughness, maintained in spite of great odds, without diversion to side issues of fame and external success, Mr. Alexander has demonstrated a new scientific principle with respect to the control of human behaviour, as important as any principle which has ever been discovered in the domain of external nature. Not only this, but his discovery is necessary to complete the discoveries that have been made about non-human nature, if these discoveries and inventions are not to end by making us their servants and helpless tools.

A scientific man is quite aware that no matter how extensive and thorough is his theoretical reasoning, and how definitely it points to a particular conclusion of fact, he is not entitled to assert the conclusion as a fact until he has actually observed the fact, until his senses have been brought into play. With respect to distinctively human conduct, no one, before Mr. Alexander, has even considered just what kind of sensory observation is needed in order to test and work out theoretical principles. Much less have thinkers in this field ever evolved a technique for bringing the requisite sensory material under definite and usable control. Appeal to suggestion, to the unconscious and to the subconscious, is in its very description an avoidance of this scientific task; the systems of purely physical exercise have equally neglected any consideration of the methods by which their faults are to be observed and analysed.

Whenever the need has been dimly felt for some concrete check and realization of the meaning of our thoughts and judgments about ourselves and our conduct, we have fallen back, as Mr. Alexander has so clearly pointed out in his writings, on our pre-existing sense of what is "right." But this signifies in the concrete only what we feel to be *familiar*. And in so far as we have bad habits needing re-education, that which is familiar in our sense of ourselves and of our acts can only be a reflection of the bad psycho-physical habits that are operating within us. This, of course, is precisely as if a scientific man, who, by a process of reasoning had been led to a belief in what we call the Copernican theory, were then to try to test this reasoning by appealing to precisely those observations, without any addition or alteration, which had led men to the Ptolemaic theory. Scientific advance manifestly depends upon the discovery of conditions for making new observations, and upon the re-making of old observations under different conditions; in other words, upon methods of discovering *why*, as in the case of the scientific man, we have had and relied upon observations that have led into error.

After studying over a period of years Mr. Alexander's method in actual operation, I would stake myself upon the fact that he has applied to our ideas and beliefs about ourselves and about our acts exactly the same method of experimentation and of production of new sensory observations, as tests and means of developing thought, that have been the source of all progress in the physical sciences; and if, in any other plan, any such use has been made of the sensory appreciation of our attitudes and acts, if in it there has been developed a technique for creating new sensory observations of ourselves, and if complete reliance has been placed upon these findings, I have never heard of it. In some plans there has been a direct appeal to "consciousness" (which merely registers bad conditions); in some, this consciousness has been neglected entirely and dependence placed instead upon bodily exercises, rectifications of posture, etc. But Mr. Alexander has found a method for detecting precisely the correlations between these two members, physical-mental, of the same whole, and for creating a new sensory consciousness of new attitudes and habits. It is a discovery which makes whole all scientific discoveries, and renders them available, not for our undoing, but for human use in promoting our constructive growth and happiness.

No one would deny that we ourselves enter as an agency into whatever is attempted and done by us. That is a truism. But the hardest thing to attend to is that which is closest to ourselves, that which is most constant and familiar. And this closest "something" is, precisely, ourselves, our own habits and ways of doing things as agencies in conditioning what is tried or done by us. Through modern science we have mastered to a wonderful extent the use of things as tools for accomplishing results upon and through other things. The result is all but a universal state of confusion, discontent and strife. The one factor which is the primary tool in the use of all these other tools, namely ourselves, in other words, our own psycho-physical disposition, as the basic condition of our employment of all agencies and energies, has not even been studied as the central instrumentality. Is it not highly probable that this failure gives the explanation of why it is that in mastering physical forces we have ourselves been so largely mastered by them, until we find ourselves incompetent to direct the history and destiny of man?

Never before, I think, has there been such an acute consciousness of the failure of all external remedies as exists to-day, of the failure of all remedies and forces external to the individual man. It is, however, one thing to teach the need of a return to the individual man as the ultimate agency in whatever mankind and society collectively can accomplish, to point out the necessity of straightening out this ultimate condition of whatever humanity in mass can attain. It is another thing to discover the concrete procedure by which this greatest of all tasks can be executed. And this indispensable thing is exactly what Mr. Alexander has accomplished. The discovery could not have been made and the method of procedure perfected except by dealing with adults who were badly co-ordinated. But the method is not one of remedy; it is one of constructive education. Its proper field of application is with the young, with the growing generation, in order that they may come to possess as early as possible in life a correct standard of sensory appreciation and self-judgment. When once a reasonably adequate part of a new generation has become properly co-ordinated, we shall have assurance for the first time that men and women in the future will be able to stand on their own feet, equipped with satisfactory psycho-physical equilibrium, to meet with readiness, confidence and happiness instead of with fear, confusion and discontent, the buffetings and contingencies of their surroundings.

JOHN DEWEY.

PART I
SENSORY APPRECIATION IN ITS RELATION TO MAN'S EVOLUTIONARY DEVELOPMENT

Inadequacy of Subconscious Guidance and Control to Meet the Rapid Changes of Civilized Life

IN the interest of readers who may not be familiar with the thesis of my earlier book, *Man's Supreme Inheritance*, I wish to point out that in the arguments therein set forth it was contended that human beings cannot progress satisfactorily in civilization whilst they remain dependent upon subconscious (instinctive) guidance and control; for the reason that in civilization, that is, in a plan of life where changes of environment have occurred and continue to occur more rapidly than in the uncivilized state, man's continued dependence upon precisely this subconscious guidance and control has resulted, either directly or indirectly, in the gradual development of imperfections and defects in the use of the human organism.

The effect of these rapid changes upon a creature, who heretofore had experienced only slow and gradual changes of environment and was still subconsciously guided and controlled, could hardly fail to be harmful, inasmuch as many of his instincts,[2] in consequence of these changes, came to survive their usefulness, whilst many of those new instincts which were developed during his *quick* attempts to meet the new demands of civilization proved to be unreliable. This degree of unreliability increased as time went on, until an observant minority became aware of a gradual but most serious deterioration, a deterioration, however, which unfortunately they recognized as a physical deterioration only, and which, at what must be considered a psychological moment in human development, they attempted to set right by the adoption of "physical exercises."

For all who are concerned with the urgency of present-day problems the point of interest in the foregoing lies in the fact that man has been and still is unable to adapt himself quickly enough to the increasingly

[2]The word "instinct" is used in this work to indicate established habits, inherited or developed. As I wrote in *Man's Supreme Inheritance* (Chapter VI): "I define instinct as the result of the accumulated subconscious experiences of man at all stages of his development, which continue with us until, singly or collectively, we reach the stage of conscious control."

rapid changes involved in that plan of life which we call civilization. It will be generally conceded, I think, that the results of man's attempts to adapt himself to this plan of life, as they are manifested to-day in the general make-up of the organism of the human creature and in the application of this organism to all the activities of life, are unsatisfactory and most disappointing. It is only necessary to read the daily papers and note the records of crime, of unbalanced human thought and activity in all spheres, of the "trial-and-error" methods of our leaders in their efforts at reform in politics, social conditions, industry, religion and education, in order to be firmly convinced of the comparative failure of our plan of life, and of the shortcomings of the different institutions which are part and parcel of it.

In order, then, to arrive at correct conclusions concerning man's comparative failure to adapt himself satisfactorily to the changing conditions of civilization, it will be necessary to make an examination and comparison of the evolutionary processes which obtained in the savage state and those which are operative in the civilized state to-day.

At this juncture I wish to make clear the sense in which I use the word *psycho-physical.* The term *psycho-physical* is used both here and throughout my works to indicate the impossibility of separating "physical" and "mental" operations in our conception of the working of the human organism. As I wrote in *Man's Supreme Inheritance*, "In my opinion the two must be considered entirely interdependent, and even more closely knit than is implied by such a phrase." Hence I use the term *psycho-physical activity* to indicate all human manifestations, and *psycho-physical mechanism* to indicate the instrument which makes these manifestations possible.

Psycho-physical activity must not, however, always be considered as involving equal action and reaction of the processes concerned, for, as I hope to shew, the history of the stages of man's development reveals manifestations of human activity which, at certain stages, shew a preponderance on what is called the "physical" side, and at other stages a preponderance on what is called the "mental" side.

I am forced to use the words "physical" and "mental" here and throughout my argument because there are no other words at present which adequately express the manifestations of psycho-physical activity present at these various stages, not in any sense because the "physical" and the "mental" can be separated as such. I wish, therefore, to make it clear that whenever I use the word "mental," it is to be understood as representing all processes or manifestations which are generally recognized as not wholly "physical," and vice versa the word "physical" as representing all processes and manifestations which are generally recognized as not wholly "mental."

Comparison of Evolutionary Processes in the Savage and Civilized States

In the first place, it is important to remember that during the animal and savage stages of evolution[3] the processes concerned with development were processes which operated very slowly; indeed, experts assure us that it took millions of years of the evolutionary process to produce the animal, not to speak of the savage. Each later stage of development was the result of the experiences undergone by the creature in the process of satisfying the new and varying needs arising during his progress from the savage to the civilized state, and years of repetition of these experiences were probably needed to establish them as part and parcel of what is understood as instinct, for, on a subconscious plane of development, continuous repetition is essential to the establishment of instinctive accuracy.

In obedience to the fundamental law of self-preservation, the animal and the savage were forced, day by day, to make use of their mechanisms in securing the food and drink necessary to their existence and in attempting to thwart the designs of their common enemies. The evolutionary processes associated with these varying experiences, essential to the continued existence and development of the organism, ensured that comparatively desirable combination in human activity, namely, an adequate and correct use of the psycho-physical organism *as a whole*, together with an adequate use at the same time of the parts of that organism.

This meant that the creature reached the stage of his development to which we shall refer as the beginning of civilization, endowed with mechanisms functioning subconsciously in accordance with the dictates of instinct, which was the product of experiences gained at an earlier stage in connexion with the evolutionary processes we have outlined. At this earlier stage the demands made upon the creature were such that he could meet them satisfactorily by the subconscious use of the mechanisms involved, for his environment rarely changed, his needs remained practically the same, and in this comparatively static environment he would be able to meet a need satisfactorily by the slowly operating forces at his command.

But the attempts of the creature to meet the demands of the civilized state called for a higher and still higher standard in the development of his potentialities. Here his most trying problem arose from the fact that

[3]In this book the word evolution is used to indicate all processes which are involved in the quickening of the potentialities of the creature at the different stages of growth and development, and which are necessary to the success of his attempts to satisfy the varying needs of an ever-changing environment, and to reach a plane of constructive conscious control of the individual organism.

his environment continued to change at an increasingly rapid pace, and that these changes brought about a more rapid development of new needs. The response to the stimuli resulting from these new needs had to be a much quicker response than any in his previous experience, for progress in growth and development under the civilizing plan involved ever-increasing needs and called for a correspondingly increasing speed in the matter of response to stimuli.

Furthermore—and this is all-important—the demands thus made upon the psycho-physical processes, generally called mental processes, which were comparatively unused in his case, were destined to increase very rapidly, whilst the demands made upon the psycho-physical processes, generally called physical processes, which were comparatively highly developed in his case, were destined to decrease, and their spheres of activity actually to become more and more limited with the advance of time. These experiences indicate that in order to meet satisfactorily the new demands of civilization, *it was essential that man should acquire a new way of directing and controlling the mechanisms of the psycho-physical organism as a whole*, mechanisms which in the savage state had been kept up, of necessity, to a high standard of co-ordination by their use in securing the creature's daily food and in meeting the great "physical" demands of this mode of life. This serves to indicate that at some period of his evolutionary progress the human creature must have reached a psychological moment to pass from the subconscious to the conscious plane of control.

The change from a subconscious to a conscious plane of control would have involved a knowledge on man's part of the *means whereby* he would be able to command a conscious, reasoning direction and control of his psycho-physical mechanisms in all activity. With this knowledge the human creature would have had some chance of meeting satisfactorily the increasing demands of his ever-changing environment, and of commanding a continuous growth and development of the organism itself, that marvellous psycho-physical instrument which holds within itself the potentialities for the satisfying of such demands.

Unfortunately, the process of reasoning out the "means-whereby" in connexion with the gaining of his "ends"[4] was not and evidently could not have been adequately established as a habit in the human creature

[4] I judge from the numerous queries received from readers of *Man's Supreme Inheritance* that many people are not quite clear as to what is meant by the expressions "means-whereby" and "end-gaining." In the endeavour to make my meaning clear, I would point out that whenever a person sets out to achieve a particular "end" (whether this "end" is the development of potentialities or the eradication of defects, peculiarities or misuse) his procedure will be based on one of two principles which I have called the "end-gaining" and the "means-whereby" principles.

at this psychological moment in his development, else a consideration of the "means-whereby" of his development under savage conditions would have led him to a due consideration of these "means-whereby" in their relation to satisfactory development under civilized conditions, and he would then have realized that the demands made upon him in the civilized state must necessarily be different in many ways from those made upon him in a savage state.

Hence, whilst it was desirable that the change from the subconscious to the conscious plane of control should have taken place, it is evident that man had not reached that advanced stage of evolution which would have made it possible for him to effect it, for experience shews that although, with the advance of civilization, conditions have continually changed and become more and more complex, man's fundamental psycho-physical method of adapting himself to these changing conditions has remained the same, with the unsatisfactory and disappointing results to which I have referred.

Complexity and Complications of Civilized Life

People attempt to account for the difficulties of civilized life by saying, "Life is so complex!" This means that though they are conscious of the presence of an undue stress and strain, they are prepared for the most part to accept the position, and consequently live on with the conviction that a growing complexity is the natural result of civilized life. What they fail to recognize is that this condition is the result of their own or others' ill-considered, end-gaining attempts to surmount the difficulties encountered during the progress of civilization. This serves to shew how the egotism of the average human being is developed out of all proportion to the degree of successful endeavour that he can legitimately claim for himself. This fact, however, rarely seems to reach his

---

The "end-gaining" principle involves a direct procedure on the part of the person endeavouring to gain the desired "end." This direct procedure is associated with dependence upon subconscious guidance and control, leading, in cases where a condition of mal-co-ordination is present, to an unsatisfactory use of the mechanisms and to an increase in the defects and peculiarities already existing.

The "means-whereby" principle, on the other hand, involves a reasoning consideration of the causes of the conditions present, and an indirect instead of a direct procedure on the part of the person endeavouring to gain the desired "end." This indirect procedure is that psycho-physical activity, associated with constructive conscious guidance and control and with the consequent satisfactory use of the mechanisms, which establishes the conditions essential to the increasing development of potentialities. Under these conditions defects, peculiarities and misuse are not likely to be present within the organism.

In this connexion I wish it to be understood that throughout this book I use the term conscious guidance and control to indicate, primarily, a plane to be reached rather than a method of reaching it.

sphere of consciousness, and hence the improbability of his awakening to his own individual shortcomings, an awakening which would lead him to attempt to reach that desirable stage of consciousness and reasoning where he would have the conviction borne in upon him that

> The fault, dear Brutus, is not in our stars,
> But in ourselves,

not in the complexity of the civilizing plan, but in our unreasoning attitude towards its demands, an attitude associated with a continued dependence upon subconscious guidance and direction in our "end-gaining" attempts to meet these demands.

The prevailing condition of stress and strain caused by these attempts is harmful to the organism as a whole, and if it continues to increase as rapidly as in the past, it is likely so to undermine our reserve forces that the most serious forms of organic derangement and kinæsthetic perversion may be predicted. Indeed, we might say that a dangerous stage of perversion and delusion has already been reached, when the attempts at solution of all the problems of life seem to call for complexity rather than simplicity in procedure. We even reach a stage when the most simple "means-whereby" in accomplishment become the most difficult. A very interesting instance in this connexion occurred in my teaching experience. A well-known man of scientific attainments had great difficulty for some days with a simple, practical problem of psycho-mechanics concerned with his re-education. When he came to his lesson one morning he said: "I know now what is the matter with us all. This work of yours is too simple for us!"

In fact, the complexity needlessly introduced into the act of living in general is equalled only by the complexity which we build up individually in our attempts at accomplishment in specific spheres, as, for instance, in the sphere of education (taking this word in its widest sense, whether in learning something or in learning to do something), and also in any process of self-instruction. All acts concerned with learning something or learning to do something call for psycho-physical activity, and the standard of efficiency in these spheres depends in every case upon the standard of the creature's satisfactory employment of his psycho-physical self in the performance of these acts. The imperfectly co-ordinated[5] child or adult, for instance, will not be likely to reach the

[5]The word *co-ordination* is ordinarily used at the present time in as narrow and limited a sense as the words relaxation, readjustment, re-education, etc. In view of this fact, I consider it necessary to give some idea of the more comprehensive sense in which it is used in this work.

I use the word co-ordination, both in its conception and in its application, to convey the idea of co-ordination *on a general and not a specific basis*. Specific co-ordination of any

standard of effective functioning enjoyed by the satisfactorily co-ordinated child or adult. The former will experience difficulties with which the latter will not be beset.

In the case of the imperfectly co-ordinated child or adult, there may be said to be serious complications in his psycho-mechanics; in other words, the mechanical working of the structures of the organism is out of order, and complications and difficulties, therefore, are inevitable. On the other hand, in the case of the satisfactorily co-ordinated child or adult, the mechanical working of the structures of the organism is not complicated but complex, in the sense that, although there are present a large number of factors or means which are related to one another (like the different parts in the mechanism of a motor car), the act of using them (like the act of driving a car or any other machine in running order) is one and simple. Satisfactory psycho-physical activity depends upon psycho-mechanical structures which are complex, but of which the mechanical working does not become complicated until the mechanisms get out of order.

Take, for instance, the simple act of learning to write. In the case of the average badly co-ordinated pupil, there will be present certain impeding factors (into the detail of which we will enter later on) on account of which learning to write becomes a comparatively complicated proceeding. However expert the teacher may be, the pupil does not possess the psycho-physical equipment which would enable him to take adequate advantage of the instructions given to him. His first attempt to carry these out will reveal defects, and the subsequent attempts new defects. Each request from his teacher to do something, and each injunction not to do something else, means a building-up of a series of specific psycho-physical acts towards the given "end," namely, learning to write. This means that although the "end" may be gained, the result *as a whole* will not be as satisfactory as it might be, for nothing will have been done in the way of re-education on a general basis to correct the mal-co-ordinated conditions connected with the use and

---

specific part of the organism, such as the muscles of the arm or leg, may be brought about by means of a direct process, during which process, however, new defects in the use of the organism in general will certainly be cultivated, whilst others already present will become more pronounced. These harmful conditions will not be cultivated if the specific co-ordination is brought about by means of an indirect process involving, primarily, the general co-ordination of the psycho-physical organism, that is to say, an integrated condition in which all the factors continue to make for satisfactory psycho-mechanical use.

This distinction between the specific and the general applies also to the terms readjustment, re-education, and relaxation as I use them in this book, for in general re-education specific defects are eradicated in process.

control of the mechanisms when employed in the act of writing. In the endeavour to overcome the impeding factors concerned, the teacher builds up for the pupil a complicated procedure in order to gain the specific "end." For the act of writing demands correct direction and control in the use of the fingers, wrist and arm, and the standard of success reached in these particulars depends upon the co-ordinated use of the mechanisms *in general.*[6]

Co-ordinated use of the organism means that there is satisfactory control of a complex mechanism. In a reasoned plan of life, the human creature would be in the enjoyment of a coordinated use of the whole organism and, comparatively speaking, there would not be any impeding factors, such as we have indicated, to be overcome. The pupil would have at command a satisfactory psycho-mechanical organism, that is, he would possess the psycho-physical equipment necessary for the ready assimilation of the teacher's instructions, and, if these instructions were correct, their assimilation would enable the pupil to reason out the "means-whereby" to the desired "end," which would then be gained in that simple and easy manner characteristic of all successful accomplishment.

Recognition and Satisfaction of Essential Needs in Relation to Evolutionary Progress

In the foregoing I have attempted to indicate the urgency of the problems concerned with the evolutionary progress of the human creature—an urgency which will be generally conceded—and a consideration of the psycho-physical "means-whereby" of such progress may be helpful at this point.

Satisfactory evolutionary progress demands a continuous advancement, in individual psycho-physical activity, from stage to stage of cultivation and development. The primary desire or need in this connexion is that individual desire or need which is the stimulus to the development of those psycho-physical potentialities which enable the creature to meet satisfactorily the demands of the processes essential to the satisfaction of the need. *The adequate development of these potentialities connotes a satisfactory standard of the co-ordinated use of the organism.*

---

[6]As I wrote in *Man's Supreme Inheritance* in connexion with drawing: "Any attentive and thoughtful observer who will watch the movement and position of these children's fingers, hand, wrist, arm, neck and body generally, during the varying attempts to draw straight or crooked lines, cannot fail to note the lack of co-ordination between these parts. The fingers are probably attempting to perform the duties of the arm, the shoulders are humped, the head twisted on one side. In short, energies are being projected to parts of the mechanism which have little or no influence on the performance of the desired act of drawing, and the mere waste projection of such energies alone is almost sufficient to nullify the purpose in view."

It is obvious that a person who is satisfied with his present position on the evolutionary plane, with his present ideas, opinions, ways of life, etc., will not have the desire or feel the need for changing conditions which, consciously or subconsciously, he deems to be satisfactory. All advancement, however, is associated with the discovery and acceptance of ideas, principles, ways of living, etc., which are new to the individual. Anyone who has established a desire to live on, influenced only by past psycho-physical experiences, and who refuses to seek consciously for and to acquire new experiences, cannot expect any real advancement on the evolutionary plane.

In such a case there are present impeding factors, such as a narrow outlook, a condition of rigidity, an undue dread of psycho-physical changes, a lack of reasoning in the sphere of guidance and control, etc., all of which tend to prevent the subject from conceiving of or seeing or accepting anything outside his present experiences, these experiences being the sum total of the experiences which he has inherited (represented by his race instincts) plus his comparatively limited individual experience in every-day life.

The establishment of psycho-physical conditions here indicated means that a number of perversions have been built up subconsciously in the human creature's use of himself in every-day activity, and, as a result, many individuals, sooner or later, become aware of the presence of some shortcoming. It is probable that only one in twenty of such shortcomings ever reaches the sphere of consciousness, and so he continues to exist within a danger zone of psycho-physical shortcomings of which he is not conscious, but which impede his progress at every turn.

Mind-Wandering Recognized as a Shortcoming—Its Relation to Self-Preservation

The shortcoming to which the individual will awaken will be one which interferes with his immediate activities outside himself, in reading, for instance, or when he is attempting to learn something, or to learn to do something, and, as a matter of fact, the shortcoming that has been recognized as interfering more than any other in this connexion is the shortcoming concerned with his inability, as he would put it, to "keep his mind" on the particular work with which he is immediately engaged; in other words, the shortcoming which is commonly known as "mind-wandering."

Now, what is "mind-wandering"? In the attempt to answer this query, we will begin with a consideration of the psycho-physical processes concerned with direction and control within the human creature in the all-important sphere of self-preservation.

In the beginning of things all growth and development must surely have resulted from a form of consciousness[7] of need. For the growth and development of the creature is and always has been associated with new experiences which involve new activities. These activities—the response to some stimulus or stimuli—result from the consciousness of some need or needs within or without the organism, the presence and recognition of need being essential to the evolutionary process.

The recognition of a need denotes a state of consciousness of a need, and the primary activity (or activities) which is the response to this consciousness of a need or needs involves new experiences in the spheres of direction and control. The process of evolution depends upon the continuous repetition of such primary experiences, or group of experiences, this repetition resulting in the establishment of a use (or what is termed habit or instinct) and in the satisfaction of the need or needs.

In connexion with the theory of conscious activity in the early stages of the creature's development, we should recall the time when a pair of eyes, for instance, became a need. It is quite conceivable that after the consciousness of this need had arisen, the growth and development of the organs of sight may have occupied a thousand or more years. It is also conceivable that when the eyes had become developed, it may have needed a conscious effort, perhaps of years, to open the eyelids[8] and likewise to close them, and that the repetition of this conscious effort, week by week, month by month and year by year, may have caused this function of the eyelids to become habitual and subconscious, and to develop to that wonderful standard of use now enjoyed by the creature.

There can be little doubt that self-preservation (taking the word in its broadest sense) was the most fundamental of the creature's needs, for, first and foremost, the creature itself needed protection and preservation during its attempts to satisfy its specific needs.

This need for self-preservation called for that satisfactory direction and control with which, in this sphere, we find wild animals and savages equipped, inasmuch as, owing to the particular circumstances which obtained in their case, the response to any stimulus arising from a need would be satisfactory in the spheres of direction and control, that is, it would be a response which would enable the creature to employ what would be for him the most satisfactory "means-whereby" to securing the essential "end," self-preservation.

---

[7]Many readers may not agree with me on this point, but it will be seen that all that is necessary to my argument is a recognition of the place of need, the requirement of a new way of linking up with environment, so that the rest of my argument is not affected by belief or disbelief on this point.

[8]I am quite aware, of course, that sensitiveness to light, likewise the eyes, developed long before there were any eyelids.

Most of us are aware of the marvellous accuracy in the use of the organism manifested by the wild animal or the savage in the various familiar spheres of activity concerned with self-preservation. The civilized creature does not manifest anything like the same standard of accuracy in the employment of the organism in the spheres of activity concerned with self-preservation. In other words, the civilized human being does not enjoy the same standard of effective direction and control as the savage and the wild animal, and it is the lack of this adequate standard in the human creature which manifests itself as a shortcoming in some spheres of activity, and, as I have said, in the sphere of learning something and learning to do something, the shortcoming most frequently recognized is that known as "mind-wandering."

Now there exists a close connexion between the shortcoming which is recognized as "mind-wandering" and the shortcoming which manifests itself as a seriously weakened response to a stimulus to an act (or acts) of self-preservation. To make this connexion clear, we have only to consider the psycho-physical processes involved in these two shortcomings to realize that in both cases these processes are the same.

For the lack underlying these two shortcomings is the lack of an adequate standard of direction and control in the human creature, manifesting itself, in the one case, in the broad sphere of self-preservation and, in the other, in the specific sphere of learning something or learning to do something.

An act of self-preservation is the response to a stimulus (or stimuli) resulting from a fundamental need, and a satisfactory response depends upon the satisfactory direction and control of the psycho-physical mechanisms which are engaged in the act or acts of self-preservation.

An attempt to learn something or to learn to do something is the natural response to a stimulus (or stimuli) resulting from a wish or need to learn something or to learn to do something, and a satisfactory response depends upon the satisfactory direction and control of the psycho-physical mechanisms which are engaged in the acts of learning or learning to do something.

It will thus be seen that the processes involved in the acts concerned with self-preservation, or with learning or learning to do something, are precisely the same, and it follows that, if in the sphere of self-preservation the direction and control are unsatisfactory, the response to the stimuli concerned with the needs of self-preservation will be unsatisfactory; and, by the same rule, if in the sphere of learning and learning to do, the direction and control are unsatisfactory, the response to the stimuli concerned with the wish or needs in connexion with the acts of attempting to learn something or of learning to do something will likewise be unsatisfactory, and this unsatisfactory response is manifested in every-day life in that shortcoming, so common in our time, called "mind-wandering."

We have now reached the point where we must consider the origin of the conception which led to our giving to this particular manifestation the name of "mind-wandering."

A person decides to learn something or to learn to do something. The conception involved in this decision immediately starts a series of activities of the psycho-physical mechanisms involved, those concerned with direction and control being of vital importance to a satisfactory result, which, in this instance, is the ability to learn something or to learn to do something.

Where a person succeeds in this connexion, he is not likely to become conscious of such a shortcoming as "mind-wandering," for the success of his attempt means that his conception of the act to be performed involves the employment of satisfactory *means whereby* he will be able to gain his desired "end." In such a case, the activities of the psycho-physical mechanisms involved in his attempt will be the result of satisfactory direction and control.

On the other hand, where a person does not succeed in his attempt to learn something or to learn to do something, the failure of his attempt means that there are defects in his conception of the act to be performed, in the sense that this conception does not involve the employment of satisfactory *means whereby* he will be able to gain his desired "end." In such a case, the activities of the psycho-physical mechanisms involved in his attempts will be the result of unsatisfactory direction and control, resulting in a *misdirected* use of the psycho-physical mechanisms, and hence his inability to keep them operating on the satisfactory *means whereby* he will be able to gain his desired "end." The whole procedure is an attempt to communicate with points of vantage along lines of communication which are unreliable, resulting in a shortcoming which reaches the consciousness of the ordinary person as an inability to attend to, or, as we say, to "keep the mind upon" the work in hand; and hence it is called "mind-wandering."

As a matter of fact, the defective use of the mechanisms which is responsible for such conditions cannot be adequately described as "mind-wandering," seeing that it is the manifestation of a harmful and misdirected action and reaction, not only in connexion with those processes commonly spoken of as "mind," but *throughout the whole psycho-physical organism.* It is the manifestation of that imperfectly co-ordinated condition which is associated with an unreliable sense of feeling (sensory appreciation) concerned with unsatisfactory direction and control, and which, in the course of its development, has gradually weakened the response of the human creature to stimuli in the sphere of self-preservation.

In this connexion it is important to remember that the savage creature depended chiefly upon the sense of feeling in the spheres of direction and control, and, as his sense of feeling (sensory appreciation) was comparatively reliable, the activities thus directed and controlled would be associated with an *increasing* response to the stimulus for self-preservation.

The civilized creature also depends chiefly upon the sense of feeling in the spheres of direction and control, but as the sense of feeling (sensory appreciation) in his case has now become harmfully unreliable, the activities thus directed and controlled are becoming more and more associated with a *weakening* response to the stimulus to self-preservation.

This all points to a general weakening in the psycho-physical directing and controlling forces of the human creature,[9] a weakening which has been brought about by the fact that man has continued to depend upon subconscious guidance in his endeavours to meet the demands of the civilizing plan, and to rely upon instincts which have survived their usefulness and upon the harmful guidance of defective sense registers (feeling).

Experience follows experience in the human creature's activities, some of these experiences satisfactory, but the majority unsatisfactory, and the creature may be satisfied for the moment, only to be again dissatisfied, however, with the varying results of attempted accomplishment; and the psycho-physical experiences involved do not make for confidence in regard to any attempts which he may be forced to make in the future to meet the demands of civilization.

When conditions such as these are present in the human creature, success is hardly possible; indeed, failure will be almost certain to result, even though he may devote to the accomplishment of his aims the time deemed necessary to ensure success. The natural result of his experiences of failure or comparative failure is that in time he will come to

[9]The fact that an individual happens to exhibit satisfactory specific direction and control in some particular activity does not confute this statement; indeed, only serves to strengthen it, as I shall endeavour to shew throughout the pages of this book.

In this connexion I have found in my professional work that too often a person will consider a psycho-physical experience to be quite satisfactory, when I, as an expert, know it to be in reality unsatisfactory. In such a case, the supposedly satisfactory experience is a delusive and harmful experience, on the part of the person concerned, of feeling and thinking he is right when he is actually wrong. In fact, the experience is really an unsatisfactory one, but he does not know it; and so, when later he becomes dissatisfied, he does not attribute his dissatisfaction to his own psycho-physical experiences, but to other people, surroundings, "something wrong somewhere," always believing the cause to be without instead of within the organism.

give consideration to the cause or causes involved in these experiences, and this consideration is of special interest to us, because it practically always leads him to the same conclusion, namely, that his failure is due to "mind-wandering."

Let us now follow out his consideration of the facts in detail. He sets out to learn something or to learn to do something and proceeds, as he would put it, to "give his mind to" his work, in accordance with his conception of this phrase. But he soon discovers that his "mind" is not "on his work," that it has become more occupied, as it were, with some other trend of thought. He therefore proceeds to make a special effort, as he would say, to "keep his mind on" the original task in hand.

Now it is highly probable that he has never given consideration to the "means-whereby" required for such a special effort, for if he had, he would probably have awakened to the fact that he did not have within his control the *means whereby* a special effort of this kind could prove satisfactory. However this may be, the fact remains that in spite of all his efforts to "keep his mind on" what he is doing, the process he thinks of as "mind-wandering" is repeated, with the result that after a certain number of repetitions of this experience, he becomes convinced that the cause of his failure is his *inability* to "keep his mind on" what he is doing.

Just think of the psycho-physical disaster that is here indicated, for it means that the human creature has reached that dangerous stage in connexion with the employment of his psycho-physical mechanisms when the response to a stimulus arising from a need is ineffective, erratic and produces a state of confusion.

The seriousness of this inability of the human creature to "keep his mind on" what he is doing is widely recognized, and this recognition has led to the almost universal adoption of what is called concentration[10] as the cure for "mind-wandering." Unfortunately, this remedy, as

[10]It is of interest to remember that the recognition of the defect called "mind-wandering" long antedated the conception of concentration as a remedy. I must refer my readers to the chapter on concentration for a fuller discussion of this important question. For the moment I wish merely to point out that I am not here objecting to concentration in the sense which implies a number of things going on, moving at the same time and converging on a common consequence, a form of concentration which is present in the processes involved in the psycho-physical manifestations of the normal child at play and of the competent artisan or artist engrossed in his work, and *which simply implies a condition of co-ordination.* On the other hand, the form of concentration to which I am objecting is that which implies fixating on one thing, "bringing the mind to bear" on one object, for just the same reason that I object to that conception in education which seems to justify people in considering the essential aim of educational procedure to be the securing of "ends" by *specific* methods ("end-gaining"), irrespective of the *means whereby* the psycho-physical mechanisms are employed *in general* during the attempts to gain these "ends."

I shall shew later, is in itself a most harmful and delusive psycho-physical manifestation, and has been adopted without any consideration being taken of its effect upon the organism in general or of the psycho-physical processes involved in what is called "learning to concentrate."

Consideration of the Mechanism of the Human Psycho-Physical Organism in Relation to the Activities called Learning and Learning To Do

The foregoing will serve to indicate that in the sphere of learning something or learning to do something (as indeed, in connexion with all psycho-physical acts) there is an important problem to be solved if we are to progress to that standard of psycho-physical functioning and use which will enable us to meet satisfactorily the ever-increasing demands of an advancing civilization. Since, as we have seen, the standard of functioning in the performance of any psycho-physical act depends upon the conception which influences the direction and control of the mechanisms involved, it is most essential to give consideration to this all-important matter of conception, in connexion, with the understanding of what we wish to learn or learn to do, and also in connexion with that psycho-physical activity by means of which we are enabled to arrive at our conceptions concerned with learning and learning to do.

We will therefore go on to consider the mechanisms of the psycho-physical organism in relation to the activity called learning something.

First, for every form of psycho-physical activity there must be a stimulus. In considering the response to this stimulus, I would remind my readers that I do not separate "mental" and "physical" operations (manifestations) in my conception of the manner ("means-whereby") of the functioning of the human organism. For how can we prove that the response to any stimulus is wholly "physical" or wholly "mental"?

On the one hand, in what would ordinarily be considered purely physical spheres (the performance of "physical" acts), the standard of functioning depends

(1) *upon the degree of correctness of the conception of the act to be performed,* and

(2) *upon the degree of co-ordinated employment of the guiding and controlling orders or directions, and of the mechanisms involved in carrying out the activities essential to the correct means whereby the act can be performed.*

On the other hand, in what would ordinarily be considered purely mental spheres, the standard of functioning depends

(1) *upon the degree of reliability of the sensory guidance and direction in the use of the mechanisms involved in conveying the stimuli primarily responsible for the psycho-physical processes concerned with conception,* and

(2) *upon the standard of co-ordination reached in the use of the whole organism.*

If the highest standard of so-called physical functioning is to be reached, there must be *co-ordinated employment of the muscular system through co-ordinated guidance, direction and control by processes so-called mental, involving action and reaction in psycho-physical unity* and an adequate standard at all times of the vital functioning of the organism.

In the same way, as I am prepared to demonstrate later, if the highest standard of so-called mental functioning is to be reached, there must be *co-ordinated employment of those processes which are involved in the coordinated use of the so-called physical self, involving action and reaction in psycho-physical unity* and an adequate standard at all times of the vital functioning of the organism.[11]

It is clear, therefore, that no human activity can be said to be wholly "physical" or wholly "mental," but that all human activity, in whatever sphere, is psycho-physical activity, *the standard of individual functioning, both mental and physical so-called, being determined by the standard of co-ordinated use of the organism in general, the standard of this co-ordinated use being determined in its turn by the standard of co-ordinated employment of the psycho-physical processes concerned.*

Now psycho-physical activity is simply the response to some stimulus (or stimuli) received through the channel of the senses, of hearing, for instance, of sight, touch, feeling, etc., and the nature of the resulting conception and of the response, or psycho-physical reaction, will be determined by the standard of psycho-physical functioning present.

It then follows that *the process of conception, like all other forms of psycho-physical activity, is a process the course of which is determined by our psycho-physical condition at the time when the particular stimulus (or stimuli) is received.* We all know that a man's conception of his present or future financial or other condition in life is quite different when he is, as we say, in a good and happy "frame of mind," from what it is when he has a "grouch." Again, the conception as to the outcome of a disaster or piece of good fortune in life will be quite different in the case of a man in enjoyment of good health from that of a man weakened by bad health.[12]

---

[11]We are all aware, for instance, that a sluggish liver does not make for the best use of the "mental" powers, and we know of people who, through bad habits of over-indulgence, have reached a stage of liver or kidney disorder when their reasoning processes have become seriously impaired and those of remembering practically ruined. If the vital functioning of the "physical" mechanisms and organs is for any reason inadequate, the organism, as a whole, becomes gradually more or less poisoned, with resulting gradual interference with the processes of remembering.

[12]The latter may usually be classed as a pessimist and the former as an optimist.

Influence of Sensory Appreciation Upon Conception in All Psycho-Physical Activity

This dependence of the process of conception upon the general psycho-physical condition is a factor of paramount importance. For if, as we contend, all so-called mental processes are mainly the result of sensory experiences in psycho-physical action and reaction, it will be obvious that in our conception of *how* to employ the different parts of the mechanism in the acts of every-day life *we are influenced chiefly by sensory processes* (feeling). Thus we may receive a stimulus through something we hear, something we touch, or through some other outside agency; in every case, the nature of our response, *whether it be an actual movement, an emotion or an opinion*, will depend upon the associated activity, in action and reaction, of the processes concerned with conception and with the sensory and other mechanisms responsible for the "feeling" which we experience. This associated activity is referred to throughout my work as *sensory appreciation.*

Sensory Appreciation

This sensory appreciation is the factor upon which the baby, like the animal, depends for guidance in his first subconscious attempts to use the different parts of the mechanism, the success of these attempts depending upon the degree of reliability of the child's sensory appreciation, and I assert that wherever we find defects, peculiarities, etc., in children at a very early age, even in their first attempts at crawling, standing, walking, etc., these defects are present because the instinctive processes of such children are unreliable. It is my purpose throughout this book to attempt to prove the truth of this contention, which is based on the results of a teaching experience of very many years; also to shew that we must be prepared, in cases where the instinctive processes are unreliable, to restore the sensory appreciation to that standard of reliability upon which the adequacy of the functioning of all psycho-physical processes depends.

A comprehensive understanding of sensory appreciation, of its enormous influence for good and evil in the development of the creature, and of its future bearing upon the progress of mankind, is therefore of the greatest importance to all, but especially to those interested in education, both in the sense of education in our schools and in the broadest sense of the word.

Sensory appreciation, from our point of view, has a much wider significance than is generally attributed to it. But it will be sufficient at this point to state that, taken even in the most limited sense, it includes all sensory experiences which are conveyed through the channels of sight, hearing, touch, feeling, equilibrium, movement, etc., and which are responsible for psycho-physical action and reaction throughout the organism.

If we raise an arm, move a leg, or if we make any other movements of the body or limbs, we are guided chiefly by our sensory appreciation or, as most people would put it, by our sense of feeling. This applies to the testing of the texture of a piece of cloth between one's fingers, or to the gauging of size, weight or distance, etc., in fact, to the employment of the "physical" mechanisms in the processes of hearing, seeing, walking, talking, and in all the other activities of life.

The Human and the Inanimate Machine Compared and Contrasted

The function of sensory appreciation will be clear to us if we stop for a moment and consider the human organism as an animate machine, and compare its mechanical processes with those of an inanimate machine. The reliability of both machines is dependent upon the standard of reliability of their controlling, propelling, motor and other mechanisms, the controlling factor taking first place as causing the other mechanical factors to work co-ordinately and to give the best results in practical use.

But the all-important difference from our standpoint between the animate and the inanimate machine lies in the quality and function of their respective controlling mechanisms. In the inanimate machine, the controlling mechanism is limited by the fixed nature of its own make-up, and by certain fixed conditions in the other mechanisms without which it cannot operate. In the animate machine, or human psycho-physical organism, the controlling mechanism is a wonderful psycho-physical process by means of which an almost unlimited use of the different units which make up the whole may be brought about, so that at one moment a correct use and at another an incorrect use may be commanded.

This psycho-physical process is that essential factor in satisfactory human development which we call sensory appreciation. When functioning adequately, this sensory appreciation has a wide field of operation, and our ability to reach the maximum of our potentialities depends upon the standard of its reliability. This being so, it will be obvious to the most casual observer that, if we are to continue to develop satisfactorily, our sensory appreciation of the working of the mechanisms concerned with the movements of our bodies and limbs in the activities of life must be reliable.

Unreliable Sensory Appreciation a Universal Defect

Unfortunately, we can prove by practical demonstration upon any person, adult or child, that the sensory appreciation of the people of our time is more or less unreliable and in the great majority of cases positively delusive.

Readers of *Man's Supreme Inheritance* will probably be convinced on this point without demonstration. If they are not, and will take the trouble, with the help of some friend, to make tests on themselves in the light of the facts given, they will assuredly be convinced.

> Take the case of a person who persists in putting his head back whenever he makes an attempt to put his shoulders back. Ask him to put his head forward and keep his shoulders still, and it will be found that, as a rule, even though he may put his head forward as asked, he moves his shoulders also. Ask him to put his head forward whilst the teacher holds his shoulders still, and the pupil, as a rule, will put his head back instead of forward. In practically every instance, be the pupil adult or child, the attempt to carry out this simple request will be unsatisfactory, owing to the pupil's harmful interference with the general adjustment and use of the organism and limbs, due to unreliable sensory appreciation.
>
> Similarly, if a pupil is asked to turn his toes out, it is my experience that, instead of taking the weight of his body on his heels in order to lift the front part of the feet to turn them out, he will, as a rule, throw the weight on to the balls of the feet and still attempt to lift the front part, or else he will move his heels in towards one another instead of turning out the toes. Point out one or other of these errors to the pupil, and he, as if aware of the delusive sensory appreciation which is responsible for these errors, at once looks down at his feet in order to try to see how to move them correctly.
>
> Again, there are very few persons who, when asked to do such a simple thing as open the mouth, will not throw the head back, with the idea, as it were, of lifting the upper jaw away from the lower. This serves to shew that they have not given any consideration to the psycho-physical use of the muscular and other mechanisms concerned with this act. If they had, they would have realized that there are subconscious processes continuously operative which keep the mouth closed, and, consequently, the first thing to do is to cause these processes to be inoperative, and so to bring about such relaxation of the muscular tension involved as would allow the jaw to drop. It does, in fact, commonly drop in the case of that type of idiot who is most often open-mouthed; whilst it is common knowledge that if a boxer receives a blow on the head, heavy enough to throw out the controlling gear, his jaw drops of itself and frequently remains dropped for a considerable time. When I ask a pupil to allow me to move his lower jaw away from the upper, he usually increases instinctively the tension that keeps the lower jaw in place.

As I have frequently pointed out, an enormous aggregate waste of energy is involved in these constant and irrational tensions.

Many who are brought for the first time face to face with the fact that the sensory appreciation of most of the people of our time is more or less unreliable become unusually disturbed, especially when they realize that this fundamental factor in human activity has been practically ignored by our experts and leaders in educational and other spheres in their attempts to effect reforms in the civilizing plan.[13]

The truth is, we have not given sufficient consideration to this essential matter. We have merely acted on the presumption, in the usual subconscious way, that if we have a potentiality such as sensory appreciation (feeling), it must as a matter of course be reliable.

Consideration of Three Stages of Man's Development in Relation to Deterioration of Sensory Appreciation

I will now endeavour to put before the reader certain facts concerning stages in the evolution of the human creature, when psycho-physical conditions became present which made for the gradual deterioration of sensory appreciation, indicating possible causes of this deterioration in our sense of feeling and in all our other senses.[14] I shall confine this consideration of man's development to three stages:

---

[13]This is indeed a fearful fact to ask the ordinary human being to face, and when in my professional sphere I have been forced to impress it upon my pupils, I have read in their faces the different ideas, opinions and feelings evoked by my statement. Very often it has been evident that they have looked upon me almost as an enemy. For instance, I was recently discussing the point with a professional friend who at once denied that our sensory appreciation was unreliable, and asked, "Why should Nature *permit* us to go wrong in such an essential?" I agreed to answer this, if he, on his part, would first explain to me why Nature *should* prevent us from going wrong, seeing that in the process of the creature's development in civilization even the simplest fundamentals of nature have been ignored. It was clear to me that my original statement had been a shock to my friend, and that his question was more an emotional reaction to this shock than the outcome of any process of reasoning, for he admitted later that until I had brought the matter up to him, he had never given thought to this question of unreliable sensory appreciation, and yet had disagreed with one who, as he knew, had not only been considering this subject for more than thirty years, but for more than twenty-five of these had been professionally engaged in demonstrating practically to his pupils the fact of their unreliable sensory appreciation.

[14]The factors which made for the establishment of reliable sensory appreciation, and for a continuously improving standard in this connexion, have been indicated in *Man's Supreme Inheritance*. The matter concerned with the technique of ploughing may suggest the kind of human experiences responsible for that early interference with the standard of functioning and use of the psycho-physical mechanisms, which lowers the standard of reliability of sensory appreciation. See *Man's Supreme Inheritance*, chapter: "Conscious Guidance and Control in Practice."

(1) the stage when he was guided chiefly by sensory appreciation;

(2) the stage when he was developing the ability to inhibit in specific spheres, and was still, as we say, "physically fit";

(3) the stage when he had still further developed this inhibitory power in specific spheres, but had recognized a lower standard of "physical" fitness which called for a remedy.

Stage I.

Uncivilized Stage: Standard of Sensory Appreciation Reliable and Satisfactory Conditions Maintained

We are all well aware of the higher standard of sensory appreciation (associated with all the sensory experiences involved in the general psycho-physical activities essential to a healthy existence) in the uncivilized as compared with the civilized state. In the stage we are considering the satisfactory condition of the savage creature was maintained by the constant use of the mechanisms in the limited spheres of activity concerned with procuring food, drink and shelter, and with preservation of life from human and other enemies. Under such conditions, and at this stage of evolution, subconscious guidance satisfactorily met his immediate needs. He was unaware, that is, of the *means whereby* he employed his mechanisms in the simplest of every-day activities, and this unawareness did not matter at this stage.

The reason for this is not far to seek. It is that, at this early period, the standard of co-ordination and of the accompanying sensory appreciation in both sexes was comparatively high, and the needs of uncivilized existence did not call for the continual adaptation to rapid changes which civilized life demands.

In fact, the physical co-ordination and development of the savage, like that of the animal which he encountered daily, had reached at that period a fine state of excellence. For if we are justified in believing that the two-footed upright creature inherited from its predecessor on four feet a well-developed and healthy organism (and surely there can be little doubt upon this point), we may assume that it reached the human stage in a condition of health which may be described as relatively high.[15]

[15]This does not exclude the possibility of the creature's experiencing occasional aches and pains or even of suffering from specific diseases, but barring such specific troubles, the usual level was a normal one. It is significant in this connexion that primitive man always thinks of disease after the analogy of wounds from arrows, stone bruises, etc., that is, as coming in specifically from without, and the technique of the medicine man is to drive out the foreign substances that have come in; if he sweats the patient, for instance, it is to expel some foreign substance.

Since then, during a slow growth of thousands of years, this human creature had been surely and gradually building up a use and development on the so-called physical side in an environment in which changes but rarely occurred, and which, when they did occur, were comparatively slow, so that his activities would generally consist of the daily repetition of the same series of acts of which the standard of difficulty remained about the same.

But on the so-called mental side his use and development had been comparatively limited in an environment where his chief daily effort would consist of hunting down the animals, birds or fish which constituted his daily food supply, an activity for which his instinct was as sure a guide as that of his prey.

With this relatively high standard of use and development on the "physical" side and the associated development of the organism in general, his experience of ill-health must have been correspondingly small, but if he ever incurred an illness or met with an injury, there can be little doubt that he would apply as a remedy some specific herb or root which he would know to possess the curative qualities he needed.[16] This act would be a subconscious reaction to the stimulus resulting from the sense of ill-being, in exactly the same way as the act of seeking his daily food was a subconscious reaction to the stimulus resulting from the sense of hunger, and as long *as he possessed a mechanical organism which worked with mechanical accuracy, instinctive procedure served his purpose.* The "specific" cure in these circumstances was in keeping with sane and natural requirements. For just as the automatic, slowly developing, subconscious process called instinct guided him in his daily life when he was well, so, when he was ill, this same mysterious but limiting process would indicate to him the necessary and specific remedy, through the agency of the only part of his organism which was as yet highly developed, namely, his sensory appreciation, which would mean that, in this case, his senses of taste and smell would be working in co-ordination with his stomach and his digestive processes.[17]

---

[16]Thus we see that the habit of "taking something" for an ill had a very early origin. This habit led naturally to the coming of the medicine-man. For one of the first channels into which man would direct his developing intelligence would be the discovery of the means of remedying or allaying his physical ills or discomforts. This was bound, sooner or later, to produce men and women who would devote themselves exclusively to the study of such remedies and of the human ills for which the remedies were needed.

[17]Incidentally, it is interesting here to draw attention to the fact that up to this day the majority of people under similar conditions are dominated more or less by their sensory appreciation, and the practical proof that this sensory appreciation has deteriorated lies in the difficulty, known only too well to workers in the curative sphere, of persuading the patient to give up some particular food or drink which he himself knows

Thus we see that, whether he were well or whether he were ill, the subconscious guidance of instinct was reliable in the practically unchanging routine of his daily life, so that, because of its association with a reliable sensory appreciation, man would have no need of recourse to the higher directive processes.

Stage II.

Early Civilizing Stage: Development of Reasoning Inhibition and the Beginning of the End of the Dominance of Instinct as a Controlling Factor

As time went on, reasoning came more and more to illumine the creature's dull and limited existence, shewn by the fact that he began to construct rude weapons and to build primitive shelters. This reasoning process was destined to grow and develop through the myriad operations of evolutionary building involved in the new and diverse experiences concerned with his progress towards a higher plane. With every advance and with every change which he made in his environment, he began to put into practice a reasoning inhibition which enabled him, within certain well-defined limits, to master or modify for his own purposes the desires and tendencies of that sensory mechanism upon which up to that time he had depended entirely for judgment and direction.

The development and use of this reasoning process marked primitive man's differentiation from the lower animals, but it also marked—and this is even more important from the point of view of man's evolutionary history—the "beginning of the end" of the dominance of instinct as a controlling factor in human activity, so that from this period onwards man could no longer satisfactorily live and move by subconscious guidance alone.

Let us see how his newly awakened processes of reasoning would work in the new sphere. In the early stages of his emergence from the savage state, any changes which took place in his environment would be but slow and gradual, and the consequent demands upon his newly developing, higher directive processes would be correspondingly light. As civilization advanced, however, slowly at first but with increasing rapidity as time went on, man must have been placed more and more

has caused and is still causing his illness.The same thing holds good in cases where a doctor recommends some food or drink which he knows will be most beneficial to his patient, but is not pleasing to the patient's sense of taste. In nine cases out of ten, the doctor's advice will be ignored, and even where it is followed, it will probably be only because he has brought considerable pressure to bear upon his patient. This means that the patient will have allowed his reasoning processes to be dominated by his deteriorated sensory appreciation.

in new and untried situations which would inevitably demand from him an increasing use of his reasoning processes. This would be exactly the opposite of what had occurred in the earlier savage state where, as we have seen, conditions had called for a relatively higher development on the so-called physical than on the so-called mental side. It is conceivable, therefore, that the new conditions of civilization would call for a relatively rapid increase in man's use and development on the "mental" as compared with the "physical" side. There can also be little doubt that at this stage he had not become dissatisfied with the results of this changing process, and that he continued to receive from within and without more stimuli to "mental" than to "physical" activities. The further he progressed from the savage state, the more frequent would become such stimuli, and the more urgent the call on him to deal with new situations, with the result that he would be forced more and more to develop his reasoning processes, in the constant inhibition of his natural desires to meet the demands of a young and developing society and to make the necessary adjustments to the complex requirements of an advancing civilization.

Man had now arrived at the stage where he had left behind him the environment with which he was familiar and to which his limited experiences had adapted him, and as the pathway of his new experiences inevitably widened out, he was confronted with one of the greatest difficulties experienced in his evolutionary progress on a subconscious basis, namely, that of adapting himself quickly to an environment which continued to change with ever-increasing rapidity, and so continually entailed new psycho-physical experiences.

He did adapt himself, of course, to these new conditions whilst his sensory appreciation was still more or less reliable, else he could not have survived, but it was only in the same way as he had always adapted himself, that is, by trusting blindly to the subconscious guidance of instinct which had served his primitive forefathers in their particular environment. Thus early, it seems, in his civilized career, man presumed subconsciously that he was equipped in every way for any new procedure in life such as sawing, for instance, ploughing, chopping, etc., and even for occupations which, with the progress of time, entailed working more and more in cramped or difficult positions.

We may remember, however, that at this early stage a man had every justification for believing that, if he received either from without or within a stimulus to carry out some new duty, perform some new evolution or adopt some new position in the carrying out of a particular piece of work, he would be able, in all probability, to accomplish his aim with impunity. As far as we can see, nothing as yet had occurred to make him suspect that his sensory appreciation was not reliable or that his standard of coordination was not satisfactory, or that, in adapting his mechanisms to new activities in a *specific* way he might be injuring them in a *general* way, and thus be paving the way for a general deterioration. In all his activities hitherto, such as, for instance, the hunting and fighting of his savage days, he had been accustomed to rely upon the subconscious guidance of his sensory appreciation, and so it was upon this same guidance in the use of himself that he continued to rely for all the new and varied occupations of civilization.

This shews that although he had developed his reasoning processes to some extent in inventing crude weapons, implements, etc., during the early stages of his progress towards the civilized state, he did not apply these reasoning processes to the direction of his psycho-physical mechanisms in the use of himself in the various activities of every-day life. With his reasoning processes thus limited in their use, and with no consciousness as yet of any sense of physical shortcoming, it is most unlikely that man could have received even a slight, subconscious hint that his instinct would be in any way affected in the new surroundings and amidst the new experiences of civilization, or that he would ever lose a fraction of that satisfactory "physical" use and development which his race had enjoyed for countless ages, which was then his inheritance, and which he never doubted he was to hand down to his successors for all time.

Had he reasoned the matter out, he would have realized that his instinct was built up from very limited experiences, gained in the uncivilized state where growth was slow and changes rare, so that this instinct could not be expected to meet the demands of a mode of life in which growth was much more rapid and changes more frequent and unforeseen. He would also have realized that many of his instincts were being used less and less in the old way, and consequently were becoming less and less reliable. *It would then have been obvious to him that in order to meet satisfactorily the requirements of his new and changing environment, he must employ new guidance and direction, and that in order to build up this new guidance with the rapidity that his necessities demanded, he must call upon reasoning to supersede instinct (the co-worker of slow development) in the use of his psycho-physical mechanisms. In other words, he would have realized that his primitive psycho-physical equipment must pass from the subconscious to the conscious plane of guidance and direction.*

The centuries passed, bringing with them an increasing scope for the use of man's reasoning processes. Unfortunately, he continued to confine this use of his reasoning processes to the consideration of the relation of "cause and effect," "means and ends" in connexion with his activities in the outside world, both social and physical, and failed to apply this reasoning to the consideration of the relation of "cause and effect," "means and ends" in connexion with the use of his psycho-physical organism. At the same time, the use of his so-called physical mechanisms was being gradually but surely interfered with, partly owing to the change from a standard of daily use to one of comparative inactivity, but chiefly owing to the failure of his instincts to meet the demands made upon them by the activities of the new life.

The results of the failure of man's instincts to meet the new and varied demands of civilization would not manifest themselves at once. For it is reasonable to suppose that as man emerged from the savage state, his instinct was still working satisfactorily and that there was little need for curative measures on account of his comparatively high standard of health. Up till then, the so-called physical self, as being more highly developed, had been the guiding and controlling factor in human activity. It is almost beyond human power to-day to realize that the experiences of millions of years had gone to the building-up of this so-called physical development. The experiences man had gained on the so-called mental side were infinitesimal in comparison.

Henceforward this restless, inquisitive creature, endowed with wonderful potentialities and developing on the so-called mental at a far greater rate than on the so-called physical side, continued to progress in the direction of what we call civilization with ever-increasing rapidity. But his race instincts had not equipped him for such a sudden psycho-physical rush, such a tremendous overbalancing on the so-called mental side, so that he arrived at the new stage breathless, dazed, at a loss, as it were, from the lack of the graduated psycho-physical experiences which had been part and parcel of his earlier growth.[18]

[18]This indicates (1) that conscious, reasoned psycho-physical activity must replace subconscious, unreasoned activity in the processes concerned with making the changes demanded by the ever-changing environment of civilization; (2) that these changes must be made more quickly than heretofore in order to meet this demand satisfactorily; and (3) that, with the advance of time, there will be a corresponding call for quickening in this sphere of psycho-physical activity.

In short, the fundamental difficulty arises from the following facts. Uncivilized man depended upon subconscious guidance and control, and probably hundreds of years were occupied in making simple changes, for subconscious activity is very slow in its response to the stimulus of the need of change. Civilized man still depends upon subconscious guidance and control just as he did in the uncivilized state—the tragedy of civilization—but although he has remained satisfied with the form of direction and control by means of which changes have hitherto been made, it would seem that he has become dissatisfied with the time occupied with making changes. It is man's supreme civilizing blunder that he has failed to realize in practice that an adequate quickening of the response to the stimuli, arising from the need for some comparatively rapid change, calls for a corresponding quickening of the spheres of direction and control in the use of the psycho-physical mechanisms involved, such as is possible only on a plane of constructive conscious control.

Stage III.

Later Civilizing Stage: Recognition of a Serious Shortcoming Which was Called Physical Deterioration

There came at last a time in the history of man when a number of people became aware of a certain serious shortcoming, and the adoption of "physical exercises" as a remedy is proof that they recognized this shortcoming as a "*physical*" deterioration. This sense of shortcoming and of general lack of well-being was more or less to accompany mankind from that time right on through the different stages of the civilizing process.

I write "was to accompany" him advisedly, because it has done so. I also write that it should not and would not have done so if man had realized that this sense of shortcoming was the signal that he had reached a psychological moment in his career, and that the time had arrived for him to come into his great inheritance, that is, to pass from the subconscious, animal stage of his growth and development to higher and still higher stages of apprehension (conscious reasoning) in connexion with the use of his psycho-physical mechanisms.

Unfortunately, man did not recognize the real significance of this danger signal, for the fact remains that he continued the experiment of guiding himself subconsciously, even though this experiment was already proving a failure, and has since so proved itself, with signs unmistakable which "he who runs may read."

There certainly was some consideration of the position. There was this recognition of a deterioration on the so-called physical side beyond any previously recognized experience of mankind, whilst on the other there may even have been a distinct sense of gain through the increased use and development of the so-called mental processes. But the point I wish to make clear is that, where this unequal development was concerned, there had been an inadequate co-ordinating process at work, a process, in fact, the very opposite of co-ordination and one which has continued, with but few exceptions, in human beings until our own time. Indeed, from its beginnings, the process of civilizing tended to widen the scope for so-called mental and to narrow the scope for so-called physical activities, and, on a basis of subconscious guidance and control, this process meant for the time being a further development on the so-called mental side, but at the cost of an equally distinct if more gradual deterioration on the so-called physical side, with an accompanying deterioration in the standard of sensory appreciation. But it must be remembered that because of the interrelation and interdependence of the mechanisms and potentialities of the organism in the process we call human life, any deterioration on the so called physical side must, in time, seriously affect the so-called mental side. Enlargement of the spheres of so-called mental activity does not necessarily denote a growth of healthy "mental" activity.[19] This has been proved by man's experiences in civilization up to the moment, a statement borne out by the events of 1914-1919. In fact, the process of civilization has gone hand in hand with a harmful interference with those co-ordinating processes upon which the satisfactory growth of man's psycho-physical organism depends.

This being so, it follows that from the time that man entered the civilized state, human growth on this subconscious basis was bound to be uneven and unbalanced, and this unbalanced development marked the beginning of a new era in human existence. It marked the beginning of an interference with the co-ordinated use of his mechanism as a whole, and particularly with those muscular co-ordinations so essential to his "physical" well-being.

Interference with the Co-ordinated Use of the Psycho-Physical Mechanism and an Associated Lowering of the Standard of Sensory Appreciation

In the savage state instinctive guidance and control was associated with a co-ordinated use of the human mechanism, and with an accompanying reliable sense of feeling (sensory appreciation) for guidance. This old instinctive guidance, as we have seen, gradually lost its sphere of usefulness under the new conditions, and so became more or less impaired, but man continued to place upon it the same implicit reliance as in his uncivilized days. The inevitable result was an interference with the coordinated use of his psycho-physical mechanism, together with a more or less continued lowering of the standard of general functioning and of the standard of sensory appreciation, the harm being intensified by the fact that by leaving himself to blind subconscious guidance in all matters connected with the use of his psycho-physical organism, he continued to depend upon a sense of feeling which was continually deteriorating, with the result that to-day he represents perhaps the most imperfectly co-ordinated type of human creature ever known in the history of mankind.

We can readily understand how this gradual interference with the co-ordination of man's psycho-physical mechanisms would cause a number of disagreeable and alarming symptoms to manifest themselves,

[19] "Mental" growth continued even after a deterioration had been recognized in the "physical" self, and this deterioration caused, as it were, one limb of the tree to grow at such a pace that it overbalanced the tree, bent it too much in one direction, seriously disturbing the roots responsible for its equilibrium and healthy growth.

and, as a matter of fact, the deterioration of the human creature at last reached a point where the need for a remedy became exceedingly urgent. Man was now faced with a situation which was new to his experience, and which demanded from him, not only a response, but a *quick* response. The problem was complicated by the fact that the human creature on whom this urgent demand was made was already badly co-ordinated and had acquired, by reason of the rapidity with which his experiences had been gained—a rapidity hitherto unknown to the human organism—the habit of reacting in a certain confident, nay, almost reckless way to stimuli.

When, therefore, this insistent, this urgent call came upon man to find a remedy for his ills, we can easily conceive of the confusion that would of necessity accompany the first experience of the human being in making a comparatively hasty decision on a new problem of psycho-mechanics, a problem, moreover, which did not present itself to him until he had reached an advanced stage of psycho-physical mal-co-ordination. We have only to imagine such an experience repeated indefinitely, (1) the increasing sense of shortcoming, (2) the urgent S.O.S. call for a remedy, (3) the hurried haphazard response, to realize that the disturbed condition involved[20] is not conducive to the employment of the reasoning processes.

We all remember Mr. Carlyle's reaction under similar circumstances to the needs of his friend Henry Taylor; how, on hearing that his friend was ill, he became confused and rushed off with a bottle of medicine which he believed had helped Mrs. Carlyle, without any consideration of the nature of his friend's trouble, or even a knowledge of the contents of the bottle. If a man of such attainments, living in a so-called advanced civilization, acted at a psychological moment in such an unreasoning way, we cannot be surprised to find that the poor subconsciously guided human being of an earlier period, when faced with the problem of his deterioration, rushed in the same unreasoning way to find a "cure." As far as we can judge, he subconsciously adopted the form of "cure" to which instinct had prompted his ancestors in the past, without recognizing that this form of "cure" was no longer suited to the circumstances of his life owing to the ever-changing demands of civilization, and without any consideration of the effect of these changes upon his organism.

So, because in an earlier stage of evolution, the form of "cure" sought

[20]It is easy to see how, under these conditions, unreliable lines of communication can become established, with the associated unsatisfactory psycho-physical actions and reactions, such as will have that general effect upon the kinæsthesia which leads in time to the cultivation of the fixed habit or phobia, so common to-day and so erroneously called nerves or neurasthenia.

by primitive man had always been a *specific* one, instinct guiding him in the choice of the specific berry or root to alleviate some specific pain or hurt, man now followed, as far as we can judge, the example of his more lowly evolved ancestors, and dealt in a *specific* way with his trouble. Recognizing that his standard of well-being was being lowered and that his muscular development was also continuing to deteriorate, he decided that his loss of health was *due* to a deterioration in his muscular development. But he saw this deterioration as a deterioration in his muscular development alone, not as a deterioration in his general psycho-physical co-ordination and in his sensory appreciation, an interference, that is, with the general adjustment of the organism together with a misplacement of the vital organs and viscera, causing serious pressure and irritation and resulting in a number of disagreeable and alarming symptoms.[21]

Specific Remedy Chosen to Counteract a General Malcondition

Owing to the limited range of the working of his reasoning processes, he must have concluded that his general shortcomings were due to specific muscular shortcomings, and this narrow and erroneous conception led directly to the idea of muscle development by means of *specific* exercises to be performed at *specific* times for the purpose of developing *specific* muscles. It will be evident that such a process could not satisfactorily check the deterioration in *general* co-ordination, and the maladjustments and misplacements to which I have referred.

By way of illustration let us begin with what might be called the "weight-lifting conception" of a remedy. This was a crude remedy indeed,[22] and one well in keeping with the stage of evolution in which instinct had become impaired and the reasoning processes were only employed as yet in limited spheres. The era of weight-lifting exercises was superseded by the crudest form of gymnasium where most strenuous exercises were performed. These primitive mechanical exercises were succeeded by others less strenuous, and then again by an increasing number of machines which were destined to become the vogue with enthu-

[21]Unfortunately, the narrow view here indicated is still held by most of our authorities on physiology and anatomy, with results which are only too evident. It is only necessary to watch the movements of many who are experts in the subject-matter of physiology and anatomy to realize the futility of their knowledge from a practical standpoint. For the knowledge of the ordinary anatomical and physiological workings of specific muscles does not enable any person to re-educate or co-ordinate them on a general basis in the acts of every-day life, and it is on this basis of common sense and practice that the value of any knowledge or principle must be judged.

[22] In *Man's Supreme Inheritance* I have pointed out the gradual modification which has taken place in these muscle-building exercises, a modification which is still going on at the present day.

siasts for muscle building. This particular form of muscle-development passed through a number of phases, but it is evident that the results were still unsatisfactory. Whether it was that they considered that the "right" remedy had not yet been found, or that the rapidly deteriorating psycho-physical condition of man was now beyond the power of the most satisfactory muscle-building machine or method to remedy, one thing at least is certain, that all concerned became aware that the results were still discouraging, and that the deterioration was continuing in spite of all efforts to check it. Hence changes in methods were made. Swedish drill became the fashion and also different types of exercisers and dumbbells which were used in the performance of muscle-tensing movements of all kinds, and succeeding experiences in connexion with posture, calisthenics, plastic dancing, deep breathing, "Daily Dozens" and other specific methods cannot evidently be considered satisfactory, as the search for the "great unknown or unrecognized" still continues.

Another set of people, convincing themselves that civilization was never meant as a mode of life for a human being, decide that in this fact they can see the light in their long "physical darkness" and come to the conclusion that *the remedy* is a "return to Nature," to the "simple life." And so we have the spectacle of these simple, lowly evolved human beings actually trying to return to the scenes of the early triumphs of their prehistoric forbears, where, as they imagine, all experiences will be sufficiently non-varied and slow in development to meet their present capacities on the subconscious plane to which they so tenaciously cling. The picture of early man in his crude but natural surroundings presents a curious but interesting study to those who have evolved beyond that state, but the spectacle of civilized man trying to return to the environment of his prehistoric ancestors would give us cause for laughter, were it not for the tragedy involved in a conception which is so uncomplimentary to our intellectual pride.

Certain Errors of Judgment in Man's Choice of "Physical Exercises" as a Remedy for a Fundamental Shortcoming

Now what I wish to emphasize is that throughout the long search for the remedy for his deterioration, man overlooked certain most important factors in the case, factors which are still overlooked to-day by the majority of people in their search for health and general uplifting.

In the first place, man completely overlooked the fact that the sensory mechanism, upon which he had heretofore entirely depended for guidance in general activity, was no longer registering accurately, and that he could no longer rely, therefore, entirely upon feeling, that is, on instinctive subconscious guidance for the satisfactory performance of the ordinary acts of life. The very fact that at some period "physical exercises" were considered necessary proves that imperfections must have developed to a very serious extent, and the reason for this, as I again repeat, is that the gradual failure of the sense registers to continue to guide men satisfactorily in the use of themselves in the activities of life had finally brought about an advanced stage of mal-co-ordination in the human psycho-physical organism.

It was clearly unreasonable, therefore, to expect "physical exercises" of whatever kind, to bring about any lasting or fundamental improvement in this unsatisfactory condition, when the person performing them would be guided by the same imperfect and delusive sensory appreciation, *dependence upon which had led originally to the very condition he wished to remedy*. What is more, during the performance of "physical exercises" under these conditions there would be an actual development of his original mal-co-ordinated condition, and he would be sure to encounter some new and very baffling psycho-physical problems in himself.[23] These problems actually arose and have become since then increasingly complicated, and I should like here to reiterate that even if they cannot be said to be wholly overlooked to-day, their real significance is still almost entirely misunderstood, in that the majority of people do not realize that human beings are still propelling an already maladjusted and damaged mechanism along the difficult road of modern life, whilst relying for guidance upon an imperfect and sometimes delusive sensory appreciation.

Secondly, in choosing "physical exercises" as a remedy for his deterioration, man did not take into consideration the fact that his body was a very delicate and highly co-ordinated piece of machinery, so that there might be many contributing causes other than muscular weakness to account for his deteriorated condition; further, that the exercises themselves were not correlated in any way to the needs of his organism, either in the practical activities of life or during those periods of rest which are such an important part of the daily round (a point constantly overlooked by enthusiasts for "physical culture").

If we ask ourselves why man overlooked these important points, the answer may throw light on many of our own problems at the present time. It was undoubtedly because he was aiming exclusively at a method of "cure," not of prevention. In the terms of my thesis, his attention was fixed on the "end" he was seeking (his "physical" amelioration), not on the reasonable *means whereby* that "end" could be brought about.

If he could have thought of his body in the terms of the very intricate-

[23]In the second part of this book I have dealt with certain of these problems as they occur in educational and other spheres of life.

ly constructed machine which it is, he would have seen in his deteriorated condition, not a deterioration in his muscular development alone, but a deterioration in his general psycho-physical co-ordination, accompanied by an interference with the general adjustment of the organism and by a general lowering of the standard of its functioning. He would then have realized that his deterioration must be merely the symptom of some failure in the working of the machinery, *and that the whole machine would need to be readjusted before it could work co-ordinately once more.*

He would have dealt with it as he would have dealt with any other machine, his watch, for instance, that was out of working order. If his watch gained half an hour one day and on the next stopped altogether, or if its small hand worked at the same speed as the big one, he would not trust to its accuracy if he wanted to catch a train, and, still more to the point, he would not start to repair it at random. He would send it instead to an expert who, through his knowledge of the correct working of the machinery, would make good any worn or broken part and readjust the mechanism once more. The watchmaker would then probably suggest, *as a preventive measure*, a periodic overhaul so that wear might be watched, and, when necessary, damaged parts repaired or new ones supplied. By this means, a reasonable endeavour would be made *to prevent* another such derangement of the mechanism as had rendered the watch an unreliable guide.[24]

We cannot be surprised, however, that man did not reason in the same way in connexion with the deterioration of his own mechanism. His reasoning processes in connexion with the care of his own mechanisms and with his general well-being had not been employed to anything like the same degree as in connexion with the mechanisms of external nature. He decided that he had discovered a "physical" defect for which he must find a remedy, and there can be little doubt that as soon as he conceived the "remedy" idea, any other possible consideration was shut off, whether of the cause or causes of the "physical" deterioration, or of the psycho-physical principles involved, or (even if the cause or causes had been discovered), of the *means whereby* the desired "end" (remedy) could be secured. His decision, in short, was the result of a subconscious and, therefore, unreasoned procedure, not of conscious reasoning reflexion. As we have already pointed out, a different

[24]We must again note the difference that exists between human and inanimate machinery. The human machine, when in a state of co-ordinated and adequate use, commands in itself the power of growth and development in each part of the muscular mechanism, and the condition approximating to wear in inanimate machinery may be prevented more or less from becoming present in the human being by nature's method of supply and repair under right conditions in the matter of used and wasted tissue.

result could hardly be expected at this early stage of man's development, seeing that even to-day in the twentieth century, the problem of psycho-physical unfitness is met with the same primeval "remedy" outlook both in theory and practice.

Man's Conscious Reasoning Processes Applied in Connexion With Outside Activities but Not in Connexion with His Psycho-Physical Organism

The stubborn but unpleasant fact must be faced that civilized man has never progressed personally, that is, in himself, as he has advanced in matters outside himself. Although he has reasoned out the *means whereby* he can control and turn to his own uses the different forces he has discovered in the outside world, he has not applied this reasoning principle where his own organism is concerned. He has left this masterpiece of psycho-physical machinery, more subtle, more delicate in its workings than the most intricate man-made machine,[25] to the subconscious guidance of his sensory appreciation, unaware that this sensory appreciation is becoming, as we have seen, more and more unreliable with the boasted advance of civilization.

We are all acquainted with the word sacrilege, and we have a knowledge of the acts which come under this category. But the word has not yet been applied, as far as I am aware, in connexion with the use of the psycho-physical organism of the human creature. Yet, is it not a sacrilege that during the experiences of civilization in the past two thousand years, the human psycho-physical organism has been directed and employed in the activities of life on a subconscious and unreasoned plan, with the result that distortions and defects have been developed and have become established? The adjustment of the wonderful psycho-physical machinery has been harmfully interfered with, likewise the co-ordinations which play the great part in the actual working of this machinery, this interference resulting in a lowered standard of general functioning of the organism.

There was a time when the body and limbs of the human being were the "mould of form," an inspiration to sculptor and painter, and a joy to look upon as "a thing of beauty" and symmetry. In our time, however, the organisms of the vast majority of people may be described as more or less misshapen, maladjusted and unsymmetrical. Awkwardness and ungainliness have superseded grace and poetry of motion, shapely limbs have become misshapen, and the psycho-physical mechanisms are employed not to advantage but to disadvantage.

[25]It is well known that a passion for mechanics exists among boys of our time. How very easy it would be to turn this desire towards an understanding of their own mechanisms!

* * * * *

To sum up, we have seen how in his choice of "physical exercises" as a remedy for what he recognized as physical deterioration, man overlooked certain important facts. Firstly, he left out of account the fact that he had developed a state of unreliability in his sensory appreciation which was therefore no longer a reliable guide in psycho-physical activity. Secondly, he did not think of his body as a co-ordinated mechanism, and was therefore misled into choosing a specific remedy for a specific malcondition, instead of laying down on broad, general lines *preventive principles*, by which a condition of co-ordination of the entire psycho-physical mechanism could be restored and maintained. Above all, he did not apply to his problem the one great principle on which I claim man's satisfactory progress in civilization depends, namely, the principle of *thinking out the reasonable means whereby a certain end can be achieved*, as opposed to the old subconscious plan of working blindly for an immediate "end."

We can now have a clear understanding of a fundamental process which has been in course of building from the early days of the human creature, and is still to-day in course of building among the great majority of people who, at certain psychological moments, still act in the same way as their forbears of the so-called Dark Ages, and, when faced with similar problems, still work subconsciously for their immediate "ends" ("cure" idea), instead of thinking out first the reasonable *means whereby* their desired "ends" can be achieved (prevention idea).

It is quite true that some modification is going on here and there. I am quite willing to admit that we have a small minority of people actually attempting to analyze their own and others' cases, where ills and imperfections are concerned, but, as I shall shew later on, they are all attempting to make "cures" by means of a *specific* remedy instead of dealing with each problem on a *general* basis.

This applies equally to the various forms of so-called mental healing, including Christian Science, Auto-suggestion, New Thought, etc., which have recently come into vogue. These are simply a reaction from the earlier idea of "physical culture," but like the reactions of all creatures who are subconsciously controlled, they are but the reaction from one extreme to another. For it would seem that in most of our attempts to progress on a subconscious plane, we tend to move from one extreme to another, and fail to recognize the danger into which we are drifting, until we are metaphorically struck on the head by some unforeseen or unknown force of Nature which makes us pause. We then retrace our steps perhaps, but only to start off just as blindly in another direction until we reach the other extreme (a process which amounts to over-compensation), when Nature again intervenes and forces us once more to cry a halt. Our progress under subconscious guidance, in other words, resembles that of a man lost in the Bush, who, becoming oblivious to those signs which, if he were not emotionally disturbed, could not escape his observation, wanders round and round in a circle, and after a long and sad experience finds himself back at the place from which he started. It is owing to this habit of rushing from one extreme to another—a habit, which, as I have pointed out, seems to go hand in hand with subconscious guidance and direction—to this tendency, that is, to take the narrow and treacherous sidetracks instead of the great, broad, midway path, that our plan of civilization has proved a comparative failure.

Harmful Concept of Division of the Psycho-Physical Organism

There is yet one other aspect of the case which I will now put forward, as it epitomizes all the errors which human beings have made in their attempts to solve the problem of living in civilization whilst relying upon subconscious guidance. In the adoption of "physical exercises" and of the various methods of "mental healing" as specific remedies for human ills, man made an arbitrary attempt to separate the psycho-physical organism into parts which he defined as body, mind and soul.[26]

Now to separate any organism into parts and then to expect it to function satisfactorily is an unreasoned proposition, as unreasoned as it would be to expect to obtain the best results from any other machine, by separating the gear mechanism, for instance, from the explosive and steering mechanism.

It is probable that this unreasoned conception had its origin in that emotional and confused condition which is responsible for the majority of unreasoned acts and beliefs, and is generally found to be associated with fear in some form or other. The confused state into which man was

[26]In *Man's Supreme Inheritance* I endeavoured to leave no room for doubt that I base my philosophy and practice on the unity of human potentialities, which, up till now, have been differentiated and represented as "body," "body and mind," or "body, mind and soul."

The words "mind" and "soul" are in as common use as the word "body," and we have all been guilty of using them. Now we do know something about the body, something tangible, but what do we really know about "soul"? And do we know anything more about "mind" as such, than we do about "soul"? Yet phrases in connexion with "mind" still remain in continual use, such as, for instance, to "hold in mind," to "keep the mind" on something, or when we speak of "improving the mind," or of "developing or making a mind," or of a person's "mental" attitude, of "mental" progress, "mental" control, "mental" habits, or of a person suffering from "mental" trouble.

The pages of *Man's Supreme Inheritance* and also of this book abound with arguments and illustrations in connexion with the harmful results which follow the efforts of people

thrown in his first attempts to find a "cure" for his psycho-physical deterioration was naturally linked up and associated with his original fears. For fear had been man's constant companion from very earliest times, and whether the fear was a healthy or an unhealthy fear depended upon the conditions involved; in either case, it was a form of illness for which the lowly evolved creature could not find a "cure." The primary law which ordains that one creature should feed upon another, the shock of new experiences, and ignorance of even simple laws of Nature were responsible for this. There was no escape. Every creature, human or otherwise, lived in constant expectation of an attack from its natural enemy. Our little canary, whose great-great-great-grandparents were caged birds, still looks from side to side with anxious rapidity after picking up each seed, just like the earliest of its kind.

It is easy to understand what would be the effect of thunder, for instance, when heard for the first time by the primitive creature, whose very existence depended upon a proper reaction to the stimulus of fear, and to imagine his terrified aspect when lightning first flashed before his

---

beset with unreliable sensory appreciation, when they attempt to follow out written or spoken instructions, with the aim of eradicating defects or peculiarities in the use of their psycho-physical mechanisms. Now of the working of these mechanisms it is possible to acquire some tangible knowledge; if, then, harmful results can follow attempts at improvement or development in a sphere where we can acquire some tangible knowledge, how much more harmful must be any attempts to follow out such specific instructions as "hold in mind," or "keep the mind" on something, when of the working of what we call "mind" we have no tangible knowledge. And when we reach the point where we can suggest the possibility of "developing or making a mind," we must surely be so far removed from concrete realization of facts as to have reached the borderland of mysticism. The history of man's efforts at every stage of his development furnishes proof of the harmful results which accrue, whenever the human creature attempts to respond to a stimulus (or stimuli) arising from his conception of a phrase which represents intangible phenomena. How can this be otherwise? How is it possible for him to come into possession of any tangible *means whereby* he may secure an intangible "end"?

It will therefore be understood that I have a special reason for giving so many concrete illustrations in my books. Here we have something demonstrable in simple, practical procedures; and free from those intangible phenomena which are too often inseparable from what is known as "mental" or "spiritual" discussion.

If it were not for the world-wide tragedy of it all, one could almost be amused at the attempts of those who are trying to pierce the veil of the "beyond," whilst they are still ignorant of the discoverable human potentialities within their grasp. Is it not reasonable to assume that the knowledge of the *means whereby* these potentialities may be continuously developed and employed to the best possible advantage should be the stepping-stone to satisfactory activities on other planes of life? Surely mankind should at least come into the great earthly inheritance—the conscious plane of evolution—before time and energy is devoted to those fields of speculation and doubt in connexion with the "undiscovered country from whose bourn no traveller returns."

eyes. There can be no doubt that from the very earliest stages man's reaction to such fears as these had been to seek refuge in the supernatural. Indeed, civilized men who have not prayed for years, who may even have ridiculed the practice of prayer, have been known in the circumstances of shipwreck to kneel down and pray instinctively. In such cases fear overrules their convictions, the old primitive subconsciousness holds sway, and they probably fall on their knees without being aware of it.

So it would be with primitive man. Dazed and terrified by the thunder and lightning, he would drop down, and hide his face in his hands, mumbling, incoherently perhaps, to "something." Sooner or later, when the paroxysm of fear had begin to pass, he would take his hands from his face, and it is conceivable that the first tree or stone to meet his terrified gaze would impress him as being the power which had rescued him from some awful fate. From this there would develop the worship of images of wood and stone, and the various religious rites with which we are familiar.

We will not stop to consider all the intervening stages in this development, but will pass on to the time of the Christian Era, and see in what form the primitive fear now manifested itself.

Here we find that though man's fears were modified in the case of thunder and lightning, and other terrors with which he had now become familiar, they were no less acute in new and unfamiliar spheres. And beyond this original fear of the unknown, a new form of fear had come upon him, associated with the one-sided development which had taken place in the human organism. For unbalanced psycho-physical development connotes unsatisfactory equilibrium in all spheres, and unsatisfactory equilibrium is ever associated with fear. As we have seen, since man's entry into the civilized state, he had been developing more rapidly on what is called the mental side, whilst on the so-called physical side there was actual deterioration. He had thus been building up within himself two forces, as it were, the one working against the other, until it was almost as if he had developed two separate entities, the "physical" and the "mental." It was the conflicting demands of these "separate entities" which caused the interference with psycho-physical equilibrium and produced in him the condition of inward fear to which I refer, and which to-day is too often called "nerves."[27]

This new fear—*actually a fear of himself*—gradually developed until its presence was recognized as an urgent problem, and it is in man's solution of this problem that we are faced with a conception which will be

---

[27]The presence of fear always means a condition of conflict. The man who is inwardly afraid puts on an outward show of bravery by an assumed manner. Similarly, it is doubtless this inward fear which induces in certain nations a mania for carrying arms and for the massed attack in accordance with their horde instinct.

seen to be a most harmful one when considered in relation to his evolutionary progress.

The conception to which I refer is that of the separation of the human organism into the parts which have been named soul, mind and body. Those who were bent on this separation attempted, in obedience to their own arbitrary and unreasoning conception, to develop each of the three parts named soul, mind and body, specifically, nay, even to make a class-distinction, as it were, between them, this last procedure being a reversion to a "habit of thought" associated with other spheres. Surely, even to those who believed in this separation, their knowledge of the process of Nature should have indicated the place which the body should occupy in order of importance, and its relationship to the other parts in the series named body, mind and soul.

Those who have followed our argument to this point will be cognizant of the following facts:

(1) that the rules of moral, social and other conduct already established at the period designated the Christian Era were the result of human conceptions;

(2) that the human beings responsible for these conceptions were themselves the product of the psycho-physical experiences involved in a subconscious attempt to pass from a very low stage in the evolutionary process, which we call the uncivilized stage, to a much higher stage, which is known to us as the civilized stage;

(3) that, during this transition, man's use and development on the so-called mental side had proceeded at a much greater rate proportionately than on the so-called physical side, and for the reason that on the so-called physical side his use and development had already reached such a high standard that the possibilities of future development on that side (as development was then understood) were not so great as on the, as yet, almost undeveloped so-called mental side. Also, in the new mode of life there was relatively less demand on the former and an increasing demand on the latter;

(4) that, in the sphere of civilization, with the new and increasing use and development on the so-called mental side, there was a correspondingly gradual decrease in use and development on the so-called physical side, as compared with those earlier periods when man roamed the plains and mountains in search of his daily food and other necessities;

(5) that this was the beginning of a new era in the experience of the creature called man. It was the beginning of an interfer-

ence with the co-ordinated use and development of the psycho-physical organism.

From all this it will be conceded that up to a certain point the so-called physical processes, as being the more highly developed, constituted the leading and guiding factor in human activity. Yet, in a comparatively short space of time, the relatively unused but more rapidly developing interdependent processes called "mind" were exalted to a higher place than the "body" in the human economy, only to be superseded by what those concerned were pleased to call the "soul," of which they knew even less than the little they knew of the "mind" and its workings.

The very conception of a separation and class distinction between "body, mind and soul" indicates the presence of a more than usually potent stimulus which could emanate only from a condition of over-balancing in some direction. As far as we can learn, the poor body came into disgrace on account of the "lusts of the flesh," themselves a natural result of a mal-co-ordinated condition, and if we may judge by the special laws and customs which were formulated, the chief results of this unbalanced condition would seem to have manifested themselves in the sexual sphere. Else why should this sphere have been particularly selected for condemnation, seeing that the satisfaction of the needs and desires of the reproductive system is as essential as the satisfaction of the needs and desires of the digestive and assimilative systems to the welfare of the individual and of the race, and that the results of satisfying the sensory desires and needs of these three systems are normal and salutary, as long as moderate use and not abuse is the rule? The evil of over-eating is only equalled by that of over-drinking, and surely in the last analysis the abuse of the sexual act is intensified by one or the other, or by both. A man or an animal placed on a low diet does not evince any particular desires in the way of sex-relations. As a matter of fact, the very reverse would prove to be the rule.

Indeed, this idea of "separation" in the human organism was a purely arbitrary conception formed to fit in with certain stultifying premisses which human beings, probably in all honesty and meekness of spirit, had laid down and made a law unto themselves in striving to fulfil what they considered were the essential demands of the religious ideal.

This led naturally to that dreadful and debasing conception which caused men and women actually to castigate the flesh, to cut, as it were, a way to Heaven through the very fundamental of their earthly being.

But the limit of the destruction wrought by this dissecting process had not yet been reached. As the process called education progressed, this principle of a class-distinction within the organism grew and developed.

Side by side with the growth of education the idea was cultivated that lack of knowledge in certain specific spheres was the factor which must determine whether a person should be classified as ignorant or otherwise. A man might be a glorified Touchstone, a person with a prodigious fund of common sense, or even a reasoning, intelligent creature, but if he did not happen to be versed in all the paraphernalia which made up the curricula of the universities, schools and colleges of his time, he would be classified as ignorant.

Next followed the most stupid of all the conceptions formed by subconsciously controlled human beings in connexion with education, a conception which was the co-mate of the idea of class-distinction, namely, a more or less growing contempt for those who, despite their natural gifts, were thus classified as ignorant, and especially for those whose work made more demands upon their so-called physical than upon their so-called mental selves (that is, from the educationalists' point of view), together with a wholly absurd and exaggerated admiration for those who worked in professions in which it was concluded the demands were almost exclusively "mental."[28]

Need for Unity and Simplicity

We have only to consider these facts to realize how far men had travelled from one of the original fundamentals of life. For as we have already indicated, in the beginning of things there must have been unity, and it was a strange lack of reasoning that permitted man to make a false division in an organism that can only be satisfactorily developed as an indivisible psycho-physical unity.

I was recently discussing this and other kindred matters with a scientific friend, who put the following query to me: "Why have we overlooked these important points for so long?" In reply I referred to the phrase now in such common use: "Life has become so complex." In my opinion we have here the crux of the whole matter, and I venture to predict that before we can unravel the horribly tangled skein of our present existence, we must come to a full STOP, and return to conscious, simple living, believing in the unity underlying all things, and acting in a practical way in accordance with the laws and principles involved.

28 This is only one of the many proofs that we possess that the idea of class-distinction lies at the very root of man's makeup, and that despite all efforts that may be made by legislation or other external means to counter this idea, it will surely remain as a conviction, in one form or another, with both its defenders and its advocates, until mankind has reached the reasoning stage of conscious guidance and control of the individual. Until this stage is reached, those ideals which we indicate by the words democracy, liberty, etc., are impossible of attainment.

In the midst of a world-wide tragedy such as we are witnessing at the present time, a tragedy which seems to have been increasing instead of decreasing in its intensity since the declaration of the Armistice and the work of the peace-makers in Paris, surely it behoves every individual to stop—and I mean this in its fullest sense—and reconsider every particle of supposed knowledge, particularly "psychological" knowledge, derived from his general education, from his religious, political, moral, ethical, social, legal and economic training, and ask himself the plain, straightforward question, "Why do I believe these things?" "By what process of reasoning did I arrive at these conclusions?"

If we are even and direct with ourselves in regard to our cherished ideas and ideals, the answer at first may prove a shock to us, to some of us, indeed, almost a knockdown blow. For the truth will be borne in upon us that much of our supposed knowledge has not been real knowledge, and too often the boasted truth a delusion. Many of us may awaken to the fact that the majority of our cherished ideas and ideals are the product, not of any process of reasoning, but of that unreasoning process called impulse, of unbalanced emotion and prejudice, that is, of ideas and ideals associated with a psycho-physical condition in the development of which unreliable sensory appreciation has played the leading part.

Need for Substituting in all Spheres the Principle of Prevention on a General Basis for Methods of "Cure" on a Specific Basis

As we have seen, unreliability of sensory appreciation has been and still is associated with a general deterioration in the standard of the health of mankind. Consequently, in the matter of making decisions, man's conceptions and thoughts have been and still are conditioned by this unreliable sensory appreciation, and still lead him, as in the past, to erroneous conclusions and decisions in the settlement of the new problems with which he has been continually confronted. Nowhere can we find a better illustration of the erroneous conceptions, leading to unbalanced judgment, which are associated with unreliable sensory appreciation, than in man's choice of a specific "cure" on the "end-gaining" principle, namely, "physical exercises." It was his erroneous estimate of the relative value of the principles of prevention and "cure" which permitted him to make this choice, and so to neglect the "means-whereby" principle which is involved in all preventive procedure.

We have evidence of similar unbalanced judgment in all other spheres where the attempted improvement of the individual is concerned, and the erroneous decisions and opinions which result from unbalanced judgment in these spheres are analogous to the error man made in choosing a specific "cure" in his attempts to stem the tide of general deterioration. Each generation has fallen into the same error in this connexion, and in this way has built up a heavy burden for the succeeding one, inasmuch as the necessity for "cure" has increased and still continues to increase at a pace which bids fair to heap upon the individuals of coming generations such a load as will be beyond the power of human endurance. If the methods which have led to this undesirable situation are ever reviewed by the individuals upon whom will devolve the onerous duty of carrying on the scheme called civilization, we shall probably be written down by them as poor, subconsciously directed human beings, rushing wildly from one extreme to another in the howling wilderness of twentieth-century wonders. Such a review will provide abundant proof of the lowered standard of reliability of sensory appreciation in the human beings of our time, which has caused them to become overbalanced in many directions, and consequently has deluded them into experimenting blindly in too many spheres. Disaster has followed such experiments in chemistry and death-dealing machines, for instance, in exactly the same way as it would follow the activities of children well-supplied with powder and matches. The historian of a century or two hence will be able to produce evidence of the psycho-physical state of the peoples of the twentieth century which will shew that in this regard they have progressed little on the evolutionary plane beyond the man of the Stone Age, whilst, on the other hand, he will only have to refer to human activities during the years 1914-1918 to convince the most sceptical that human beings of our time have developed a new form of devilry and brutality that surpasses the best efforts of prehistoric man.

Should we decide, however, at the present time upon a retrospection such as I have suggested, we can hardly fail to see that a psychological moment in man's experience has undoubtedly arrived for a widespread consideration of the principle of prevention in its fullest application to human needs (in all "physical," "mental" or "spiritual" spheres), as they are presented to us at this present world crisis. Investigation will shew that the proportion of human energy devoted to prevention and "cure" in the twentieth century in all these spheres may fairly be said to be as nine to one in favour of "cure." That this is so after some thousands of years of supposed civilization gives food for reflexion. For the idea of seeking and adopting a specific "cure" had its origin, as we have seen, in the experiences of a lowly evolved type of human creature belonging to an earlier period of human development. It goes with a view of life which is narrow and limited, since it represents an attempt on man's part to gain an immediate "end" without consideration of larger issues.

We are, therefore, faced with the fact, hitherto almost unrecognized, that our adoption of the principle of "cure," with its associated "end-gaining" procedures, as the basis of our attempted reforms in all spheres, means that the foundation of too many of our cherished ideals and beliefs to-day is the same as that from which were built up the instinctive procedures of our earlier ancestors when they sought a "cure" in some specific herb or berry.

On the other hand, a scheme of life in which prevention is the leading principle does not involve working for an immediate "end"; its application, rather, is on a broad, constructive basis, without limits, humanly speaking, and is the product of a consciously conceived and consciously executed plan; in short, it is the conception of a highly evolved type of human creature.

Illustration I.

I need not detain my readers with the many obvious illustrations of the lack of reasoning associated with all methods of "cure." I will give three instances, beginning with what is called the "liver cure."

A man feels out of sorts and has suffered from certain symptoms for a year or more. He at last consults his medical adviser and is told that his liver is sluggish. He is ordered to take some grains of calomel or some such drug, and goes home with the conviction that all will now be well. He has his "remedy" and the plan is so simple. If the symptoms recur, all he has to do is to swallow the prescribed number of grains of his drug. This applies to the whole list of such "cures."

At this point I would beg my reader not to judge my standpoint until I have placed my evidence before him. We, the people of the twentieth century, pride ourselves that we are a reasoning race; at any rate, that we have employed the processes of reasoning in far more spheres than our forbears of several centuries ago. This being so, why have the reasoning processes been so comparatively little employed in connexion with those problems on the solution of which our present and future well-being depends?

Let us consider, for instance, how the person of our illustration reasons in connexion with his sluggish liver and his calomel remedy. It is quite understandable that, on the occasion of an acute attack, he should follow the instructions of his doctor, take his grains of calomel and so get clear, as he considers it, of a crisis. But why does the matter end there, as far as he, personally, is concerned? He has probably been aware of trouble for quite a long time, and now he has it on his doctor's authority that his liver is unduly inactive. As a matter of fact, he has suspected this himself, led to the conclusion by the presence of certain symptoms and by the knowledge that his sedentary life and his over-indulgence in certain foods and drinks, which are particularly gratifying to his none too reliable sensory appreciation (in this case, particularly the sense of taste) are liable to have caused the trouble. This being so, one would expect him to shew some intelligent recognition of the real situation. It would not require any special degree of reasoning to enable him to grapple successfully with the obvious facts of his case. But unfortunately he does not think beyond the crisis of the moment. He is set only on being "cured" of his specific ill, and so, in the twentieth century, he continues to act on the "end-gaining" principle, a procedure which was excusable in his forbears of four thousand years ago. He has never applied either to himself, or to the difficulties encountered in the sphere of his psycho-physical well-being, any other principle than that of working for an immediate "end." In these spheres he has never adopted the plan of reasoning out first the common sense *means whereby* an "end" may be secured. Why should he do it now? He is simply a subconsciously controlled person in whom, in this connexion, the processes of reasoning are in abeyance.

An interesting fact, however, is that the drug devotee, on discovering that calomel, say, does not relieve his liver trouble, will try another drug and yet another, and so on, in spite of numerous failures. This serves to shew that within one narrow groove he is prepared to make changes, actually to reason out, for instance, that even if calomel fails, podophyllin may prove to be the liver elixir. But he is held down to the "cure idea" of the Stone Age by his confidence in drugs, and thus remains true to one of the most harmful habits which he has inherited as race instincts. Think for a moment of the harmful nature of the building process indicated in the foregoing illustration, where you have a man, supposedly advanced, still clinging to primitive methods of "cure," instead of adopting the only principle a highly evolved, reasoning human creature could conceive of or tolerate, the great comprehensive principle of prevention. If in all his decisions his reasoning processes had not been limited within such a narrow groove, it must have dawned upon him that his liver trouble was the sign that something had gone wrong with the machinery of the whole organism, a conception which would have tended to cause him to consider the guiding and controlling processes involved.

For when a machine, animate or inanimate, has developed mechanical defects, that machine is not functioning at its maximum, and, with the continued use of the machine, these defects not only become more and more pronounced, but actually increase in number. It is obvious, then, that as soon as the mechanical defects are recognized, all possible means should at once be employed to restore the maximum standard of mechanical functioning. In order to accomplish this, a knowledge of the motive, adjusting, guiding and controlling principles of the mechanism is needed. In the case of the human mechanisms, a knowledge of the psycho-mechanical principles involved is necessary to their co-ordinated use, and this knowledge implies the possession of a sensory appreciation which is reliable.

For in all cases of so-called mental and physical shortcomings there are present imperfections and defects in the use of the psycho-physical organism. If the sense registers in connexion with this organism had continued in civilization to be reliable, how could these imperfections and defects have developed in a satisfactorily co-ordinated person? And if the sense registers are so unreliable and deceptive that a person can develop imperfections and defects in the ordinary activities of life, what may be expected as a result of his activities in remedial and other spheres,[29] if he continues to be guided by the same imperfect sense registers which have deceived and are still deceiving him at every turn?

The time is not far distant when these facts will be widely recognized, and it will then be obvious that immediately we decide to do something to remove a psycho-physical imperfection or defect, the first thing is to acquire gradually a reliable sensory appreciation during a process of re-education, readjustment and co-ordination on a basis of constructive, conscious guidance and control.

Illustration II.

This important point is unfortunately overlooked in all curative spheres, so that palliative and "end-gaining" specific methods prevail, and a good illustration of this may be found in the field of surgery. In all that follows on this point, however, I wish to make it clear that I am not lacking in the fullest appreciation of the value of surgery in special spheres or of the good results that may accrue from skilful surgery within these spheres. But I should like, if I may, to suggest that it is possible for the surgeon to confer in the future far greater benefits on humanity than those which he is conferring at the present time, if he will extend both his field of operation and his outlook to include the wider plan of

[29]Many of my readers may object to these arguments and refer to some defect or imperfection which at some time they have removed, with or without aid as the case may be. I am quite ready to admit this, but I assert that several other defects and imperfections will have been cultivated in the process. As a matter of fact, I am prepared to prove this, if the objector will submit himself or herself for examination whilst he or she demonstrates the process adopted for the "cure." Incidentally, I may mention that these examinations are made whilst the subject remains dressed.

prevention. Take, for instance, the major operations of the removal of the appendix or of the colon. The surgeon's business is to remove these organs in cases where he finds a condition of deterioration which justifies him in concluding that the presence of these organs is harmful or even dangerous. It will be seen, therefore, that to this extent the sphere of surgery is confined within narrow limits. The surgeon is asked to examine an organ which is functioning imperfectly, and if he concludes from this examination that a certain stage of deterioration of the particular organ has been reached, he performs an operation.

Under this method of procedure, little consideration is given to the cause or causes of the general interference with the functioning of the whole organism, an interference of which the *specific* deterioration in the appendix, or colon, is merely a symptom. Nor do I find that consideration is given, as a rule, to the fact that the operation, however skilfully performed, does not restore that standard of reliable sensory appreciation necessary to the readjustment and co-ordinated use of the mechanisms, by means of which adequate vital activity will be restored and the dropped viscera caused to resume their normal and healthy position in the torso.

This point is in no way affected by the fact that an operation may be entirely successful from the standpoint of the successful removal of an organ which, being in a state of deterioration, is a danger to the patient. The patient recovers from his operation, but, even so, what is implied by this? The patient, it is true, has escaped the result of a crisis which might have proved fatal, but we are still face to face with the same old "end-gaining" principle. The appendix was diseased, the appendix was removed, and the patient recovers from the operation. Nothing, however, in all this has been done to introduce such a change in the working of the psycho-physical mechanisms and general functioning as would prevent a continuance of the imperfect working and imperfect functioning which caused the specific trouble necessitating the operation. This original imperfect functioning not only continues, but is bound to become more and more imperfect as time goes on, and, sooner or later, some other dangerous symptom (due to increasingly imperfect functioning) is almost certain to supervene, when the same palliative remedy—surgery—will again have to be called upon to give relief in a new direction. In the recognition of these facts lies the surgeon's opportunity to pass from the narrow sphere of curative work to the greater achievements that are awaiting him in the broad and comprehensive field of prevention.

Illustration III.

Another form of treatment to which I should like to draw attention in this connexion is psychoanalysis. This method has enjoyed a certain publicity in recent years, but in spite of the "cures" which are claimed for it, I am prepared to demonstrate that it is based on the same specific "end-gaining" principle as the less modern methods which it is claimed by some to supersede. By way of illustration I will take the case of a person who suffers from some unreasoning fear, and goes to a psychoanalyst for help in overcoming it. We will suppose that in the course of the analysis, long or short as the case may be, the teacher and the pupil together unravel the knot and decide that the origin of the fear lies in some event, or train of events, which took place in the past and unduly excited the patient's fear reflexes and established a "phobia." For the sake of our illustration, we will say that a "cure" is made. What does this "cure" indicate, however? Wherein lies the fundamental change in the patient's psycho-physical condition?

Before we can answer these questions, we must take into consideration the all-important fact to which I drew attention at the very outset of this book, namely, that all so-called mental activity is a process governed by our psycho-physical condition at the time when the particular stimulus is received. This being so, it is obvious that the reason a person falls a victim to some unreasoning fear is that his condition of general psycho-physical functioning at the time when he receives the stimulus, to which the fear is the reaction, is below a normal and satisfactory standard.[30] For, if his condition of general functioning were normal, his reaction to the particular sensory stimulus would be a normal reaction, not an unreasoning "phobia."

It follows, therefore, that the patient of our illustration must have been below the standard of normal psycho-physical functioning at the time of the establishment of the "phobia," that is, he must have been beset with a condition of debauched kinæsthesia, the result of imperfect co-ordination, imperfect adjustment, and unreliable and delusive sensory appreciation. The question, then, I must again ask is, What can be done by the "unravelling" procedure of psychoanalysis to remedy these serious defects of general psycho-physical functioning? Will psychoanalysis as practised restore a reliable sensory appreciation to the patient, and co-ordinate and re-educate his psycho-physical mechanisms on a general basis? Certainly not. The psycho-physical condition which permitted the establishment of the first phobia will permit the establishment of another. All that is needed is the stimulus.

The method of psychoanalysis, therefore, like other methods of treatment on a subconscious basis, is an instance of an "end-gaining"

[30]It is common knowledge that a person is more subject to infections (colds, etc.) when he is, as we say, run down, that is, in a more or less lowered psycho-physical condition.

attempt to effect the "cure" of a specific trouble by specific means, without consideration being given to the necessity of restoring a satisfactory standard of general psycho-physical functioning and of sensory appreciation.

Fundamental Defect in Our Plan of Civilization a Lack of Recognition of the Importance of the Principle of Prevention on a General Basis

It is the recognition in practice of the principle of prevention which makes possible man's advancement to higher and higher stages of evolution and opens up the greatest possibilities for human activities and accomplishment. I have illustrated and insisted upon this point thus fully, because I wish to emphasize what in my opinion constitutes a fundamental defect in a plan of civilization at least two thousand years old, namely, that in all attempts at reform or improvement in spheres where the well-being of the creature is concerned, human energy has been and still is expended mainly on the adoption of plans based upon methods of specific cure, instead of upon the principle of prevention. For many years past I have endeavoured to put this point of view before those who have consulted me, for I have found that in the case of a new pupil, even after I have made my diagnosis of the malconditions present, explained their actual cause or causes and described the practical procedures I should adopt to remedy such malconditions, I am still generally asked, "Have you ever 'cured' a case like mine?" In answer I point out that I do not undertake to "cure" anything or anyone.[31] I merely look at the subject before me as a damaged machine, as it were, note the badly used mechanisms, the imperfect sensory direction and control, and in the light of my experience ask myself, "Can one restore this machine, improve the mechanical working, build up a new and satisfactory sensory direction and control, restore a well-co-ordinated condition of the psycho-physical organism as a whole?" In other words, instead of trying to remove specific symptoms directly (method of "cure"), I endeavour to bring about such a readjustment of the organism as a whole that the symptoms in question disappear in the process

[31]As I write these words, I can imagine my readers, sooner or later, asking this question, "Why, then, if you advocate a plan of life founded on the principle of prevention, have you yourself continued to work in a more or less curative sphere?" The answer to this is simple. In the first place, the principle of prevention should be applied to children at a very early age; and, secondly, up to the present it has proved impossible to create a sufficient demand for fundamental psycho-physical re-education to induce young men and women to study it with a view to professional teaching in the preventive sphere. This implies that their work must be confined to children, and the reader will at once see the difficulty in which we are placed. We are faced with the inevitable law of supply and demand. Parents must first be themselves convinced *(continued on next page)*

and are not likely to recur if the new conditions are maintained (principle of prevention).

This implies in the case of some pupils a long process, for it means a gradual building-up of new and satisfactory psycho-physical use, and the pupils' co-operation in this process must be based upon a reasoning, rather than a blind acceptance of the principles involved. If, at the end of our talk, I consider that there is any doubt on the part of the prospective pupil, I beg him to read my book, study the principles therein set down, and then, if he comprehends and believes in these principles, I suggest that he should come to me for help, but not otherwise. In all seriousness, I beg of him not to come simply because he believes that I can "cure" him of something. I am ready to admit that anything will sometimes effect a "cure," as "cure" is generally understood, but the case of the exceptional "cure," by whatever means, whether by a course of medical treatment, by suggestion, transfer, or by any other method—accompanied as these "cures" are by thousands of fail-

---

of the need for fundamental psycho-physical re-education, and of the value of the technique I have to offer, before they will entrust their children for the time necessary and in sufficient numbers to create a demand that will make it possible for young men and women to take up the work on a sound professional and financial basis. Up till now what the parents have said is, "We will first come to you ourselves; then, if you are able to 'cure' our psycho-physical defects, we will consider the matter in relation to our children."

It is in vain that I protest that I do not set out to "cure" anything. "You see," they reply, "for us to accept your work as the basis of our children's education means such a complete change in all our views and methods; it means practically beginning afresh, and giving up so much that we have been taught is true up till now, that we cannot interfere with our children's education without first having the proof of your work in ourselves." Some of my scientific supporters are no less insistent on these points. Under these circumstances, my reader will understand that I am forced to work in a so-called curative sphere with adults, in the hope that they may help me in my efforts to gain a wide recognition of the necessity for re-education on a general basis and for preventive measures for the children. For once we have created amongst parents a demand for teachers of the work in the interests of the children, the first part of the problem will have been solved, for the supply, the material will be there, and will in time bring the right type of man and woman into the work. I am anxious and ready to devote the rest of my life, and the experience I have gained, relatively small though this may be, to preparing teachers to teach the children. To this end we need to establish a school for the education of teachers. Such a plan, however, is not without its difficulties, if the right type of man or woman is to be induced to take up the work. A number of people in England and America have been working with me to the end of establishing such a school. We are all aware of the harm we can do to the cause, if we attempt to gain this end quickly, at the cost of training only those people who are able to bear the financial burden involved during the necessary years of training, irrespective of the standard to which those psycho-physical potentialities, which go to the making of a teacher, have been developed in their case. Such an attempt could end only in comparative failure, and in the long run do much to delay the wide acceptance of the principles involved.

ures—cannot justify any reasoning person in attempting or promising a continuance of "cures" on these lines. I hold that we have reached a stage in our development when all attempts to remove the cause or causes of suffering which do not come within the scope of reasoned, practical procedure must, with the broader view, be definitely abandoned, and that we should ere now have passed that stage of ignorance and narrowness which permits the human creature to entertain for a moment the idea of a miracle.

The miracle worker and the advocates of "cure" methods have had free scope for over two thousand years, but despite this fact there has been a gradual increase in malconditions and in the symptoms and complications connected therewith, and therefore a correspondingly increasing need for "cure."

I would even state that in my opinion the fact that man has not been guided by his reasoning processes in connexion with the problems of his well-being is responsible for the tragedy of his progress in civilization. The crisis of 1914 serves to shew us that he has released forces which he is not capable of controlling, and by means of which millions of his fellow-beings have been swept from the earth, and it would seem that man is simply preparing the way for his own extinction unless those energies, which in the past have been directed into harmful channels in the outside world, are in future directed and controlled by reasoning processes which have been primarily employed in connexion with the use of his psycho-physical organism.

This horrible recrudescence of barbarity is for the moment held in check, but, like a fire whose white-heated embers have been cooled by water on the outside—a process which has merely served to intensify the degree of heat of the embers which this drenched crust encloses—it will sooner or later burst once more into flame. Every ember, which in our analogy represents an individual human being, must be dealt with singly and separately, and if we wish to prevent another fierce outbreak we must treat each ember in such a way that it will be as difficult to fire it, as it is to fire a piece of stone.

Similar treatment of the individual human creature on a basis of constructive conscious control will bring nearer that stage of evolutionary development where the masses, when thrown together, will no longer exhibit the inflammable traits associated with the horde instinct.

It is clear, then, that our first efforts to enable man to rise above the depths in which he is now struggling, and from which many people today believe he cannot extricate himself, should be devoted to the establishment in the individual of a reliable sensory appreciation by means of conscious, reasoning guidance, so as to prevent the recurrence of the disasters which have hitherto been associated with the activities of men and women whose judgments, opinions and policies have been based more upon a deteriorated sense of feeling than upon reasoning.

Just stop for a moment and think, for instance, of the lack of reasoning associated with the continuance of a plan of life under which the child, the adult of the future, is permitted gradually to develop imperfections and defects, so that long ere the age of adolescence is reached, some curative method of treatment has to be adopted in an attempt to eradicate imperfections and defects which, under a reasoning plan of life, would never have been permitted to become present. Under such a reasoning plan of life, the principle of prevention would be the fundamental underlying the child's education, which means that *from the beginning* preventive measures would be adopted where the well-being of the child is concerned.

The attempt to deal with a form of education based on a principle of prevention will lead into many fields of discussion, and probably force me, by way of illustration, to set down descriptions of technical evolutions, a procedure which, on the face of it, would seem to be an encouragement to people to cling to the "curative" and to neglect the preventive plan of life. But I wish here to free myself from responsibility for any such serious harm as invariably follows the attempt of the ordinary subconsciously controlled human being to follow written instructions for some exercise, drill, etc., with the aim of eradicating a defect or imperfection. I have already pointed out in *Man's Supreme Inheritance* that even though a person may succeed by this means in eradicating some specific defect or imperfection, he will be cultivating in the process quite a number of other defects, and in what follows I hope to make clear the reason for this generally unrecognized fact.

For the fundamental shortcoming underlying all human psycho-physical defects, imperfections and peculiarities is an imperfect and often delusive sensory appreciation, and until those conditions are restored in which the sensory appreciation (sense register) becomes again a more or less reliable guide, *all exercises are a positive danger.* A reliable sensory appreciation, therefore, is an essential and we will proceed to consider the part which this invaluable human endowment must play in any reasoned and satisfactory plan of education.

I shall therefore devote the rest of this volume to an examination of the part played by sensory appreciation in the process called education, taking this word in its broadest sense, for it is clear from tragic evidence all around us that, despite the influence of our past education, we have not been enabled to stem the rapid progress of human psycho-physical deterioration.

I shall attempt by practical illustrations to demonstrate that the establishment of a reliable sensory appreciation must be the foundation of education of children and of adults in what we call the act of learning and learning to do, or in the performance of all the activities which make up the daily round of occupations and recreations.

PART II
SENSORY APPRECIATION IN ITS RELATION TO LEARNING AND LEARNING TO DO

CHAPTER I

EDUCATION AND RE-EDUCATION

AT no time in our history has the same general interest been shewn in education (taking this word in its widest sense) as is manifested at the present day. The experiences of the War and of the world-wide unrest which has followed it have caused all thinking men and women to put to themselves searching questions as to the validity of long-cherished beliefs in every sphere, and nowhere has the searchlight been more vigorously used than in the sphere of education. Articles dealing with defects in educational methods appear with regularity in our newspapers, and because of this prevalent dissatisfaction all kinds of new methods are being advocated, so that the state of confusion and uncertainty, of which we are all so conscious in the world outside, is equally apparent in the educational world.

This state of confusion and uncertainty, experienced in the practical application of educational theories, has its parallel in that which is experienced in our attempts to decide as to the merit or demerit of any particular system, and for the reason that such decisions have remained till now within the doubtful range of individual opinion, which is too often formed subconsciously and based chiefly upon results.

In the endeavour to make plain what, in my opinion, constitutes the fundamental cause of this generally chaotic condition, I should like to begin by drawing attention to a fact which, though well-known, has been practically disregarded in all forms of past and present education, and, indeed, in all our dealings with our fellow-beings in every sphere. This fact is that whenever we wish to convey to anyone a new idea, whether by the written or spoken word, or, in other words, to teach him something, the person wishing to make use of it by that psycho-physical activity which we call learning something must first get his or her conception of what is indicated by those written or spoken words, and his practical use of the new idea will be conditioned by this conception. This applies equally when similar attempts are made by any process of self-instruction (auto-education). It then follows that in the sphere of acquiring knowledge, especially psycho-physical knowledge, this matter of the particular person's conception of written or spoken words is all-important, for it is the construction which the learner, adult or child, places upon what he hears or reads, which determines the course of his actions or the trend of his opinions. Yet the ordinary teacher acts and the ordinary teaching methods are based on the assumption that the pupil's conception of a new idea is identical with that of the teacher, the words teacher and pupil being here used in the widest possible sense. Anyone who has had practical dealings with children will know how frequently disappointment and failure in their studies, or anything else, is due to their not understanding exactly what is required of them. The daily experiences of life are studded with instances of misunderstanding, not only in trivial matters, but also in matters of great importance, and if the broad view is taken, I think we may justly say that the great majority of these experiences constitute one long series of specific and general misunderstandings and lead us to the conclusion that, where misunderstanding occurs, there is present some impeding factor (or factors) which interferes with the process of reasoning, a process inseparable from what is called understanding or "mental conception."

The significance, however, of the fact that a person's attempt to make practical use of a new idea is conditioned by his conception of the written or spoken word, cannot be fully realized until we connect it with the further fact, that this conception, in its turn, is conditioned by the standard of the psycho-physical functioning of the individual, this standard again being influenced by the standard of sensory appreciation; in other words, that *the accuracy or otherwise of the individual conception depends upon the standard of psycho-physical functioning and of sensory appreciation present.* It is our total disregard of this fundamental fact that, in my opinion, is at the root of all the confusion and uncertainty so prevalent to-day in the sphere of education, and, for that matter, in every sphere of practical life.

For, if the foregoing is true, we can see at once how essential it is that in the matter of conveying and imparting knowledge, in other words, in education, we should be able to command a high standard of psycho-physical functioning in the whole organism, associated with that growth and development which makes for the continuous raising both of this standard and of the standard of sensory appreciation; and, further, that in order to arrive at sound conclusions concerning the fundamentals upon which any scheme of education should be based, we must first take into consideration the standard of psycho-physical functioning of the human being whom we are to educate, both to-day and in what we hope is to be a progressive future.

Unfortunately, a satisfactory standard of psycho-physical functioning has not been considered an essential either in the early or subsequent schemes of education which man, whilst depending mainly upon subconscious guidance and control, has adopted in the attempt to make what is known as "mental" progress. Even to-day this essential factor does not seem to be considered an essential, for in this regard modern methods of education are as lacking as those which have been obtained for generations.

The seriousness of this position is at once apparent when we take into consideration the fact that, during the past two hundred years, the standard of sensory appreciation in the great majority of people has become harmfully lowered with the result that mankind has generally become more and more imperfectly co-ordinated and has developed serious defects. Yet, in spite of this, the teachers and originators of modern systems, like those of an earlier date, are still trying to help individuals to progress towards a higher stage of "physical" and "mental" development, whilst leaving them dependent on subconscious experiences for guidance and control, without any consideration or, indeed, understanding of the harm that results from attempts to obey instructions made by people who are guiding themselves by an unreliable and often delusive sensory appreciation.

The problem, then, with which we are faced is that the human beings to be educated to-day are already saddled with a more or less debauched kinæsthesia, a condition in which psycho-physical reactions are abnormal and harmful. Satisfactory education is incompatible with abnormal and harmful reactions, and a teaching technique, therefore, to be satisfactory, must be one that will meet the needs of those who are beset with the varying and more or less serious defects in the employment of the psycho-physical mechanisms which are responsible for unsatisfactory and harmful reactions. We shall now attempt to outline some of these defects and to indicate the difficulties they present to both teacher and pupil in any attempt to teach or to learn something, and we will start by considering them in connexion with the child's activities at school.

I should first like to point out that, though there may be a large increase in the number of parents who do not need compulsion in the matter of sending their children to school, the idea that a child should go to school is too often a preconceived idea with them, not a reasoned conviction. It is probable that very few parents have given due consideration to the effect of sending a child to school, other than that it should be educated. To most people the educational process is one by means of which the child is to acquire knowledge and be put right in all matters where he is judged to be wrong. This judgment is usually the outcome of the combined experience of his teacher and parents, the former being influenced by the latter, as all parents have more or less fixed ideas in regard to the present and future needs of the child, and choose the school in accordance with their ideas in this particular.[32] They also have very definite ideas concerning the processes which should be involved, in spite of the fact that they have never had the experience that might have justified them in holding these fixed opinions. Further, it occurs to very few of them to consider whether, in this process of "education" (i.e., in certain specific directions) the child's fear reflexes will not be unduly and harmfully excited by the injunction that it must always try to "be right,"[33] indeed, that it is almost a disgrace to be wrong; that the teachers concerned do not even know how to prevent the child from acquiring the very worst psycho-physical use of itself whilst standing or sitting at its desk or table, pondering over its lessons, or performing its other duties; that on account of the methods of cramming and other means adopted in the act of learning, there is being cultivated a harmful psycho-physical condition—one result being recognized in a loss of memory—which in our time has developed to such a serious point that it has paved the way for the exploitation of educated people by means of various methods, such as "memory systems," etc.[34]

---

[32] Incidentally, I should like to say that in a properly constituted civilization based on a principle of conscious control, parents would be qualified by training and experience to know their child's needs, and, what is more to the point, they would know how to satisfy these, if need be.

[33]The idea of "right" is almost always associated with *product* or result, not with *method* of operation. We have only to listen to any lesson from this point of view to realize that the directions the child receives, such as "sit up straight," "speak out," "take a deep breath," "see how quietly you can walk," etc., are all specific "end-gaining" instructions which rarely include the correct *means whereby* he can carry them out. It is only when instructions include the correct "means-whereby" that the process of carrying them out involves the satisfactory use of the psycho-physical mechanisms concerned.

[34]All these systems being framed, however, on the "specific" or "end-gaining" principle, are devoid of the fundamentals of satisfactory psycho-physical development. Incidentally, in connexion with failing memory, the following is exceedingly interesting. We are all aware that a sluggish liver does not make for the best use of the "mental" powers, and we know people who, through bad habits of over-indulgence, have reached a stage of liver and kidney disorder when their reasoning processes are seriously interfered with, and they are conscious of a temporary comparative loss of memory. Facts such as these serve to remind us of the interdependence of "mental" and "physical" activity. If the vital functioning of the "physical" mechanisms and organs is inadequate, the organism becomes gradually more or less poisoned, and the "mental" machinery gradually less and less efficient. In such a case it is very difficult to understand in what mysterious way the ordinary memory system can enable one to remedy the "physical" disorders indicated, and if it does not, a successful result is highly improbable.

See, further, Chapter on "Memory and Feeling."

In this matter of sending children to school, we must realize that any undue excitement of the fear reflexes in the daily routine of school work has a very serious effect upon the respiratory processes,[35] which are so closely linked up with the emotions, and when in addition we consider the detrimental effect upon these processes of the defective use of the organism[36] during study at school desks and in school chairs (for in study, as in deep sleep, the respiratory processes are reduced to their minimum of activity), in standing, walking, and, in fact, during the assumption of any ordinary posture, we are faced with a problem which no scheme on a subconscious basis will solve. For when harmful conditions such as have been mentioned are present in the child, they will be found to constitute an impeding factor in all its general activities. In the attempt to improve its handwriting, for instance, new faults will be developed in the general use of the psycho-physical mechanisms, and the established defects will tend to become more pronounced. It is obvious that knowledge, acquired in this way, is being acquired at a cost represented by an interference with the general control, and particularly with the use of those psycho-physical mechanisms upon which respiratory control depends. With these conditions present, the child lacks the psycho-physical equipment essential to the best efforts in learning something. The gradual lowering of the respiratory and other vital processes during study is undoubtedly one of the impeding factors which make for the dreamy condition—often amounting almost to stupor—into which people of the student and orthodox "thinking class" drift.

I am ready to admit that there is a steadily growing minority of parents who want more for their children than for them to read and write, do sums, etc., and who will say that what they desire for them is a "complete and all-round development." I also admit that there have been changes and modifications in certain spheres of education, whilst in others attempts have been made to counter supposed evils or defects. These attempts, unfortunately, are too often merely a reaction from one extreme to another. But beyond this, the fatal defect in all such instances of attempted reforms on a subconscious plane is that they have been, and still are, based on the principle of a specific, not

[35] As Byron wrote: "Breathless as we stand when feeling most."

[36] This defective use will be even more pronounced when the arms are employed in the ordinary acts of life, particularly in the acts of writing, drawing, etc. The arm resting on the table or desk will be wrongly employed as a support for the body, and the arm, hand and fingers engaged in the movements necessary for the act of writing will also come in for criticism, the result being harmful to the child's organism *as a whole*, thereby seriously impeding progress in the act of learning penmanship, and, in many cases, making a satisfactory result practically impossible.

of a general development, and that whatever form the attempt may take in a particular school, we shall find that it has been worked out neither in relation to the child's organism *as a whole*, nor with any recognition of the fact that the child of to-day does not start life with the standard of co-ordination and sensory appreciation enjoyed by the children of, say, two hundred years ago.[37] Its psycho-physical mechanisms are not nearly as reliable, nor its ingenuity at a given age as great as theirs in relation to most psycho-physical acts in the practical way of life. As a result, by the time the ordinary child reaches school age, certain wrong uses of the psycho-physical mechanism have become established, constituting a serious condition which baffles the most thoughtful teachers.[38]

Anyone having a doubt in this connexion will be convinced by visiting any school with an expert capable of pointing out the defects of which we speak, and of indicating the influence of these defects upon the whole organism in daily activity. The head of an important preparatory school came to consult the writer in the hope that some solution might be found for what she rightly considered *the problem* of the school. She said that although all the most recent methods providing satisfactory environmental conditions, outdoor activity and opportunity for "free expression" had been adopted in this school, the problem still remained unsolved, whilst the urgency for its solution became more and more apparent to all concerned. She admitted that, until she had read *Man's Supreme Inheritance*, she could not understand why the active outdoor life did not serve to prevent or eradicate the physical defects and shortcomings in the children which gave cause for such serious consideration. But of what avail are good hygienic conditions, an outdoor life, a greatly-improved environment, "free activities" and "physical exercises," whilst the child that is to be given an "all-round development" under these conditions is actually allowed to use himself during his activities in ways which interfere to such an extent with the psycho-mechanics of his respiratory processes that these are working nearer to their minimum than to their maximum capacity, and this in spite of the fact that his teachers would unanimously agree that the proper working of these processes is the

---

[37]I have drawn attention to this fact in *Man's Supreme Inheritance.*

[38]As one teacher wrote: "No one who observes carefully the predominant characteristics of the present generation can fail to note:

"(1) Alarming imperfections of physique, i.e., defects of spine, wrong posture, lack of correct co-ordination of muscles in bodily acts, depressed stature, etc.

"(2) No less great limitations in the purely mental field, e.g., domination by a fixed idea, inability to apprehend and to respect other points of view, failure to grasp the essentials of freedom, etc. All this is symptomatic of some underlying cause."

most vital element in the child's development? [39]

The almost universal call for physical drill, or physical exercises, in schools, for training in posture, breathing exercises, etc., coming from parents, teachers and all concerned, is an admission that there is a great need in this direction, but, unfortunately, these methods will not give the necessary help. The harmful effects of the child's psycho-physical experiences, gained whilst at study, cannot be remedied by the performance of the movements involved in any forms of exercises, drill, posture, calisthenics, etc., for the defects resulting from these daily psycho-physical experiences are the manifestations of a badly adjusted and imperfectly co-ordinated machine, guided and controlled by a delusive sensory appreciation and therefore functioning much nearer to its minimum than to its maximum capabilities.

The problem is further complicated in that there has been and still is a continual increase in the educational demands which are being made upon the child, unavoidably, it is supposed, in the present stage of civilization. For the increase in the degree of mal-co-ordination present in the child continues in the same ratio as the difficulties to be overcome in any attempt to eradicate defects, whilst at the same time the degree of difficulty which the child will encounter in connexion with its lessons or other activities will be in accord with the degree of imperfect general functioning. This again means that the child, to ensure success, must of necessity devote more and more time to these subjects, with the result that increasing demands are being made upon him, involving longer hours of work and increased effort, and the increasing complications these imply. How can the psycho-physical mechanisms of the children meet these demands satisfactorily, when they are functioning much nearer to their minimum than to their maximum possibilities? And what is to happen if the educational demands continue to increase, whilst the psycho-physical possibilities of the children continue to decrease, as they surely will, unless the defects which make for badly co-ordinated use of the psycho-physical self are eradicated, and instead there is set in motion a process of genuine development on a plane of conscious control in the use of the organism?

We must remember also that every attempt on the part of the child to do something or to acquire knowledge makes a psycho-physical demand, and that the child's efforts, *when judged on a general and not a specific basis*, will always be in accordance with the standard of psycho-

[39]I must refer my reader to *Man's Supreme Inheritance* in regard to the failure of "physical exercises" and drill to eradicate such defects as are present. It is possible to prove by demonstration that even if a specific defect should chance to be eradicated, several others, often more harmful, will be cultivated during the process of eradication.

physical functioning of its organism. Where harmful conditions such as those we have indicated above are present in a child, the teacher, in any attempt to remedy *specific* defects (such as, for instance, defects in a child's handwriting) must take into account the standard of the general psycho-physical use of the child, otherwise the attempt will result not only in the development of new faults in this use, but also in a tendency to strengthen any old-established imperfect uses.

It follows, therefore, that in those cases where the psycho-physical mechanism is imperfect and functioning more or less inadequately, we cannot expect the best results in the conveyance or the acquisition of knowledge. There is a lack of co-ordination of the parts of the organism involved in the process called education, so that any attempts made to learn something or to learn to do something (and this applies equally to all processes of self-instruction) must tend to the cultivation of new psycho-physical defects and cannot fail to exaggerate the old ones. The child's early efforts in learning any simple subject which forms part of the curriculum are on a *specific* basis; that is, the child's work is planned for him from the beginning on "end-gaining" lines of teaching him to do specific things in specific ways, and of teaching him to try to get these specific things "right," and long ere the stage of adolescence is reached, this "end-gaining" procedure will have become established, associated with a bad psycho-physical attitude towards the acceptance of new ideas and new experiences, and too often with a serious deterioration in memory. When these defects and shortcomings are present, they constitute two impeding factors which could account for the general lack in the majority of adults to link up knowledge.[40] Knowledge is of little use in itself; it is the linking up of what we know with that which comes to us daily in the shape of new ideas and new experiences which is of value, and this ability to link up is inseparable from the processes concerned with remembering. In other words, the value of knowledge lies in our power to make use of it in association with the greater knowledge which should come to us as we increase in years of experience, and as we substitute reasoning for instinct and for what Professor Dewey calls "emotional gusts."

Our first consideration, therefore, in all forms of education must be

[40]I fully realize that efforts are being made to link up and correlate subjects in the school curriculum which were formerly taught as separate subjects, or to group various subjects round one central idea, as the teaching of history in connexion with drama, mathematics and carpentering, nature with the drawing lesson, etc. But this again is *specific* correlation, and does not affect the point I have raised as to the need for co-ordination of the child's organism as a whole and for the co-ordinated use of this organism in every activity and interest in life.

in regard to securing for the child the highest possible standard of psycho-physical functioning during his attempts to master the different processes which make up the educational scheme. In this way the child will make a fair start, and, what is more to the point, he will continue to improve the conditions involved, hand in hand with his efforts as a pupil in all other spheres of activity.

The plan of education we advocate is a comprehensive one, such as will not only meet the needs of the human creature at the present stage of his evolution, but will also meet his future needs, as he passes from this present stage of subconscious guidance and control through the progressive evolutionary stages which lead to a higher and still higher state of civilization. The test of man's advance in this connexion demands a consideration of

(1) the plane of consciousness reached in his recognition of incorrect psycho-physical use within the organism, and in the employment of that organism in all psycho-physical activity in every-day life;

(2) the standard of his ability to accept readily a new and expanding idea, when once he has become convinced of its value and of its superiority to older and long-cherished ideas, associated with a keen desire for the new experiences which go hand in hand with new and expanding ideas, and for that standard of psycho-physical development which will enable him to profit by the experiences;

(3) the standard of his ability to adapt himself to the rapid changes of environment in civilization with benefit, instead of detriment or injury, to his psycho-physical self;

(4) the standard of his ability to hold in abeyance the fear of giving up his job, in whatever profession, trade or calling this may be, and boldly to make the necessary change, should he find that the fundamental principles concerned are defective; and to make the necessary adjustments which are essential to the acceptance and assimilation of new and approved knowledge whilst going on with his job.

The foregoing serves to outline principles which are worthy of first consideration in all forms of education which are to meet satisfactorily the present and future needs of the human creature. There can be little doubt that the knowledge of the satisfactory and adequate use of the organism is of first importance, for it is upon this satisfactory and adequate use that the degree of our success depends in meeting the demands made upon us in educational and all other spheres of activity.

The consideration of principles in connexion with any plan of education leads naturally to the consideration of the technique, the *means whereby* these principles are to be carried out, and in the pages of this book we are concerned with the technique to be employed in putting the principles I have outlined to practical use in the work of re-education, co-ordination and readjustment on a conscious plane.

At this point it is necessary to remember that all teaching methods on the subconscious basis are formulated on the principle that if a pupil suffers from some defect, imperfection or peculiarity that needs to be eradicated, he must at once *do something* (usually with the help of a teacher) to eradicate the defect or defects. The teacher on a subconscious basis believes in this system for dealing with defects. It is his business to teach the pupil to do something to eradicate his defects, the "doing" in this connexion meaning to the pupil simply *the performance of a series of physical movements to be carried out in accordance with the pupil's conception of the teacher's instructions.* The fact that the teacher fails in this attempt in the great majority of cases may disturb him, but does not undermine his faith in his methods or change his attitude towards his original premiss. He may point to some successes, but unfortunately he lacks that keenness of observation, he has not reached that desirable state of awareness, which would reveal to him the fact that his success is merely a *specific* one and that, in the process of eradicating the particular defect, he has permitted the pupil to cultivate several others more harmful than the original, and of which teacher and pupil alike remain in blissful ignorance.

On the other hand, the whole procedure of teaching on a plane of constructive conscious control is based on the opposite principle, namely, that those who have developed a condition in which the sensory appreciation (feeling) is more or less imperfect and deceptive, cannot expect to succeed in remedying this condition by relying upon this same deceptive feeling for guidance in their efforts in re-education, readjustment and co-ordination, or in their attempts to put right something they know to be wrong with the psycho-physical organism. For immediately the child or adult attempts to perform any psycho-physical act, that use of himself which is the manifestation of his inherited and cultivated instincts (i.e., of his habits), becomes the dominating factor. It then follows that if a pupil is more or less badly co-ordinated, the use of his psycho-physical self will be imperfect and therefore more or less harmful. This means that he will be beset with defects, that his sensory appreciation (feeling) of what he is doing will be deceptive, and that immediately he makes any attempt to correct these defects, he will be at a still greater disadvantage in consequence of the lack of correct guidance through reliable sensory appreciation.

The significance of this in relation to education comes out fully if we follow our argument a step further. For if the foregoing is true (and I assert that it is capable of practical demonstration), it follows that in the case of a child who is found to experience difficulty in carrying out some simple activity, or to be suffering from certain defects and imperfections, it is of no use, indeed, it is unreasoning for its teachers to ask it to *do anything itself* with the aim of helping it over its difficulty, or of eradicating its defects, because (and this is the point that is overlooked in all schemes of reform or remedial work with which I have come in contact), *the only guidance the child has to rely upon in doing anything to carry out the teacher's instructions is the very same delusive subconscious guidance (unreliable sensory appreciation) that was instrumental in causing the defects to develop and become established in the first instance.* For all defects and imperfections are symptoms of a condition of mal-co-ordination and of maladjustment, a condition which will always be found to go hand in hand with the possession of an unreliable sensory appreciation. In the same way, we shall find that where a condition of unreliable sensory appreciation exists in the child or adult (and all that is written here applies with even greater force to the adult), there will also be present a condition of mal-co-ordination, in some form or other, and some incorrect adjustment. Any attempt, then, made by the child that is imperfectly co-ordinated to use its unreliable sensory appreciation as a guide in its efforts to do something in obedience to directions in order to correct a defect, is bound to result in some form of misdirected activity, accompanied by an increase of the original defect or imperfection, and by the undue development of the fear reflexes.

This brings us face to face with the demand for a teaching technique which will meet this difficulty, and such a technique involves correct manipulation on the part of the teacher in the matter of giving the pupil correct experiences in sensory appreciation, in the spheres of re-education, readjustment and co-ordination. Furthermore, in order to give these satisfactory sensory experiences, the teacher must himself be in possession of a reliable sensory mechanism and have gained the experience in re-education and co-ordination that is required for a satisfactory readjustment of the organism.

But in this connexion it must always be clearly understood that the correct sensory experiences to be acquired by means of this technique cannot be described in writing or by the spoken word in such a way as to be of practical value. As a friend of mine, a well-known scientific man, replied to a query in this connexion, "We cannot write a kinæsthesia, any more than we can write the sense of sound. We can only write the symbols of sound, notes of music, for instance."

It is necessary to emphasize this point, as it is one that is so constantly overlooked. Many people have said to me, for instance, with quite a friendly knowing look, "You know, that book of yours, *Man's Supreme Inheritance*, is quite a clever piece of work." When I ask them for their reason, the same answer is always forthcoming:—"Because you give us enough to make us interested in your theory and just lead us to the point where we realize we must go to you for lessons." It has happened in my experience over and over again that, after I have carefully explained to a pupil that he needed re-education because of his lack of reliable sensory appreciation, and have even shewn him by practical demonstration that he was actually developing harmful defects, because he was guiding himself in his movements by a deceptive "feeling," the pupil has turned to me and said, "Please give me some exercise that I can practise at home." Beyond this I have emphasized in my book the point that manipulation is necessary for the development and establishment of reliable sensory appreciation in the case of individuals who have developed defects, because in everything they are doing *themselves* by the usual methods to remedy these defects, they are guiding themselves by an unreliable sense of feeling, thus adding to the incorrect experiences which must always result from guidance by unreliable sensory appreciation. Yet in spite of all that I have written on this point, I have been criticized for "keeping things back," because I would not give in my book instructions and set exercises that people could *do* at home by themselves! In all such instances, I point out that I will not be guilty at this stage of my teaching experience of adding to the mass of literature on the subject of exercises, or take the grave responsibility for the harmful consequences which are certain to result from the practice of exercises, according to written instructions, by people whose sensory appreciation is unreliable and often positively delusive. The technique, therefore, in which we are interested has been developed throughout from the premiss that, if something is wrong with us, it is because we have been guided by unreliable sensory appreciation, leading to incorrect sensory experiences and resulting in misdirected activities.

These misdirected activities manifest themselves in the use of the psycho-physical mechanism in connexion with all the general activities of life, and in many varying ways according to our individual idiosyncrasies. They are influenced by and associated with our incorrect conceptions, our imperfect sensory appreciation, our unduly excited fear reflexes and uncontrolled emotions and prejudices, and our imperfectly adjusted mechanisms. These psycho-physical derangements in the process of formation are the forerunners of a psycho-physical attitude towards the conduct of life in general which must be considered perverted, and because these misdirected activities are so closely connected with this perverted attitude, they present a problem of great difficulty to both teacher and pupil in any endeavour to convey or acquire knowledge, particularly in regard to the satisfactory use of the psycho-physical mechanisms. I shall now go on to consider this problem in its relation to incorrect conception.

CHAPTER II

INCORRECT CONCEPTION

In the matter of conception, the first step is to convince the pupil that his present misdirected activities are the result of incorrect conception and of imperfect sensory appreciation (feeling).

Now, in this regard, I would at once warn those who are inexperienced in this matter that the pupil, as a rule, will not be convinced on this point by discussion and argument alone. A pupil will, indeed, often assure his teacher that he sees the argument, and, from his standpoint this statement may be true. But, in my experience, there is only one way by which a teacher can really convince a pupil that his sense of feeling is misleading him when he starts to carry out a movement, and that is *by demonstration upon the pupil's own organism.* A mirror should be used so that the pupil, as far as possible, can have ocular demonstration as well.

The next point of importance to be impressed upon the pupil is the necessity for listening carefully to the teacher's words, and for being quite clear as to the meaning that these words are intended to convey *before he attempts to act upon them.* This may seem a truism, but, as a matter of fact, it is at this point that we come up against a rock on which even a highly experienced teacher may make shipwreck. For, in every case, the pupil's conception of what his teacher is trying to convey to him by words *will be in accordance with his (the pupil's) psycho-physical make-up.*[41]

If, for instance, the pupil has fixed ideas in some particular direction, these fixed ideas must inevitably limit his capacity for "listening carefully" (a capacity which we are apt to take so much for granted), that is, for receiving the new ideas *as the teacher is trying to convey them to him.* In this connexion, therefore, a teacher in dealing with the shortcomings of a particular case must give due consideration to the pupil's fixed conceptions, otherwise these will greatly complicate the problem for both teacher and pupil. Certain of these fixed ideas are encountered in the

[41] In this sense it can be truly said that a pupil hears only what he wants to hear, because what he wants is decided by the standards fixed by his present habits.

case of almost every pupil; fixed ideas, for example, as to what constitutes the right and what the wrong method of going to work as a pupil; fixed ideas in regard to the necessity for concentration, if success is to attend the efforts of pupil and teacher; also a fixed belief (based on subconscious guidance), that, if a pupil is corrected for a defect, he should be taught *to do something* in order to correct it, instead of being taught, as a first principle, *how to prevent (inhibition) the wrong thing from being done.*

The teacher experienced in the work of re-education can diagnose at once, by the expression and use of the pupil's eyes, the degree of influence upon him of such conceptions, and at each step in the training he should take preventive measures to counteract this influence. It is absurd to try to teach a person who is in a more or less agitated or even anxious condition. We must have that calm condition which is characteristic of a person whose reasoning processes are operative.

The list of fixed conceptions given above might be increased a hundredfold. The peculiarities of fixed conceptions, like peculiarities of handwriting, differ greatly in different people, and the form they take depends, as in the case of handwriting again, upon the individual psycho-physical makeup.[42]

A teaching experience of over twenty-five years in a psycho-physical sphere has given me a very real knowledge of the psycho-physical difficulties which stand in the way of many adults who need re-education and co-ordination, and, as the result of this experience, I have no hesitation in stating that the pupil's fixed ideas and conceptions are the cause of the major part of his difficulties.

I will now take certain of these fixed conceptions from my teaching experience, because they are so wide-spread and have such far-reaching and harmful effects upon life in general, and I will begin with the habit which has become established in most pupils trained on a subconscious basis, and to which we have already referred, viz., *that of trying to correct one defect by doing something else.*

Illustration 1. "Doing It Right"

Let us suppose that a person decides that he will take lessons in re-education from a certain teacher and comes for the first lesson. The teacher proceeds to indicate to the pupil, firstly, the results of his diagnosis of the pupil's psycho-physical peculiarities, delusions and defects which he proposes to attempt to eradicate; and, secondly, the *means whereby* the eradication is to be effected.

[42]All that is written here about fixed conceptions applies equally to the teacher as to the pupil.

It invariably follows that by the time the teacher has concluded his statement, the pupil will have formed his own conception (often diametrically the reverse of his teacher's) of the facts disclosed, and unless he is a very unusual person, he will already have come to a decision in accordance with his preconceived ideas,

(1) as to the cause or causes underlying the facts disclosed;
(2) as to the ends that will be gained by the removal of these causes; and, most important of all,
(3) as to the means he will adopt in order to gain these ends.

In this last decision he will be influenced by his fixed belief that in order to secure the end he desires his first duty is *to do something* (as he understands "doing"), and *to do it right* (as he understands "doing it right"). This is not surprising, as it is probable that all his former teachers will have instilled into him from his earliest days the idea that when something is wrong, he must do something to try and get it right. Beyond this, he will have been told that, if he is conscientious, he will always try to be right, not wrong, so that this desire to "be right" will have become an obsession in which, as in so many other matters, his conscience must be satisfied.[43]

As soon as the teacher observes that the pupil (following out his fixed idea) is setting out to do something he thinks right to bring about the end he desires, he will point out to the pupil that, in trying to remedy his defects by "doing something" himself he is relying upon his own judgment, but that *his (the pupil's) judgment cannot be sound in this respect, based as it is on his previous incorrect sensory experiences.* The teacher will therefore advise the pupil to stop relying on his own judgment in these mat-

---

[43]If we think the matter out, we shall be forced to admit that in such matters a person's insistence on satisfying conscience is too often merely an attempt to unload responsibility. He is aware of certain orthodox ways of dealing with his difficulties. His own experience of these ways is that they have mostly ended in failure. Still he argues that if he tries them and they fail, he at least has done his best. In other words, he tries to satisfy his conscience, not his reasoning intelligence. He embraces this way of going to work because it is the easy way. If he once stopped to reason the thing out, and based his judgment on the experience gained from the knowledge of his previous failures, he would have to discard these orthodox plans and seek new ones. This would not be the easy way. It would be the difficult way. It would mean, among other things, a painful dissection of his psycho-physical peculiarities, defects, prejudices, sensory excesses, and these are to him just as much a manifestation of his malconditions as the diseased liver and kidney are in the case of the drunkard. To give his liver and kidneys a chance, the drunkard would have to give up drinking wine, but he has not the control to do this. So with the pupil in our illustration. He knows that certain psycho-physical habits are responsible for his condition, but these habits have become a part of him; they appeal to his perverted sense of feeling and so he will not make the effort to give them up.

ters, and, instead, to listen to the new instructions, and to allow the teacher to give him by means of manipulation the new correct sensory experiences.

The idea, however, of ceasing to do the wrong thing (as a preliminary measure in re-education) makes little or no appeal at first to the average pupil who, in most cases, goes on trying to "be right" in spite of his experience and of all that his teacher may say.[44]

There are many reasons for this, chief among them being, in my opinion, the fact to which I have already drawn the reader's attention, namely, that in our conception of *how* to employ the different parts of our mechanisms, we are guided almost entirely by a sense of feeling which is more or less unreliable. We get into the habit of performing a certain act in a certain way, and we experience a certain feeling in connexion with it which we recognize as "right." *The act and the particular feeling associated with it become one in our recognition.* If anything should cause us to change our conception, however, in regard to the manner of performing the act, and if we adopt a new method in accordance with this changed conception, we shall experience *a new feeling* in performing the act which we do not recognize as "right." We then realize that what we have hitherto recognized as "right" is wrong.

For instance, suppose the teacher, in trying to change some malcondition in the pupil, asks him to bend his knees. The pupil, thinking only of what his teacher asks him (the "end") and desiring to do it right (as he understands "doing it right" in connexion with the act of bending his knees) bends his knees, and bends them as he has always bent them, that is, with a great amount of unnecessary tension and pressure, interfering with his equilibrium, shortening his spine[45] (by increasing the curve, etc.), stiffening his neck, and so attains his end (the bending of his knees), but at the cost of undue strain and disadvantage in the use of the organism. I do not mean, of course, that the pupil is conscious of all this. He has probably never thought out how (the "means-whereby") he has performed such acts as "bending his knees," and though he knows in a general way that something is wrong with him (else it is improbable that he would be coming to a teacher at all), he has not associated this "something wrong" with anything that *he has been doing himself*, that is, with his own misdirected activities. Therefore, when he bends his knees in response to his teacher's request, he is not conscious of anything being wrong in his manner of doing it. He bends them as he has

[44]He is so possessed with the idea of "specific cure" that the principle of prevention (inhibition) is accepted by him at such a low valuation that, in ninety-nine cases out of a hundred, it will be ignored.

[45]See Chapter: "Illustration."

always been accustomed to bend them. This satisfies him, *it feels right to him.*

Now suppose that the teacher, after drawing the pupil's attention to the very disadvantageous manner in which he has been using himself during the process of bending his knees, gives him some help (into the details of which we will enter in the following chapters), and succeeds in inducing him to bend his knees to the best advantage in the general use of his mechanisms. When this occurs, the act of bending the knees *becomes, as far as this pupil is concerned, to all intents and purposes, a new act, bringing with it a new feeling.* This time the act is not what he is accustomed to, and so it *feels wrong* to him.

Henceforward, whenever the conception of bending the knees comes to this pupil (whether in response to his teacher's directions or through his own initiative), the choice lies before him of bending them in the old way (i.e., at great disadvantage to himself) and "feeling right," or of changing the manner in which he performs the act and "feeling wrong." As a little girl said quaintly when this point was explained to her in connexion with something she was doing, "Oh, I see! If I feel at all, I must feel wrong. If I don't feel wrong, I mustn't feel." Unfortunately, the average adult pupil, unlike the little girl, does not "see," or, if he does, he will not act accordingly. Indeed, we have to face the fact that the adult, as a rule, does not like a new feeling; in some cases he is positively *afraid* of it. A new "feeling" gives him a sense of insecurity when he experiences it in connexion with acts that he has been accustomed to associate with a different feeling all his life. This sense of insecurity is particularly marked in connexion with the maintenance of his equilibrium in the acts of standing, walking, etc., in accordance with the newly acquired feeling.[46] And so it comes about that, when a pupil is faced with the alternative of using his mechanisms badly and "feeling right," or of using them well and "feeling wrong," he is apt, as we say, to lose his head, does not stop, therefore, to consider (that is, inhibit) and falls back upon "feeling right."

This is only one example of the difficulty which a pupil's incorrect conceptions and misdirected activities in certain directions will present both to him and his teacher in any endeavour to convey or acquire knowledge in the psycho-physical sphere. In such a case as the one we have cited, the pupil's fixed ideas as to what constitutes "right" and what

---

[46]Incidentally, I would point out that, in cases where a person develops a "phobia" in connexion with crossing streets, travelling by train, crossing bridges or open spaces, being alone in a room, being unduly alarmed by ordinary noises etc., there is already present in that person a serious condition of unsatisfactory psycho-physical equilibrium, which accounts for the susceptibility to the particular stimulus responsible for the "phobia."

"wrong" in certain conditions will produce a deadlock. For how can new and correct experiences be given to a pupil who, in all the movements he makes, is working subconsciously to reproduce certain feelings that he has grown used to and likes? The situation is one that no teacher, be he ever so expert, can deal with satisfactorily, one from which the pupil cannot possibly be extricated, until he stops trying to get things right, stops, that is, working blindly for his *ends*, and gives thought instead to the new *means*[47] given to him by his teacher, *whereby* his ends can be attained.

Illustration 2. Doing Things "His Way"

I will now take an equally fixed and unreasoning conception which is common to most pupils who need re-education and co-ordination, namely, their fixed ideas *as to what they can and cannot do.*

Their judgment on these points, of course, can only be based on their previous misleading experiences, but in spite of this fact they are not ready to change their ideas, even when their teacher has given them practical proof that their judgment on these points is not to be relied on. Now, it would seem reasonable that any pupil who decides to take lessons of a certain teacher because he believes him able to help him to overcome some difficulty would take that teacher's word for it as to whether he is capable or not of doing what he is asked to do at a particular point. But too often the opposite is the case. For if a teacher during a lesson should ask a pupil to do something which happens to be among the things which, in the days before he came for lessons, he was convinced he could not do (i.e., his difficulty), the pupil will immediately baulk. He may not openly refuse to follow out the new instructions given to him, but, what amounts to the same thing, he will make a "mental reservation," as we say, when he receives them. The reason for this is that he subconsciously believes that he knows more than his teacher about the things he can or cannot do. So that when he receives the instructions, he starts to carry them out on a plan of his own, that is, in "his way," and so intent is he on this plan that the new instructions do not reach his consciousness, that is, they do not make upon him that due impression which is required for carrying them out satisfactorily, or even for remembering them accurately.

Curiously enough, a pupil's confidence in "his way" of doing things is not in the least disturbed by the fact that "his way" has never worked well in the past, and, as his teacher is careful to point out to him, can never work well in the future, for the simple reason that *"his way" is essen-*

[47]The matter of these new means will be dealt with in the next chapter.

tially wrong for his purpose, that, in fact, what he thinks of as a "difficulty" is not a difficulty in itself, but simply the result of "his way" of going to work.

Further, the teacher will point out that any reason he may have had in the past for clinging to "his way" of doing things no longer exists, because the practical help that the teacher is able to give him places him in a totally new position in regard to his "difficulty"; so that all he has to do is to stop trying to overcome his difficulty "his way," and, instead, to remember and follow out the new instructions, by which means he will obtain the result he desires.

This cannot be called an unreasonable proposition, if we have once allowed that a teacher should be trusted to know more than his pupil about the particular matter in hand. In my experience, however, the pupil who has been brought up on subconscious methods is not attracted, as a rule, by this form of reasoning when faced with a "difficulty."

And so it comes about that, although a teacher may demonstrate to a pupil over and over again that he will never be able to do what he is trying to do *unless he changes his "means-whereby"* (gives up, that is, "his way" of doing it), the pupil will still go on trying to overcome his difficulty "his way."[48]

Similarly, although a teacher may assure his pupil over and over again, that, if only he will adopt the new means given to him, *he will be able to do quite easily the thing he has always believed he cannot do*, the pupil will not make any attempt to adopt the new means. He will go on, in fact, trying to be right "his way," and always being wrong. More unreasonable still, after a certain time he will actually begin to worry because he finds that he is not getting on, that "his way" is not working. Could anything be more unreasonable?

Suppose a man starts out to reach a certain destination and comes to a place where the road branches into two. Not knowing the way, he takes the wrong road of the two and gets lost. He asks the way of someone he meets and is told to go straight back to the crossroads and take the other road, which will lead him directly to the place he wants to reach. What should we say if we heard that the man had gone back to the crossroads as directed, but had there concluded that he knew better after all than his adviser, had taken again his old road, and again got lost, and had done this thing not once or twice, but over and over again? Still more, what should we say if we heard that he was worrying dread-

[48]It must be pointed out that in such instances as the one we are discussing, the pupil's "right way" is the wrong way. The right way (that is, the teacher's right way) is the very last that would ever be recognized by the pupil as the "right way," because this right way has never yet come within the pupil's experiences.

fully because he kept getting lost, and seemed no nearer to getting to his destination?

I can see the reader's look of scepticism as he reads this and assures himself that he, at any rate, could not be guilty of the crime of *not really attempting to do* that which he knows he *can* do, or *of not ceasing to try and do* that which the experience of hours, days, nay, of years, has proved to be *the impossible* in his particular case. Yet this is more or less what happens in the case of every pupil, even of those who are accounted the most intelligent, the most highly educated, the most scientifically trained, and this serves to strengthen my conviction that the principles underlying present methods of education are erroneous. Indeed, it would seem that our educational systems, our methods of training in scientific and professional spheres, have tended actually to cultivate and establish the defect to which I have referred. To call it a defect is to use a word that is inadequate to express what really amounts to the loss of one-half of our original psycho-physical endowment by the gradually decreasing use of the invaluable process called inhibition. And I repeat that the comparative loss of this most valuable potentiality is chiefly due to the erroneous principles which underlie our teaching methods in all spheres. Those who are responsible for these methods have not realized the importance of holding the balance true in every sphere of life between the desire to do (volition) and the ability to check that desire (inhibition).

The words volition and inhibition are in constant use in these pages and I wish at this point to make it clearly understood that they are used merely as names for two respective acts, volition standing for the act of *responding* to some stimulus (or stimuli) to psycho-physical action (doing), and inhibition standing for the act of *refusing to respond* to some stimulus (or stimuli) to psycho-physical action (not doing). In other words, volition is used to name *what we intend to do*, and inhibition to name *what we refuse to do*, that is, to name what we wish to hold in check, what we wish to *prevent*.

We are not interested here in any controversy concerned with the problem as to whether or not volition and inhibition are different manifestations of the same force, or even as to what this force is, any more than the engineer who is using electricity as a power to a particular end is immediately interested as to what electricity is. We prophesy, however, that before we have acquired accurate knowledge as to the latter, we may possibly have solved the former by means of that consciously acquired knowledge which is coming to us through the practical understanding of our psycho-sensory potentialities upon which a higher and higher standard of human psycho-physical functioning depends.

In the sense, then, implied by a process enabling one to stop, a process concerned not with "ends," however good in themselves, but with the *means whereby* these "ends" can be brought about, I maintain that there is a lack of inhibition in all spheres. In no sphere, however, has the lack of inhibitory development been fraught with such danger as in matters concerned with the actual use of the psycho-physical mechanism in the activities of every-day life, for the lack of this development tends to produce in the individual a state of unbalanced psycho-physical functioning throughout the whole organism. Indeed, all our methods of educational training make for rigidity rather than mobility in educational use. Small wonder, then, that adults in whom such psycho-physical conditions have become established in childhood, manifest, where their activities are concerned, an almost total lack of the most ordinary common sense, associated with unreliable sensory appreciation.

Illustration 3. Not Seeing Ourselves as Others See Us

Perhaps the most striking and at the same time the most pathetic instance of human delusion is to be found in the human creature's attitude towards his own psycho-physical defects, disadvantages, peculiarities, etc., on one hand, and towards his merits, advantages and natural gifts on the other. "To thine own self be true," is an inspiring incentive when the human creature's co-ordinated psycho-physical development has reached a point where that self cannot be duped by its sensations.

As a striking instance in this field of human delusion, we will take the attitude of the stutterer towards the things he thinks of as "right" or "wrong" in himself, when he is faced with the practical problem of speaking in every-day life. The case to which I refer is just one instance of many that have come within the writer's experience during investigations made in the past thirty years. The pupil, in this particular case, was what is generally called a bad stutterer, but he made rapid progress during his lessons, and in an unusually short space of time was able to speak without any sign of stuttering as long as he spoke slowly. He reached a point where he could carry on a conversation with his teacher without being troubled with the old defects, provided that he enunciated the words slowly and deliberately.

The teacher then said, "I want you to speak in the way that you are speaking to me now, during your conversations throughout the whole day." The pupil at once became agitated, thus disturbing temporarily his new and developing control, and relapsed into his old way of stuttering, as he replied, "Oh! I couldn't do that; everyone would notice me!"

Now, if we try to analyse the condition of a person who can seriously make a remark like this (and the pupil was quite sincere, he meant it), we shall see that his agitation caused him to revert to a condition associated with his previous mal-co-ordination, in which he had been accustomed to hypnotize himself where the facts of his shortcomings and peculiarities were concerned. We may try to explain his remark by saying that he had become so used to the conditions of his stuttering, that he no longer cared what "the other fellow" thought about it, or else that he had determined to ignore the disagreeable fact that he stuttered, and in this way had deluded himself into thinking that the "other fellow" did not notice his contortions.[49] The fact remains that he had reached such a stage of defective sensory appreciation and self-hypnotic indulgence that his whole outlook was topsy-turvy. He no longer saw things as they were, and was out of communication with reasoning, where his consciousness of his defects was concerned. He was therefore able to persuade himself that *the normal condition would be conspicuous, whilst the abnormal would pass unnoticed. In this he was relying almost entirely on his perverted sense of feeling.* The point on which we should lay particular stress is that the condition of delusion and self-deception indicated in this illustration will be found to be more or less present in all people who are imperfectly co-ordinated and have an unreliable sensory appreciation.

Illustration 4. "Out of Shape"

In connexion with unreliable sensory appreciation and with perverted ideas or conceptions of what is "right" or "wrong," where the human creature's uses of his own mechanisms are concerned, the following is a most significant illustration.

A little girl who had been unable to walk properly for some years was brought to the writer for a diagnosis of the defects in the use of the psycho-physical mechanisms which were responsible for her more or less crippled state. When this had been done, a request was made that a demonstration should be given to those present of the manipulative side of the work (the child, of course, to be the subject to be manipulated), so that certain readjustments and co-ordinations might be temporarily secured, thus shewing, in keeping with the diagnosis, the possibilities of

[49]This is the opposite delusion of that of the person who becomes self-conscious over a comparatively unnoticeable peculiarity. For example, a pupil will exaggerate to himself a minor, and comparatively unnoticeable, peculiarity to such a degree that he becomes self-conscious about it and imagines that everywhere he goes people are looking at him on account of it, whereas the defect is so slight that it would not be noticed by outsiders. I have pointed out in the chapter entitled "Individual Errors and Delusions," in *Man's Supreme Inheritance*, the harmful effects that may follow a person's misguided attempts to conceal or change characteristics which they believe to be very serious drawbacks to their appearance, but which, compared with other very serious defects which they completely overlook, are relatively minor peculiarities.

re-education on a general basis in a case of this kind. The demonstration was successful from this point of view. For the time being the child's body was comparatively straightened out, that is, without the extreme twists and distortions that had been so noticeable when she came into the room. When this was done, the little girl looked across at her mother and said to her in an indescribable tone, "Oh! Mummie, he's pulled me *out of shape*."

Here, indeed, is food for reflection for all who are concerned in any attempt to eradicate psycho-physical defects! In accordance with this poor little child's judgment, her crookedness was straightness, her sensory appreciation of her "out-of-shape" condition was that it was "in shape." Imagine, then, what would be the result of her trying to get anything "right" by doing something herself, as she had always tried and had always been urged to try to do, whilst practising remedial exercises according to the directions and under the guidance of a teacher. Small wonder that all attempts to teach her had resulted in failure!

Consideration of the foregoing cannot but lead us to a full realization of what would have been the psycho-physical condition of such a child when she reached adolescence, if the orthodox methods of teaching in all spheres had been employed to help her. The child's remark is proof positive that, where her defects were concerned, her ideas and conceptions were dominated by her sensory appreciation, and that this sensory appreciation was not only unreliable but actually delusive. Her experiences in connexion with the functioning of her organism were consequently incorrect and harmful experiences, and as her judgment in these spheres was the result of these experiences, little wonder that her judgment of what was right and what wrong in her case was not only practically worthless, but constituted a positive danger to her future development. Unless in such cases a child is re-educated and co-ordinated on a basis of conscious control, it cannot acquire a new and reliable sensory appreciation, and, lacking this, it will grow up employing guiding sensations which are delusive and which tend to become more and more so with the advance of time. Incorrect experiences and bad judgment will be associated with this delusive guidance of the mechanisms in the functioning of the organism, and all its efforts in the different spheres of the activities of life will be in accordance with this functioning.

* * * * *

The point that comes out clearly in all these illustrations is *that conceptions which are mainly influenced by unreliable sensory appreciation, acting and reacting subconsciously and harmfully on the processes involved, are incorrect con-*

ceptions, and that in these cases unreliable sensory appreciation goes hand in hand with incorrect and deceptive experiences in the psycho-physical functioning.

And when we remember that (as we saw in the case of the little girl of the last illustration) our judgment is based on experience, we must also see that where this experience is incorrect and deceptive, the resulting judgment is bound to be misleading and out of touch with reality. *We have to recognize*, therefore, *that our sensory peculiarities are the foundation of what we think of as our opinions, and that, in fact, nine out of ten of the opinions we form are rather the result of what we feel* [50] *than what we think.*

Our emotional defects also are linked up with our sensory peculiarities, so that, given the slightest disturbance in these directions, we must be temporarily thrown into a danger zone[51] where serious and uncontrolled psycho-physical conditions prevail.

We can now see how far this line of thought has brought us. For the fact that emerges from all these considerations is that our approach to life generally, our activities, beliefs, emotions, opinions, judgments in whatever sphere, *are conditioned by the preceding conceptions, which are associated with the individual use of the psycho-physical mechanisms and conditioned by the standard of reliability of our individual sensory appreciation.*

This is the great fact which must be realized by our leaders in educational, religious, moral, social, political, and all other spheres of human activities before there can be any "uplifting" of the human creature out of the present chaotic conditions. We all think and act (except when forced to do otherwise) in accordance with the peculiarities of our particular psycho-physical make-up. We read a particular paper each morning because the policy of that paper is the one we believe in, and we can read there what we want to read; we cultivate friendships with people who think as we think, and we ignore or are antagonized by those who do not; the preacher attracts to church only those who want to go to church; we start to read a book, but immediately we reach a

---

[50] It is only reasonable to conclude that it is because the opinions of most people are much more the manifestation of their sensory peculiarities (feeling) than of their reasoning processes that we find so many varied and conflicting opinions held by people about a single simple point, or serious subject. It is positively alarming that reasoning plays so small a part in most of the opinions we hold, and in our judgment with regard to things that matter. It is for this reason that we find ourselves in such a fearful muddle after two thousand years of struggle towards a better standard of psycho-physical functioning, struggle which it was hoped would bring in an era of goodwill, universal unity, tolerance and mutual understanding.

[51] It only needs a certain number of repetitions of harmful experiences, such as are alluded to above, to produce one or other of the different phases which we place within the borderland of insanity. Many phases of this development of temporary insanity are accompanied by violent physical manifestations.

point with which we disagree, our more or less debauched kinæsthesia cannot control the impulses which, when set in motion, put us out of communication with our reasoning. Yet in spite of all this, books are written, lectures given, sermons preached, speeches made in the belief that ideas which are given out by these means can be satisfactorily assimilated by hearers or readers, and that good ideas may thus be passed on for the uplifting of mankind in social, religious, political and other spheres of activity.

Here we have a great delusion. For, as we have shewn, our degree of ability to assimilate a new and unfamiliar idea, or to overcome our prejudices in connexion with our cherished ideas and beliefs, depends upon our individual conception of such ideas and beliefs, and this conception is conditioned by the standard of individual psycho-physical co-ordination and of reliability of the sensory appreciation. Had this fact not been overlooked, writers, lecturers, preachers, orators, etc. would long since have shewn some practical interest in the *means whereby* their hearers and readers could reach such a standard of functioning of the psycho-physical organism that they would be able to assimilate satisfactorily new ideas and teachings. For how, I ask, can those who have developed a condition of unreliable sensory appreciation (with all the incorrect experiences, beliefs, and judgments that we now know to be inevitably associated with this condition) assimilate satisfactorily ideas that do not fit in with these experiences? Correct apprehension and reliable sensory appreciation go hand in hand.[52]

The mass is made up of individuals, and reliable sensory appreciation cannot be given on the mass-teaching principle or by precept or exhortation. This can only be done by individual teaching and individual work. Moreover, people who are massed together are apt to be governed by the "herd-instinct," and we need to help man to evolve beyond that influence as soon as possible, and to this end we must have conscious and individual development.

---

[52]As a friend, a member of the medical profession, wrote to me recently: "I am getting more and more convinced that people can learn only what they know."

CHAPTER III

IMPERFECT SENSORY APPRECIATION

THE problem, then, before us is to find a *means whereby* a reliable sensory appreciation can be developed and maintained throughout the organism, and the basis for my argument is that both in education and in re-education this must be brought about in every case by the reliance of the individual, not upon subconscious, but upon *conscious, reasoning* guidance and control.

For we find that the human creature, subjected to the present processes of civilization, develops defects and imperfections in the use of the organism, even in cases where a reliable sensory appreciation *has already existed* on a subconscious basis, whilst in the much larger number of cases, where defects have already been developed, we find that satisfactory results cannot be secured unless during the process a new and reliable sensory appreciation is being gradually acquired. Almost all civilized human creatures have developed a condition in which the sensory appreciation (feeling) is more or less imperfect and deceptive, and it naturally follows that it cannot be relied upon in re-education, readjustment and co-ordination, or in our attempts to put right something we know to be wrong with our psycho-physical selves. The connexion[53] between psycho-physical defects and incorrect sensory guidance must therefore be recognized by the teacher in the practical work of re-education. This recognition will make it impossible for him to expect a pupil to be able to perform satisfactorily any new psycho-physical act *until the new correct experiences in sensory appreciation involved have become established.*

I will now endeavour to outline as clearly as possible the general scheme which I advocate in connexion with the development of reliable sensory appreciation, first setting out the principles on which the scheme is based, then giving an illustration which will shew the appli-

[53]The recognition of this vital connexion marks the point of departure between methods of teaching on a conscious and on a subconscious basis.

cation of these principles to the practical work of co-ordination and re-education.

First, then, this scheme demands in particular on the part of the teacher a recognition of the almost alarming dominance of the pupil's psycho-physical processes by an incorrect sensory appreciation during the attempted performance of any psycho-physical activity. It is therefore of primary importance that the teacher should recognize and endeavour to awaken his pupil to the fact of his (the pupil's) unreliable sensory appreciation, and that during the processes involved in the performance of the pupil's practical work, he should cultivate and develop in him the new and reliable sensory appreciation upon which a satisfactory standard of co-ordination depends.

To this end the mode of procedure is as follows. The teacher, having made his diagnosis of the cause or causes of the imperfections or defects which the pupil has developed in the incorrect use of himself, uses expert manipulation to give to the pupil the new sensory experiences required for the satisfactory use of the mechanisms concerned, the while giving him the correct guiding orders or directions which are the counterpart of the new sensory experiences which he is endeavouring to develop by means of his manipulation.

This procedure constitutes the *means whereby* the teacher makes it possible for the pupil to *prevent* (inhibition) the misdirected activities which are causing his psycho-physical imperfections. In this work the inhibitory process must take first place, and remain the primary factor in each and every new experience which is to be gained and become established during the cultivation and development of reliable sensory appreciation upon which a satisfactory standard of co-ordination depends.

With this aim in view, that is, the prevention of misdirected activities, the teacher from the outset carefully explains to the pupil that his part in this scheme is very different from that which is usually assigned to pupils under other teaching methods. He tells the pupil that, on receiving the directions or guiding orders, he must not attempt to carry them out; that, on the contrary, *he must inhibit the desire to do so in the case of each and every order which is given to him.* He must instead project the guiding orders as given to him whilst his teacher at the same time, by means of manipulation, will make the required readjustments and bring about the necessary co-ordinations, in this way performing for the pupil the particular movement or movements required, and giving him the new reliable sensory appreciation and the very best opportunity possible to connect the different guiding orders before attempting to put them into practice. This linking-up of the guiding orders or directions is all-important, for it is the counterpart of that linking-up of the parts of the organism which constitutes what we call co-ordination. The aim of re-education on a general basis is to bring about at all times and for all purposes, not a series of correct positions or postures, but *a co-ordinated use of the mechanisms in general.*

The second point to be noted in connexion with the technique we are advocating is that the directions or guiding orders given to the pupil are based in every case on the principle of ceasing to work in blind pursuit of an "end," and of attending instead to the *means whereby* this "end" can be attained. We have already considered this principle in its general application, but I am anxious to lay stress upon it again at this point, because it is of the utmost importance that the pupil should both accept this principle and apply it to his work in the sphere of re-education, for by no other method can he get the better of his old subconscious habits, and build up consciously the new and improved condition which he is anxious to bring about.

If we consider for a moment, we shall see the reason for this. For if the pupil thinks of a certain "end" as desirable and starts to pursue it directly, he will certainly take the course of action in regard to it that he has been accustomed to take in like conditions. In other words, he will follow his habitual procedure in regard to it, and should that procedure happen to be a bad one for the purpose (and the fact that he needs re-education proves this to be the case), he only strengthens the incorrect experiences in connexion with it by using this procedure again. If, on the other hand, the pupil *stops himself* from going to work in his usual way (inhibition), and proceeds to replace his old subconscious means by the new conscious means which his teacher has given him, and which he has therefore every reason to believe will bring about the desired result, he will have taken the first and most important step towards the breaking-down of a habit, and towards that constructive, conscious and reasoning control which tends towards a mastery of the situation.[54]

It is therefore impressed on the pupil from the beginning that, as the essential preliminary to any successful work on his part, *he must refuse to work directly for his "end" and keep his attention entirely on the means whereby this end can be secured.*

In the illustration which will shortly be given, it will be noticed that it is left to the teacher's discretion whether, in the case of a particular evolution, the pupil shall or shall not be told beforehand what the "end" is for which he and the teacher are working. But in either case everything possible is done to convince him that the "end" does not matter, because given:—

[54]This applies equally to the breaking of habit in every sphere of activity.

(1) The teacher's knowledge of the correct means whereby the particular "end" can be secured,

(2) The pupil's correct apprehension and conscious repetition of the guiding orders or directions relating to these "means-whereby,"

(3) The manipulation by the teacher who, with his expert hands, gives to the pupil the reliable sensory appreciation which should result from such directive orders, it is then merely a matter of time[55] before the desired end will be secured. In other words, the pupil is asked to take care of the "means," and the "end" will take care of itself.

In this way all responsibility for the final result is taken off the pupil. He has no "end" to work for, and therefore nothing to get right. All that is asked of him is, when he receives a guiding order, to *listen and wait*; to wait, because only by waiting can he be certain of preventing himself from relapsing into his old subconscious habits, and to listen, so that he learns to remember gradually and connect up the guiding orders which are the counterpart of the *means whereby* the teacher is employing to bring about the desired "end." In other words, he is asked to adopt consciously a principle of prevention as the basis of his practical work, and in every other way to leave the teacher a free hand.

Now it would seem that this procedure, by relieving the pupil from all responsibility as to results, should, from any common-sense point of view, relieve him also from strain and anxiety; and those pupils who are satisfied that they do not know how to put themselves right, and are therefore willing to remain quietly giving themselves certain guiding orders or directions at the prompting of the teacher, but leaving to him all responsibility in the matter of enabling them to bring about the desired result, are able to gain the new and correct experiences without strain and with a gradually increasing sense of power and control.

But the teacher experienced in the work of re-education on a general basis is well aware of the difficulties which pupils actually make for themselves in this procedure, for the immediate call of instinctive habit is so insistent that unless the pupil learns to resist that call by bringing into use and developing his power to inhibit, he is almost certain to fall

[55]In this connexion the length of time that may be required in the process of re-education before the new and correct experiences can become established has proved a stumbling-block to some enquirers; but here again, if we reason the matter out, we shall see that the ability to break with habits that are sometimes very long-established must depend upon certain natural aptitudes and qualities in the pupil, and especially upon the standard of acuteness of his sense perceptions, and of the development of his ability to inhibit.

back into his old and harmful habit of blindly pursuing his "end," which means that he forgets to project his directive orders (the "means-whereby") and falls back again for guidance upon his unreliable and delusive sensory appreciation (feeling).

And it is rare in my experience to find adult pupils who are awake to the necessity of *preventing* themselves from falling back into their old subconscious habits, even though the necessity for this is proved to them over and over again. Very few, again, have any idea of giving themselves a guiding order or direction without making an attempt to carry it out. They do not separate the order they are asked to give from the act or acts of which it is the forerunner. Therefore, as soon as they are asked to give a certain continuous order, they rush impulsively into action according to their habitual subconscious use of the parts concerned. This relapse into old habits is exactly what the teacher asks the pupil to prevent, because it renders a successful result impossible from the outset, and reinforces all the incorrect experiences associated by the pupil with this use of the parts, the very experiences that the teacher is endeavouring to replace by new and correct ones.

Let us take, for example, the case of a pupil who has been accustomed to stiffen the muscles of his neck in all his daily activities. His teacher points this out to him, and explains that this habit of stiffening his neck has come about because he is endeavouring to make his neck perform the functions of other parts of his psycho-physical mechanism, so that it is not an isolated defect, but connected with other harmful imperfections in the use of himself. His stiffened neck, in fact, is merely a symptom of general mal-co-ordination in the use of the mechanisms, and any direct attempt to relax it means that he is dealing with it as a "cause" and not as a "symptom," and such an attempt will result in comparative failure unless a satisfactory co-ordinated use of the mechanism in general is restored. The teacher further explains that, as the pupil's sensory appreciation is unreliable,[56] it is unlikely that he will be able to do anything himself to remedy these defects, but that if he will inhibit his desire to stiffen his neck, and give himself the guiding orders or directions to relax it, the teacher will be able by means of manipulation to bring about such a general readjustment of his body that, as a result, his neck will be relaxed.

[56]In this regard, it is significant that the pupil whose sensory appreciation in connexion with the use of his organism is most unreliable (the pupil, for example, who "feels" that his head is going forward when he is carefully putting it back) is the one who is most unwilling to believe that he really does not know what he is doing with himself, and who, in spite of all remonstrances, will persist in trying to carry out the orders himself, instead of inhibiting this desire and allowing the teacher to assist him in carrying them out.

If, after this explanation, the pupil gives himself the order to relax his neck (i.e., inhibits his desire to stiffen it), his teacher, provided he has the necessary knowledge and experience, will be able to assist him to bring about *those general conditions upon which relaxation of the neck depends.* If, on the other hand, the pupil forgets to inhibit, and so, when he is asked to order his neck to relax, tries to relax it *by direct means* (i.e., according to his own idea of relaxing it), he will in this attempt either do exactly what he has always done with his neck (i.e., stiffen it), or else bring about in one or more parts, or perhaps in the whole organism, a more or less collapsed condition, and until he stops trying to relax it by direct means, the teacher, be he ever so expert, will be able to do little towards bringing about those conditions which make for a satisfactory state of relaxation of the neck.

Another difficulty which pupils make for themselves is in connexion with the giving of guiding orders or directions. They speak sometimes as if it were a strange and new thing to ask them to give themselves orders, forgetting that they have been doing this subconsciously from their earliest days, else they would not be able to stand up without help, much less move about. The point that is new in the scheme we are considering is that the pupil is asked consciously to give himself orders, evolved from a consideration of the requirements, not of a subconscious, but of a conscious, reasoning use of the organism, orders and directions, moreover, the satisfactory employment of which depends on the pupil's clear understanding (1) as to which of these orders are primary, to be given, but not to be carried out (inhibition), and (2) as to which are to follow and to be actually carried out.

To make this clear let us suppose that a pupil is asked by his teacher to sit down. Now if he obeys this order at once and sits down, he will be guided in doing so by the unreliable sensory appreciation established in connexion with the performance of the act in his case; that is, he will simply repeat his usual faulty subconscious manner of sitting down. The object of his re-education is to eradicate such psycho-physical faults, and so, as soon as he is asked to sit down, he immediately says "No," *and gives himself the order not to sit down*, thereby inhibiting the misdirected activity hitherto connected with the act, a procedure which prevents indulgence in the old subconscious faults.

The old faulty activity being prevented by the processes just indicated, the pupil will then proceed to give his attention to the different guiding or directing orders which the teacher considers essential to the correct direction and control of those psycho-mechanics (the correct "means-whereby") concerned with the satisfactory use of the organism as a whole in the act of sitting down. *These are the orders to be ultimately carried out by the pupil.*

It follows, then, that the orders which are to be given, but not to be carried out, are those which, if carried out, would result in the habitual faulty use of the mechanisms. They can therefore be referred to as "preventive orders." All orders which follow preventive orders are to be carried out (at first by the teacher), for if the teaching technique is reliable, such orders will be concerned with the correct *means whereby* the new and co-ordinated use of the mechanism can be secured.

I have already pointed out that children from the first moment of school life onward manifest a lack of inhibitory development, and the fact that in most cases they learn to obey orders at once,[57] without stopping to consider the "why and the wherefore" is a contributing factor to this harmful condition.

As a result of this early training, many pupils have become so accustomed to react quickly and subconsciously to any directions they receive, or to any idea that comes to them, that this quick and unthinking reaction has become a habit with them that they find hard to break.

And so, when pupils insist that giving orders is a difficulty, what they really mean is that because of their long-established habit of reacting quickly and unthinkingly to a direction, a habit fostered by years of training, they find it difficult to stop, to wait, to be content just to give orders and to say "No," when the impulse comes to carry the orders out. In other words, they find it difficult not to want to be obedient, not to want to be right, not to work directly for their end. The difficulty, however, as in the case of most human difficulties, lies, not in the thing itself, but in the "breaking of a habit," the indulgence of which not only impedes the pupil's progress, but, if persisted in, makes it impossible for him to achieve his desired end.

It will be found that in every case a pupil's success in achieving an end will depend upon his practical recognition of the fact that only by continually attending to the "means-whereby" essential to the successful achievement of his "end" can a satisfactory result be secured. This applies equally,

> (1) whether the pupil is in the early stages of his work, where he is asked merely to give orders and to leave the carrying-out of these orders to the teacher;

[57]I know that I shall be told that if children are to be taught to inhibit in the sense in which I use the word, i.e., the prevention of misdirected activities, so much time will be taken up in this part of the work that they will not be able to get through their studies. Children have said to me more than once in this connexion: "I could not stop like this at school. They tell us to hurry." In answer I can only say that time spent in teaching children to inhibit impulses to unreasoning activity to which otherwise they must later on become slaves is time not lost, but actually saved.

(2) whether he has reached a later stage where, under his teacher's supervision, he is gradually developing a reliable sensory appreciation upon which he can rely in carrying out the orders himself; or

(3) whether he is working by himself at his ordinary activities outside.

Our discussion of inhibition in the foregoing leads us to the consideration of the individual's ability to wait (inhibit)[58] before reacting to a stimulus (or stimuli) to pursue some "end" in the ordinary way of life, and it may be of interest to give some facts in regard to the experiences in this connexion of people taking lessons in speaking, breathing, singing, etc.

Most people who need lessons in speaking have a tendency to speak too quickly, and they fail to pause, to wait between their sentences. This tendency, of course, has to be checked, but in the work of re-education on a conscious plane we do not try to check the tendency directly, but rely instead on the use of certain "means-whereby" which will indirectly bring about the desired result. Therefore, instead of telling the pupil directly to pause at certain places, the teacher points out to him that he is gasping at the end of his lines or sentences, and that he is sniffing or "sucking in air" through the mouth, and he endeavours to make the pupil realize that these bad habits are the result of his incorrect subconscious conceptions in connexion with the act of breathing, and with the incorrect use of the psycho-physical mechanisms upon the correct use of which satisfactory breathing depends. From this it follows that in all vocal use the pupil must have a correct conception as to the nature of the respiratory act, associated with a conscious, reasoned understanding of the principles underlying the correct use of the psycho-mechanics involved in the act of breathing, before he makes any attempt to put these principles into practice.

When this point has been reached, the teacher will be justified in asking the pupil to stop, to wait at the end of each sentence in speaking or reading (or at the end of each phrase in singing), and to refuse to take another breath until he has inhibited the habitually incorrect, subconscious guidance and direction concerned with the act of taking a breath (which, in his case, is responsible for the imperfect use of the mechanism as diagnosed by his teacher), and, further, has substituted for these imperfect uses the new, correct conscious orders which make for increasingly satisfactory use. The teacher therefore asks him

[58]This "wait" is to give himself time to comprehend and consciously rehearse the orders which are the counterpart of the correct means whereby he is to attain his end.

to perform:—

> (1) *An inhibitory act*, by inhibiting "his way" of taking breath, in other words, by *preventing* or holding in check, in connexion with the act, the wrong subconscious guidance and direction, which constitutes the bad habit he has formed when taking breath at the end of each sentence.
>
> (2) *A volitionary act*, by giving himself certain orders which are the *means whereby* a more satisfactory act of inspiration may gradually be cultivated *before he attempts to go on to the next sentence.*

Now, in connexion with the latter act, the pupil will very likely raise the objection that if he stops to give the new orders before going on to speak, he will attract unpleasant attention to himself, because he will have to wait so long between his sentences that his way of speaking will appear slow and stilted. This objection only means, however, that he has not realized that his old habit of breathing audibly through the mouth, instead of through the nostrils, and of running his sentences into one another were noticeable defects to other people, however little he may have been aware of them himself. He is quick enough to object to the new way of speaking which, he believes, will draw unpleasant attention to himself, and also to the new instructions because, in carrying these out he is forced to break with habits which are familiar and therefore satisfying to him; but he is not so quick to observe defects in his own old way. Once, however, he has been taught to act in accordance with the new instructions, his defects will gradually disappear, because he will have learned to prevent the wrong use of the mechanisms responsible for these defects. The time taken to give, first, the preventive order to stop and wait at the end of the vocal effort and, secondly, the correct directing and controlling orders in connexion with the processes concerned with the respiratory act will constitute the necessary pause between the sentences. After this, it is merely a matter of time before the activities, which result from the series of psycho-physical experiences detailed above, become continuously operative, and, because they are now consciously directed, they will be henceforth under the pupil's constructive, conscious guidance and control.

The same difficulty is encountered in any pupil who breathes imperfectly, immediately he begins the actual practice of singing. This pupil also is so intent on his "end" (singing) that he finds it irksome to wait to take breath properly. He also "sniffs" and "sucks in air" through the mouth instead of through the nostrils, and, as a rule, audibly.

It is unlikely that such defects as these can be eradicated or that the cultivation of new defects can be prevented by those processes which we find associated with "breathing exercises" or lessons in "deep-breathing." But if the pupil attacks his difficulties—i.e., his general condition of mal-co-ordination—by means of re-education on a plane of constructive, conscious control, he can be helped to overcome them by learning, firstly, to hold in check his subconscious desire to "take breath" at the end of each phrase (inhibitory act), and, secondly, to give the guiding orders and directions in connexion with the correct psycho-mechanics of respiration (volitionary act).

This pupil also will probably make the objection that he cannot pause, giving as his reason that, if he pauses, he cannot keep time in his song. This objection, of course, will not hold any more than the previous one, for when once the necessary control has been gained, the pause required for inhibition and for giving the necessary orders will only be momentary.

But even if we suppose, for the sake of argument, that the objection holds, of what avail can it be to keep time, if thereby the primary principles which are essential to good singing, namely those concerned with the correct and adequate use of the psycho-physical mechanisms connected with respiration, are treated in practice as secondary factors, and are being actually perverted in use?

In all these considerations we must bear in mind that, in the sphere of acquiring satisfactory psycho-physical functioning, though speed will follow as the result of the necessary experience in the correct use of the parts concerned, a correct use can hardly follow a speed which has been achieved at the cost of an incorrect use of those parts.

Now that I have indicated the principles which underlie the general scheme which I advocate in connexion with the development of a reliable sensory appreciation, I will go on to describe in detail one of the technical evolutions[59] which I use in my teaching. It is given as an illustration of what should be the attitude of the pupil towards the practical work in connexion with the cultivation and development of the new sensory appreciation during the processes involved in the performance of the evolution, *but more particularly as an illustration of the means whereby we may develop a reliable sense appreciation of the minimum of so-called "physical tension"*; for in this sphere of sensory appreciation, the most difficult problem to be solved, in most cases, is concerned with the matter of developing a correct register of the *due and proper amount of so-called "muscular tension" necessary at a given time.*

It is not possible, of course, to tell the pupil in terms of relativity the

[59]A description of this evolution was first published in 1910.

degree of muscular tension which will be his or her required minimum at any particular moment. Furthermore, even if this were possible, what chance is there that the pupil will be able to register this minimum accurately, when the very factor upon which he will rely for guidance in this connexion (viz., his sensory appreciation) is unreliable, inaccurate and often positively delusive? I have known cases where a pupil failed to recognize a difference in muscular tension, whether his arms were hanging loosely at his sides, as in the act of walking, or were being used for the performance of an act requiring extreme tension.

The question, then, of dealing with the matter of a correct or incorrect degree of "physical tension" is probably, from the teacher's point of view, the most difficult problem to be solved in the scheme that we are considering. It is clear that this problem cannot be solved by the technique involved in the performance of "physical exercises" as such, and the chief danger involved in the performance of exercises associated with systems of physical culture, posture, etc., lies in the fact that this fundamental difficulty concerned with muscular tension has been ignored. If ever a plan of development by means of exercises to be performed according to written or spoken instructions—minus manipulative help—is to be evolved, this problem will have to be satisfactorily solved. I claim, however, that in its particular application to the evolution about to be described, this problem has been solved, and in a very practical way, and the unfolding of this part of the technique should prove of great interest to the student. Special attention is directed in this connexion to the instructions given in the following illustration to the pupil in regard to the work to be done with his hands and arms, associated with a more or less co-ordinated body, and particularly to the position of his fingers, wrists and elbows when placed on the chair as directed.

I would add that the correct performance of this evolution calls for the co-ordinated use of the body, legs and arms, and of the muscular system in general; it calls, in particular, for their co-ordinated use during the movement of bringing the body forward, and during the act of placing the hands in position on the top rail of the chair, also during the final work to be done with the hands and arms in this position. I want it to be very clearly understood that when I write of the arms, legs, hands, feet, etc., *I always imply their co-ordinated use* with the body as a co-ordinated support. Indeed, we might say that in this sense the body represents the trunk of a tree and the arms the limbs.

It must be clearly understood that in what follows it is taken for granted that the pupil gives special attention to the primary principles laid down for him by his teacher, before he attempts to carry out any instructions given him.[60] If this is done, the majority of the experiences that the pupil receives should be correct experiences, thus making for the development of confidence and for the continuance of the processes involved in the eradication of defects.

[60]It is not possible, of course, to give here all the detailed instructions that would meet every case, because these instructions naturally vary according to the tendencies and peculiarities of the particular pupil. An experienced teacher, however, should be able to supply these instructions in the practical application of the technique to meet the needs of the individual case. We must learn in this connexion to differentiate between the variations of a teacher's art and the principles of the teaching technique which is being employed.

CHAPTER IV

ILLUSTRATION

In the technical evolution about to be set down, it is necessary to use certain phrases employed in the teaching technique, phrases which I consider call for comment, seeing that they do not always adequately express my meaning and that, furthermore, they cannot be defended as being demonstrably accurate.

My reader may justly ask, then, why I use them. Readers of *Man's Supreme Inheritance* will remember that when I used the phrase "position of mechanical advantage," I pointed out that I did so because a better one was not forthcoming, and I mentioned then that I had called to my aid a number of scientific and literary friends.

I have pursued the same course in regard to the phrases which will follow. As I have already stated, I think them inadequate, but with a teacher present to demonstrate in person what he means by them, they serve their purpose. The phrases are:

1. Shortening the Spine

An objector might justly say that this is practically impossible, but we are dealing with the *use* of the spine, and one of the most common defects amongst human beings to-day is an undue curving of the spine in the use of the self in the acts of every-day life, and naturally this causes a shortening in stature. As a practical demonstration, take a piece of paper, and after placing it flat on another sheet, draw a line along the extreme ends of the top piece, thereby recording the length by the pencil marks on the paper underneath. Now lift the top piece and curve it slightly and replace it with one end touching one line, and without interfering with the curve. It will then be seen that the other end of the paper does not reach the other line.

2. Lengthening the Spine

The foregoing will serve to shew that if we modify the curve in the spine, we tend to lengthen it. For instance, to go back to our illustration, if we take the curve out of the top piece of paper, and replace it as in the first instance, it will reach both lines, shewing that during this experiment a lengthening process has been operative.

3. Relax the Neck

There is considerable confusion on the part of the pupil when he attempts to obey directions to relax some part of the organism. In ordinary teaching, pupils and teachers are quite convinced that if some part of the organism is too tense, they can relax it, that is, *do the relaxing by direct means*. This is a delusion on their part but it is difficult to convince them of it. In the first place, if they do chance to get rid of the specific tension it will be by a partial collapse of the parts concerned, or of other parts, possibly even by a general collapse of the whole organism. In the second place, it is obvious that if some part of the organism is unduly tensed, it is because the pupil is attempting to do with it the work of some other part or parts, often work for which it is quite unsuited.

4. Head Forward and Up

This is one of the most inadequate and often confusing phrases used as a means of conveying our ideas in words, and it is a dangerous instruction to give to any pupil, unless the teacher first demonstrates his meaning by giving to the pupil, *by means of manipulation*, the exact experiences involved.

5. Widen the Back

This instruction rivals the last one in its shortcomings, when considered as a phrase for the conveyance of an idea which we expect a pupil to construe correctly, unless it is given by a teacher who is capable of demonstrating what he means by readjusting the pupil's organism so that the conditions desired may be brought about.

What really occurs is that there is brought about a very marked change in the position of the bony structures of the thorax—particularly noticeable if a posterior view is taken—also a permanent enlargement of the thoracic cavity, with a striking increase in thoracic mobility and the minimum muscle tension of the whole of the mechanisms involved.

6. Support the Body with the Arms

This instruction is given to the pupil when he is holding the back of a chair, whilst sitting or standing, in order to give the teacher the opportunity to secure more quickly and easily for the pupil certain experiences essential at a particular stage of his work in co-ordination. The varying details of the *means whereby* the use indicated of the arms and body is to be gained could not be set down in writing to meet the requirements of each pupil, for they vary with each slight stage of progress. It is for this reason that "correct positions" or "postures" find no place in the practical teaching technique employed in the work of re-education advocated in this book. A correct position or posture indicates a fixed position, and a person held to a fixed position cannot grow, as we understand growth. The correct position today cannot be the correct position a week later for any person who is advancing in the work of re-education and co-ordination.

7. *Widen the Arms Whilst Supporting and Raising the Body*

This is the most deceptive of the list of instructions set down in these pages. In the first place, if carried out without manipulative assistance, it is a contradictory instruction, seeing that if you widen the arms as the act is generally understood, the body would be lowered, not raised. The tendency of the pupil in this movement is to contract unduly the inner muscles of the upper part of the arms, a procedure which interferes with the work the teacher has in view. This must be prevented and a skilful teacher can employ the above instructions successfully to this end.

We will now pass on to our illustration.

THE PUPIL IS ASKED TO SIT IN A CHAIR IN ACCORDANCE WITH THE PRINCIPLES AND TECHNIQUE SPECIALLY SET DOWN FOR THE ACT OF SITTING AND STANDING IN *Man's Supreme Inheritance*. When he is seated, his body being supported by the back of the chair on which he is sitting, another chair is placed before him with its back towards him.

THE PUPIL IS THEN ASKED TO GIVE THE FOLLOWING PREVENTIVE ORDERS.

In the way of correct direction and guidance, HE IS ASKED TO ORDER THE NECK TO RELAX, TO ORDER THE HEAD FORWARD AND UP TO LENGTHEN THE SPINE.

It must here be clearly understood that in the previous manipulative and other work done in connexion with the technique, the pupil will have been made familiar in theory and practice with Order 1. He is able to give certain orders correctly and also to put them into effect. In the present instance, it is explained to him that the order given is to be merely preventive—a projected wish *without any attempt on the pupil's part to carry it out successfully.*

THE TEACHER REPEATS THE ORDERS AND WITH HIS HANDS HE PROCEEDS TO BRING THE PUPIL'S BODY GENTLY FORWARD FROM THE HIPS.

It is important to note here that the imperfectly co-ordinated person tends to *shorten* the stature and *pull the head back* in making this movement forward. Unless, therefore, the pupil remembers this subconscious tendency to shorten, and attends to the new directive orders which will counteract this subconscious tendency, his old habit will prove too strong for him, and at the first touch from the teacher to bring his body forward, though this touch may be so light that it would not move an inch-thick pineboard of the same length and width as the torso of the pupil, the latter will start to move forward at a ratio of, say, seventy-five per cent subconscious response to his old habit, and only twenty-five per cent conscious response to the new directive and guiding orders. This latter estimate is, in most cases, too liberal a one, for, as a rule, the slightest touch releases the old sensory activities associated subconsciously in the pupil's conception with the act of "moving forward," this being an "end" which the pupil, in spite of all warnings to the contrary, has already decided upon, and he becomes so dominated by the idea of "moving forward" (his "end"), that the new conscious directive orders are no longer projected. Instead, the old subconscious directive orders associated with his bad habits and with his unreliable sensory appreciation hold sway, and so, in the place of ordering his neck to relax, his head forward and up, in order to secure the necessary lengthening, he will actually throw his head back, stiffen his neck, and tend to shorten his spine by unduly curving it, in accordance with his old fixed habit in moving forward. These particular faults are accompanied, more or less, by an undue and incorrect tension of the legs and other parts of the organism, and also by a stiffening at the hip joints, the defective use of the parts culminating in an expenditure of energy out of all proportion to the requirements of the evolution.

When this happens, the teacher must point out to the pupil that he has not quite comprehended what is required of him, and he must again place the whole position before the pupil, and from as many angles as possible, until he is certain that the pupil understands that the primary orders which he is asked to give are *preventive orders*, and that if he gives these preventive orders (inhibition of the old misdirected activities), and then proceeds to give the new ones, *his spine will be kept at its greatest possible length* (not shortened), whilst the body will be moved forward from the hips easily and satisfactorily, without interfering with the general relative position of the torso (except in the matter of angle) just as a door moves on its hinges.

THE TEACHER WILL THEN RENEW THE REQUEST TO THE PUPIL TO GIVE THE ORDERS, AND WITH HIS HANDS WILL COMMAND FOR HIM THE ACTUAL PERFORMANCE OF THE MOVEMENT, of which these orders are the counterpart. Sometimes it may be suggested that the pupil shall himself request the teacher to move his body forward for him whilst he (the pupil) gives his orders or directions.

When the teacher is satisfied that the pupil is giving due attention to the directive orders up to this point, and has gained a due appreciation of their relative value as primary, secondary and following factors; when, also, the correct sensory experiences, made possible by the teacher's help in the way of readjustment and re-education, have been sufficiently repeated, the pupil can be taken a step further in the evolution.

At every step in the work it is essential that the pupil should rehearse his orders from the beginning, because these earlier orders constitute the *means whereby* a further step may be successfully taken. In giving himself orders, the pupil must on every occasion begin with the primary orders before going on to the secondary orders, and so on.

THE PUPIL MUST NOW AGAIN ORDER THE NECK TO RELAX, THE HEAD FORWARD AND UP, WHILST THE TEACHER WITH HIS HANDS SECURES THAT POSITION OF THE TORSO IN WHICH THE BACK MAY BE SAID TO BE WIDENED. These orders should be repeated several times and be *continued* WHILST THE TEACHER TAKES THE PUPIL'S RIGHT ARM WITH HIS HANDS, AND MOVES IT FORWARD UNTIL THE PUPIL'S HAND IS ABOVE THE TOP RAIL OF THE BACK OF THE CHAIR. THE PUPIL SHOULD THEN BE REQUESTED TO REPEAT THE ORDERS SET DOWN AT THE BEGINNING OF THIS PARAGRAPH, AND THEN TO TAKE THE WEIGHT OF THE ARM ENTIRELY, AS THE TEACHER DISENGAGES HIS HANDS FROM THE SUPPORTED ARM.

Great care must be taken to see that the pupil has not interfered with the mechanism of the torso in the effort to take the weight of the arm. This interference can take place in various ways, but it always implies that the pupil has forgotten his orders and has harked back to one or other of his subconscious habits. What is essential here is a *co-ordinated use* of the arms and the only way by which he can secure this is, first, by giving the necessary preventive orders, and then by rehearsing the series of new orders given by the teacher, in which the movement of the arms is *linked up* with the use of the other parts of the body.

If the pupil has not interfered with the mechanism of the torso in the effort to take the weight of the arm, HE SHOULD NEXT BE REQUESTED TO GRASP THE TOP RAIL OF THE BACK OF THE CHAIR GENTLY AND FIRMLY, KEEPING THE FINGERS AS *straight* AS POSSIBLE AND QUITE FLAT AGAINST THE WOOD OF THE FRONT PORTION OF THE TOP RAIL OF THE CHAIR, THE THUMB ALSO TO BE KEPT AS STRAIGHT AS POSSIBLE, BEING CALLED UPON TO DO DUTY ON THE BACK PORTION OF THE TOP RAIL OF THE CHAIR, WITH THE WRIST CURVED SLIGHTLY INWARDS TOWARDS THE LEFT. The teacher will, of course, as far as possible, assist the pupil with these hand movements.

If, however, as is too often the case, the pupil fails to continue to give his orders, and so interferes with the mechanisms of the torso during the movement of the arm towards the chair, *the pupil must be requested to begin once more at the very first step in the evolution, and this must be continued until a satisfactory result has been secured. This principle must be applied in every instance* in this work of re-education and readjustment. It should be realized here that, during the course of this work, a process of building is going on, fundamental sensory building, on a general and not a specific basis. It will perhaps make this clearer if we use the analogy of building with bricks, for the processes concerned with this fundamental sensory building calls for the use of directive orders, just as the process of ordinary building calls for the use of bricks.

THE PUPIL MUST THEN BE ASKED AGAIN TO ORDER THE NECK TO RELAX, THE HEAD FORWARD AND UP, AND THE TEACHER WILL REPEAT HIS PREVIOUS EFFORT TO ESTABLISH THAT CONDITION OF THE TORSO AND BACK ESSENTIAL TO SATISFACTORY ARM WORK, WHILST HE REPEATS WITH THE PUPIL'S LEFT ARM THE EVOLUTION JUST PERFORMED WITH THE RIGHT, SO THAT THE PUPIL WILL BE GRASPING THE BACK OF THE CHAIR WITH THE LEFT HAND IN THE SAME WAY AS HE HAS BEEN HOLDING IT WITH THE RIGHT, the teacher giving such assistance in this movement as he deems necessary in the light of his experience.

It will be found that at this, as at every other step in the work, one pupil will need more assistance than another. One pupil will need help in one part of the movement, the next will need it at another part, and so on. It may even, in some cases, be necessary for the teacher to give a pupil as much assistance in bringing forward the left arm as he gave him in bringing forward the right arm. In all these matters the decision must be left to the discretion of the teacher. *To command success, correct experiences in sensory appreciation must follow the giving of correct directive and guiding orders. By the repetition of this process the pupil reaches a stage where he can depend on himself with confidence.*

At this point THE PUPIL SHOULD BE ASKED TO RECONSIDER THE DIFFERENT *means whereby* HE HAS BEEN ENABLED TO REACH THIS STAGE OF HIS WORK, AND TO REPEAT ORALLY THE DIRECTIONS AND GUIDING ORDERS EXACTLY IN THE SEQUENCE IN WHICH THEY HAVE BEEN GIVEN TO HIM BY HIS TEACHER, AS PRIMARY, SECONDARY, AND FOLLOWING FACTORS. In this way the teacher will be able to test the pupil's accuracy or otherwise in this connexion. *Whilst the pupil repeats the orders, he must remain in the co-ordinated condition which has been secured during the performance of the evolution.*

When the teacher is satisfied that his pupil has succeeded up to this point, he may go on to give him the additional guiding orders, and proceed to help him to put them into practical effect during the completion of the evolution.

The following are the new directive orders:—

The pupil is asked:—

(1) TO CONTINUE TO HOLD THE TOP OF THE CHAIR BY KEEPING THE FINGERS QUITE STRAIGHT FROM THE FIRST JOINTS OF THE FINGERS TO THEIR TIPS, WITH THE THUMBS AND FINGERS KEPT FLAT AGAINST THE TOP RAIL OF THE CHAIR AS PREVIOUSLY INDICATED.

(2) TO ALLOW THE WRIST OF THE LEFT ARM TO BE CURVED INWARDS TOWARD THE RIGHT, AND THE WRIST OF THE RIGHT ARM TO BE CURVED INWARDS TOWARDS THE LEFT.

(3) TO ALLOW THE ELBOW OF THE LEFT ARM TO BE CURVED OUTWARDS TOWARDS THE LEFT, AND THE ELBOW OF THE RIGHT ARM TO BE CURVED OUTWARDS TOWARDS THE RIGHT.

In order that the pupil may hold the rail of the chair, keeping the fingers and wrists in the position indicated above, HE SHOULD REHEARSE ALL THE DIRECTIVE ORDERS PREVIOUSLY GIVEN TO HIM AND WHICH HE HAS ALREADY ORALLY REPEATED TO HIS TEACHER.

The teacher's aim is now to give the pupil the experiences necessary to a gentle forearm pull from the fingers, and to this end HE WILL TAKE HOLD OF THE PUPIL'S ELBOWS AND DIRECT THEM OUTWARDS AND SLIGHTLY DOWNWARDS, and, following this, will give the sensory experiences required in DIRECTING THE UPPER PARTS OF THE ARMS (ABOVE THE ELBOW) AWAY FROM ONE ANOTHER (THE RIGHT ARM TOWARDS THE RIGHT AND THE LEFT ARM TOWARDS THE LEFT), IN SUCH A WAY THAT THE PUPIL WILL BE SUPPORTING THE TORSO WITH HIS ARMS.

THE PUPIL WILL NOW BE ASKED TO CONTINUE TO SUPPORT THE TORSO IN THIS WAY, CONTINUING TO REHEARSE HIS ORDERS, whilst the teacher so adjusts the torso that the large "lifting" muscles of the back will be employed co-ordinately with the other parts of the organism in bringing about such use of the respiratory mechanisms that they will function to the maximum at the particular stage of development reached from day to day. Success in this part of the evolution will bring about a change in the condition of the back which would be described by the ordinary observer as a "widening of the back."

These orders are the *means whereby* such use of the mechanisms may be brought about, associated with a satisfactory readjustment of the back, as will cause the floating ribs to move freely, and also tend to develop the maximum intra-thoracic capacity and to establish the most effective use of the respiratory mechanism during the sleeping as well as the waking hours.

In my opinion, it is expedient here to set down some of the impeding conditions which, in my teaching experience, will be found present, more or less, in the case of every pupil during the attempt at co-ordination at this stage of the movement. The muscular tension, for instance, employed in the use of the fingers and arms is almost always a harmful and unnecessary one. Very frequently this undue tension of the arm muscles will actually prevent the pupil from using his fingers to anything like the best advantage in holding the chair. I have even known instances in which the fingers would actually be kept away from the wood without the pupil's knowing it. This undue tension is particularly noticeable in the case of the contractor muscles of the arm in the region of the biceps and in that of the pectoral muscles in the front of the chest, whereas, in a satisfactory state of sensory appreciation these muscles would remain more or less relaxed during the movement, and the greater part of the work would fall on the muscles of the opposite side of the arm and the back (chiefly on the latissimus dorsi). These would thus be the chief factors in the act, factors which make both for the maximum activity of the respiratory processes, with the minimum of effort, and also for an increased intra-thoracic capacity accompanied by a broadening of the costal arch (increased vital capacity).

Other impeding conditions are apt to occur at the pupil's first attempt to pull gently with the arms. In his attempt to do this, either one or other or all the fingers will become bent and the wrists will be curved outwards, *exactly the reverse of the action indicated by the orders* or of the one desired. *This failure to carry out the given orders is due chiefly to the fact that the pupil's sensory appreciation in the matter of due and proper muscular tension is sadly inadequate.*

This leads us directly to a consideration of the means we have adopted whereby a new and reliable sensory appreciation can be developed in the pupil, the *means whereby* he will be enabled to perform this evolution with the *minimum of muscular tension.* In this connexion the reader's attention is specially directed to the following:

If the pupil will carry out the act of the forearm pull and attend to the widening of the upper parts of the arms, whilst continuing to recognize as factors of primary importance the keeping of the fingers straight and the wrists curved inwards, *the minimum tension will be exerted.* Immediately the pupil interferes with the position of the fingers or wrists (in the latter case, tending to curve them outwards instead of inwards), this will indicate that *the point of minimum muscular tension has been passed.*

It should be remembered here that the pupil's position in this act is an ideal one for watching the hands and wrists. Therefore, if the pupil will watch carefully any tendency to the incorrect movements described above, these can be checked as soon as they shew themselves. But here again we have one of the numerous instances where a person will refrain from doing the thing he knows he can do (in this instance, to watch the hands—"means-whereby") and will prefer to depend instead on the old haphazard method of "trying to do it right" guided by his feeling, and this despite the fact that in every experience in which he has taken "feeling" for a guide, he has found it to be unreliable and even delusive.

* * * * *

There has just come to my knowledge an interesting objection to the importance which I attach to the process of inhibition as a primary and fundamental factor in the technique of the scheme I advocate, and the objection is made on the ground that this use of inhibition will cause harmful suppression in the individual concerned. I shall proceed to shew that such an objection is the outcome of a total misunderstanding of the fundamental psycho-physical processes concerned with the application of the preventive principles employed in my technique.

There has been and still is a growing tendency to attempt to free children from undue external restraint, both at home and at school, with the idea of preventing those harmful suppressions supposed to be the result of the inhibitions associated with the imposition of the restraint characteristic of less modern methods. The idea concerned is conceived on a specific and curative basis and is generally accepted, particularly in schools where an effort is being made to create conditions of environment and occupation to meet the pupil's needs. The points I wish to emphasize in this connexion are (1) that the process of inhibition involved is employed in connexion with ideas directly associated with the gaining of "ends," these ideas being the response to a stimulus (or stimuli) arising from some primary desire or need, and (2)—and this is all-important—that the stimulus (or stimuli) to inhibit this response comes from without, and the process of inhibition is *forced* upon the pupil. This means that his desire is thwarted in consequence of compliance with a command from an outside authority, and this could account for the disturbed emotional conditions associated with what is known as suppression.

Now the inhibitory process involved in my technique has little in common with that to which reference has just been made. For the idea concerned with inhibition in my technique is conceived on a general and preventive basis, and the process of inhibition involved is employed primarily in connexion with ideas which are dissociated from any direct attempt to gain an "end," but associated instead with that indirect procedure inseparable from the practical application of the principles concerned with the *means whereby* an end may be gained. These ideas are the response to a stimulus (or stimuli) arising from a reasoned, constructive conscious understanding and acceptance by the pupil of the principles concerned with the "'means-whereby," and as the procedure concerned with the application of these principles involves the prevention of "end-gaining" acts, the performance of which is associated with misdirected activities, it follows that the pupil's acceptance of the need for and efficacy of such procedure includes also his acceptance of the principle of inhibition of primary desires concerned with such "end-gaining" acts. This, again, really means that in the application of my technique the process of inhibition, that is, *the act of refusing to respond* to the primary desire to gain an "end" *becomes the act of responding* (volitionary act) to the conscious reasoned desire to employ the *means whereby* that "end" may be gained.

The stimulus to inhibit, therefore, in this case comes from within, and the process of inhibition is not forced upon the pupil. This means that the pupil's desire or desires will be satisfied, not thwarted, and that there will be present desirable emotional and other psycho-physical conditions which do not make for what is known as suppression in any form.[61]

---

[61]There are many persons who pride themselves on self-control who are really victims of enslavement to a fixed "end," that is, they do not control themselves by stopping to think out the "means-whereby" to their "ends," but by excluding *(continued on next page)*

The tendency of people on a subconscious plane to speak and act without adequate thought or consideration is a particularly marked manifestation, when there is present an unusually potent stimulus to those processes concerned with what are known as prejudice and emotional disturbances. We are all familiar with the phrases, "Why don't you think before you act?", "Think before you speak," and so on. When the human creature's activities are on a plane of constructive, conscious control, he will have reached a standard of development and use of the processes of inhibition (as outlined in the technique which I advocate), which will enable him to apply in practice to his activities in the outside world the very principles concerned with the processes of inhibition which he has applied to the use of his psycho-physical self, with accruing benefit in both spheres of application.

In this connexion I will now give an incident which I think is of particular interest and pertinence as shewing the application of the technique employed in the work of re-education on a general basis to the practical ways of life, and also the analogy which exists between the process of "linking-up" (association of ideas) during the lessons, and the process of linking up what has been gained during those lessons with the experience of every-day life. I also give it in proof of the fundamental value of the principle of inhibition involved.

A pupil of mine, an author, had been in a serious state of health for some time, and had at last reached the point where he was unable to carry on his literary work. After finishing his latest book he passed through a crisis which was described as a "breakdown," with the result that even a few hours of work caused him great fatigue and brought on a state of painful depression. From the outset of his lessons, therefore, I expressly stipulated that he should *stop* and make a break at the end of each half-hour's writing, and should then either do fifteen minutes' work in respiratory re-education, or take a walk in the open air before resuming his writing.

One afternoon he came to his lesson unusually depressed and enervated, and, in response to my enquiries, he admitted that he had been indulging in his literary work that morning from nine till one without a break, in spite of my express stipulation that he must make frequent breaks. I pointed out to him that if he had been continuing his work for

everything which does not agree with the "ends" which they have set up as right and proper. They themselves may contend that their control is purely self-imposed and not externally imposed, but to other persons it manifests itself as a form of rigidity. On the other hand, control which results from stopping to reason out the *means whereby* desired ends may be secured is unassociated with that rigidity which is inseparable from enslavement to pre-conceived and unreasoned ideas and beliefs, or to hard and fast rules in regard to what is right and proper in conduct and procedure.

four hours without a break, we could not be surprised at the unfortunate result, for, as I explained to him, during deep thought, as in sleep, the activity of the respiratory processes is reduced to a minimum, a very harmful minimum in his case, owing to the inadequacy of his intra-thoracic capacity, this latter condition being one of the symptoms of his breakdown. "But I am unable to stop when once I get into my work," said my pupil. I suggested that if this were so, it must come from some lack of control on his part. "But surely," my pupil objected, "it must be a mistake to break a train of thought?" I answered that my experience went to shew that this was not the case, that, on the contrary, as far as I could see, it should be as easy to break off a piece of work requiring thought, and take it up again, as it is to carry on a train of thought, whilst taking a walk with all its attendant interruptions, and that this should be possible not only without loss of connexion, but with accruing benefit to the individual concerned.

In all this I was really preparing the way to a special end, namely, the attempt to shew my pupil the analogy that existed between the point in question and his difficulty in accomplishing certain simple parts of the technique in his lessons through his disinclination to stop. I wished to convince him that *the gaining of control in the simple psycho-physical evolutions in which we were engaged during the lessons meant sooner or later the gaining of control in the practical spheres of his daily life.* My pupil had failed to make this all-important connexion between his work in re-education and his outside activities, and therefore the connexion between the difficulty he experienced in "stopping" in his lessons and "stopping" in the midst of his literary work had completely escaped him.

In this, however, he was only in like case with thousands of other well-educated and intelligent people who, in dealing with a situation, fail to make an obvious association of ideas, and so miss most important connecting links between different factors in a case. In this particular instance, had my pupil made the necessary connexion between the difficulty he had in "stopping" in his lessons and "stopping" in his activities outside, this recognition would have given a new meaning, a0.nd therefore an added stimulus to the psycho-physical effort upon which the successful working-out of the technique depends.

CHAPTER V

RESPIRATORY MECHANISMS

WE shall probably find the best practical illustration of the need for correct sensory experiences in guidance and control if we consider sensory appreciation in its connexion with the psycho-mechanics of respiration. It is universally admitted that there are harmful defects in the use of the respiratory mechanisms and a corresponding deterioration in the chest capacity and mobility of the great majority of people. The scientific medical man describes certain types of children as born with a "low respiratory need," and this really means that when the child is born, it is more or less imperfectly co-ordinated and its organism is functioning much nearer to its minimum than to its maximum capacity. This condition of inadequate vital functioning is present in the greater number of men, women, and children of to-day, and is one that is commonly associated with what we speak of as "bad breathing." For we say that a person is a "bad breather," or that he "breathes imperfectly." But we must remember that this so-called "bad breathing" is only a symptom and not a primary cause of his malcondition, for the standard of breathing depends upon the standard of general co-ordinated use of the psycho-physical mechanisms. What we ought to say, therefore, in such a case is not that a person "breathes badly," but that he is badly co-ordinated. The truth is that when we refer to this mal-co-ordinated condition as "bad breathing," we are mistaking a general malcondition for a specific defect, and the conception of the respiratory act which makes this error possible, and which affects even our way of expressing it, provides yet another instance of the dominance of our general attitude by the "end-gaining" principle.

This "end-gaining" principle is again dominant when it is decided that a person who is spoken of as a "bad breather" needs specific "breathing exercises" or "lessons in breathing." We shall see that in this, as in so many other spheres, a vicious circle is developed.

In the attempt to make this clear we must give consideration to the fundamental principles upon which these breathing exercises (usually called "deep-breathing" exercises) or "lessons in breathing" are based. Take any book on breathing, whether written by a scientific author or by an expert in vocal or "physical culture," and read the written instructions in connexion with the exercises therein advocated. Take the opportunity also, when possible, to be present when the unfortunate children or adults in a gymnasium are being given a lesson in breathing or are performing their breathing exercises. You will then have proof that the whole of the processes concerned are directed towards specific and not general improvement, and though the people who are guilty of teaching "breathing exercises" may differ in detail of method, they all base their work alike on the same specific "end-gaining" principle. I shall now proceed to detail the processes involved.

The pupil is asked to take a deep breath. He may also be asked to perform some "physical" movement at the same time as he takes the deep breath, the idea behind this request being that the performance of the movement may help to increase the chest expansion. Yet it is a scientific fact that all "physical" tension tends to cause thoracic (chest) rigidity and breathlessness (lack of respiratory control), two conditions which should be avoided as far as possible by such pupils during their attempts to pass from conditions which are symptomatic of bad breathing to those which ensure satisfactory respiratory functioning.

It will be necessary for the layman to watch the pupil (or pupils) carefully during their attempts to carry out their written or spoken instructions in connexion with "deep breathing." Specific defects and peculiarities to be noted during the process have already been set down in *Man's Supreme Inheritance.* Here we wish to refer only to the defective *general* use of the psycho-physical organism during these attempts. In order to make the point, we must refer to the fact that the pupil or the teacher, or both, must have recognized certain harmful manifestations which called for some remedial procedure on the lines of "deep-breathing," etc. Hence the decision to employ "deep-breathing" as a remedy. These harmful manifestations would be the result of certain incorrect psycho-physical uses of the organism. This would indicate that the sensory appreciation in the sphere of guidance and control of the psycho-physical mechanisms concerned must have become unreliable and defective, and in the present instance, so far as the observation of the teacher and pupil is concerned, certain defects must have been particularly noticeable in the use of the breathing mechanisms.

Here we have a clear case of certain established incorrect uses of the mechanisms, associated with a condition of unreliable sensory guidance and control, and any effort to remedy these incorrect uses by means of such processes as "deep-breathing" or "lessons in breathing" is merely an attempt to correct a *general* defective condition of psycho-mechanics by a *specific* remedial process. In other words, it is an attempt to correct the imperfect uses by the performance of exercises, the guidance and direction in such performance being associated with the same imperfect sensory appreciation which was already established when the lessons began. This means that with the continued practice of the exercises, the original defects in the general use of the mechanisms will become more and more pronounced and, what is more, increase in number.

It may be argued that, as the result of the lessons, the pupil's chest measurements are increased, that he "feels better," and so on. We are quite ready to admit that this may be so, but owing to the unreliability of his sensory appreciation, what he feels is as likely as not to be a delusion. Of what avail, therefore, is it for the pupil to "feel better," if he is still left with a defective sensory appreciation to guide him in all his activities during his waking moments as well as his sleeping hours? It is only a matter of time before the unfortunate pupil will be awakened from his dream by discovering that he has developed certain other serious conditions. I should like here to point out that these serious conditions must result, sooner or later, from the lack in such cases of a reliable guiding sensory appreciation, also from the lack of psycho-physical co-ordination which is associated therewith, and which continues to increase whilst these conditions are present. We have all known people who tell of the improvement in their chest measurement from the practice of exercises. The writer has examined many such in the course of thirty years' professional investigation. In the majority of these cases, the supposed increase in chest capacity has been chiefly due to muscular development on the outside of the bony chest, in other cases to some distortion or distortions cultivated during the processes involved, rather than to that co-ordinated use of the psycho-physical system which is associated with a real increase in the intra-thoracic (inner chest) capacity.[62] And it is the same in the case of those who tell you that they "feel better" as the result of these exercises, for to the expert observer it is obvious that the habit of "sniffing" (sucking in air), the contraction of the alae nasi, the depression of the larynx, and all the accompanying defective use of the organism associated with the practice of the exercises must, sooner or later, cause serious nose, ear, eye, and throat troubles. In other words, the exponents of these breathing exercises act in direct pursuance of their "end," remaining oblivious to the harmfulness of the *means whereby* they are attempting to bring this "end" about, and

[62]An interesting delusion prevalent with teachers of breathing exercises is that of mistaking an increase in the muscle development on the outer walls of the chest for increase in intra-chest (thoracic) capacity.

to the many wrong uses they are cultivating during the process.

This method of procedure, as we have seen, is the very opposite of that which underlies the process of re-education, readjustment and co-ordination on a conscious, general basis, and we will consider the application of this process to a satisfactory use of the psycho-physical mechanisms.

We will begin by a consideration of the fundamental psycho-physical principles underlying the act of breathing. In the course of this consideration it will be found that breathing is many times removed from the primary principle concerned, and that, therefore, it is incorrect and harmful to speak of "teaching a person to breathe," or of "giving lessons in breathing or deep-breathing." Such a stimulus to the subconsciously controlled person at once induces projections of all the established incorrect guiding orders associated with imperfect or inadequate breathing processes; in other words, this stimulus sets in motion all our bad habits in breathing.

Breathing is that psycho-physical act by means of which air is taken into and expelled from the lungs of the creature. The lungs are an extremely interesting part of our anatomy. They consist of two bags containing a network of cells capable of contraction and expansion, with air passages and blood-vessels so associated and constituted that the oxygen contained in the air, when taken into the lungs, can be absorbed through the tissue of the blood vessels and cells and air passages, whilst carbonic acid gas (poison) passes through this tissue from the bloodvessels into the lung cells to be expelled from the lungs. The thorax (chest) has a bony structure, made up of the vertebrae of the spine, the different ribs and the sternum (breast-bone), those ribs which are attached to the sternum as well as to the spine being much less mobile than those which are not attached to the sternum, the most mobile being known as "floating ribs." The lungs are enclosed within the cavity of this bony thorax of which the diaphragm is the floor, and the only entrance to which is through the trachea (windpipe). From the very first breath there is a more or less constant air pressure (atmospheric pressure) within the lungs, but not any air pressure on the outside of the lungs. Air pressure is sufficient to overcome the elasticity of the tissue of the air-cells, and to increase their size, when not held in check by the pressure of the walls of the thorax upon the lung-bag itself. The lungs are subject, however, to this pressure exerted by the walls of the thorax during the contraction, and to the release of this pressure during the expansion of the thoracic cavity. The pressure that can be exerted by the walls of the thorax on the outside of the lung-bag is much greater than that which results from the atmospheric pressure (air pressure) within the lungs. Therefore, when we wish, as we say, to "take a breath" (inspiration), all we have to do is to reduce the pressure exerted upon the lungs by the chest walls, and to employ those muscular co-ordinations which increase the intra-thoracic capacity of the lungs (increased chest capacity), thereby causing a partial vacuum in the lung cells of which atmospheric pressure takes advantage, by increasing the size of the cells and thus the amount of air in the lungs. It then follows that if we wish to exhale breath (expiration), we merely have to increase the pressure on the lungs by contracting the walls of the thorax, thereby overcoming the atmospheric pressure exerted within the lungs, and thus forcing the air out of them. It must be remembered that in all these contractions and expansions, the floor of the cavity (diaphragm) plays its part, moving upwards or downwards in sympathy with the particular adjustment of the bony thorax.

Consideration of the foregoing will serve to convince the reader that if anyone desires, either by his own effort or with the help of a teacher, to secure the maximum control and development in breathing, all that he has to do is to be able to command the maximum functioning of the psycho-physical mechanisms concerned with the satisfactory expansion and contraction of the walls of the thoracic (chest) cavity. *It is not necessary for him even to think of taking a breath*; as a matter of fact, it is more or less harmful to do so, when such psycho-physical conditions are present as call for re-education on a general basis.

The crux of the whole matter, then, is how to gain this control in expanding and contracting the chest, as we say, and thus permanently to increase its capacity and mobility. The answer to this question calls for a comprehensive consideration of the primary, secondary and other psycho-physical factors involved.

Naturally, the most potent stimulus to the use of the respiratory mechanisms is the necessity for an adequate supply of oxygen, and for the elimination of carbonic acid gas (poison) from the blood. But we must not overlook the fact that in any attempt to gain for a pupil the desired control and the increased thoracic capacity, the pupil's incorrect use of the mechanisms involved is an impeding factor, and so, in attempts to correct such imperfect use, the first consideration must be to *prevent the psycho-physical activities which are responsible for this defective use* by the development and employment of the pupil's ability to inhibit. This demands from the teacher a correct diagnosis of the pupil's numerous bad habits in connexion with the act of respiration in every-day life, and a comprehensive understanding of the imperfections in sensory appreciation, conception, adjustment and co-ordination which are manifested in these bad habits.

As a result of the diagnosis, the teacher will go on to explain to the pupil why certain readjustments and improved co-ordinations are necessary in his case, and will then give him a reasoned consideration of the *means whereby* these readjustments and improved co-ordinations may be secured. To this end the teacher will first name the preventive guiding orders or directions which the pupil is to give to himself in the way of *inhibiting* the deceptive guiding sensations concerned with the defective use of the mechanisms responsible for what we call bad habits in breathing. The teacher must make certain that the pupil remembers these guiding orders or directions *in the sequence in which they are to be employed*. When this has been done, the pupil may begin the practice in connexion with the work of prevention. This means a series of repeated experiences on the part of the pupil in refusing to try for the "end," and in positively pausing to think of the original faults pointed out by the teacher, and refusing to repeat them.

For instance, suppose that a pupil has a special desire to increase his chest capacity. This desire acts as a stimulus to the psycho-physical processes involved and sets in motion all the unreliable guiding and directing sensations associated with his established idea of chest expansion. The only way, then, by which he can *prevent* the old subconscious habits from gaining the upper hand is for him to *refuse to act* upon this idea. This means that as soon as the idea or desire comes to him *he definitely stops* and says to himself: "No. I won't do what I should like to do to increase my chest capacity, because, if I do what I feel will increase it, I shall only use my mechanisms as I have used them before, and what is the good of that? I know I have been using them incorrectly up to now, else why do I need these lessons?" In other words, he inhibits his desire to act.

The teacher, of course, must decide when the pupil can proceed from the preventive to the next stage of his work. He must then proceed to name for the pupil the new orders in connexion with the satisfactory guiding sensations concerned with the correct use of the mechanisms involved. The pupil should recall and give himself these new guiding orders, whilst the teacher, by means of his manipulation, assists him to secure the correct readjustment and co-ordination (the desired "end"), thus ensuring a series of satisfactory experiences which should be repeated until the bad habits are eradicated and the new and correct experiences replace them and become established.

Repetition of these correct experiences is all that is required to establish a satisfactory use of the co-ordinated psycho-physical mechanisms concerned, when an increase or decrease in the intra-thoracic (chest) capacity can be secured at will, with the minimum of effort and with a mathematical precision. The increase in the intra-thoracic (chest) capacity indicated decreases the pressure on the outside of the lung-bag and causes a momentary partial vacuum in the lungs. This vacuum is promptly filled with air, in consequence of the atmospheric pressure exerted upon the inside of the lung cells, and this process increases the amount of air in the lungs, constituting the act of what we call "taking a breath" (inspiration). The marvellous efficiency of the respiratory machine, when properly employed, becomes apparent when we realize that we have only to continue to employ the same *means whereby* we secure the increase (expansion) to secure the decrease (contraction) of the intra-thoracic capacity, which means that in process the contracting chest walls exert such increased pressure on the lungs that the air-pressure within is overcome, and the air consequently expelled, this process constituting "expiration"; the expiration and previous inspiration being the completed act of breathing. When a satisfactory, co-ordinated use of the mechanisms concerned with the acts of inspiration and expiration is established, the teacher may then proceed to help the pupil to employ this co-ordinated use in connexion with all vocal effort. As has been pointed out in *Man's Supreme Inheritance*, this should begin with *whispered* vocalization, preferably the vowel sound "Ah," as this form of vocal use, being so little employed in every-day life, is rarely associated with ordinary bad psycho-physical habits in vocalization.

For this reason, the teacher will begin by helping the pupil to make the expiration on a whispered "Ah." This calls for a knowledge of the psycho-physical "means-whereby" of the use of the organism *in general*, and of the acts of opening the mouth, using the lips, tongue, soft palate, etc., with freedom from stress and strain of the vocal mechanisms, and to this end a definite technique is employed. The process involved prevents sniffing and "sucking in air," undue depression of the larynx and undue stiffening of the muscles of the throat, vocal organs and neck. It also prevents the undue lifting of the front part of the chest during inspiration, its undue depression during expiration, and also many other defects which are developed by any imperfectly co-ordinated person who attempts to learn "breathing" or "deep-breathing," etc., guided by the unreliable sensory appreciation which is always associated with an imperfectly co-ordinated condition of the psycho-physical mechanism.

CHAPTER VI

UNDULY EXCITED FEAR REFLEXES, UNCONTROLLED EMOTIONS AND FIXED PREJUDICES

THERE can be little doubt that the process of reasoning tends to develop more quickly and to reach a higher standard in a person whose attitude towards life might be described as calm and collected. In such a person, the psycho-physical processes called "habits" are governed by moderation, and his inhibitory processes are adequately developed in all spheres of activity. Their use is not limited to those comparatively few spheres where it was considered necessary to establish taboos during the early and later periods of man's struggle with the problems which arose in the various stages of the civilizing process. In these spheres there has been a harmful and exaggerated development of the inhibitory processes, often causing virtues to become almost vices, whilst in other spheres there has been a correspondingly harmful lack of the development of inhibition, particularly in those spheres connected with the use of the psycho-physical mechanisms in practical activity. This represents an unbalanced use of this wonderful process of inhibition, and tends to produce, as a general result, a state of unbalanced psycho-physical functioning throughout the whole organism, and to establish what we shall refer to as "the unduly excited reflex" process.

This unbalanced psycho-physical condition of the civilized human creature is apparent in most spheres of activity, and the child of to-day is more predisposed to the factors which make for this condition than his parents or their ancestors. This child, therefore, starts his school career with a comparatively poor equipment on the inhibitory side. Now volition and inhibition are invaluable birthrights of the human creature and should be developed equally, as it were, hand in hand, but from the first moment of a child's school life right on to adolescence the training[63] he

[63]The fact of the great number of "don'ts" to which some children are subjected, and the implicit obedience expected of them at school and at home, does not affect my contention that the children of to-day manifest a serious lack on the inhibitory side in all activity involving the use of the psycho-physical organism.

receives tends to interfere with his balanced development, and so is another factor in the cultivation of those psycho-physical defects and abnormalities which make for the unbalanced condition to which we have already referred.

Unduly excited fear reflexes, uncontrolled emotions, prejudices and fixed habits, are retarding factors in all human development. They need our serious attention, for they are linked up with all psycho-physical processes employed in growth and development on the subconscious plane. Hence, by the time adolescence is reached, these retarding factors have become present in a more or less degree, and the processes thus established in psycho-physical use will make for the continued development of such retarding factors. This is particularly the case when a person endeavours to learn something calling for new experiences.

It is only necessary to watch adult pupils at their lessons to realize that, in the great majority of cases, more or less uncontrolled emotions are a striking feature in their endeavours to carry out new instructions correctly. Watch the fixed expression of these pupils, for instance, their jerky, uncontrolled movements, and their tendency to hold the breath by assuming a harmful posture and exerting an exaggerated strain such as they would employ in performing strenuous "physical" acts. In many cases there will be a twitching of the muscles of the mouth and cheeks, or of the fingers. In each case, the stimulus to these misdirected activities is the pupil's idea or conception that he must try to do *correctly* whatever the teacher requests, and, as we have seen, on the subconscious plane the teacher insists upon this. The teacher of re-education on a conscious plane does not make this demand of his pupils, for he knows by experience, and has to face the fact that in cases where there is an imperfect functioning of the organism, *an individual cannot always do as he is told correctly*. He may "want" to do it, he may "try and try again" to do it, but as long as the psycho-mechanics by which he tries to carry out his teacher's directions are not working satisfactorily, every attempt he makes to carry out his teacher's directions "correctly" (trying to be right) is bound to end in comparative failure. For in making these attempts, as we point out elsewhere, the pupil has only his own judgment to depend on as to what is correct, and since his judgment is based on incorrect direction and delusive sensory appreciation, he is held within the vicious circle of his old habits as long as he tries to carry out the directions "correctly." Paradoxical as it may seem, the pupil's only chance of success lies, not in "trying to be right," but, on the contrary, in "wanting to be wrong," wrong, that is, according to any standard of his own. In this connexion, it is most important to remember that every unsuccessful "try" not only reinforces the pupil's old wrong psycho-physical habits associated with his conception of a particular act, but involves at the same time new emotional experiences of discouragement, worry, fear, and anxiety, so that the wrong experiences and the unduly excited reflex process involved in these experiences become one in the pupil's recognition; they "make the meat they feed on," and the more conscientious the teacher and the pupil are on this plan, the worse the situation becomes for both.

It is for this reason that the teacher on a conscious plane does not expect a pupil, as I have pointed out, to perform "correctly" a new act calling for new experiences, but instead, by means of manipulation, gives to the pupil the new experiences, repeating them until they become established. We have seen, indeed, in Chapter III that he asks his pupil not to make any attempt to gain the "end" at all, but instead to learn gradually to remember the guiding orders or directions, which are the forerunners of the *means whereby* the end may one day be gained. This may not be to-day, tomorrow or the next day, but it will be, and then the pupil will be able to repeat the act with mathematical precision at all times and under all circumstances, for such retarding factors as unduly excited fear reflexes, uncontrolled emotions and fixed prejudices will not have been developed in the process just outlined. Indeed, a process which does not involve a pupil's being asked to perform any act, until his teacher has prepared the way by raising the standard of the pupil's sensory appreciation and psycho-physical co-ordination to that satisfactory state which will enable him to perform the act, as we say, easily, will be a process which ensures that the pupil's experiences will be, with rare exceptions, satisfactory experiences, which make for confidence and are not associated with those emotional disturbances which tend towards the minimum instead of the maximum functioning.

The relation of all this to the very important question of the ability to "keep one's head" at critical moments is clear, and it may be interesting to apply the points we have raised in the foregoing to such activities as playing games and to other performances in which skill and so-called "presence of mind" are required. We constantly hear in this connexion remarks like the following: "I didn't do so badly at it at first, but the longer I play the worse I play." One writer in the public Press remarks that it is a curious feature of golf that "the more one knows about it . . . the more difficult it seems to become"; and another writes that a well-known professional had "confessed . . . that golf had become almost too much for him." All this applies equally, of course, to other games, but I have chosen golf for my illustration because it happens that writers on golf, commenting on some of the incidents that have occurred at matches during the past two years or so, have unwittingly emphasized the existence of *the problem* which underlies these admissions and with which I am dealing in the present book. For instance, they have commented on the failure of certain experts to perform some simple stroke when under an unusual stress, and at a moment when success depends on their not throwing a chance away; they have pointed to the tendency of some players to become confused and to hurry their strokes through anxiety to "get it over"; "truly heart-breaking" is the description of one such incident, words that will be echoed by many who have had similar discouraging experiences in other matters besides golf.

We are told that this is all a matter of "nerves" and so forth. It is undoubtedly a case of the undue excitement of fear reflexes on the player's part, fear, for instance, that he may miss a shot which he knows he is not in the habit of missing and ought not to miss. As a pupil once said to me at a first interview, "I am always coming up against things that I know I can do, and yet when it comes to the point, I can't do them." The fact is that in all our processes of learning things, the fear reflexes are unduly and harmfully excited by the teaching methods employed, according to which demands are made upon us that we are not able to fulfill. So, for a time, we get bad results, with the undue and harmful development of emotional reflex processes which, as we have seen, inevitably accompanies these unsuccessful attempts. We continue to practise on wrong lines, so that our successful experiences are few and our unsuccessful experiences many. We attempt on a subconscious basis to develop a particular stroke, and in any failure to make the stroke satisfactorily the imperfect use of the psycho-physical mechanisms plays more than its fair share. It is experiences like this which cause disappointment and undue excitement of fear reflexes and serious emotional disturbances, and nothing whatever is done at this later stage of the process to nullify these effects of the psycho-physical experiences cultivated during the earlier stages. These emotional disturbances were part and parcel of an unbalanced psycho-physical condition, of a state of anxiety and confusion, and there can be little doubt that any circumstance that is more or less unusual is likely to bring about a recurrence of the same disturbed psycho-physical condition as was experienced by the subject during his early efforts to make the stroke.

But, beyond this, we must remember that it is only the small minority of experts in any line who really know *how* they get their results and effects,[64] in the case of golf, for instance, *how* they perform their most

[64]The same thing applies to the expert singer who does not know how he sings, any more than the political and social leaders of our time know how much more they are influenced in their decisions and actions by their prejudices and "emotional gusts" by their reasoning processes.

successful strokes. Therefore directly anything puts them "off their game," they experience considerable difficulty, at any rate, in getting on to it again. It is only by having a clear conception of what is required for the successful performance of a certain stroke or other act, combined with a knowledge of the psycho-physical *means whereby* those requirements can be met, that there is any reasonable possibility of their attaining sureness and confidence during performance.

I would here refer my readers to my earlier volume, where this point was dealt with at some length in connexion with golf, and I have the less hesitation in doing so, as what I have written there has since had the endorsement of such a distinguished golfer as Mr. John Duncan Dunn,[65] a matter, naturally, of great gratification to me. I there attempted to make clear that the success of any particular process in golf, such as, for instance, "following through," must depend, primarily, on the *general* condition of psycho-physical development and control present, because a player whose sensory appreciation is in any way at fault cannot satisfactorily carry out directions given to him. For the indispensable preliminary to success is a reliable sensory appreciation which will guide the particular player in his efforts to reach and maintain *during the stroke* an adequate standard of co-ordination in the general use of his mechanism. This satisfactory *general* use is essential to satisfactory *specific* use. By chance or good luck a man may make a good stroke without having attained to a good standard in the general use of himself, but he can never be reasonably certain of repeating it, and the experiences associated with this state of uncertainty do not make for the growth of confidence, but rather for the development of undue fear reflexes and serious emotional disturbances.[66]

We must realize that if an individual is to reach that satisfactory stage

---

[65]Author of *ABC of Golf. Intimate Golf Talks* (Dunn and Jessup).

[66]The following quoted from the *Times*, October 29th, 1921, is a delightful little parable showing the fallacy of expecting pupils to be able to put right some defect unless the *means whereby* they can correct it is first given into their hands.

> 'Wandering a little farther along the course, I came across two elderly gentlemen playing a short hole. The first hit a good shot on to the green. The second did not. "Would any sane man," he exclaimed, "believe that such things could be?" "I could put you right in a minute," said complacent No. 1. "I wish you would," replied humble No. 2. "Well, I will," said No. 1. And I waited, breathless, thinking that at last I was going to find out the secret of all hitting. "You don't follow through." It was yet one more disappointment in a bitterly disappointed life, *for I knew that I, and most other people in the world, very often "don't follow through," and that knowledge does not make one play any better.* "Oh No. 1, No. 1," I murmured, "what the devil is the good of telling me that? You must tell me *what I do with my confounded arms and legs on the way up, that they behave so ill on the way down.* You are not such a good coach as I thought you, No. 1," and I went away sorrowful.' [The italics are mine.—F. M. A.]

of progress where he can be reasonably certain of success in achieving his "ends," those principles must be observed which imply reliance in all activities upon the *means whereby* an "end" may be gained, irrespective of whether, during the progress of the activities concerned, the performance is correct or incorrect. The application of these principles in any sphere of learning means that the teacher during lessons must be able to supply the pupil's needs in the matter of reliable sensory appreciation, by giving him from day to day the necessary experiences until they become established. No technique which does not meet the demands herein indicated will prove satisfactory as a means of re-educating a pupil on a general basis to a reliable plane of conscious activity. When this plane is reached, the individual comes to rely upon his "means-whereby," and does not become disturbed by wondering whether the activities concerned will be right or wrong. Why should he, seeing that the confidence with which he proceeds with his task is a confidence born of experiences, the majority of which are successful experiences unassociated with over-excited fear reflexes? This confidence is further reinforced by his confidence in the reliability of his sensory appreciation which ensures that any interference with the co-ordinated use of himself will come to his consciousness as soon as it occurs (awareness). This consciousness is really a state of acute awareness which has been developed in him during the processes of re-education and co-ordination on a general basis, and the confidence associated with it is not likely to desert him in moments of crisis. It is true that he may be put off the right track, but he knows that it will only be momentarily, as he is certain that his awareness, associated as it is with reliable sensory appreciation, will not fail him in such situations or crises, but will prove his protector and reliable guide; for this state of awareness means that he will be able at such moments to remember, reason and judge (that is, to size up the situation, as we say), and the resultant judgment, based as it is upon experiences associated with reliable sensory appreciation and unassociated with unduly excited fear reflexes, will be in its turn a sound and reliable judgment.

This matter of unduly excited fear reflexes has been referred to in the chapter on education and here I wish to discuss processes used in tests made on children in this connexion.

In some schools special mechanical tests are made in order to discover the potentialities and qualities of the children and to grade them accordingly. The young and undeveloped organism of the child's "mental apparatus" is, as it were, put upon the rack, and his intellectual status and probably his educational fate depend upon the result of these tests which are supposed to be a reliable guide, not only as to the line of procedure to be taken in regard to the details of his school education, but also as to the particular career for which he will be best adapted when the state of adolescence is reached.

A teacher recently told me of an interesting personal experience in this connexion. She visited a modern school where a psychologist was engaged in testing the children for such qualities as accuracy, muscular control, observation, etc. She was taken into a small room set apart for the purpose of such tests. A boy of seven was waiting there to be tested for "control." He had shewn various symptoms which were described as "nervous," and the test to be taken was to enable the school authorities to prescribe a curriculum to meet his special needs. The test was made as follows. An apparatus, electrically worked, was placed in front of the child. It consisted of a metal tray in which were sunk two rows of shallow circular holes decreasing gradually in size from that of a shilling to a very small size. The boy was told to touch the centre of each hole with a small metal rod tapering to a point like a pencil. If he made a mistake and touched the side of a hole in his effort to get the centre, an electric flash would be the result.

The child, so I was told, was already in a state of nervous dread, and when he received the instruction, "Now you must try and touch the centre of each hole, and do not touch the side of any hole or else you will make a flash," he at once became so excited *through the fear of making a mistake* that his hand shook and he stiffened and tensed his whole body unduly in making the first try. He was therefore unable to control his hand to find the centre of the first hole, touched the side and produced a flash. Still more frightened by this, still more anxious not to do the wrong thing again, he proceeded from hole to hole, making flash after flash, realizing that every mistake he made was being noted by the "tester," against him, as he thought, so that, by the time he had reached the last hole his condition was one of undue excitement. It is obvious that a test taken with such emotional conditions present was not a reliable test of his control or a trustworthy guide to anyone wishing to estimate his potentialities and general qualities. Indeed, I am prepared to prove by demonstration that nine out of ten of the children now being submitted to tests are imperfectly co-ordinated, and that a great number are beset with very serious psycho-physical defects.

Now in this matter of tests, because the human organism is an animate machine, I wish to carry the reader on to a consideration of an inanimate machine, say a motor car. Would any sane person attempt to test a motor car on the road, if he were certain that a number of the important parts of the mechanism were imperfectly adjusted? And if he happened to be foolish enough to do this with his badly adjusted machine, could he expect to judge of the standard of functioning of that particular make of car by the result of these tests? These are unreasonable propositions such as no mechanic would entertain for a moment. But unfortunately, in the field of education, the same idea in regard to mechanics does not prevail. The "end-gaining" principle holds sway and in the sphere of psycho-physical activity under consideration the process of reasoning takes little part. If it had done so, the psychological expert in tests would have demanded that a child should be in a satisfactory state of co-ordination and adjustment before he would consent to make tests as to the child's potentialities. He would then be dealing with a psycho-physical organism functioning satisfactorily and tests made with these conditions present could probably be of some assistance to those concerned with the child's growth and development and future career.

Where the imperfectly co-ordinated child is concerned, its first need is to be readjusted and co-ordinated on a plane of conscious control, until the standard of functioning in psycho-physical use of the organism is adequate. The organism will then function as near to the maximum as is possible, and the potentialities for improved functioning will continue as the child gradually develops to that standard of conscious guidance and control in psycho-physical use, which makes for the conditions essential to the fullest development of latent potentialities.

* * * * *

We have all heard instances advanced of wonderful feats being performed by people in an emotional state, of "faith cures" being effected when the subjects of these "cures" are in that uncontrolled and harmful psycho-physical state which is akin to conditions associated with drunkenness, and which at times approximates to mild insanity. For instance, the writer was acquainted with a man who never accomplished anything worth mentioning in his particular sphere of life until he was half crazed with alcohol. He also knows of a carriage painter who is unable to put in the straight lines satisfactorily unless he is well under the influence of alcohol. We can all point to instances of men and women who have performed remarkable acts whilst in an uncontrolled emotional state, in which they have been a danger to themselves and to those around them. Men are sent into battle in a half-drunken condition in order that their "controls" may be temporarily released, and for centuries bands of musicians have been employed in warfare to induce this emotional condition of lowered control. "Muddling through by instinct" is unintelligent enough, but deliberately to induce in human beings by artificial means (such as the processes involved in methods of "faith cure," auto-suggestion, religious revivalism, etc.), a condition of lowered control, where intelligence and reasoning are superseded by uncontrolled emotions, is a procedure which may be described as an insult to even a very lowly evolved intelligence. All concerned reach the borderland of insanity through the use of such means for the accomplishment of their aims, and the psycho-physical experiences involved have only to be repeated sufficiently to bring madness in their train. In all these instances, the "end-gaining" principle is in operation, and the people subjected to these unnatural and harmful experiences are more or less influenced by them in after life, for the uncontrolled forces which run riot on these occasions are rarely mastered again, and recur more or less in other spheres of activity, frequently developing into dangerous manifestations, culminating often in tragedy. Small wonder that after the experience of 1914-1918 we are confronted with dangerous uncontrolled forces in human activity which, before the War, were manifested only by a small minority! When the individual is dominated by his uncontrolled emotions, even a weak stimulus will often cause him to indulge in dangerous activities, leading him temporarily to experiences which are well within the psycho-physical state which we call "insanity." The repetition of such experiences is the beginning of the formation of what we call a habit, in this case, the habit of unbalanced psycho-physical activity, and unfortunately, as we all know, it does not take long to establish a bad habit.[67] So-called "mental" tricks are more common than purely "physical" tricks, and we are well aware that, when indulged in, they soon become a habit, and that the indulgence of one bad habit tends to the development of others, with a rapid increase in the degree of indulgence.

In this matter of bad habits, and the lack of control which they connote, we must recognize the fact that the human creature cannot be expected to exercise control in the different spheres of his activity in civilization, unless he is in possession of reliable sensory appreciation and of a satisfactory use of the psycho-physical mechanisms involved. People who are lacking in control will be found to be imperfectly co-ordinated, and their sensory appreciation to be unreliable, and no form of discipline or other outside influence can secure that satisfactory standard of psycho-physical functioning without which the individual cannot com-

[67]Worry is one of these bad habits which, once established, are very hard to break. A curious feature of this habit is that, in certain cases, though you may remove the cause for worry, and the subject may admit that the cause has been removed, the removal of the cause does not remove the "mental" state which the subject declared was the cause of the worry. The fact is, the person has developed the worry habit, a state in which he manufactures the stimulus to worry.

mand a satisfactory standard of control within or without the organism.

Where the human being manifests this lack of control, he needs to be re-educated on a general basis so that reliable sensory appreciation may be restored, together with a satisfactory employment of the psycho-physical mechanisms. The processes of this form of re-education demand that the "means-whereby" to any "end" must be reasoned out, not on a specific but on a general basis, and with the continued use of these processes of reasoning, uncontrolled impulses and "emotional gusts" will gradually cease to dominate, and will ultimately be dominated. The organism will not then be called upon to satisfy those unhealthy cravings which we find associated with unreliable and delusive sensory appreciation (debauched kinæsthesia).

The fact is, the principle of reasoning out on a general basis the *means whereby* we shall command our "ends" simply implies a common-sense procedure. Common sense is a very familiar phrase and we all have our particular conception of what it means. We know many people who will point out that individual opinion can differ as much in regard to the meaning of common sense, as in regard to religious, political, social, and educational matters. We will therefore put our point of view in regard to common sense by giving an instance in which we consider the human creature does not evince common sense. The man who is convinced that he is suffering from digestive and liver disorders, and knows that this has been caused by his indulgence in alcohol, or by excessive eating, and still continues to indulge in either of these habits, despite the depression and suffering which result, and despite the assurance of his medical adviser that moderation will put him on the road to good health once more, cannot be said to act in accordance with common sense.

My reader may say that the man cannot refrain from taking alcohol or from over-eating, and it may be advantageous to consider this man's inability to act in accordance with the dictates of common sense. In the first place, it is clear that he had recognized the fact that he was ill. The fact that he had consulted his medical adviser is proof that the stimulus (or stimuli) in this connexion had reached his consciousness, and no doubt he was quite ready to take the medicine or carry out the form of treatment prescribed, provided that these did not interfere with his habit of indulging in alcohol or in over-eating. But, of course, the desired return to health could not be secured by such an unreasoning procedure. The habit is always the impeding factor and, in this case, the medicine and the treatment were of little importance unless the bad habit of over-indulgence in alcohol, or of excessive feeding, could be eradicated.

This leads us to the consideration of the psycho-physical activities within the organism of which habit, so-called, is a manifestation. In the case of a person who is blessed with a satisfactory standard of psycho-physical co-ordination, moderation will be the rule and excess the exception to that rule. With the person who is badly co-ordinated, the reverse will be the case, in a more or less degree, in one or more spheres, for the habit of excess will gradually become more firmly established with too frequent repetition of the indulgence of the debauched sensory desires connected, in the case given, with eating and drinking, thus making indulgence the rule and not the exception.

In the continuance of our consideration we will trace the cultivation of the alcohol habit, where the subject of our illustration is concerned. That we speak of the cultivation of this habit presupposes a time in the history of the man when he did not make a habit of taking alcohol in such quantities as would cause liver and other internal disorders. The facts concerned with his reasons, however, for beginning to take alcohol to excess at some particular time of his life would not help us very much, even if we could be certain of them. The important point for us to remember is that his sensory appreciation was unreliable and perverted, and his psycho-physical organism in an unsatisfactory state of co-ordination, so that he gradually became dominated by that sensory debauchery which results from excessive alcoholic and other indulgence, and by the depressing and enervating conditions which follow. These latter conditions are among the most potent of the stimuli which make for the repetition of the excesses at more and more frequent intervals, this repetition counteracting again for a time the depressing and enervating conditions brought about by the renewed indulgence. Unfortunately, the process is one that "makes the meat it feeds on," so that the degree of sensory debauchery increases rapidly until the functioning of the organism becomes utterly demoralized.

It is almost certain that in the early stages of his alcoholic experiences, the subject was unaware of his lack of satisfactory co-ordination and sensory appreciation. As a matter of fact, it is unlikely that he had ever given consideration to his psycho-physical condition. He had simply taken alcohol occasionally, as he had taken many other things in the way of food and drink, never for a moment meaning that it should become a habit, or even suspecting that he lacked the ability either to continue taking it only occasionally, or to discontinue taking it altogether if he so wished. This reveals the degree to which egotism may be subconsciously developed in the human creature, until it becomes a potent factor in influencing the processes associated with subconscious and unreasoned conclusions, such as the one arrived at by the subject of our illustration in regard to his ability to continue to drink occasionally or to discontinue drinking altogether. If he had consciously attempted to search out the correct premisses from which to make his deductions, and if his effort had been attended with success, he would have discovered the unsatisfactory standard of his general functioning, and this would have brought a realization that he must, by some means, make certain that his standard of psycho-physical co-ordination and sensory appreciation was satisfactory, before he allowed himself to entertain even mildly egotistical conclusions regarding his ability to fight his bad habits. If such an analysis of the psycho-physical factors involved had been made, he must have been led to the conclusion that *in the matter of the breaking of habit, the standard of sensory appreciation is the all-important factor.* His increasing desire for alcohol probably came very gradually, as also the corresponding decline in his standard of co-ordination and sensory appreciation. Thus the gratification experienced in satisfying the already abnormal desire would soon dominate psycho-physical processes which otherwise might have been exercised in the field of reasoning and common sense, and he might then have been led to a consideration of the consequences of permitting himself to become a victim of the alcohol habit.

In all such experiences, there comes a time at last when the person concerned is forced to recognize the harmful effects of such a habit, and then very often makes an effort to fight the desire and to eradicate the habit. But too frequently it happens that the effort is a feeble one or that it is made along impossible lines. Some well-meaning friend, for instance, may urge the man to use what is called "will-power" to fight and control his desire, *but the desire is a sensory desire and the processes called "will-power" have in this case long since been dominated by the debauched sensory appreciation associated with this desire*, and therefore his hope of salvation lies in the restoration of his sensory appreciation to that normal condition which we do not find associated with abnormal and unhealthy desire. In *Man's Supreme Inheritance* we have referred to that degenerate state of the organism when the human creature will desire a form of sensory satisfaction through actual pain. In the case of alcoholic excesses, each occasion of indulgence is followed by suffering, often intense suffering, but even this does not act as a deterrent. We must therefore realize the enormous influence of perverted sensory desire on the human creature, and recognize that satisfactory development in the control of his psycho-physical processes is impossible without that reliable sensory appreciation which goes hand in hand with normal sensory desires.

One point more. Fundamental desires and needs must be satisfied; if they are not, serious results must follow sooner or later, and the fact that the attempt to satisfy desires and needs leads many individuals to indulge in abuse and excess does not affect this conclusion. Abuse and excess are always associated with abnormality, and abnormality is due to abnormal conditions in the psycho-physical functioning of the organism, and this applies in the matter of abuse and excess in eating, as well as in drinking and in connexion with any other needs and desires. Abuse or excess is an attempt to satisfy a need or desire, which, originally normal, has become abnormal, and as long as this abnormal desire or need remains, it is useless to deny a man the "means-whereby" to his excesses and abuses. Our energies should instead be applied to attempts to eradicate the abnormal conditions responsible for the excess and abuse, and so to restore the normal psycho-physical functioning of the organism and the reliable sensory appreciation which ensures the maintenance of normality in our desires and needs.

CHAPTER VII

PSYCHO-PHYSICAL EQUILIBRIUM

THE lack of a satisfactory condition of psycho-physical equilibrium in all human activities is one of the most striking manifestations of imperfect functioning of the organism. The present faulty subconscious use of the psycho-physical mechanism, in our educational and other spheres, makes for the gradual increase of this condition of defective equilibrium. It would seem that this fact is generally taken for granted, seeing that we expect defective equilibrium at a certain age, just as we expect the development of a flabby and protruding abdomen. This is surely the end of our contention that practice makes perfect; it also seems evident from this that there must be something wrong with the practice in the act of walking.

The fact is that people walk without any clear understanding of the guiding and controlling orders which command the satisfactory co-ordination and adjustment of the psycho-physical mechanism in the act of walking. Hence when one or more defects become present in the functioning of these mechanisms, even though the persons concerned may be aware of their cause or causes, they are incapable of establishing once more that standard of reliable sensory appreciation which would enable them to eradicate these defects. This needs a process of re-education on a general basis, which will restore satisfactory functioning throughout the organism, and so ensure a continued raising of the standard of psycho-physical equilibrium right on through life.

In what follows I shall endeavour to shew that with almost every attempt to correct some supposed or real psycho-physical imperfection, new defects are developed which tend to lower the standard of psycho-physical equilibrium. In this connexion, it is an interesting but very unfortunate fact that this unsatisfactory condition develops in the subject hand in hand with the desire to hurry unduly, this being a subconscious endeavour to compensate for the growing lack of equilibrium and lack of control. In extreme cases of lack of equilibrium this manifestation is most pronounced. The subject becomes conscious, first, of a weakness or difficulty which affects his general equilibrium in walking, and, without making any attempt to discover the cause or causes of this newly recognized weakness or difficulty, proceeds, as he would put it, to try to "walk properly," i.e., to walk without the slight unsteadiness of which he is conscious. But the fact that this weakness or difficulty has developed is proof that the subject's guiding sensations and general psycho-physical co-ordinations of the organism are defective. It is therefore obvious that any subconsciously directed efforts on his part to "walk properly," i.e., more steadily, will be carried out according to these same defective guiding sensations and imperfectly co-ordinated mechanisms, and cannot therefore succeed.

It must be remembered that during all these "trial-and-error" experiences the fear reflexes are being unduly excited by the fear of falling, and by the general unreliability and uncertainty of the psycho-physical processes which are employed during such subconsciously directed efforts. Taking this process as a whole, we shall find that most harmful psycho-physical conditions will be developed, which soon manifest themselves in other spheres of psycho-physical functioning, and very often culminate at last in some serious crisis.

It is easy to trace the development of this lack of equilibrium in what is usually considered the "purely physical" sphere. Let us take by way of illustration the case of a boy who, in the ordinary way, would be classed as a good walker. We will assume that he has been injured at the age of, say, thirteen by being thrown from a horse or by a fall downstairs, or has met with some other accident which has necessitated his being treated by a doctor and being confined to his bed for some time. It is obvious that his injury and the cessation of his ordinary activities will produce in the patient a more or less weakened condition generally, and also definite specific difficulties in connexion with the injured parts of the organism. The result is that at the psychological moment when the patient makes the first attempt to resume walking, certain impeding factors will manifest themselves which he will immediately proceed to overcome by "trying to walk properly" as he understands it. His attempt to walk "properly" must necessarily be on the subconscious plan of "trial-and-error," for it is almost certain that he has never known HOW he walked, never had the least idea of the guiding orders concerned with the co-ordinations essential to the act of walking and to the development of satisfactory equilibrium.[68]

[68]My reader will probably think of the case of some friend who made an attempt to "walk properly" after an injury, and who is now walking about to HIS OWN satisfaction. My point is, that the subject is not capable of judging whether his use of his psycho-physical mechanisms in walking is satisfactory or not. It is quite certain that anyone

It will be necessary here to analyse the psycho-physical processes involved in his effort, for success in such efforts demands quite a high standard of co-ordinated functioning of the organism. Experience has proved to us that this standard of functioning is not at the command of a person who has been through the experiences connected with such an injury, and with the subsequent treatment and gradual recovery to the point when what we call the convalescent stage has been reached. Real success is practically impossible and for the reasons which follow.

These attempts to walk would be made at a time when the subject was conscious of a weakness throughout the whole organism, of a comparative loss of control, of an interference with the psycho-physical equilibrium, of a lack of confidence, together with a whole series of hopes and fears in regard to what he will or will not be able to do, associated, again, with fears which have their origin in the pain which results from his incorrect subconscious attempts to use parts that have been injured. This whole combination of psycho-physical conditions constitutes a set of experiences which are new as compared with those present at the time of the accident. Each subconscious attempt to walk awakens consciousness of shortcomings, of strange and often alarming sensations, and tends to increase the real difficulties, viz., those concerned with that correct use of the psycho-physical organism in general upon which "walking properly" depends.

It will thus be clear that the attempt to walk properly by subconscious guidance would merely be an attempt to revert to the habit or habits established in the act of walking before the accident. This way of walking was instinctive, and a particular instinctive process is the result of certain psycho-physical conditions operating, as we say, by instinct. Change those conditions quickly and you interfere with the reliability of the working of the particular instinct.

This illustration furnishes us with a splendid practical instance of a definite need calling for new experiences in psycho-physical use. The boy wishes to walk. The stimulus to do so produces an immediate response involving the processes concerned with subconscious guidance and control which are habitual, but which depend for efficiency upon a given standard of co-ordinated functioning of the organism. Unfortunately, this standard has been lowered by his experiences associated with the accident, and the psycho-physical machinery does not

---

with an expert knowledge in this connexion could point to certain harmful defects in the subject's use of himself which are the combined result of the injury, the varied experiences in treatment and recovery, and the attempts "to walk," all of which are indicative of comparative weakness, a sense of interference with equilibrium and a general loss of control.

work as satisfactorily as before; in fact, in the majority of such cases, it works very unsatisfactorily. The subject is able to compare the result of his present efforts with those he made before his injury. They compare very badly, and he is conscious of the fact. This merely causes him to "try harder," as he would put it, "to walk properly," and, on a subconscious basis, he has no alternative but to continue the unintelligent method of "trial-and-error."

We will now outline the experiences which the procedure based on the principles of re-education on a conscious general basis would have ensured in the foregoing case. In the first place, we should not allow the subject to try to "walk properly" until he had been given, by expert manipulation, correct experiences in the general use of the psycho-physical mechanisms, and had become well acquainted with the correct guiding and controlling orders which would assist in the securing of the *means whereby* he should use the mechanisms in any attempt to walk properly.

The recognition of weakness or difficulty would be the signal for an examination of the psycho-physical mechanisms involved in the use of the organism as a whole, which in time would enable us to note the defects and peculiarities in the use of these mechanisms in the specific act of walking. The technique we advocate would demand in practice that the subject should cease to try to improve his walking. We would therefore endeavour to convince him by demonstration that his efforts to improve his walking by "muddling through by instinct" are not only futile but quite absurd. By the same process (demonstration) he would be shewn that as soon as he receives the stimulus to walk, he must begin his remedial work by employing his inhibitory powers to prevent the use of the wrong subconscious guidance and direction associated with his conception of "walking." In this connexion it is explained to him that it is the use of the incorrect, subconscious guiding orders to the mechanisms concerned with the act of walking, associated with unreliable sensory appreciation, which has caused the mechanisms to be used imperfectly, resulting in the weakness and difficulties with which we are contending.

When the subject is more or less familiar with these inhibitory experiences, we go on to give him a knowledge of the new and correct directive and guiding orders which, with the aid of manipulation, are to bring about the satisfactory use of the mechanisms in a sitting, prone, or other position. These experiences must be repeated until the new and reliable sensory appreciation becomes established, by which time there will have taken place an actual change in the use of the psycho-physical mechanisms of the organism in general, making for a satisfactory condition of co-ordination and adjustment. When the required improvement in the general co-ordinations and adjustments has been secured, the processes we have outlined will be more or less in conscious operation, and a corresponding improvement in equilibrium in walking will be the result.

The reader must understand that the details involved in such processes (differing as these do in each case) cannot be set forth here, and that, moreover, from the very first lessons the teacher's aim would be to cause the pupil to be conscious of what he should or should NOT do, and to give such help to the pupil as would enable him to begin at once to apply the principles involved, not only to his attempts at walking, but more or less to all the acts of his daily life. In other words, the pupil is not taught to perform certain new exercises or to assume new postures for a given time each day, whilst continuing to use his faulty mechanisms and unreliable guiding sensations in his old way during his other activities, but he is shewn HOW he may at once check, more or less, the faulty use of these mechanisms in the general activities of his daily life.

An increase in lack of equilibrium in what is called the "physical" sphere, will be found, in every case, to go hand in hand with a corresponding lack of equilibrium in so-called "mental" spheres. And in any consideration of "mental" and "physical" phenomena, it must be remembered that in our present stage of evolution on the subconscious plane, the response to any stimulus or stimuli is at least seventy-five per cent subconscious response (chiefly feeling) as against twenty-five per cent any other response, this estimate of the ratio of subconscious response being probably too low.

When these facts are fully realized by all those who are interested in education and in the conduct of life generally, there may be some chance of the realization of those commendable ideals for the uplifting of mankind cherished by leaders in the social, religious and political spheres.

PART III
SENSORY APPRECIATION IN ITS RELATION TO MAN'S NEEDS

CHAPTER I

"KNOWING ONESELF"

THOSE who give thought to the present trend of human endeavour in political, social, industrial and other spheres will recognize that our times are "out of joint," and many of them will admit that the masses living in this disjointed time are more or less out of communication with their reasoning. In the midst of this unrest and uncertainty, the individuals composing the masses are struggling blindly for their individual betterment, without any clear understanding of the cause or causes of their difficulties, or of the fundamental principles which constitute in application the satisfactory *means whereby* these difficulties may be prevented or overcome.

"Man, know thyself" is an old axiom, but in my opinion the more fundamental one is "Man, know thy needs." Of course, it may be contended that he who knows himself knows his needs, and that to know one's needs implies knowing oneself, but the contention does not apply to that great majority of human beings whose sensory appreciation is unreliable. We have seen that reliable sensory appreciation is essential to that co-ordinated psycho-physical growth and development of the individual which is fundamental to the satisfactory psycho-physical growth and development of the mass, and this being so, in order to secure this growth and development of the mass, it is essential to command the "means-whereby" of recognizing and supplying the real needs of the individual.

Unfortunately, our attempts to supply and satisfy these needs in the educational, social, political, economic, industrial, religious and other spheres, have proved, up to now, more or less of a failure, and this is due in a great measure to the fact that our efforts on a subconscious basis have been directed chiefly to evolving methods of teaching, treatment, conduct, guidance and control to meet the demands of the mass, instead of making the primary application of the principle or principles involved an individual application on a conscious basis. The foregoing leads us to a consideration of plans for human development and endeavour on the conscious and subconscious planes of life, and of the relative possibilities for advancement on each of these planes.

On the subconscious plane, the orthodox plan has been and still is to attempt to eradicate "physical" defects and peculiarities by means of physical culture, exercises, etc., "mental" shortcomings and idiosyncrasies by means of the different cults for "mental" training, specific systems for the development of memory, will, and so on. Investigation will shew that the deductions concerned with the adoption of such methods were made from wrong premisses, the fundamental principle of conscious guidance and control in the development and growth of the creature being ignored. Furthermore, it will be found that where "physical" and "mental" methods are employed, any apparent gain will be a specific sphere, and accompanied by harmful cultivated defects of which the teachers and pupils are ignorant, but which, sooner or later, reveal themselves and gradually become established as habits.

The progress made in recent years in what is called "psychological" knowledge leaves no room for doubt that human beings are too often unaware of their most striking psycho-physical defects, peculiarities and tendencies which, in such cases, have not risen, as we say, to the sphere of consciousness. Before we can make any real attempt to reach a satisfactory state of awareness in this connexion, that is, to know ourselves, we must cultivate, in connexion with our psycho-physical development, an increasing use of the process of reasoning in conscious endeavour, and having reached a satisfactory standard of readjustment and co-ordination through the establishment of a new and reliable sensory appreciation, we must proceed to put into practice this satisfactory, conscious use of the psycho-physical mechanism in every act of daily life.

The reader who becomes familiar with the principles of the special technique which has been evolved to meet these demands will realize that "knowing oneself" is part and parcel, as we say, of the process, and a knowledge which will increase and keep pace with the development in conscious psycho-physical guidance and control. This knowledge should be the foundation of the act of living in all spheres, and will be so when the education and general development of children is built upon the principles of constructive, conscious control. On this principle we can continue to raise the standard of "knowing oneself," and this is the surest way of raising the standard of everything else we know, and of securing satisfactory results in all spheres of learning.

A friend of mine who wanted to impress me with his right to be considered an authority on up-to-date psychology admitted that he based his claim on his intimate knowledge of human history, which he had acquired by a long and careful study of the works of eminent historians.

This belief gave him such satisfaction that I could not find it within me to suggest to him that the real history of human endeavour, as a guide to up-to-date psychology, has not been written by the historians, in fact, that it has yet to be begun, and that one does not dare to speculate as to the date of its possible completion.

When I write of human endeavour, I mean individual human endeavour in connexion with individual development and growth, and, therefore, from any real history of human endeavour we must eliminate the record of man's activities in wars and other spheres in which he is swayed chiefly by the herd instinct, where the example, good or bad, or the command of one person, is immediately followed by the rest as an unthinking, unintelligent, automatic mass. I am quite prepared to admit that the history of human beings in wars and other spheres of massed activity is of great interest to many people, but it is of infinitesimal interest or value, particularly where man's future is concerned, as compared with that of the individual effort of the human creature struggling daily to find a solution of the flesh-and-blood difficulties which directly concern his well-being. These difficulties are the natural consequences of his endeavours to adapt himself to ever-changing psycho-physical conditions and of his attempts to evolve from the uncivilized to the civilized state in accordance with his early established subconscious conception of educational and general development.

This is equally true of the every-day development and general experiences of ordinary men and women in every sphere of human activity, for we are beset with contending and disorganizing forces in the working of the psycho-physical organism of each individual, inasmuch as we are developing so-called "mental" processes at a rapidly increasing pace never before experienced, whilst attempting to employ them side by side with so-called "physical" processes which for years have become less and less satisfactorily controlled and directed, the result being a lowering of the standard of psycho-physical co-ordination.

The long line of daily difficulties with which we are now beset is only equalled by the series of shattered hopes that have followed each subconsciously directed, specific "end-gaining" attempt to bring about a solution of these difficulties. Each failure makes "the meat it feeds on," and the "trial-and-error" method of the ape has been persistently adhered to, despite the fact of its failure in most civilized spheres.

I will now deal from this point of view with certain systems of education and development which hold public attention at the moment, and which were designed to meet certain difficulties and defects, and I will endeavour to shew that the hopes of those concerned cannot be justified, because these systems were conceived on a specific basis, and because the processes involved in their practical application call for reliance only upon subconscious experience for direction and control. We have reached a stage in our evolution when we should refuse to consider the merits or demerits of any new system of education or development which is not built upon a conscious basis.

One of these systems has been taken up in recent years by a number of people in England and America as a new and valuable form of education, but as the principles involved are simply those which were employed by the circus trainers of our grandfathers' time, in training horses to perform evolutions to music and at the change of music to change the step, etc., in a discussion of general psycho-physical development on a basis of reasoning control, it can be put out of court and dismissed without further comment.

Another system has been hailed as a new and progressive movement and is well known for the special claim that is made for it in connexion with its value in the development of the young child's senses of sight, feeling, taste, hearing, touch, etc. An organized series of materials, or educative toys, provides the technique for this attempted sense cultivation, but it will be realized by anyone who has watched the classes of children at work that it is again a *specific* and not a general development that is aimed at in this technique, a fatal mistake when we consider the interdependence of what have been differentiated as "mental" and "physical" in the human organism. It is quite possible that a child, by using this material, may gain a certain facility in the use of its hands, or a specific development, say, of the sense of touch. But if, in making the movements necessary to the particular occupation in which he is engaged, he is relying upon the guidance of an imperfect sensory appreciation in the general use of his organism, it must follow that any specific improvement in the sense of touch will be accompanied by a use of his psycho-physical mechanism which, faulty to start with, will become more and more faulty, the harder he tries or the more absorbed[69] he becomes in working subconsciously for his end. Although a specific improvement may take place in one direction, many more serious defects in the use of his mechanism *as a whole* will be cultivated in the process. It has been my experience that children who have had a specialized training such as this in their early years, have exhibited more than the usual number of psycho-physical defects and imperfections, that their sensory appreciation has been more than usually unreliable, and anyone who has followed my argument through the earlier pages will see that this must be the case where any specific development has been sought and achieved on a subconscious basis.

[69]See Chapter on Concentration.

The interdependence of the "mental" and "physical" and of the muscular mechanism in general in psycho-physical acts has long since been recognized in theory, and yet methods of education aiming at specific development remain the vogue.[70]

As a matter of fact, in connexion with this very question of the specific development of a particular sense, it is now a well-recognized fact that the sense of sight, for instance, is greatly affected by the "muscle-pulls" of the organism in general, and this applies where all the senses are concerned. For many years past we have had practical proof of the improvement that can be effected in the sense of sight of pupils, who have been re-educated and co-ordinated on a general basis of conscious control. In every case this improvement has followed a general improvement in the co-ordinated use of the whole organism.

This is the point which must always be emphasized by those advocating the claims of re-education and co-ordination on a general as against the claims of re-education and co-ordination on a specific basis. The person with defective sight will have quite a number of other psycho-physical defects, and re-education on a general basis must precede any attempt at specific re-education. This applies in the case of the person with defective use of the organs of speech, defective use of the arms or legs or any other defect, peculiarity or shortcoming.

In the case of children, if they were re-educated and co-ordinated on a plane of conscious control, seventy-five per cent of the ordinary sense imperfections and difficulties with technique would never be encountered by the teachers working in educational and other spheres. It does not require any special degree of intelligence to realize the tremendous amount of time and energy that would be saved if we adopted the comprehensive and constructive principle herein involved and applied it to all forms of human development and general growth in our attempts to ensure a progressive civilization.

The satisfactorily co-ordinated child on a plane of conscious control will be possessed of a psycho-physical mechanism which will tend to function to the maximum in all spheres in accordance with the standard of co-ordination reached. With such conditions present, the teacher can draw from the child the very best that the particular psycho-physical

[70]A striking instance may be mentioned in connexion with re-education. Some forty years ago well-known scientific men in France recognized the value of re-education and adopted forms of re-education on a specific instead of a general basis, and I am informed that this obtains even today. The principle involved has been dealt with in *Man's Supreme Inheritance*, and those acquainted with the facts and arguments employed will appreciate the relative value of general as against specific development or treatment of any kind.

organism, functioning adequately, is capable of giving, and can also be confident of a more or less increasing improvement, without the undue excitement of the fear reflexes and without undue effort.

Think, on the other hand, of what will be the harmful psycho-physical effect on a child, beset with all the impeding factors resulting from a condition of bad co-ordination, if, when learning to write, for instance, it takes up its pencil to use it for the first time and holds it with strained and cramped fingers, this being the result of a harmful condition of stress and strain in the general use of the psycho-physical organism. Even if the teacher does not point out directly to the child that its use of the pencil is not what it should be, the child will probably be conscious of a lack of control and of being below the ordinary standard of success with its writing. Sooner or later, however, the teacher will endeavour to improve the child's writing, and he may succeed up to a point, but it will be a very poor result as compared with the standard that might be attained, if the child were first re-educated and readjusted, and thus enabled to hold the pencil without the general imperfections to which I have referred.

I have already stated that I am prepared to prove that when the usual methods on a subconscious basis are employed to establish a condition, or to eradicate a fault or defect, quite a number of others, often more harmful than the one in process of eradication, are developed. At recurring stages, therefore, of our attempted progress and development, we are confronted with new and increasing difficulties calling for eradication, which we have actually cultivated in educational and other processes. I shall now point out different attempts that have been made in the educational process to counteract by specific means the retarding influences of certain peculiarities and defects, manifestations which have themselves been developed by this same educational process. A little thought will enable the reader to discern the developing complications inseparable from such a process.

In fact, this process becomes operative as soon as the child goes to school, for the experiences gained at school too often lead to complications, if from the beginning the child is functioning nearer to its minimum than to its maximum. The methods of training, etc., actually make for complications, in consequence of the numerous specific attempts which are made to remedy the many defects or shortcomings which are recognized in the child's efforts, most of which defects, however, would not have manifested themselves if the child's psycho-physical functioning had been satisfactory when it entered the school. The establishment, therefore, of this condition should be the first consideration in any sound educational plan. To attempt to educate an imperfectly co-ordinated child by dealing in a specific way with specific defects or shortcomings is an unreasoning process, especially when we take into consideration the important part which is played in a child's life by the process of imitation. We will now go on to consider this point.

CHAPTER II

IMITATION

THE psycho-physical process called imitation would seem to be one that is operative in most people to a high degree, as compared with other fundamental processes. We are all aware of this aptitude, as we call it, in our fellow-beings, and subconscious imitation of the characteristics of others is a factor which plays a great part in the development and growth and also in the use of our individual psycho-physical selves. Overwhelming proof is forthcoming in regard not only to the natural aptitude and subconscious inclination to imitate, but also in regard to the harmful consequences which may result from imitation, and we will now consider some of the chief factors responsible for the disappointing results accruing from the exercise of this natural aptitude in civilization.

This book deals with the defects, peculiarities, imperfect uses, etc. of the human psycho-physical organism; furthermore, it is herein contended that the majority of people are more or less beset with these shortcomings, whilst in a certain number these shortcomings are so extreme that they may be said to constitute a condition of deformity in the human creature. Herein lies the cause of the disappointing and harmful results which follow imitation. For the process of imitation remains inoperative unless there is something striking to be imitated, and the chief stimulus to imitation comes from our perception, subconscious or conscious, of some characteristic or striking manifestations of another human creature, and such manifestations are as a rule the manifestations of psycho-physical defects or peculiarities. In all spheres of present-day life the dangers from the individual imitation of others' defects or peculiarities are very great, and it is therefore of the utmost importance that these dangers should be eliminated, or at least minimized, in all our activities in learning or learning to do, particularly where people are associated as teachers and pupils, as, for instance, in schools and gymnasiums, in fact, wherever teachers and pupils are in that close contact which makes possible the operation of the process of imitation.

Most children at school manifest defects in the use of themselves in the ordinary acts of life, in a large number of cases, very serious defects, and all kinds of drills and remedial exercises are employed in the attempt to eradicate these defects. Yet, except in very rare instances, the teachers employed in these remedial and other spheres in our schools are too often themselves beset with exaggerated forms of the same or other defects or peculiarities. If teachers are worthy of the name, it is certain that their pupils will be influenced by them in more ways than one, and that most pupils will tend subconsciously to imitate them. Now as has already been pointed out, the most striking manifestations of these teachers will prove the most potent stimuli to the pupils' processes of imitation. Such manifestations, for instance, as peculiarities in the quality of a voice, in the manner of opening the mouth, of using the arms, or in defective utterance, vocal production, or use of the different parts of the organism in standing, walking, sitting, etc., in fact, all defects or peculiarities manifested as striking characteristics of the teachers will be found to be the most potent stimuli to the pupil's aptitude for imitation. A realization of the serious consequences involved in the foregoing will bring conviction that all teachers who manifest defects and peculiarities which are the result of their own unreliable sensory appreciation and unsatisfactory use of their psycho-physical organism, are a bad example, indeed, a positive danger to their pupils, and that the possibility of satisfactory psycho-physical results accruing to both pupil and teacher is seriously minimized by this impeding factor, viz., the acquisition of defects and peculiarities by imitation.

In any sphere of learning on a subconscious basis, we have to face the fact that pupil and teacher are imbued with the erroneous idea that the pupil, by observing the teacher doing something successfully, will be able to copy it and succeed also. The pupil is quite convinced as to this and the teacher is certain that if he teaches the pupil to do as he (the teacher) believes[71] he does himself, he will succeed in enabling the pupil to succeed.

---

[71]Take the case of a singer who, in consequence of throat trouble, is forced to retire from the public platform and becomes a teacher of singing. I can recall two such instances in which singers were forced to retire through this cause, and having listened to their vocal efforts on several occasions prior to their retirement, one did not need to be a prophet to be sure that this would happen. For no human throat and accessories could withstand indefinitely the abuse to which they were subjected in the matter of strain and larynx displacement and chest and abdominal distortion, through the imperfect use of the psycho-physical mechanisms upon the satisfactory use of which depends the normal condition of the specific parts named. When these same people took up teaching, they at once proceeded to impart to their pupils, as far as they were able, the methods of singing or breathing in which they themselves believed. *(continued on next page)*

Yet most of us are aware that if a pupil in some art is sent to watch a great artist, as is so often done, in order that he may learn something which will assist him in his particular art, the pupil is almost invariably more impressed by some characteristics of the artist that may be classed as faults than by his "better parts."

These characteristics are seized upon by the pupil as factors essential to his own improvement in performance, but experience constantly proves this belief to be mistaken. In the first place, the characteristics may be faults which the genius of the particular artist enables him to defy. It is possible that the artist succeeds *in spite of them* rather than because of them.[72] But even if the characteristics seized upon by the pupil for imitation were of value, the only way by which the pupil could make practical use of them would be, firstly, by a study of the general employment of the organism of the person to be imitated, of which the characteristics named are but special manifestations, and, secondly, by being himself re-educated so as to be able to command the same general use of the organism for good or ill, according to the standard of such use as that enjoyed by the expert he tries to copy.

We can only suppose that they believed their methods were correct ones, because they were the ones they had themselves adopted during their days of learning to sing, and had continued to practise up to the time that they took up teaching, and that the fact that they had both lost their voices by remaining faithful to these very methods had not even reached their consciousness. Otherwise, how could they have ventured to try and pass on to others the methods that had been the cause of so much injury to themselves? The power of the human creature to hypnotize himself is nowhere more apparent than in such instances of human idiosyncrasy as this.

[72]Unfortunately, this tendency may be noticed in all spheres of learning. Take the point in connexion with games, for instance. S. H. Smith indulged in a crouch and whirlwind drive; Gore was noted for his forehand drive; Doherty for his use of the unchanged grip, and so on. These characteristics have been imitated by other players with the idea of improving their own game, but again experience has constantly proved this idea to be mistaken, and for the reasons given above.

CHAPTER III

CONCENTRATION AND THE SUSTAINED (CONTINUOUS) PROJECTION OF ORDERS

A CONSIDERATION of the experiences outlined in the last chapter in connexion with the conscious use of the process of imitation leaves little doubt that this conception of the employment of imitation involves specific attempts to gain an "end," in other words, *specific* manifestations are selected for *specific* imitation, and thus the process of imitation becomes one of "fixating on specific points or objects," that is, of what is known as "concentration."

This conception of concentration is a disastrous and narrowing one, if we may judge by the use of the word as revealed in practice, and by the harmful manifestations which follow the intention of a person to "concentrate"; these harmful manifestations becoming more and more exaggerated according to the degree with which the teacher finds it necessary to urge the pupil to develop this doubtful acquisition.

Whence came this idea of "concentration"? At what stage in the process of education was it considered necessary?

There can be little doubt that the conception and use of concentration sprang from a desire for the ease, spontaneity and healthy enjoyment, associated with that use of the organism which is considered a successful one, and which is characteristic of people who are said to "give their attention" to whatever they wish to do. What has not been realized in this connexion, however, is that only those children whose psycho-physical organisms are functioning imperfectly and inadequately manifest such symptoms of "mind-wandering" as lack of spontaneity of observation, of curiosity, etc., granted, of course, a reasonable approach by the teacher. There is little doubt that the child of, say, two hundred years ago, was born with comparatively reliable instincts, adequate respiratory need, and all the necessary psycho-physical equipment which would have made for satisfactory development, if the educational process adopted had been on a plane of conscious control, that is, worked out on the principle of the "means-whereby." Unfortunately it was worked out on a subconscious basis, that is, on the "end-gaining" principle, and the harmful effects of the employment of this "end-gaining" principle grew very rapidly, until at a certain stage in the educational process the child exhibited amongst other shortcomings a lack of attention, or, as they say, "mind-wandering." When this shortcoming called "mind-wandering" increased to the extent that it called for a remedy, what was more natural than that the educational experts, subconsciously directed and controlled, and dominated, therefore, by the "end-gaining" principle, should attempt to counteract it by some idea which would "hold the mind" (attention) to one subject or to one plan.[73] The word "concentrate," according to the Students' English Dictionary, means "to force or cause to move to a common centre; to bring to bear on one object," the latter being the general acceptance of the word.

Here, then, was the remedy. As we all know, it has been applied for many, many years, and to-day it makes a universal appeal in accordance with a universal belief in what the particular person conceives of as "concentration." Make a search for a person who does not believe in concentration, and the results of your investigation will convince you of the truth of the foregoing statement. Introduce the subject to a friend and for the sake of argument tell him that you do not believe in concentration, that, in fact, you believe the practice to be harmful in its effects. You will almost certainly be met with such remarks as, "But surely we should concentrate our minds on what we are doing! How can we keep our minds on what we are doing unless we concentrate?" "One is naturally anxious to do one's best, and surely one's degree of success depends upon one's power of concentration." And so on.

Again, people will tell you that they cannot work successfully except in perfect quiet, that any interruption breaks the train of thought, and many other points will be brought forward to support the speaker's belief in concentration. There is only one satisfactory way to end such arguments as this. The teacher who has worked on a basis of conscious control employs psycho-physical demonstration in his attempts to convince, and in this particular sphere we are prepared to convince anyone who can and will trust his or her eyes during such a demonstration. Statements and arguments in connexion with psycho-physical activities should not be accepted unless the persons making them can give a practical demonstration of their truth, whilst evidencing at the same time that they themselves are in communication with their reasoning. By way of proof by demonstration, then, note the psycho-physical manifesta-

[73]The recognition of the defect of "mind-wandering" and the remedy adopted for it has its parallel in the first recognition of "physical" deterioration and the remedy applied. The false principle underlying both remedies is the same.

tions of the person who believes in concentration during the act of reading, writing, thinking, or during the performance of any other of the numerous daily activities. First observe the strained expression of the eyes, an expression of anxiety and uneasiness, denoting unduly excited fear reflexes; in some cases the eyes may be distorted, and the whole expression one that is recognized as the self-hypnotic stare. Then turn your attention to the general expression of the face, and pass on to the manifestations of the body and limbs. You will notice that there is an undue and harmful degree of tension throughout the whole organism. How could it be otherwise when the subject, instead of consciously reasoning out the cause (or causes) which has tended to develop his defect, is making a subconscious effort (on the method of "trial-and-error") to overpower one set of imperfect so-called "mental" projections and "physical" tensions by a still more powerful set?

For example, suppose a person is in the habit of performing a certain act, the act of sitting in a chair, for instance, with a great deal of unnecessary tension, and suppose his teacher points this out to him, and reasons out with him the *means whereby* the act can be performed without this unnecessary strain, giving him the necessary directions (series of orders) to this end, and the reliable sensory appreciation which the satisfactory carrying-out of the orders demands. Suppose, further, that the pupil, instead of following these directions quite simply in the order in which they are given to him, starts, as he calls it, to "concentrate" upon them. What will he really be doing? In a specific way, he will be concentrating upon one order and comparatively neglecting the others, whilst, in a general way, he will be overpowering the new set of conscious orders which he is asked to give in connexion with the act of sitting in a chair, by a still more powerful set of orders which are in accordance with his conception of the requirements of *the act of concentration.* This last proceeding being an unreasoned one on his part, all he accomplishes by it is to reinforce all the old misdirected activities subconsciously connected with the act of sitting down, whilst the new reasoned directions concerned with the act go by the board. He sets up what I have described elsewhere as a state of civil war within the organism, with the greatly added tension and strain that always accompanies this condition. The point is most clearly brought out in the case of the pupil who is asked to sit quietly and do nothing whilst the teacher moves some part of his body for him. In my experience, as soon as the pupil is asked not to do anything, he will immediately shew all those signs of strain and fixity of attention that he shews when he is asked to do something, and which we have learned to associate with any attempt at concentration. Point this out to the pupil, and he will answer, nine times out of ten, "I am trying to do nothing!" He actually believes that he has something *to do* to do nothing. To such a point can we be led by our belief in concentration!

This whole matter is most instructive, as shewing the danger of applying a specific remedy to a psycho-physical defect like "mind-wandering," which has its basis in an imperfect use of the psycho-physical mechanism in general. When a person has developed "mind-wandering," there is present a condition of unreliable sensory appreciation and that undue stress and strain during psycho-physical activities, which is always associated with imperfect co-ordination. To a subject in this condition any attempt to supply a specific remedy is fraught with danger. On a plane of conscious control such dangers can be escaped, but practically never on a subconscious basis.

Now as to the narrowing effect of so-called "concentration." Those who are fortunate, or unfortunate enough, to undertake to act as teachers are well aware of the difficulty of finding an adult who can, as we say, think of more than one thing at a time, or perform satisfactorily any evolution requiring the co-ordinated use of even two parts of the organism. Co-ordinated use of the different parts during any evolution calls for the continuous, conscious projection of orders to the different parts involved, the primary order concerned with the guidance and control of the primary part of the act being *continued* whilst the orders connected with the secondary part of the movement are projected, and so on, however many orders are required (the number of these depending upon the demands of the processes concerned with a particular movement). Ordinarily, in attempts to use two or more parts in remedial work, the primary projection *ends* with the correct or incorrect use of the parts concerned with the primary movement. This applies to all other projections concerned with other parts of the movement, and is another instance of concentrated effort connected with a procedure based on the "end-gaining" principle. The projection of continued, conscious orders, on the other hand, calls for a broad, reasoning attitude, so that the subject has not only a clear conception of the orders essential ("means-whereby") for the correct performance of a particular movement, but he can also project these orders in their right relationship one to another, the co-ordinated series of orders resulting in a co-ordinated use of the organism.

It follows that an imperfectly co-ordinated use of the human organism is not associated with the broad, reasoning attitude and the accruing benefits just indicated. And as most people have developed a more or less imperfectly co-ordinated use of the mechanism, which involves reliance upon the "end-gaining" principle, it is not surprising that so many pupils have the habit of projecting unconsidered and *disconnected* orders, orders, that is, that have not been reasoned out from the point of view of the co-ordinated use of the different parts concerned, *and which therefore result in a mal-co-ordinated movement.* When, therefore, such a pupil comes for remedial work on a plane of conscious control, and is asked to project a series of connected orders continuously, he naturally finds great difficulty in breaking the habit he has formed of discontinuous attention and of haphazard and subconscious guidance and direction. In fact, it will be found that, as a rule, a pupil has no conception of linking up the different parts of the movement and the orders relating to these. He may, as I say, give the primary orders or directions required for the first part of the movement, but as soon as that point is reached, he no longer attempts to carry on the primary order in association with that required for the secondary part of the movement, although the essential connexion between these two parts may be pointed out to him over and over again. The chief reason is that he believes that he cannot "bring his mind to bear" on more than one point at a time. As he expresses it, "I cannot think of so many things at once." This is entirely in line with the definition of concentration given above, but it represents a delusion on his part, because, of course, he has been "bringing his mind to bear" on several things at once subconsciously all his life, else he could not have carried out the simplest of his daily activities.

A simple illustration will make this clear. Suppose a person who has been sitting down rises to speak to a friend who comes into the room. The stimulus to rise from the sitting position comes to him and his response to this is his decision to stand up. Immediately this decision is made, the orders connected with the well-established habit of rising from the sitting to the standing position are projected to the psycho-physical mechanisms involved, and the act of rising is performed, ending in the assumption of what is called the "standing position." Suppose, further, that this person engages at once in an ordinary conversation or a scientific discussion with his friend for, say, half an hour. As far as our subject is concerned, he is absorbed by the requirements of the discussion; in fact, he will tell you that he must concentrate on the matter of the discussion in order to do his best. The point of interest for us is the consideration of the *means whereby* he remains standing, and *of which he is not and never has been conscious.* We have already referred to the projections which were associated with his decision to stand up, and these projections must be sustained until he makes a different decision, as, for instance, to move to some other position. It will be clear, therefore, that during the process of subconscious development, the human creature has also developed the ability to sustain continuous projections of orders. Insistence, therefore, on the necessity and importance of sustained projections in the work of co-ordination and re-education is based, not on a new, but on a very old and fundamental principle in human development.

The point of interest in all these considerations lies in the fact that this prevalent belief in concentration goes hand in hand with the acceptance of the "end-gaining" principle, as against the principle of thinking out clearly and *connectedly* the *means whereby* an "end" can be secured, and of "bringing the mind to bear" on as many subjects (continuous projections of orders) as is necessary for the purpose. The whole psycho-physical tendency of the person who believes that concentration is essential to success, and adopts and develops it as a practice in his efforts in different spheres of activity, is "to bring the mind to bear on one object." This exactly fits the "end-gaining" principle, and is antagonistic to the "means-whereby" principle which calls for the ability "to bring to bear on" a dozen or more objects if necessary, and which implies a *number* of things, all going on, and converging to a common consequence (continuous projection of orders).

In the sphere of every-day life it will be found that in the opinion of ninety-nine persons out of a hundred, the consideration of "means-whereby" in connexion with the use of the psycho-physical self will prove a hindrance or an interference. These people are confident that they cannot attend to two things at once, that is, to themselves and to their work, business or profession at the same time. It never seems to occur to them that their psycho-physical self is the instrument or machine by means of which they carry on their business or profession, and that their standard of success, therefore, in this sphere of their business or professional activity will be in accordance with the standard of functioning of this instrument or machine. This instrument or machine being the *means whereby* they will be able to carry on their business or profession successfully, it follows that due attention to the functioning of this instrument or machine is essential to the due and satisfactory attention to their business or profession. The confession, therefore, that they are incapable of carrying on, hand in hand, as it were, these two all-important and interdependent psycho-physical processes is tantamount to an admission that due attention to the *means whereby* they can gain their "ends" will render them unable to attend to these "ends"; which is absurd! Such a confession, indeed, fixes the stage on the evolutionary plane where mankind, as a mass, stands to-day. It certainly is not a very high stage, when we take into consideration the potentialities of the human creature and the fact that in the development of the animal and the savage the two processes concerned with the use of the creature's self and the use of that self in the activities of life were interdependent.

In a world where the ordinary person not only believes in but practises what is called "concentration," the conception of the word itself and of its practical application will be in accordance with the psycho-physical defects of the individual concerned, who, on becoming conscious of certain defects, believes that what he understands as "concentration" will remove them. Once he has adopted this narrowing process, it is not surprising that he finds it impossible to do or think of more than one thing at a time. The harmful psycho-physical condition thus established does not make for a satisfactory condition of all-round functioning.

On the other hand, those of us who have watched the progress of pupils who have been re-educated on a general basis, have had conclusive proof that it is possible for a person to learn to give due attention continuously to, i.e., to "keep the mind" on the "means-whereby" of the satisfactory use of the psycho-physical mechanisms, whilst employing these mechanisms in the round of daily life, whether this be a business or professional life or any other, and with the desirable result of a continuous development in general psycho-physical health. The human machine is capable of doing many things at the same time, and in those cases where a condition of unified psycho-physical co-ordination is operative (a condition in which the process of true concentration is present), the subject is as unaware of the operation of the process of concentration as he is of that of the process of co-ordination. As a matter of fact, it is unlikely that such a person will have given thought to the necessity for concentration; he will not have recognized the need for it, and, this being so, he will not have considered it in the light of a process requiring special attention in its application.

The satisfactory conditions of co-ordination and the manifestations of the co-ordinated creature to which I have referred represent a form of concentration which cannot be secured by "thinking of concentration" or by telling another to think of it (which also means that one cannot be "concentrated" in that sense of the word). This whole book is devoted to the exposure of the fallacy of asking any imperfectly co-ordinated person to attempt to eradicate a defect or peculiarity by some written word or spoken instructions. It is certain that any person who fails to concentrate, in the sense of giving due attention to the matter in hand, is an imperfectly co-ordinated person. To ask such a person to overcome his failure to concentrate by "concentrating" or "by learning to concentrate" in accordance with his conception of these acts, is to cause a harmful and artificial division of personality. What is needed is the restoration of a satisfactory condition of psycho-physical co-ordination on a general basis which will involve the use of the true processes of concentration.

CHAPTER IV

MEMORY AND FEELING

TEACHERS in most schools of to-day, if we are to judge by the opinions they express, are fully awake to the growing lack of attention on the part of the children; they seem to be unusually disturbed by this lack of attention, that the children, as they say, "cannot concentrate"; but they do not seem to be so disturbed by the increase in what is called "loss of memory." Possibly they are not yet as aware of it as they should be. Be this as it may, there can be little doubt that these teachers are not aware of the fact that learning to "concentrate," and the subsequent psycho-physical efforts in connexion with the act of "concentrating" tend to interfere with the processes of remembering (taking this word in its broadest sense), with the result that unequal, narrowing and often inadequate impressions are registered.

Many people now-a-days acknowledge their growing "loss of memory" and many attempts are being made by means of memory systems, courses of of mental training," etc., to help educated people to make good a certain loss in this connexion. Here again the point of interest for us lies in the fact that all these systems are based on the "end-gaining" principle, and that no attempt has been made in any of them (any more than in the case of "mind-wandering") to associate the particular defective manifestation, in this case, "bad memory," with other psycho-physical defects which will be found to be associated with it.

At a stage of our development when what we call "loss of memory" is more or less a general defect, it behoves us to consider the psycho-physical conditions involved and also the various imperfect uses of the psycho-physical mechanisms which make for the development of these conditions.

Memory is the impression which is registered as the result of some stimulus or stimuli. The lasting quality of the impression depends upon certain psycho-physical processes concerned with registering impressions, and the effectiveness of these processes in their turn upon the general psycho-physical condition, and especially upon the standard of sensory appreciation present in the particular case. Environment also influences these conditions in accordance with the standard of psycho-physical functioning present at the time of the registration of the impression, whilst a further factor in the case is the degree of ability possessed by the individual concerned to link up the knowledge or the experience, conveyed by a given stimulus or stimuli, with the knowledge and experiences already acquired. As we are aware, our habits of life are the manifestations of our psycho-physical functioning, and this functioning governs our habits in the matter of registering impressions in connexion with memory, just as it influences all our other activities.

There can be little doubt that the growing habit of newspaper reading and light literature, and the accompanying decline in the reading of books or matter which is to be retained as valuable knowledge, has been accompanied by harmful psycho-physical habits which to-day are seriously affecting the human memory, in a more or less degree in accordance with the standard of psycho-physical functioning of the individual concerned. People study and commit to memory printed matter contained in certain books, because by this means they hope to acquire lasting knowledge. As a rule, they merely read hastily the printed matter in newspapers, magazines, etc., without making any attempt to memorize it. In the same way, they simply glance at the news of the day and register only the faintest impression. This probably serves them for that day or a week, but in a month's time they will probably be hazy about it, and in a year's time the impression may be completely effaced. This habit of taking faint impressions in reading is repeated daily by millions of people who rarely read a book in the way of study, a form of reading which would make for the registering of definite and lasting impressions. "Skimming," that is, receiving only faint impressions of what is read, is a harmful habit which, if indulged in, rapidly becomes established, and very soon the person concerned is aware of a growing loss of memory in all spheres.

We are all aware that what we term "loss of memory" is a more or less general defect in the process of remembering and recalling knowledge which has become more and more marked during the past twenty or thirty years, and it would seem that, like insanity and other besetting evils, it is a defect which, unless checked in time, must undermine the usefulness of our psycho-physical processes.

For reasoning is dependent upon the association of remembered facts with other facts, which are the stimulus or stimuli to the processes concerned; hence, when the memory fails, the process of satisfactory reasoning will be suspended.

As we are to deal with the effects of certain sensory habits in connexion with memory, it will be useful to consider the interdependence and the action and reaction of sensory appreciation and so-called "mental" activity. The idea conveyed by the voice of one person reaches the consciousness of another through the sense of hearing, the written word through the sense of sight; then we have all the stimuli received through the senses of touch (feeling), taste, smell, etc. In a general way it will be seen that our senses play the leading part in all the processes of remembering and reasoning, in fact, in the great round of psycho-physical activity. The standard of functioning in the foregoing processes of reasoning and remembering depends, therefore, directly or indirectly, upon the standard of functioning of sensory appreciation.

My readers may, of course, point to instances of remarkable feats of memory performed by people in specific spheres but the writer's experience of these cases is that excellence in one sphere will be found to be equalled by lack of it in all others. In fact the cases to which I refer are simply abnormal.

One of the most interesting in my experience was that of a young man whose abnormality was manifested in dealing with time-tables and the like. If you asked him to look up a train to a particular place at, say, three o'clock, he would turn up the page, look for the particular train by running his eyes up and down the list of times of departures, and during this apparently cursory glance at the time-table he would memorize the whole list. Three months later, if you asked him to name the trains in the list departing between any two hours you liked to name, you would be certain to receive a correct answer. But this same young man would continually leave his umbrella in the bus, go out to purchase some ordinary article for domestic use, and, forgetting what he had gone to fetch, return without it. In fact, in the general way of life, and judged by the ordinary standard of human intelligence, he was quite a hopeless person.[74] We have here a fine instance of a remarkable feat of memory in a specific sphere accompanied by defective remembering and reasoning in general activity, a condition which, as I am able to state, in consequence of personal acquaintance, was, in this case, associated with delusive sensory appreciation.

[74]I should like to urge here that we must beware of placing an exaggerated value upon intelligence which manifests itself only in some specific sphere. Judgment must always be made upon the human creature's intelligent activities on a general basis in the process of living and all-round usefulness. The genuine specialist, for instance, must always be primarily a proficient general practitioner in the sphere of trade, profession or general activity, for satisfactory growth as a specialist demands a continuous growth and development of those experiences which only the general practitioner can command. This important matter of correct relative values is of the utmost importance, and if we are to establish a sound basis for judgement in the future, we must first give consideration to the "means-whereby" of the act rather than to the act itself. What useful part does the performance of an act play in a man's so-called "intellectual" or "physical" development, if the man is injured thereby?

There is little doubt that most of the early bad habits, which result in what we call "loss of memory," are actually cultivated during the different processes in all forms of education. This cultivation is most marked in those teaching processes where the pupil is called upon to perform some "physical" act. Therefore, now that we have been unreasoning enough to force every unfortunate school child, irrespective of his individual standard of sensory appreciation, to learn "physical" drill or to perform exercises, we must expect among the majority a more rapid development of "loss of memory" than during the previous years. As the writer is prepared to demonstrate the truth of these statements before any scientific or intelligent body of men and women, he has decided to take his illustration from this sphere of teaching.

If the reader takes the trouble to be present in the school or gymnasium or during any outdoor teaching in connexion with exercises, drill or games, he will note, if he observes carefully, that each of the children or adults is occupied chiefly in endeavouring to learn the teacher's instructions by the "physical" performance of some small part of these instructions which has specially appealed to him, and is so concentrated and absorbed in this part of the performance that he is oblivious to any other part of the instructions that are being given by the teacher. He will only have to question the pupil to find that this is true; an expert in psycho-physical re-education has only to observe the expression in the pupil's eyes, and certain other manifestations, to be quite certain.

The following is an incident in this connexion which occurred recently during a lesson in re-education in the writer's own experience. The pupil was asked to listen to certain simple instructions which involved the use of the lips, tongue, and jaw, in the order named. (Of course, the necessary work in regard to the general co-ordinated use of the organism during such teaching had already been given.) The first time the instructions were given it was obvious that, before the teacher had finished speaking, the pupil was trying to memorize them, as they were given, by a "physical" (sensory) process, i.e., by trying to "feel" the instructions as they were spoken, rather than to acquire them by a process of remembering ("committing to memory," as we say).

The pupil was again asked to listen to the instructions, and not to attempt to make any movements of the parts concerned. He was asked merely to concern himself with the process of remembering the instructions. Before the instructions had been given to him a second time, however, the pupil was again very busily engaged in making certain movements of the neck, lips and jaw. He was then asked why he was making these movements. He promptly answered, "I am trying to make certain of the instructions." It was then explained to him that the method he was pursuing was not the correct and satisfactory way of making certain of instructions; that, instead, the instructions should first be memorized, and that only when this had been done would there be any chance of his carrying them out in the psycho-physical sphere, and then, only provided that the instructions included the correct *means whereby* the act was to be performed.

Spoken instructions reach our consciousness through the sense of hearing, written instructions through the sense of sight, the resulting action and reaction being influenced by the standard of general psycho-physical functioning of the organism. But as the standard of psycho-physical functioning in the ordinary child or adult of our time is inadequate, the creature is brought within a danger zone directly as he attempts to carry out any activities which call for new psycho-physical experiences. In a very large number of cases the standard of this functioning has been so lowered that the individuals concerned may be said to be perpetually within this danger zone, for their guiding sensations are unreliable and often harmfully delusive.

It is quite conceivable that any stimulus, as it is conveyed by sensory appreciation to the consciousness, is influenced by the psycho-physical conditions present, and there is not the least doubt as to this influence on the reaction which follows. We are all aware of the different reactions of different people to the same stimulus or stimuli. Now, where the psycho-physical conditions are such as we find associated with unreliable defective or delusive guiding sensations (sensory appreciation), we cannot surely expect a proper standard of psycho-physical functioning in the general round of so-called "mental activities." Sound and comprehensive reasoning is rare in a person whose sensory appreciation is unreliable, in other words, whose kinæsthesia may be said to be debauched.

To return to our illustration. The facts set down serve to shew that the pupil, in going to work in the way he did, was following out a preconceived plan in regard to the attempt to memorize instructions. In his conception, the act of memorizing was much more a "physical" than a "mental" act, and if in his case the psycho-physical functioning had been up to that standard which commands a reliable sensory appreciation, the pupil's plan might have proved successful; and in this connexion the most interesting fact in the whole experience remains to be stated. For on the morning following the lesson, when he was asked to repeat the instructions, he said, "I can't recall them now." Here, then, was the proof that the pupil's preconceived plan of memorizing his instructions by trying to feel them had failed, as how could it be otherwise, considering the very imperfect sensory appreciation that he had at his command? The habit of attempting to perform an act before the directing and guiding orders concerned have been memorized is, in such a case, associated with an inadequate use of the processes of inhibition as compared with those of volition; therefore, when the pupil is brought face to face with the new psycho-physical experiences, his inhibitory processes are ineffective. This means that he is gradually cultivating within himself an unbalanced psycho-physical condition in which the so-called "mental" impressions he receives during the act of learning are unduly faint and unreliable.

In order to restore balance in such a case, it is necessary first to develop a conscious, reasoning inhibition (prevention). To this end, the person concerned must learn to say "No" to every stimulus to psycho-physical activity until he has taken time to consider what are the reasonable *means whereby* the end he desires can be achieved, and he must then repeat and memorize the orders relative to these means before employing them in guiding and directing the mechanisms essential to the particular psycho-physical act to be performed.[75]

[75]We have recently seen the rise and fall in reputation of a system which, it was claimed, could restore failing memory and by specific means bestow "mental" blessings which were, however, quite beyond the most sanguine expectations of any person who still enjoyed even a temporary state of sanity or who possessed even a reasonable knowledge of the fundamentals of the psycho-physical processes which are essential to satisfactory memorizing. In this particular instance, the rapid rise and fall of this system affords food for reflection in connexion especially with the eulogies which the proprietors of this system published from time to time from the pens and over the names of men and women, some of whom are recognized leaders of thought in our time. It is unfortunate that we cannot call these men and women to account and force them to justify these eulogies of a system, which was after all but a piece of "mental gymnastics" or series of gymnastics carried out in accordance with definite instructions, which totally ignored those general psycho-physical conditions of the person concerned, which were the cause or causes of the "mental" shortcoming and of which these leaders of thought were themselves totally ignorant. The blind continue to lead the blind in the twentieth century as in the days of the cave-man, but the process brings with it more disastrous results in our time than was possible in those early days of man's more limited spheres of psycho-physical activities.

CHAPTER V

COMPLEXITY AND COMPLICATIONS IN RELATION TO STRESS AND STRAIN

VERY frequently we are told that the cause of most of our difficulties is the increasing complexity of the demands of living in the present stage of civilization. It is much more to the point to say that our real difficulties arise from the almost universal adoption in practical life of the lowly evolved "end-gaining" principle in our attempts to meet these demands, the result being that we cultivate within ourselves a condition of stress and strain (which in our ignorance we look upon as something apart from ourselves), in a subconscious, unintelligent effort to adapt ourselves to the ever-changing environment of what we designate as an advancing civilization.

First, we have stress and strain within ourselves, that is, in the functioning of the psycho-physical mechanisms as we employ them to satisfy the needs of the organism in the maintenance of health conditions and in general activity. The errors and defects in the sphere of psycho-mechanics indicated by the foregoing are the result of the dependence upon unsound and misleading principles concerned with our individual development and growth.

Then we have the stress and strain of what we so often describe as the "fight for life," "the complexity of life," and so on; in other words, the stress and strain occasioned by our endeavour to make the wheels of the complex man-made machinery of life go round in social, industrial, political, educational, religious and moral spheres.

These two spheres of stress and strain, which we have indicated, must always be considered as inseparable, seeing that our social, educational, industrial, political, religious and moral life depends for its being on the experiences of our individual psycho-physical life. The false principles which are applied to the act of living in both instances are entirely responsible for these harmful conditions of strain and for the unsettled state which holds sway at this very moment. Had the prophets, philosophers, and leaders of the past recognized this fact, they would have shewn proof of clear analysis and foresight. That they did not do so is most unfortunate, and to this fact we may attribute the growing tendency towards disunion instead of unity, towards dissatisfaction instead of satisfaction, towards enmity and discord instead of good-fellowship and peace, the sum total of these present conditions constituting an unsatisfactory instead of a satisfactory stage in human evolution. We have unrest everywhere, unrest in men, women and children, which is attributed to "nerves" or some such symptom, and the alarming feature of it all is that it is an increasing unrest. The venomous and penetrating roots of the cancer of disunion continue to spread and have already caused to deteriorate and, in many instances, have actually demoralized the vital parts of our psycho-mechanical life as well as our social and industrial life, and the dffficulties in application of the principles which make for unity are already alarming. It is universally contended that we need unity in all spheres, and we are all familiar with the cry "united we stand, divided we fall," and this has a universal application to satisfactory human endeavour. Yet in almost every sphere of human activity, in religion, in education, in the social plan, in politics, in trades unionism, etc., we find a growing tendency to disunion. Review the history of human endeavour during the past few hundred years, and consider the cause or causes of the increase in the number of different sects in the sphere of religion, in the number of different systems of education, social reform, in the number of political parties, and, probably most striking of all, in the increase in the tendency to adopt, under the banner of trades unionism, measures and principles which impede unity. Surely it is fair to conclude that the cause or causes of the growing disunion in all these spheres is due to some serious defect or defects in the fundamentals of these man-made institutions. If the principles involved had been sound, their application would have tended towards unity, and the fact that the people immediately concerned failed to remain in agreement as to the relative value of the principles they had decided to apply, is surely an admission of their unsoundness. Be this as it may, we cannot fail to recognize the important fact that an alarming growth of disunion leading to complications in human activity is herein indicated and complications are ever associated with misdirected activity. If we keep to our present system of life, living will be still more complicated in a hundred years from now, and so on, until possibly such a degree of complication will be reached that we shall not even have time to live!

The foregoing serves to indicate that the unreasoned processes which lead to harmful complications in the educational sphere are paramount in every other sphere of life. The parallel to the failure in our teaching methods is to be found in our attempts to progress in social, political, industrial, religious and other spheres, where the remedy is often more harmful than the disease. How absurd, for instance, are the attempts for the "uplifting of man" in the industrial sphere, when these are associated with that demoralizing conception which has led to the lowering of the standard of man's daily efforts to that of the less capable and so to the lowering of the standard of individual psycho-physical functioning in the sphere of labour. We are all aware of the psycho-physical effect of giving our best in our daily labours, and there is little hope for the person who is no longer able to gain satisfaction and happiness from this source. Again, in the sphere of politics, what can be more stupid than the ordinary party attitude leading, as it does, to undesirable individual manifestations of deception, prejudice, egotism and "emotional gusts?" It is an unreasonable and dishonest course to withhold support from or denounce measures which one believes to be right and of value to humanity, simply because they chance to be advocated by the political party to which one does not belong. Under the present plan politics and deception are interdependent. The individual seeking re-election will resort to forms of deception, to which he would not stoop in other walks of life, particularly in the matter of making promises which he has not the least hope of fulfilling, and which his electors, if they used their reasoning powers, would often know he cannot fulfil. They are still at a stage of evolution where reasoning is dominated by the herd-instinct, and so they are carried away by his oratory or personality or both. The harmful effects of the activities of individuals beset with serious and often abnormal psycho-physical defects are present in every sphere of life, and we have to face the fact that it is not the people who are out to do harm to their fellow-beings who are setting back the clock of civilization to-day, but, on the contrary, those misguided people who are devoting themselves to the uplifting of their fellow-men, whilst remaining themselves under the influence of perverted emotions and prejudices. The history of our social plan in the spheres of industrialism, politics, religion, education, medicine, etc., for the past three hundred years is of the greatest interest in this matter of the attitude of those concerned with attempts at reform, organization, advancement and unity, for these attempts will invariably be found to be specific and "end-gaining" attempts, resulting, even where the specific "end" is gained, in new complications leading to social conflict and harmful diversity. If we are to check the present overbalancing in these directions, and to advance satisfactorily, we must gradually raise the standard of individual psycho-mechanical co-ordination, and pass to a stage of constructive conscious control which would be associated with the establishment of "means-whereby" principles instead of "end-gaining" principles.

PART IV
SENSORY APPRECIATION IN ITS RELATION TO HAPPINESS

THE characteristic note of true happiness is struck when the healthy child is busily engaged in doing something which interests it. It may be the little girl washing and wiping her tea-cups, or dressing and undressing her doll, or the little boy setting to work to make a toy train or cart with the aid of a piece of wood and a string, or piecing together some modern toy which, when completed, will be a house, or a bridge, or a working model of some machine. The child is always attracted by machinery; indeed, to find out "how it works" is the natural desire of every healthy child, and it is therefore very significant that in schools where experiments have been made in re-education on a general basis, the children have become more interested in this work than in any other of their school activities. They are not slow to recognize that they are themselves the most interesting machines, and their natural interest in mechanics finds full scope in the process of their own re-education. Our experience has been that this interest, an intelligent interest in the working of their own psycho-physical mechanisms, is one that grows steadily and comprehensively. For the psycho-physical processes which precede and accompany the child's desire to acquire a knowledge of the mechanical working of inanimate machinery are the same as those which are called into activity in connexion with the acquisition of the knowledge of the satisfactory use of its own mechanisms. It should be obvious to all concerned that in any process of growth or development of the child or adult, experience in employing the mechanics of the psycho-physical organism should precede all other mechanical experience, and that any experiences gained later in the sphere of inanimate mechanical experimentation would thus be materially increased in value.

One can recall the expression of interest, happiness and satisfaction exhibited by the child when one has enabled him to understand[76] for the first time that his unduly stiffened neck—with perhaps his head too far pulled back—is really not the fault of his neck at all, but is due to the fact that he is trying to do with the muscles of his neck what should be done by other mechanisms.

[76]Of course the teacher's manipulation will have given him previously the reliable sensory appreciation in this connexion. For a detailed statement, see Chapter "Imperfect Sensory Appreciation."

One cannot forget either the unfamiliar but satisfactory manifestations of the child when he becomes able to inhibit[77] that is, to say "No" to some stimulus to misdirected activity (which in the case of the last illustration would be to say "No" to his subconscious desire to throw back his head and stiffen his neck), and then, with an expression born of confidence, to give the orders or directions, which are the result of a reasoned conception of his correct "means-whereby," the whole process tending to prevent the over-excitement of the fear reflexes. Experience has proved to us that children are unusually interested in the working of their own psycho-physical machinery when the processes employed are concerned with re-education on a general and conscious basis. They find a new interest in all activities to which they can apply an improving use of themselves, and their happiness in finding, for instance, that they can improve their games by a conscious *general* direction of themselves (a very different thing from the usual *specific* directions they receive in coaching lessons) is a happiness which increases with their psycho-physical improvement.

I shall now endeavour to shew that the lack of real happiness manifested by the majority of adults of to-day is due to the fact that they are experiencing, not an improving, but a continually deteriorating use of their psycho-physical selves. This is associated with those defects, imperfections, undesirable traits of character, disposition, temperament, etc., characteristic of imperfectly co-ordinated people struggling through life beset with certain maladjustments of the psycho-physical organism, which are actually setting up conditions of irritation and pressure dur-

[77]The demeanour of the child changes when he learns to inhibit his desire to respond to a certain stimulus, before going on to give the new orders or directions which are the forerunners of the new *means whereby* the particular "end" he desires can be achieved. This change of expression was very noticeable in the case of a little girl who had developed the most pronounced bad habits in the use of her psycho-physical organism, and had what we call a "dour" expression when her lessons started. At a certain stage in her re-education she developed a conscious recognition of the new and correct experiences secured by the teacher's manipulation, and she became able to inhibit, i.e., to say "No" to the stimulus which had previously started up the whole train of movements that were incorrect and harmful. When she discovered this, viz., that by saying "No" to herself she could PREVENT her troublesome and long-established bad habits from gaining the upper hand, her whole demeanour changed, and, with a confidence that was quite new to her she proceeded to give herself the directions which would enable her to make in the new and co-ordinated manner (correct "means-whereby") the very movement which she had stopped herself from making in her old mal-co-ordinated manner. The fact that she could not only think out but CONTROL THE MEANS WHEREBY she could attain her "end" (instead of rushing at it blindly in her old subconscious way) robbed her of the diffidence which had been such an overdeveloped trait in her case, and with the gradual development of control the old "dour" expression gave place to one of confidence and happiness.

ing both sleeping and waking hours. Whilst the maladjustments remain present, these malconditions increase day by day and week by week, and foster that unsatisfactory psycho-physical state which we call "unhappiness." Small wonder that under these conditions the person concerned becomes more and more irritated and unhappy. Irritation is not compatible with happiness, yet the human creature has to employ this already irritated organism in all the psycho-physical activities demanded by a civilized mode of life. It stands to reason that every effort made by the human creature whose organism is already in an irritated condition must tend to make the creature still more irritated, and, therefore, as time goes on, his chances of happiness diminish. Furthermore, his experiences of happiness become of ever shorter duration, until at last he is forced to take refuge in a state of unhappiness, a psycho-physical condition as perverted as that state of ill-health which people reach when they experience a perverted form of satisfaction in the suffering of pain, that is, in "the enjoyment of bad health," as we say. This perversion links up with those purely animal traits which are apt to accompany morbid conditions, and which become unduly and harmfully manifested in those states of unusual excitement and marked depression, when the individual's reasoning is in abeyance, and he is dominated by his emotional impulses.

We have merely to consider the experiences of the human creature, afflicted with the conditions of the irritation and pressure already referred to, in his attempts to employ this irritated organism in a general way in the activities of life, to recognize that even his occasional experiences of happiness will be of unduly short duration, and will tend to become more so with the progress of time. It matters not whether these experiences are gained in the sphere of rest, work, recreation, pleasure, games or general education; in all these activities impeding factors, such as irritation and pressure, remain more or less unchanged. This means that experiences that would only tend to irritate a person in possession of a comparatively high standard of sensory appreciation and of satisfactorily co-ordinated psycho-physical mechanisms, would be certain to irritate most harmfully a person who is already beset with irritation and pressure, in consequence of the harmful condition of unreliable sensory appreciation in the use of the organism which we have indicated. Furthermore, such a person will be irritated by experiences which would not have the least effect upon one whose sensory appreciation is reliable.

The psycho-physical condition of the person afflicted with irritation and pressure is such that all his efforts in any direction will be more or less of a failure as compared with the efforts of those who are not so afflicted, and there is probably no stimulus from without which makes more for irritability of the person concerned than failure (either comparative or complete) in accomplishment, nothing which can have a worse effect upon our emotions, self-respect, happiness or confidence, in fact, upon our temperament and character in general. Just note the expression and general demeanour of one who is a success in life, then of one who is a failure; of one who has just succeeded in some simple act, in work, games or learning something, then of one who has failed comparatively or completely. If we note any of these people on days when comparative success has attended their efforts, the least observant among us must be convinced of the striking influence of success and of how conducive it is to happiness. Watch the child in its earliest efforts before and during school days, or the experiences of adults in the activities of daily life in any sphere, and it will be observed that when either is employing his organism successfully, happiness and satisfaction rule supreme. Confidence is born of success, not of failure, and our processes in education and in the general art of living must be based upon principles which will enable us to make certain of the satisfactory *means whereby* an end may be secured, and thus to command a large percentage of those satisfactory experiences which develop confidence, as against a small percentage of those unsatisfactory experiences which tend to undermine our confidence and make us unhappy.

A well-known medical specialist sent one of his patients to me for a diagnosis. He then called upon me to discuss the details of my conclusions, and when I pointed out to him that his patient would be a difficult pupil to re-educate, in consequence of his unusually unbalanced emotional condition and state of harmful irritability, he remarked, "I must tell you that he has been soured by comparative failure in his professional work."

In order to illustrate these points, we will deal with the practical experiences of the human creature in the fields of recreation and games, because we may assume that here, at any rate, he will be acting in accordance with the dictates of his own wishes and desires, in the anticipation of those psycho-physical experiences which make for happiness.

We are all aware of the pleasurable anticipation, and even joyous mild excitement, associated with the early experiences of our men and women friends who take up golf, tennis, cricket, football and other games and forms of recreation. This pleasurable anticipation arises from the fact that they associate the manifestations which we call happiness with indulgence in these activities, and there can be little doubt that we should be able to command a continuance of happiness, and an increasing satisfaction with the increase of our experience in any game or form of recreation, as far as our personal efforts, at any rate, in the practice of the game are concerned. But despite this fact we know that in the great majority of cases, manifestations of happiness, contrary to expectation, tend to decrease rather than increase with the accumulation of practical experiences in these forms of recreation. That this is the case with most of us is surely proof that something is radically wrong with the use of our psycho-physical mechanisms, and with the application of these mechanisms to the demands of the particular game or recreation.

The reason for this will be clear if we try to set down the psycho-physical experiences in action and reaction which result from a person's decision to play, say, golf. Let us take the case of any ordinary person (not some person exceptionally well-equipped for golf) and watch him at his first lesson with his teacher, professional or otherwise. It is safe to conclude, firstly, that this pupil's sensory appreciation is more or less unreliable, and associated with an imperfectly co-ordinated use of his psycho-physical mechanisms, and, secondly, that he has never been re-educated on a general basis. Unfortunately, this applies equally to the teacher, and means that, in both cases, their knowledge of the use of the psycho-physical mechanisms which they are about to employ in the lesson is the result of unsatisfactory and even harmful subconscious experiences. It is safe to assume that they have little conscious knowledge of the use of these mechanisms either in the field of theory or in that of practice, and even that little will be on a specific basis. The true relation of "cause and effect" on a general basis in connexion with the working of these mechanisms, will not be given due consideration and, as we shall see, the majority of effects (symptoms of some "cause" or "causes") that they chance to recognize will not be treated by them as such, but as "causes," and dealt with in accordance with the "end-gaining" principle.

We are all familiar, for instance, with the type of instructions which the teacher will give to the pupil in regard to "holding the club," "keeping his eye on the ball," and all the other things which the pupil should or should not do with the different parts of his organism at a particular time. Now it will be clear to any spectator with a knowledge of the satisfactory employment of the psycho-physical mechanisms on a general basis that the particular pupil will be psycho-physically incapable of carrying out satisfactorily quite a number of the specific instructions given to enable him to meet his difficulties, and, indeed, that any attempt on his part to carry out these instructions on the "end-gaining" principle will result with practice in an increase, not in a decrease of his difficulties. It is a matter of common knowledge that the majority of players fail to keep their eye on the ball, but neither the pupil nor the teacher is aware of the fundamental impeding psycho-physical factors concerned with this failure.

It is impossible, within the scope of this book, to discuss these factors in detail in relation to golf, and I intend instead to deal with the pupil's attempt to carry out the teacher's instructions from the standpoint of reliability of sensory appreciation and of co-ordination on a general basis. And as a preliminary, I want to point out that in the teaching plan, of which the lesson we are watching is an example, nothing is given in the way of practical help to the pupil in these directions. The teacher is certainly unable to make a satisfactory diagnosis in the matter of reliable sensory appreciation, and probably does not know whether a pupil is well co-ordinated on a general basis or not; in any case, it is a fact that he does not attempt to make a diagnosis in either connexion. He merely assumes that if he gives the pupil certain instructions, tells him what to do and what not to do, he has conscientiously carried out his duties as a teacher. Yet, he should know perfectly well that in the course of the "up and down swing" of the club, for instance, quite a number of separate instructions that he has given his pupil have to be carried out by quite a number of different parts of the organism. Further, he should know that all these instructions must be linked together (that is, the pupil must be able to think of and put into practice more than one thing at a time), and that all the different parts of the organism must be employed "sympathetically"; must, as he would say, "work together." In other words, the teacher should know that there must be co-ordination in the employment of all the mechanisms involved, yet he gives his pupil no *means whereby* he can achieve this necessary co-ordination on a *general* basis in the use of his psycho-physical self.

Now, we have already pointed out and we are prepared to prove that the great majority of people of our time are more or less imperfectly co-ordinated. If this is so, how is it possible for a pupil to co-ordinate this psycho-physical organism on a general basis for the carrying-out of the golf teacher's specific instructions, on that first day or any subsequent day of lessons, until he has been restored to a satisfactory standard of general co-ordination by some process of re-education which will restore a reliable standard of sensory appreciation?

It is clear, therefore, from the foregoing that the pupil whose lesson we are watching is ill-equipped to carry out the teacher's instructions successfully, and we will now follow him through the experiences which result from the different efforts he makes to carry out these instructions in his ill-equipped condition.

It will be safe to assume that after the performance of the first stroke the teacher will have noted some particular fault or faults, to which he will draw the attention of the pupil, and it is equally safe to assume that the pupil (working on the "end-gaining" plan, and indulging in that process which he calls "concentration") will start to concentrate upon the different corrections suggested by the teacher in connexion with the fault or faults pointed out to him, after which he will make another shot, i.e., "try again." It will be found that in this attempt the pupil has already decided that one or other of these corrections is the all-important one, and so he will proceed to concentrate specially upon it, to the practical exclusion of the others, and he will repeat this process with each subsequent attempt.

Now, although it is quite possible that by this plan of concentrating on the corrections he may succeed in eradicating some specific fault or faults, the point I wish to emphasize again is that he will have gained this end at the expense of overlooking some other equally important corrections in consequence of his having concentrated upon one at a time. By this process of concentration, therefore, as we have pointed out in an earlier chapter, he will probably have added to his list of faults. Not only this, but the psycho-physical process involved is inseparable from the over-excitement of the fear reflexes, and gradually builds up an emotional state which impedes the pupil's progress in the game, and becomes an established phobia which will not only influence his play harmfully, but will impede him in all his other activities. One thing is certain, that if an imperfectly co-ordinated person makes a subconscious effort to carry out such specific instructions as we are now dealing with, the result *as a whole* must be unsatisfactory. The majority of his psycho-physical experiences will be harmful experiences, inasmuch as they must tend to undermine his confidence in himself, and this lack of confidence, arising from a consciousness of complete or comparative failure, will serve to add still another impeding factor to the situation, in the over-exciting of the fear reflexes and the development of harmful emotional conditions which are associated with a state of comparative unhappiness.

One of the greatest factors in human development is the building up of a form of confidence which comes as the result of that method of learning by which the pupil is put in possession of the correct *means whereby* he can attain his end before he makes any attempt to gain it. By this method, the attempt he makes will be more or less successful from the outset, and a series of satisfactory instead of unsatisfactory psycho-physical experiences will follow, and with them that intelligent confidence and state of happiness associated therewith which is the "consummated conquest" of the human being on a conscious plane.

In a civilization such as ours, where unrest, unhappiness and lack of interest in the real things of life are strikingly manifested by mankind, all our efforts should be to enable the human creature to retain the interest and satisfaction exhibited by the healthy child when employing his organism successfully; further, to create conditions in which satisfactory growth, with all that this process connotes in fundamental psycho-physical manifestations, will continue right on through life, and in which the stagnation which accompanies fixed psycho-physical habits and specific "end-gaining" uses of the psycho-physical organism will be impossible.

Conscious employment of the psycho-physical mechanisms on a basis, not of a specific, but of a general co-ordination in all the acts of living constitutes a real and never-ending intellectual problem of constructive control, which, instead of destroying, develops the interest and general intellectual pleasure in even such ordinary acts as those of "sitting down" and "standing up."

Take, for instance, the oft-repeated act of "sitting down." In this act, the subconsciously controlled person, as soon as he touches the chair, instead of allowing it to support him, proceeds, as he would say, to "sit down," that is, to make certain unnecessary movements and alterations in the adjustment and general condition of the organism, involving that imperfect use of the mechanisms which he subconsciously employs in order to seat himself ("sit down").

This means that he has performed the act of "sitting down" in accordance with his subconscious conception of it. In other words, he has "slumped," as we say, and when this imperfectly co-ordinated condition is brought about, the process of seating himself is completed, as far as his awareness is concerned. He remains oblivious to the misuse of the mechanisms involved and to the irritation and pressure associated with the harmful posture which he has subconsciously assumed, and which, unfortunately for him, *feels* natural and comfortable. Likewise, when he stands up, he "feels" the way to stand up, and repeats the same subconscious indulgence of his automatic habits connected with the act of standing up, and once he has "stood up," the process again is completed, as far as his awareness is concerned. In both instances, he ends a psycho-physical process which, in reality, should never be finished. His standard of awareness, indeed, in such connexions is as inadequate as his sensory appreciation is unreliable, and the psycho-physical conditions here indicated are inseparable from lack of interest and lack of general pleasure in the ordinary acts of life.

On the other hand, when a person sits down or stands up in accordance with the demands of constructive conscious control, the process involves an adequate and continuous state of increasing awareness in regard to the use of the mechanisms, so that immediately there is a wrong use of these mechanisms, the person concerned becomes aware of it, and at once substitutes a satisfactory for the unsatisfactory use.

Increasing awareness in this connexion makes more and more for successful accomplishment in accordance with reasoned and satisfactory "means-whereby," and connotes a continuous process which introduces a special interest and pleasure into the most ordinary acts of life.[78]

Conscious fundamental psycho-physical processes do not end; they are continuous and therefore connote real growth and development. This applies to all the acts of life, and the establishment of the psycho-physical uses which are associated with the processes of constructive control and continuous growth herein involved is inseparable from that psycho-physical manifestation which we call "happiness." They are processes which result from the application of "means-whereby" principles, and not from the application of "end-gaining" principles associated with those specific attempts which are characteristic of human endeavour on a subconscious plane and which are adopted in the pursuit of what we call "pleasure." Here we have the explanation of the growing need amongst subconsciously controlled people for *specific* pleasure, with all its attendant shortcomings of unrest and excess, as compared with that enduring happiness, with its accompanying sense of satisfaction and contentment, which is associated with moderation and general control.

Unfortunately, we have been taught that all the ordinary, most necessary, and therefore most oft-repeated acts of life should be automatic and unconscious; for this reason they have become indifferent. The psycho-physical condition here indicated is one that induces stagnation in the organism, and, as it is a condition which becomes more and more pronounced with advancing age, we gradually lose the capacity to take conscious interest in and derive pleasure from those normal and useful activities of life in the sphere of doing, hearing, seeing, etc. Small wonder then that, sooner or later, we seek satisfaction in less normal and less useful activities, and create an undue and harmful demand for specific excitements and stimulations or for some other *specific* pleasure!

All our efforts in the way of education should be to create conditions in which growth will continue through life, conditions in which the stagnation which accompanies fixed habits will be impossible. We shall not then find men and women, as we do now, actually afraid to retire from the business or profession in which they have gained their livelihood and earned a competence, because they have no interest in doing anything else, and cannot adapt themselves to a new way of life. This tragedy is

[78]As I wrote in *Man's Supreme Inheritance*, "When real conscious control has been obtained a 'habit' need never become fixed. It is not truly a habit at all, but an order or series of orders given to the subordinate controls of the body, which orders will be carried out until countermanded."

one of the most common and most poignant features of our modern life, and it will be found that, in such cases, the individuals concerned have so little control over their psycho-physical mechanisms (except within certain limited spheres), that they cannot employ them in an entirely new sphere without experiencing the most distressing forms of psycho-physical functioning.

A study of this question will shew us that the processes of reasoning and of action in the ordinary subconsciously controlled person who has reached the age when he is about to retire from his business or professional work, reveal a tendency to fall back and depend more and more upon automatic methods of procedure. By the time that the greater number of men and women have reached this age, they have become mere automatons, repeating day by day the same round of psycho-physical activities, and gradually limiting themselves, more and more as time goes on, within certain specific spheres of activity, whilst, at the same time, the defects and imperfections in the general use of the mechanisms upon which this activity depends become more and more pronounced. This means that with the approach of age a condition of deterioration and stagnation is being gradually cultivated throughout the organism generally, the very worst possible preparation for the new way of life which is entailed[79] when a man or a woman retires from his or her business or profession. This explains why so many people break down when they stop work.

Someone has said, in referring to the monotony of the environment in which the human creature lives and moves, that monotony is the deathbed of existence. But what of the monotony *within* the human creature's psycho-physical self, a monotony caused by the gradual cessation of those sensations concerned with new experiences which have accompanied growth and mobility within the organism since birth? This is, indeed, monotony in its most harmful form, for it goes hand in hand with an increasing degree of stagnation throughout the whole psycho-physical organism. We recognize, for instance, the danger of stagnation in our cells, when the processes concerned with repair of wasted tissue cease to be operative; when this occurs the stagnation which ensues is analogous to that which follows the cessation of sensations concerned with new experiences referred to above, both forms of stagnation making for monotony and unhappiness.

---

[79]One has only to note the attitude of people in general towards circumstances, even within the domestic sphere, which enforce changes in their habits of life, to realize what an exaggerated and even harmful conception they have of the sufferings or discomforts they are called on to endure on account of this disturbance of the automatic round of their domestic existence.

Yet another form of monotony results from "knowing," from having grown up; from the consciousness that we have ceased to grow. When a man reaches the point where he concludes that he "knows" his subject, he decides, consciously or subconsciously, that he has nothing more to learn, and he promptly begins to lose what he does know; when he becomes aware that he has "grown up," he has reached a stage where he has already begun to stultify those potentialities for growth which once were his, and which might have been his to the end. Boredom, monotony and discontent follow swift upon the establishment of this condition.

We also find that the people who are satisfied that they "know" are the least observant people, and at the same time the most unhappy and discontented. Most people will admit that realization too often is not equal to anticipation, but this again is in consequence of the psycho-physical conditions present. If realization is not only to equal but even sometimes to surpass anticipation, our psycho-physical plan of development must be fundamentally one of continuous growth and of new experiences, and consequently we never reach the point when we may be said to finish learning. This connotes a continuous anticipation of new experiences in growth and development, so that the realization of some new experience in psycho-physical functioning does not bring a sense of finality, with the consequent loss of interest, but is a clear indication that a step forward has been made in growth and development, which is again a stepping-stone to the next stage of advancement, and so on.

The new experiences concerned with the gradually improving functioning of the human creature, indicated in the foregoing, are primarily dependent upon a growing understanding, *consciously developed*, of the operations concerned with the direction and control of the psycho-physical organism in general during the waking and sleeping hours.

William James suggested to us that we should get up every morning looking for health. We hope to go further, for we have a technique to offer in this connexion which will command for the human creature an increasingly high standard of that condition of psycho-physical functioning which makes for health, and the experiences resulting from the use of this technique bring conviction that the all-important duty of the human creature, in our present stage of evolutionary vicissitudes, is that of the *continuous* individual cultivation of fundamental, constructive conscious control of the human psycho-physical organism and its potentialities.

It is true that man has made a specific application of so-called conscious control in the employment of his powers of reasoning in relation to "causes and effects," "means and consequences" outside of the human organism, but this attempt at specific control of environment has not resulted in a really reliable control of actual consequences; our experiences seem to shew, rather, the longer we continue to apply this form of unreliable "conscious control," the worse off we are likely to be. My experience in connexion with the practical application of the technique I have described convinces me that if we are ever to command a reliable constructive control of environment and satisfactory reasoning in relation to "causes and effects," "means and consequences" in this connexion, we must be able primarily to command fundamental constructive conscious control of the individual psycho-physical organism. This calls for a higher and higher standard of psycho-physical functioning, which in turn demands a satisfactory and growing understanding and conscious use of the wonderful mechanisms concerned. This process provides the human creature with a sphere of psycho-physical activity, almost unlimited in its possibilities, where hitherto he has evidenced the worst forms of unreasoned and subconsciously directed activity.

CONCLUSIONS

PSYCHO-PHYSICAL ATTITUDE

In the course of this book I have dealt with various human defects, peculiarities, shortcomings and imperfect uses of the psycho-physical organism, which tend to increase during the process of growth and development, and too often become established as "bad habits" long ere adolescence has been reached, the sum total of the experiences involved being the foundation of what is called "mental attitude."

The attitude of the human creature towards the functioning of his psycho-physical self, and towards the employment of this self in the activities of daily life is the "be all and end all," and only those who possess the key to this storehouse of their psycho-physical experiences, inherited or acquired, can reach that stage of understanding of their psycho-physical reactions to stimuli which justifies an optimistic view of any efforts that may be made for man's uplifting.

The understanding to which I refer is that understanding of the psycho-physical processes, present at the varying stages of the human creature's growth and development, which are responsible for manifestations, the proper understanding of which is essential to any satisfactory consideration of "cause and effect," primarily, in connexion with the activities concerned with the development of the human creature himself and, secondly, in connexion with his activities outside himself when applied to the act of living in the complex round of social, religious, political, moral, educational, industrial and other experiences in civilization. The human creature continues to rush from one extreme to another on the "end-gaining" principle in his attempts at reform or "physical" improvement, and the point just made as to what is necessary for the primary and secondary understanding of "cause and effect" is of the utmost importance in this connexion, and in any estimate of schemes for the uplifting of the human creature that are likely to prove permanently satisfactory. What probability is there that any one of these schemes of reform will do anything but make conditions more chaotic, until the individuals concerned have been re-educated on a general basis and reorganized as a psycho-physical unity? For in the last analysis, it is the creature's individual reaction to the stimuli resulting from the individual conception of that scheme of reform that matters, even if the scheme, taken by itself, might be considered a satisfactory one.

This leads us back to the theme of conception which has been outlined, and in connexion with which we have endeavoured to shew that only in a state of *co-ordinated activity*, in which the organism is functioning near its maximum, can we hope for anything approaching a satisfactory conception of new and unfamiliar ideas or experiences. Hence the necessity of having an understanding of "cause and effect," primarily, in connexion with the functioning of the organism itself.

For it is only after we have solved this problem in the individual that we can safely pass on to the secondary consideration of "cause and effect" in connexion with the problems of every-day life. Only then shall we be justified in asserting that individual reactions to stimuli will be the reactions of a controlled human creature, whose employment of the processes of reasoning in the activities of life prevents the undue and harmful excitement of the fear reflexes and emotions, especially when he is called upon to deal with those new and unfamiliar situations or problems which are the natural outcome of all processes tending towards advancement on the evolutionary plane.

THE USE OF THE SELF

Its Conscious Direction in Relation to Diagnosis, Functioning and the Control of Reaction

With an Introduction by
PROFESSOR JOHN DEWEY

DEDICATED TO ALL THOSE WHO BY THEIR INTEREST AND PARTICIPATION IN MY WORK HAVE HELPED ME TO GAIN THE EXPERIENCE SET DOWN IN THIS BOOK

PREFACE

SINCE the publication of my last book I have been much encouraged to receive written recognition of the value and scope of my technique from members both of the medical and educational professions, and as we are finishing the preparation of the subject matter of this book, I have received from Mr. J. E. R. McDonagh, F. R. C. S., a copy of the third volume of his book *The Nature of Disease* (Heinemann), in which he has devoted Chapter I, entitled "Mal-coördination and Disease," to a review of my work. Mr. McDonagh's opening lines may be of interest to the reader.

> In the epilogue to the second part of *The Nature of Disease* the author announced his intention to correlate with medicine Mr. F. M. Alexander's work on the conscious control of the individual. The announcement was made because it became apparent to the author after meeting Mr. Alexander and watching his technique, that the wrong use of the body plays an important role in disease. Now that the time has come to fulfil the promise the author is less sanguine of success. This is partly because Alexander's view is possibly even more fundamental than the author's view that there is only one disease, partly because the written word can neither convey the whole idea nor satisfactorily describe the technique, and partly because to link any subject with medicine it is necessary to commit the basic error of practising differentiation instead of correlation.

Other medical men are giving me their support as will be seen from what they have written in the Open Letter in the Appendix of this present book, and I believe that in Chapter V I have indicated how medical diagnosis may be made more complete by the inclusion in medical training of the principles and procedure that I advocate.

It has been suggested to me by a friend and pupil who has read the manuscript of the first chapter of this book, that some readers may conclude from it that my technique is limited in its usefulness to dealing with serious difficulties such as those which I describe. This is not the case, however, for pupils free from any such difficulties have frequently come to me because they believed—and results justified this belief—that however well endowed they might be with health or other gifts, they would derive benefit from learning how to direct and control the use of themselves consciously in their daily activities.

Readers of my former books are aware of my special interest in the training of children, and what I have just written applies particularly to their early training. In this connexion I would refer to the benefits derived by the children and young people in our little school where they learn to put into practice the technique for the direction of an improved use of themselves in all their "doings," in their reading, writing, etc.

I am also pleased to be able to state that the first course for the training of teachers of my work was inaugurated in March this year, and I wish to take this opportunity to thank Mr. Rugg-Gunn, F. R. C. S., for his article entitled "A New Profession" which he recently wrote for *Women's Employment* (June, 1931), in which he pointed out the advantages for young people of taking up this work as a professional career and also referred to the work done in the little school. The publication of this article has brought so many enquiries that I have decided to include in an Appendix a reprint of the Open Letter to Intending Students of the Training Course and also a special reference to the work being done in the little school where the children are helped to put into practice the principles and procedures inherent in my technique during their school work, whatever the subject that is engaging their attention.

The results of the series of experiences I have outlined in Chapter I seem to me to imply that in the process of acquiring a conscious direction of the use of the human organism, a hitherto "undiscovered country" is opened up, where the scope for the development of human potentialities is practically unlimited, and anyone who chooses to take the time and trouble to carry out the procedures necessary for acquiring a conscious direction of use can put this to the test.

I would venture to suggest that even the meagre amount of knowledge of the use of the self contained in these pages may be sufficient to enable workers in all fields of investigation, whether in biology, astronomy, physics, philosophy, psychology or any other, to realize that in their researches they have passed over a field of experience which, if explored, would add new material to the premises from which to make their several deductions. After all, the self is the instrument through which all these workers must express themselves. If, therefore, a knowledge of how to direct consciously the use of the psycho-physical mechanisms of the self were made the common starting-point of their researches, this would surely tend both to unite and amplify the results of their several labours more than anything that has so far been done.

I wish to take this opportunity to thank Professor John Dewey for giving me once more his invaluable support and for writing the introduction to this book. He has also kindly allowed me to quote from his book, *Experience and Nature.* I also wish to thank Dr. Peter Macdonald for reading the manuscript and for making his valuable criticisms and suggestions, and Miss Ethel Webb and Miss Irene Tasker for preparing the subject matter for publication. I am especially indebted to Miss Webb and Miss Tasker for their valuable and untiring help, without which the publication of the book would have been delayed. I am further indebted to Miss Mary Olcott and Miss Edith Lawson for their careful revision of the proofs, to Miss Evelyn Glover for her help with the final preparation of the typescript, and to two of my students, Mr. George Trevelyan and Mr. Gurney MacInnes, for undertaking the task of making the Index. I also desire to thank Sir Arthur Eddington for his permission to quote from his lecture on "Science and Religion," Dr. A. Murdoch for permission to quote from his Address to the St. Andrew's (James Mackenzie) Institute, Sir Edward Holderness for allowing me to quote from his article, "The Fearful Foozler," and Mr. David Low for permission to reproduce one of his well-known cartoons on the jacket cover of this book.

F. MATTHIAS ALEXANDER.
24th July, 1931.

CONTENTS

INTRODUCTION
by
PROFESSOR JOHN DEWEY

In writing some introductory words to Mr. Alexander's previous book, *Constructive Conscious Control of the Individual,* I stated that his procedure and conclusions meet all the requirements of the strictest scientific method, and that he has applied the method in a field in which it had never been used before—that of our judgments and beliefs concerning ourselves and our activities. In so doing, he has, I said in effect, rounded out the results of the sciences in the physical field, accomplishing this end in such a way that they become capable of use for human benefit. It is commonplace that scientific technique has for its consequence control of the energies to which it refers. Physical science has for its fruit an astounding degree of new command of physical energies. Yet we are faced with a situation which is serious, perhaps tragically so. There is everywhere increasing doubt as to whether this physical mastery of physical energies is going to further human welfare, or whether human happiness is going to be wrecked by it. Ultimately there is but one sure way of answering this question in the hopeful and constructive sense. If there can be developed a technique which will enable individuals really to secure the right use of themselves, then the factor upon which depends the final use of all other forms of energy will be brought under control. Mr. Alexander has evolved this technique.

In repeating these statements, I do so fully aware of their sweeping nature. Were not our eyes and ears so accustomed to irresponsible statements that we cease to ask for either meaning or proof, they might well raise a question as to the complete intellectual responsibility and competency of their author. In repeating them after the lapse of intervening years, I appeal to the account which Mr. Alexander has given of the origin of his discovery of the principle of central and conscious control. Those who do not identify science with a parade of technical vocabulary will find in this account the essentials of scientific method in any field of inquiry. They will find a record of long continued, patient, unwearied experimentation and observation in which every inference is extended, tested, corrected by further more searching experiments; they will find a series of such observations in which the mind is carried from observation of comparatively coarse, gross, superficial connections of causes and effect to those causal conditions which are fundamental and central in the use which we make of ourselves.

Personally, I cannot speak with too much admiration—in the original sense of wonder as well as the sense of respect—of the persistence and thoroughness with which these extremely difficult observations and experiments were carried out. In consequence, Mr. Alexander created what may be truly called a physiology of the *living* organism. His observations and experiments have to do with the actual functioning of the body, with the organism in operation, and in operation under the ordinary conditions of living—rising, sitting, walking, standing, using arms, hands, voice, tools, instruments of all kinds. The contrast between sustained and accurate observation of the living and the usual activities of man and those made upon dead things under unusual and artificial conditions marks the difference between true and pseudoscience. And yet so used have we become to associating "science" with the latter sort of thing that its contrast with the genuinely scientific character of Mr. Alexander's observations has been one great reason for the failure of many to appreciate his technique and conclusions.

As might be anticipated, the conclusions of Mr. Alexander's experimental inquiries are in harmony with what physiologists know about the muscular and nervous structure. But they give a new significance to that knowledge; indeed, they make evident what knowledge itself really is. The anatomist may "know" the exact function of each muscle, and conversely know what muscles come into play in the execution of any specified act. But if he is himself unable to co-ordinate all the muscular structures involved in, say, sitting down or in rising from a sitting position in a way which achieves the optimum and efficient performance of that act; if, in other words, he misuses himself in what he does, how can he be said to *know* in the full and vital sense of that word? Magnus proved by means of what may be called *external* evidence the existence of a central control in the organism. But Mr. Alexander's technique gave a direct and intimate confirmation in personal experience of the fact of central control long before Magnus carried on his investigations. And one who has had experience of the technique *knows* it through the series of experiences which he himself has. The genuinely scientific character of Mr. Alexander's teaching and discoveries can be safely rested upon this fact alone.

The vitality of a scientific discovery is revealed and tested in its power to project and direct new further operations which not only harmonize with prior results but which lead on to new observed materials, suggesting in turn further experimentally controlled acts, and so on in a continued series of new developments. Speaking as a pupil, it was because of this fact as demonstrated in personal experience that I first became convinced of the scientific quality of Mr. Alexander's work. Each lesson was a laboratory experimental demonstration. Statements made in advance of consequences to follow and the means by which they would be reached were met with implicit scepticism—a fact which is practically inevitable, since, as Mr. Alexander points out, one uses the very conditions that need re-education as one's standard of judgment. Each lesson carries the process somewhat further and confirms in the most intimate and convincing fashion the claims that are made. As one goes on, new areas are opened, new possibilities are seen and then realized; one finds himself continually growing, and realizes that there is an endless process of growth initiated.

From one standpoint, I had an unusual opportunity for making an intellectual study of the technique and its results. I was, from the practical standpoint, an inept, awkward and slow pupil. There were no speedy and seemingly miraculous changes to evoke gratitude emotionally, while they misled me intellectually. I was forced to observe carefully at every step of the process, and to interest myself in the theory of the operations. I did this partly from my previous interest in psychology and philosophy, and partly as a compensation for my practical backwardness. In bringing to bear whatever knowledge I already possessed —or thought I did—and whatever powers of discipline in mental application I had acquired in the pursuit of these studies, I had the most humiliating experience of my life, intellectually speaking. For to find that one is unable to execute directions, including inhibitory ones, in doing such a seemingly simple act as to sit down, when one is using all the mental capacity which one prides himself upon possessing, is not an experience congenial to one's vanity. But it may be conducive to analytic study of causal conditions, obstructive and positive. And so I verified in personal experience all that Mr. Alexander says about the unity of the physical and psychical in the psycho-physical; about our habitually wrong use of ourselves and the part this wrong use plays in generating all kinds of unnecessary tensions and wastes of energy; about the vitiation of our sensory appreciations which form the material of our judgments of ourselves; about the unconditional necessity of inhibition of customary acts, and the tremendous mental difficulty found in not "doing" something as soon as an habitual act is suggested, together with the great change in moral and mental attitude that takes place as proper co-ordinations are established. In re-affirming my conviction as to the scientific character of Mr. Alexander's discoveries and technique, I do so then not as one who has experienced a "cure," but as one who has brought whatever intellectual capacity he has to the study of a problem. In the study, I found the things which I had "known"—in the sense of theoretical belief—in philosophy and psychology, changed into vital experiences which gave a new meaning to knowledge of them.

In the present state of the world, it is evident that the control we have gained of physical energies, heat, light, electricity, etc., without having first secured control of our use of ourselves is a perilous affair. Without control of our use of ourselves, our use of other things is blind; it may lead to anything.

Moreover, if our habitual judgments of ourselves are warped because they are based on vitiated sense material—as they must be if our habits of managing ourselves are already wrong—then the more complex the social conditions under which we live, the more disastrous must be the outcome. Every additional complication of outward instrumentalities is likely to be a step nearer destruction: a fact which the present state of the world tragically exemplifies.

The school of Pavloff has made current the idea of conditioned reflexes. Mr. Alexander's work extends and corrects the idea. It proves that there are certain basic, central organic habits and attitudes which condition *every* act we perform, every use we make of ourselves. Hence a conditioned reflex is not just a matter of an arbitrarily established connection, such as that between the sound of a bell and the eating-reaction in a dog, but goes back to central conditions within the organism itself. This discovery corrects the ordinary conception of the conditioned reflex. The latter as usually understood renders an individual a passive puppet to be played upon by external manipulations. The discovery of a central control which conditions all other reactions brings the conditioning factor under conscious direction and enables the individual through his own co-ordinated activities to take possession of his own potentialities. It converts the fact of conditioned reflexes from a principle of external enslavement into a means of vital freedom.

Education is the only sure method which mankind possesses for directing its own course. But we have been involved in a vicious circle. Without knowledge of what constitutes a truly normal and healthy psycho-physical life, our professed education is likely to be mis-education. Every serious student of the formation of disposition and character which takes place in the family and school knows—speaking without the slightest exaggeration—how often and how deplorably this possibility is realized. The technique of Mr. Alexander gives to the educator a standard of psycho-physical health—in which what we call morality is included. It supplies also the "means whereby" this standard may be progressively and endlessly achieved, becoming a conscious possession of the one educated. It provides therefore the conditions for the central direction of all special educational processes. It bears the same relation to education that education itself bears to all other human activities.

I cannot therefore state too strongly the hopes that are aroused in me by the information contained in the Appendix that Mr. Alexander has, with his coadjutors, opened a training class, nor my sense of the importance that this work secures adequate support. It contains in my judgment the promise and potentiality of the new direction that is needed in all education.

CHAPTER I

EVOLUTION OF A TECHNIQUE

> "First, then, I must request men not to suppose that . . . I wish to found a new sect in philosophy. For this is not what I am about; nor do I think that it matters much to the fortunes of men what abstract notions one may entertain concerning nature and the principles of things; and no doubt many old theories of this kind can be revived and many new ones introduced; just as many theories of the heavens may be supposed, which agree well enough with the phenomena and yet differ with each other.
>
> "But for my part I do not trouble myself with any such speculative and withal unprofitable matters. My purpose, on the contrary, is to try whether I cannot in very fact lay more firmly the foundations, and extend more widely the limits, of the power and greatness of man."
>
> FRANCIS BACON ("NOVUM ORGANUM"—CXVI).

MY two earlier books, *Man's Supreme Inheritance* and *Constructive Conscious Control of the Individual*, contain a statement of the technique which I gradually evolved over a period of years in my search for a means whereby faulty conditions of use in the human organism could be improved. I must admit that when I began my investigation, I, in common with most people, conceived of "body" and "mind" as separate parts of the same organism, and consequently believed that human ills, difficulties and shortcomings could be classified as either "mental" or "physical" and dealt with on specifically "mental" or specifically "physical" lines. My practical experiences, however, led me to abandon this point of view and readers of my books will be aware that the technique described in them is based on the opposite conception, namely, that it is *impossible* to separate "mental" and "physical" processes in any form of human activity.

This change in my conception of the human organism has not come about as the outcome of mere theorizing on my part. It has been forced upon me by the experiences which I have gained through my investigations in a new field of practical experimentation upon the living human being.

The letters I receive from my readers shew that a large majority of those who accept the theory of the unity of mental and physical processes in human activity, find difficulty in understanding what the practical working of this theory of unity implies. This difficulty is always coming up in my teaching, but it is possible during a course of lessons to demonstrate to the pupil how the mental and physical work together in the use of the self[1] in all activity. Repeated demonstration of this kind brings conviction, but since the number of pupils one can take, even in a large teaching practice, is naturally limited, the opportunities for giving this demonstration are comparatively few, and I have therefore decided in this book to start at the beginning and relate the history of the investigations which gradually led to the evolution of my technique. I shall give as fully as possible the actual details of the experiments I made, telling what I observed and experienced during the process, as I believe that by so doing I shall be giving my readers the opportunity to see for themselves the train of events which finally convinced me

(1) that the so-called "mental" and "physical" are not separate entities;

(2) that for this reason human ills and shortcomings cannot be classified as "mental" or "physical" and dealt with specifically as such, but that all training, whether it be educative or otherwise, i.e., whether its object be the prevention[2] or elimination of defect, error or disease, must be based upon the indivisible unity of the human organism.

If any reader doubts this, I would ask him if he can furnish any proof

[1]I wish to make it clear that when I emply the word "use," it is not in that limited sense of the use of any specific part, as, for instance, when we speak of the use of an arm or the use of a leg, but in a much wider and more comprehensive sense applying to the working of the organism in general. For I recognize that the use of any specific part such as the arm or leg involves of necessity bringing into action the different psycho-physical mechanisms of the organism, this concerted activity bringing about the use of the specific part.

[2]I use the word "prevention" (and this applies equally to "cure") not because I consider it adequate or wholly suitable for my purpose, but because I cannot find another to take its place. "Prevention" in its fullest sense implies the existence of satisfactory conditions which can be prevented from changing for the worse. In this sense prevention is not possible in practice today, since the conditions now present in the civilized human creature are such that it would be difficult to find anyone who is entirely free from manifestations of wrong use and functioning. When, therefore, I use the terms "prevention" and "cure," I use them in a relative sense only, including under "preventive" measures all attempts to prevent faulty use and functioning of the organism generally as a means of preventing defect, disorder and disease, and under "curative" measures those methods in which the influence of faulty use upon functioning is ignored when dealing with defects, disorder and disease.

that the process involved in the act, say, of lifting an arm, or of walking, talking, going to sleep, starting out to learn something, thinking out a problem, making a decision, giving or withholding consent to a request or wish, or of satisfying a need or sudden impulse, is purely "mental" or purely "physical." This question raises a great many points, and I suggest that a lead may be given towards meeting them if the reader will follow me through the experiences which I will now relate.

From my early youth I took a delight in poetry and it was one of my chief pleasures to study the plays of Shakespeare, reading them aloud and endeavouring to interpret the characters. This led to my becoming interested in elocution and the art of reciting, and now and again I was asked to recite in public. I was sufficiently successful to think of taking up Shakespearean reciting as a career, and worked long and hard at the study of every branch of dramatic expression. After a certain amount of experience as an amateur, I reached the stage when I believed that my work could stand the severer test of being judged from the professional standard, and the criticisms I received justified me in deciding to take up reciting as a profession.

All went well for some years, when I began to have trouble with my throat and vocal cords, and not long after I was told by my friends that when I was reciting my breathing was audible, and that they could hear me (as they put it) "gasping" and "sucking in air" through my mouth. This worried me even more than my actual throat trouble which was then in its early stages, for I had always prided myself on being free from the habit of audibly sucking in breath which is so common with reciters, actors and singers. I therefore sought the advice of doctors and voice trainers in the hope of remedying my faulty breathing and relieving my hoarseness, but in spite of all that they could do in the way of treatment, the gasping and sucking in of breath when I was reciting became more and more exaggerated and the hoarseness recurred at shorter intervals.[3] The treatment I was receiving became less and less effective as time went on, and the trouble gradually increased until, after a few years, I found to my dismay that I had developed a condition of hoarseness which from time to time culminated in a complete loss of voice. I had experienced a good deal of ill-health all my life and this had often been a stumbling-block to me,

[3]The medical diagnosis in my case was irritation of the mucous membrane of the throat and nose, and inflammation of the vocal cords which were said to be unduly relaxed. My uvula was very long and at times caused acute attacks of coughing. For this reason two of my medical advisers recommended it should be shortened by a minor operation, but I did not follow this advice. I now have little doubt that I was suffering from what is sometimes called "clergyman's sore throat."

so that with the additional burden of my recurring hoarseness, I began to doubt the soundness of my vocal organs. The climax came when I was offered a particularly attractive and important engagement, for by this time I had reached such a stage of uncertainty about the conditions of my vocal organs that I was frankly afraid to accept it. I decided to consult my doctor once more, even though the previous treatment had been disappointing. After making a fresh examination of my throat, he promised me that if, during the fortnight before my recital, I abstained from reciting and used my voice as little as possible and agreed to follow the treatment he prescribed, my voice by the end of that time would be normal.

I acted on his advice and accepted the engagement. After a few days I felt assured that the doctor's promise would be fulfilled, for I found that by using my voice as little as possible I gradually lost my hoarseness. When the night of my recital came, I was quite free from hoarseness, but before I was halfway through my programme, my voice was in the most distressing condition again, and by the end of the evening the hoarseness was so acute that I could hardly speak.

My disappointment was greater than I can express, for it now seemed to me that I could never look forward to more than a temporary relief, and that I should thus be forced to give up a career in which I had become deeply interested and believed I could be successful.

I saw my doctor next day and we talked the matter over, and at the end of the talk I asked him what he thought we had better do about it. "We must go on with the treatment," he said. I told him I could not do that, and when he asked me why, I pointed out to him that although I had faithfully carried out his instruction not to use my voice in public during his treatment, the old condition of hoarseness had returned within an hour after I started to use my voice again on the night of my recital. "Is it not fair, then," I asked him, "to conclude that it was *something I was doing that evening in using my voice that was the cause of the trouble?"* He thought a moment and said "Yes, that must be so." "Can you tell me, then," I asked him, *"what it was that I did* that caused the trouble?" He frankly admitted that he could not. "Very well," I replied, "if that is so, I must try and find out for myself."

When I set out on this investigation, I had two facts to go on. I had learned by experience that reciting brought about conditions of hoarseness, and that this hoarseness tended to disappear, as long as I confined the use of my voice to ordinary speaking, and at the same time had medical treatment for my throat and vocal organs. I considered the bearing of these two facts upon my difficulty, and I saw that if ordinary speaking did not cause hoarseness while reciting did, there must be something different between what I did in reciting and what I did in ordinary speaking.

If this were so, and I could find out what the difference was, it might help me to get rid of the hoarseness, and at least I could do no harm by making an experiment.

To this end I decided to make use of a mirror and observe the manner of my "doing" both in ordinary speaking and reciting, hoping that this would enable me to distinguish the difference, if any, between them, and it seemed better to begin by watching myself during the simpler act of ordinary speaking, in order to have something to go by when I came to watch myself during the more exacting act of reciting.

Standing before a mirror I first watched myself carefully during the act of ordinary speaking. I repeated the act many times, but saw nothing in my manner of doing it that seemed wrong or unnatural. I then went on to watch myself carefully in the mirror when I recited, and I very soon noticed several things that I had not noticed when I was simply speaking. I was particularly struck by three things that I saw myself doing. I saw that as soon as I started to recite, I tended to pull back the head, depress the larynx and suck in breath through the mouth in such a way as to produce a gasping sound.

After I had noticed these tendencies I went back and watched myself again during ordinary speaking, and on this occasion I was left in little doubt that the three tendencies I had noticed for the first time when reciting were also present, though in a lesser degree, in my ordinary speaking. They were indeed so slight that I could understand why, on the previous occasions when I had watched myself in ordinary speaking[4] I had altogether failed to notice them. When I discovered this marked difference between what I did in ordinary speaking and what I did in reciting, I realized that here I had a definite fact which might explain many things, and I was encouraged to go on.

I recited again and again in front of the mirror and found that the three tendencies I had already noticed became specially marked when I was reciting passages in which unusual demands were made upon my voice. This served to confirm my early suspicion that there might be some connexion between what I did with myself while reciting and my throat trouble, a not unreasonable supposition, it seemed to me, since what I did in ordinary speaking caused no noticeable harm, while what I did in reciting to meet any unusual demands on my voice brought about an acute condition of hoarseness.

From this I was led to conjecture that if pulling back my head, depressing my larynx and sucking in breath did indeed bring about a

[4] This could hardly have been otherwise, seeing that I then lacked experience in the kind of observation necessary to enable me to detect anything wrong in the way I used myself when speaking.

strain on my voice, it must constitute a misuse of the parts concerned. I now believed I had found the root of the trouble, for I argued that if my hoarseness arose from the way I used parts of my organism, I should get no further unless I could prevent or change this misuse.

When, however, I came to try to make practical use of this discovery, I found myself in a maze. For where was I to begin? Was it the sucking in of breath that caused the pulling back of the head and the depressing of the larynx? Or was it the pulling back of the head that caused the depressing of the larynx and the sucking in of the breath? Or was it the depressing of the larynx that caused the sucking in of breath and the pulling back of the head?

As I was unable to answer these questions, all I could do was to go on patiently experimenting before the mirror. After some months I found that when reciting I could not by direct means prevent the sucking in of breath or the depressing of the larynx, but that I could to some extent prevent the pulling back of the head. This led me to a discovery which turned out to be of great importance, namely, that when I succeeded in preventing the pulling back of the head, this tended indirectly to check the sucking in of breath and the depressing of the larynx.

> *The importance of this discovery cannot be overestimated, for through it I was led on to the further discovery of the primary control of the working of all the mechanisms of the human organism, and this marked the first important stage of my investigation.*

A further result, which I also noted was that with the prevention of the misuse of these parts I tended to become less hoarse while reciting, and that as I gradually gained experience in this prevention, my liability to hoarseness tended to decrease. What is more, when, after these experiences, my throat was again examined by my medical friends, a considerable improvement was found in the general condition of my larynx and vocal cords.

In this way it was borne in upon me that the changes in *use* that I had been able to bring about by preventing the three harmful tendencies I had detected in myself had produced a marked effect upon the *functioning* of my vocal and respiratory mechanisms.

> *This conclusion, I now see, marked the second important stage in my investigations, for my practical experience in this specific instance brought me to realize for the first time the close connexion that exists between use and functioning.*

My experience up till now had shewn me

(1) that the tendency to put my head back was associated

with my throat trouble, and

(2) that I could relieve this trouble to a certain extent merely by preventing myself from putting my head back, since this act of prevention tended to prevent indirectly the depressing of the larynx and the sucking in of breath.

From this I argued that if I put my head definitely forward, I might be able to influence the functioning of my vocal and respiratory mechanisms still further in the right direction, and so eradicate the tendency to hoarseness altogether. I therefore decided as my next step to put my head definitely forward, further forward, in fact, than I felt was the right thing to do.

When I came to try it, however, I found that after I had put my head forward beyond a certain point, I tended to pull it down as well as forward, and, as far as I could see, the effect of this upon my vocal and respiratory organs was much the same as when I pulled my head back and down. For in both acts there was the same depressing of the larynx that was associated with my throat trouble, and by this time I was convinced that this depressing of the larynx must be checked if my voice was ever to become normal. I therefore went on experimenting in the hope of finding some use of the head and neck which was not associated with a depressing of the larynx.

It is impossible to describe here in detail my various experiences during this long period. Suffice to say that in the course of these experiments I came to notice that any use of my head and neck which was associated with a depressing of the larynx was also associated with a tendency to lift the chest and shorten[5] the stature.

As I look back I realize that this again was a discovery of far-reaching implications, and events proved that it marked a turning-point in my investigations.

This new piece of evidence suggested that the functioning of the organs of speech was influenced by my manner of using the whole torso, and that the pulling of the head back and down was not, as I had presumed, merely a misuse of the specific parts concerned, but one that was inseparably bound up with a misuse of other mechanisms which involved the act of shortening the stature. If this were so, it would clearly be useless to expect such improvement as I needed from merely preventing the

[5]Although it would probably be more correct to use the phrases "*increase* the stature," "*decrease* the stature," I have decided to use the phrases "lengthen the stature," "shorten the stature," because the words "lengthen" and "shorten" are those most commonly used in this connexion.

wrong use of the head and neck. I realized that I must also prevent those other associated wrong uses which brought about the shortening of the stature.

This led me on to a long series of experiments in some of which I attempted to prevent the shortening of the stature, in others actually to lengthen it, noting the results in each case. For a time I alternated between these two forms of experiment, and after noting the effect of each upon my voice, I found that the best conditions of my larynx and vocal mechanisms and the least tendency to hoarseness were associated with a *lengthening* of the stature. Unfortunately, I found that when I came to practise, I shortened far more than I lengthened, and when I came to look for an explanation of this, I saw that it was due to my tendency to pull my head down as I tried to put it forward in order to lengthen. After further experimentation I found at last that in order to maintain a lengthening of the stature it was necessary that my head should tend to go upwards, not downwards, when I put it forward; in short, that to lengthen *I must put my head forward and up.*

As is shewn by what follows, this proved to be the primary control of my use in all my activities.

When, however, I came to try to put my head forward and up *while reciting*, I noticed that my old tendency to lift the chest increased, and that with this went a tendency to increase the arch of the spine and thus bring about what I now call a "narrowing of the back" This, I saw, had an adverse effect on the shape and functioning of the torso itself, and I therefore concluded that to maintain a lengthening it was not sufficient to put my head forward and up, but that I must put it forward and up in such a way that I prevented the lifting of the chest and simultaneously brought about a widening of the back.

Having got so far, I considered I should now be justified in attempting to put these findings into practice. To this end I proceeded in my vocal work to try to prevent my old habit of pulling my head back and down and lifting the chest (shortening the stature), and to combine this act of prevention with an attempt to put the head forward and up (lengthening the stature) and widen the back. This was my first attempt to combine "prevention" and "doing" in one activity, and I never for a moment doubted that I should be able to do this, but I found that although I was now able to put the head forward and up and widen the back as acts in themselves, *I could not maintain these conditions in speaking or reciting.*

This made me suspicious that I was not doing what I thought I was doing, and I decided once more to bring the mirror to my aid. Later on

I took into use two additional mirrors, one on each side of the central one, and with their aid I found that my suspicions were justified. For there I saw that at the critical moment when I tried to combine the prevention of shortening with a positive attempt to *maintain a lengthening and speak at the same time*, I did not put my head forward and up as I intended, but actually put it back. Here then was startling proof that I was doing the opposite of what I believed I was doing and of what I had decided I ought to do.

I break my story here to draw attention to a very curious fact, even though it tells against myself. My reader will remember that in my earlier experiments, when I wished to make certain of what I was doing with myself in the familiar act of reciting, I had derived invaluable help from the use of a mirror. Despite this past experience and the knowledge that I had gained from it, I now set out on an experiment which brought into play a new use of certain parts and involved sensory experiences that were totally unfamiliar, without its even occurring to me that for this purpose I should need the help of the mirror more than ever.

This shews how confident I was, in spite of my past experience, that I should be able to put into practice any idea that I thought desirable. When I found myself unable to do so, I thought that this was merely a personal idiosyncrasy, but my teaching experience of the past thirty-five years and my observation of people with whom I have come into contact in other ways have convinced me that this was not an idiosyncrasy, but that most people would have done the same in similar circumstances. I was indeed suffering from a delusion that is practically universal, the delusion that because we are able to do what we "will to do" in acts that are habitual and involve familiar sensory experiences, we shall be equally successful in doing what we "will to do" in acts which are contrary to our habit and therefore involve sensory experiences that are unfamiliar.

When I realized this, I was much disturbed and I saw that the whole situation would have to be reconsidered. I went back to the beginning again, to my original conclusion that the cause of my throat trouble was to be found in something I was doing myself when I used my voice. I had since discovered both what this "something" was and what I believed I ought to do instead, if my vocal organs were to function properly. But this had not helped me much, for when the time came for me to apply what I had learned to my reciting, and I had tried to do what I ought to do, I had failed. Obviously, then, my next step was to find out at what point in my "doing" I had gone wrong.

There was nothing for it but to persevere, and I practised patiently month after month, as I had been doing hitherto, with varying experiences of success and failure, but without much enlightenment. In time, however, I profited by these experiences, for through them I came to see that any attempt to maintain my lengthening when reciting not only involved on my part the prevention of the wrong use of certain specific parts and the substitution of what I believed to be a better use of these parts, but this attempt also involved my bringing into play the use of all those parts of the organism required for the activities incident to the act of reciting, such as standing, walking, using the arms or hands for gesture, interpretation, etc.

Observation in the mirror shewed me that when I was standing to recite I was using these other parts in certain wrong ways which synchronized with my wrong way of using my head and neck, larynx, vocal and breathing organs, and which involved a condition of undue muscle tension throughout my organism. I observed that this condition of undue muscle tension affected particularly the use of my legs, feet and toes, my toes being contracted and bent downwards in such a way that my feet were unduly arched, my weight thrown more on to the outside of my feet than it should have been, and my balance interfered with.

On discovering this, I thought back to see if I could account for it, and I recalled an instruction that had been given to me in the past by the late Mr. James Cathcart (at one time a member of Mr. Charles Kean's Company) when I was taking lessons from him in dramatic expression and interpretation. Not being pleased with my way of standing and walking, he would say to me from time to time, "Take hold of the floor with your feet." He would then proceed to shew me what he meant by this, and I did my best to copy him, believing that if I was told what to do to correct something that was wrong, I should be able to do it and all would be well. I persevered and in time believed that my way of standing was now satisfactory, because I thought I was "taking hold of the floor with my feet" as I had seen him do.

> *The belief is very generally held that if only we are told what to do in order to correct a wrong way of doing something, we can do it, and that if we* feel *we are doing it, all is well. All my experience, however, goes to shew that this belief is a delusion.*

On recalling this experience I continued with the aid of mirrors to observe the use of myself more carefully than ever, and came to realize that what I was doing with my legs, feet and toes when standing to recite was exerting a most harmful general influence upon the use of myself throughout my organism. This convinced me that the use of these parts involved an abnormal amount of muscle tension and was indirectly associated with my throat trouble, and I was strengthened in this conviction when I reminded myself that my teacher had found it necessary in the past to try and improve my way of standing in order to get better results in my reciting. It gradually dawned upon me that the wrong way I was using myself when I thought I was "taking hold of the floor with my feet" was the same wrong way I was using myself when in reciting I pulled my head back, depressed my larynx, etc., and that this wrong way of using myself constituted a combined wrong use of the whole of my physical-mental mechanisms. I then realized that this was the use which I habitually brought into play for all my activities, that it was what I may call the "habitual use" of myself, and that my desire to recite, like any other stimulus to activity, would inevitably cause this habitual wrong use to come into play and dominate any attempt I might be making to employ a better use of myself in reciting.

The influence of this wrong use was bound to be strong because of its being habitual, but in my case it was greatly strengthened because during the past years I had undoubtedly been cultivating it through my efforts to carry out my teacher's instructions to "take hold of the floor with my feet" when I recited. The influence of this *cultivated* habitual use, therefore, acted as an almost irresistible stimulus to me to use myself in the wrong way I was accustomed to; this stimulus to general wrong use was far stronger than the stimulus of my desire to employ the new use of my head and neck, and I now saw that it was this influence which led me, as soon as I stood up to recite, to put my head in the opposite direction to that which I desired. I now had proof of one thing at least, that all my efforts up till now to improve the use of myself in reciting had been misdirected.

It is important to remember that the use of a specific part in any activity is closely associated with the use of other parts of the organism, and that the influence exerted by the various parts one upon another is continuously changing in accordance with the manner of use of these parts. If a part directly employed in the activity is being used in a comparatively new way which is still unfamiliar, the stimulus to use this part in the new way is weak in comparison with the stimulus to use the other parts of the organism, which are being indirectly employed in the activity, in the old habitual way.

In the present case, an attempt was being made to bring about an unfamiliar use of the head and neck for the purpose of reciting. The stimulus to employ the new use of the head and neck was therefore bound to be weak as compared with the stimulus to employ the wrong habitual use of the feet and legs which had become familiar through being cultivated in the act of reciting.

Herein lies the difficulty in making changes from unsatisfactory to

> *satisfactory conditions of use and functioning, and my teaching experience has taught me that when a wrong habitual use has been cultivated in a person for whatever purpose, its influence in the early stages of the lessons is practically irresistible.*

This led me to a long consideration of the whole question of the direction[6] of the use of myself. "What is this direction," I asked myself, "upon which I have been depending?" I had to admit that I had never thought out how I directed the use of myself, but that I used myself habitually in the way that *felt natural* to me. In other words, I like everyone else depended upon "feeling" for the direction of my use. Judging, however, from the results of my experiments, this method of direction had led me into error (as, for instance, when I put my head back when I intended to put it forward and up), proving that the "feeling" associated with this direction of my use was untrustworthy.

This indeed was a blow. If ever anyone was in an impasse, it was I. For here I was, faced with the fact that my feeling, the only guide I had to depend upon for the direction of my use, was untrustworthy. At the time I believed that this was peculiar to myself, and that my case was exceptional because of the continuous ill-health I had experienced for as long as I could remember, but as soon as I tested other people to see whether they were using themselves in the way they thought they were, I found that the feeling by which they directed the use of themselves was also untrustworthy, indeed, that the only difference in this regard between them and myself was one of degree. Discouraged as I was, however, I refused to believe that my problem was hopeless. I began to see that my findings up till now implied the possibility of the opening up of an entirely new field of enquiry, and I was obsessed with the desire to explore it. "Surely," I argued, "if it is possible for feeling to become untrustworthy as a means of direction, it should also be possible to make it trustworthy again."

The idea of the wonderful potentialities of man had been a source of inspiration to me ever since I had come to know Shakespeare's great word picture:

> "What a piece of work is a man! how noble in reason! how infinite in faculty! in form and moving how express and admirable! in action how like an angel! in apprehension how like a god! the beauty of the world! the paragon of animals!"

---

[6]When I employ the words "direction" and "directed" with "use" in such phrases as "direction of my use" and "I directed the use," etc., I wish to indicate the process involved in projecting messages from the brain to the mechanisms and in conducting the energy necessary to the use of these mechanisms.

But these words seemed to me now to be contradicted by what I had discovered in myself and others. For what could be less "noble in reason," less "infinite in faculty" than that man, despite his potentialities, should have fallen into such error in the use of himself, and in this way brought about such a lowering in his standard of functioning that in everything he attempts to accomplish, these harmful conditions tend to become more and more exaggerated? In consequence, how many people are there today of whom it may be said, as regards their use of themselves, "in form and moving how express and admirable"? Can we any longer consider man in this regard "the paragon of animals"?

I can remember at this period discussing with my father the errors in use which I had noticed both in myself and in others, and contending that in this respect there was no difference between us and the dog or cat. When he asked me why, I replied, "Because we do not *know* how we use ourselves any more than the dog or cat *knows*." By this I meant that man's direction of his use, through being based upon feeling, was as unreasoned and instinctive as that of the animal.[7] I refer to this conversation as shewing that I had already realized that in our present state of civilization which calls for continuous and rapid adaptation to a quickly changing environment, the unreasoned, instinctive direction of

---

[7]It may be contended that the athlete who successfully performs a complicated feat does consciously control his movements. It is true, of course, that in a great many cases he is able by practice on the "trial and error" plan to acquire an automatic proficiency in performing the specific movements necessary for this feat, but this does not in any way prove that he is controlling these movements consciously. And even in those rare instances where the athlete consciously controls and coordinates certain specific movements, it still cannot be said that he consciously controls the use of himself as a whole in his performance. For it is safe to conclude that he does not *know* what use of his mechanisms as a whole is the best possible for making the specific movements he desires, so that should anything happen, as it often does, to cause a change in the familiar habitual use of his mechanisms, his proficiency in making these specific movements will also be interfered with. Practical experience shews that once he has lost this original standard of proficiency, he cannot easily regain it, and this is not surprising seeing that he lacks the knowledge of how to direct the general use of himself which alone would enable him to restore the familiar use of his mechanisms which gave him his proficiency. (In this connexion, many cases have been known of people who, having purposely imitated the peculiarities of a stutterer, have themselves developed the habit of stuttering, and in spite of all their efforts have failed to regain their original standard of proficiency in speaking.)

Because he lacks this knowledge, the athlete, like the animal, has to depend upon his feeling for the direction of the working of his mechanisms, and as that feeling has become more or less untrustworthy in the majority of athletes (a fact that can be demonstrated), the mechanisms which he employs for his activities are bound to be misdirected. Such direction, being as unreasoned as that of the animal, cannot be compared with that conscious reasoned direction which is associated with a primary control of the mechanisms of the self as a working unity.

use such as meets the needs of the cat or dog was no longer sufficient to meet human needs. I had proved in my own case and in that of others that instinctive control and direction of use had become so unsatisfactory, and the associated feeling so untrustworthy as a guide, that it could lead us to do the very opposite of what we wished to do or thought we were doing. If, then, as I suspected, this untrustworthiness of feeling was a product of civilized life, it would tend, as time went on, to become more and more a universal menace, in which case a knowledge of the means whereby trustworthiness could be restored to feeling would be invaluable. I saw that the search for this knowledge would open out an entirely new field of exploration and one that promised more than any that I had yet heard of, and I began to reconsider my own difficulties in the light of this new fact.

Certain points impressed themselves particularly upon me:

(1) that the pulling of my head back and down, when I *felt* that I was putting it forward and up, was proof that the use of the specific parts concerned was being misdirected, and that this misdirection was associated with untrustworthy feeling;

(2) that this misdirection was instinctive, and, together with the associated untrustworthy feeling, was part and parcel of my habitual use of myself;

(3) that this instinctive misdirection leading to wrong habitual use of myself, including most noticeably the wrong use of my head and neck, *came into play as the result of a decision to use my voice; this misdirection, in other words, was my instinctive response (reaction) to the stimulus to use my voice.*

When I came to consider the significance of this last point, it occurred to me that if, when the stimulus came to me to use my voice, I could inhibit the misdirection associated with the wrong habitual use of my head and neck, I should be stopping off at its source my unsatisfactory reaction to the idea of reciting, which expressed itself in pulling back the head, depressing the larynx, and sucking in breath. Once this misdirection was inhibited, my next step would be to discover what direction would be necessary to ensure a new and improved use of the head and neck, and, indirectly, of the larynx and breathing and other mechanisms, for I believed that such direction, when put into practice, would ensure a satisfactory instead of an unsatisfactory reaction to the stimulus to use my voice.

In the work that followed I came to see that to get a direction of my use which would *ensure* this satisfactory reaction, I must cease to rely upon the feeling associated with my instinctive direction, and in its place employ my reasoning processes, in order

(1) to analyse the conditions of use present;
(2) to select (reason out) the means whereby a more satisfactory use could be brought about;
(3) to project *consciously* the directions required for putting these means into effect.

In short, I concluded that if I were ever to be able to react satisfactorily to the stimulus to use my voice, I must replace my old instinctive (unreasoned) direction of myself by a new conscious (reasoned) direction.

> *The idea of taking the control of the use of the mechanisms of the human creature from the instinctive on to the conscious plane has already been justified by the results which have been obtained by applying it in practice, but it may be many years before its true significance as a factor in human development is fully recognized.*

I set out to put this idea into practice, but I was at once brought up short by a series of startling and unexpected experiences. Like most people, I had believed up to this moment that if I thought out carefully how to improve my way of performing a certain act, I should be guided by my reasoning rather than by my feeling when it came to putting this thought into action, and that my "mind" was the superior and more effective directing agent. But the fallacy of this became apparent to me as soon as I attempted to employ conscious direction for the purpose of correcting some wrong use of myself which was habitual and therefore *felt right* to me. In actual practice I found that there was no clear dividing line between my unreasoned and my reasoned direction of myself, and that I was quite unable to prevent the two from overlapping. I was successful in employing my reasoning up to the point of projecting the directions which, after analysing the conditions of use present, I had decided were required for the new and improved use, and all went well as long as I did not attempt to carry these directions out for the purpose of speaking. For instance, as soon as any stimulus reached me to use my voice, and I tried in response to *do* the new thing which my conscious direction should bring about (such as putting the head forward and up), and *speak at the same time*, I found I immediately reverted to all my old wrong habits of use (such as putting my head back, etc.). There was no question about this. I could see it actually happening in the mirror. This was clear proof that at the critical moment when I attempted to gain my end by means which were contrary to those associated with my old habits of use, my instinctive direction dominated my reasoning direction. It dominated my will to do what I had decided was the right thing to do, and although I was trying (as we understand "trying") to do it. Over and over again I had the experience that immediately the stimulus to speak came to me, I invariably responded by doing something according to my old habitual use associated with the act of speaking.

After many disappointing experiences of this kind I decided to give up any attempt for the present to "do" anything to gain my end, and I came to see at last that if I was ever to be able to change my habitual use and dominate my instinctive direction, *it would be necessary for me to make the experience of receiving the stimulus to speak and of refusing to do anything immediately in response.* For I saw that an immediate response was the result of a decision on my part to do something *at once*, to go directly for a certain end, and by acting quickly on this decision I did not give myself the opportunity to project as many times as was necessary the new directions which I had reasoned out were the best means whereby I could attain that end. This meant that the old instinctive direction which, associated with untrustworthy feeling, had been the controlling factor up to that moment in the building up of my wrong habitual use, still controlled the *manner* of my response, with the inevitable result that my old wrong habitual use was again and again brought into play.

I therefore decided to confine my work to giving myself the directions for the new "means-whereby,"[8] instead of actually trying to "do" them or to relate them to the "end" of speaking. I would give the new directions in front of the mirror for long periods together, for successive days and weeks and sometimes even months, without attempting to "do" them, and the experience I gained in giving these directions proved of great value when the time came for me to consider how to put them into practice.

This experience taught me

(1) that before attempting to "do" even the first part of the new "means-whereby" which I had decided to employ in order to gain my end (i.e., vocal use and reciting), I must give the directions preparatory to the doing of this first part very many times;

(2) that I must *continue* to give the directions preparatory to the doing of the first part while I gave the directions preparatory to the doing of the second part;

(3) that I must *continue* to give the directions preparatory to the doing of the first and second parts while I gave the directions

---

[8]The phrase "means-whereby" will be used throughout this book to indicate the reasoned means to the gaining of an end. These means included the inhibition of the habitual use of the mechanisms of the organism, and the conscious projection of new directions necessary to the performance of the different acts involved in a new and more satisfactory use of these mechanisms.

preparatory to the doing of the third part; and so on for the doing of the fourth and other parts as required.

Lastly, I discovered that after I had become familiar with the combined process of giving the directions for the new "means-whereby" in their sequence and of employing the various corresponding mechanisms in order to bring about the new use, I must continue this process in my practice for a considerable time before actually attempting to employ the new "means-whereby" for the purpose of speaking.

The process I have just described is an example of what Professor John Dewey has called "thinking in activity," and anyone who carries it out faithfully while trying to gain an end will find that he is acquiring a new experience in what he calls "thinking." My daily teaching experience shews me that in working for a given end, we can all project one direction, but to continue to give this direction as we project the second, and continue to give these two while we add a third, and to continue to keep these three directions going as we proceed to gain the end, has proved to be the pons asinorum of every pupil I have so far known.[9]

The time came when I believed I had practised the "means-whereby" long enough, and I started to try and employ them for the purpose of speaking, but to my dismay I found that I failed far more often than I succeeded. The further I went with these attempts, the more perplexing the situation became, for I was certainly attempting to inhibit my habitual response to the stimulus to speak, and I had certainly given the new directions over and over again. At least, this is what I had intended to do and thought I had done, so that, as far as I could then see, I should have been able to employ the new "means-whereby" for the gaining of my end with some degree of confidence. The fact remained that I failed more often than not, and nothing was more certain than that I must go back and reconsider my premises.

This reconsideration shewed me more clearly than ever that the occasions when I failed were those on which I was unable to prevent the dominance of my wrong habitual use, as I attempted to employ the new "means-whereby" with the idea of gaining my end and speaking. I also saw (and this was of the utmost importance) that, in spite of all my preliminary work, the instinctive direction associated with my habitual use still dominated my conscious reasoning direction. So confident was I, however, that the new means I had chosen were right for my purpose, that I decided I must look elsewhere for the cause of my unsatisfactory

[9]The phrase "all together, one after the other" expresses the idea of combined activity I wish to convey here.

results. In time I began to doubt whether perhaps my failures were not due to some shortcoming in myself, and that I personally was unable to do a thing with satisfactory "means-whereby" when someone else might have been successful. I looked all round for any other possible causes of failure, and after a long period of investigation I came to the conclusion that it was necessary for me to seek some concrete proof whether, at the critical moment when I attempted to gain my end and speak, I was really continuing to project the directions in their proper sequence for the employment of the new and more satisfactory use, as I thought I was, or whether I was reverting to the instinctive misdirection of my old habitual use which had been associated with all my throat trouble. By careful experimentation I discovered that I gave my directions for the new use in their sequence right up to the point when I tried to gain my end and speak, but that, at the critical moment when persistence in giving the new directions would have brought success, I reverted instead to the misdirection associated with my old wrong habitual use. This was concrete proof that I was not continuing to project my directions for the new use for the purpose of speaking, as I thought I was, but that my reaction to the stimulus to speak was still my instinctive reaction through my habitual use. Clearly, to "feel" or think I had inhibited the old instinctive reaction was no proof that I had really done so, and I must find some way of "knowing."

I had already noticed that on the occasions when I failed, the instinctive misdirection associated with my old habitual use always dominated my reasoning direction for the new use, and I gradually came to see that this could hardly be otherwise. Ever since the beginning of man's growth and development the only form of direction of the use of himself of which he has had any experience has been instinctive direction, which might in this sense be called a racial inheritance. Was it then to be wondered at that in my case the influence of this inherited instinctive direction associated with my old habitual use had rendered futile most of my efforts to employ a conscious, reasoning direction for a new use, especially when the use of myself which was associated with instinctive direction had become so familiar that it was now part and parcel of me, and so *felt right and natural*? In trying to employ a conscious, reasoning direction to bring about a new use, I was therefore combating in myself not only that racial tendency which causes us all at critical moments to revert to instinctive direction and so to the familiar use of ourselves that feels right, but also a racial inexperience in projecting conscious directions at all, and particularly conscious directions in sequence.

As the reader knows, I had recognized much earlier that I ought not to trust to my feeling for the direction of my use, but I had never fully realized all that this implied, namely, that the sensory experience associated with the new use would be so unfamiliar and therefore "feel" so unnatural and wrong that I, like everyone else, with my ingrained habit of judging whether experiences of use were "right" or not by the way they *felt*, would almost inevitably balk at employing the new use. Obviously, any new use must feel different from the old, and if the old use felt right, the new use was bound to feel wrong. I now had to face the fact that in all my attempts during these past months I had been trying to employ a new use of myself which was bound to feel wrong, at the same time trusting to my feeling of what was right to tell me whether I was employing it or not. This meant that all my efforts up till now had resolved themselves into an attempt to employ a reasoning direction of my use at the moment of speaking, while for the purpose of this attempt I was actually bringing into play my old habitual use and so reverting to my instinctive misdirection. Small wonder that this attempt had proved futile!

Faced with this, I now saw that if I was ever to succeed in making the changes in use I desired, I must subject the processes directing my use to a new experience, the experience, that is, of being dominated by reasoning instead of by feeling, particularly at the critical moment when the giving of directions merged into "doing" for the gaining of the end I had decided upon. This meant that I must be prepared to carry on with any procedure I had reasoned out as best for my purpose, even though that procedure might *feel wrong*. In other words, my trust in my reasoning processes to bring me safely to my "end" must be a genuine trust, not a half-trust needing the assurance of *feeling right* as well. I must at all costs work out some plan by which to obtain concrete proof that my instinctive reaction to the stimulus to gain my end *remained inhibited*, while I projected in their sequence the directions for the employment of the new use at the critical moment of gaining that end.

After making many attempts to solve this problem and gaining experience which proved to be of great value and interest to me, I finally adopted the following plan.[10]

Supposing that the "end" I decided to work for was to speak a certain sentence, I would start in the same way as before and

(1) inhibit any immediate response to the stimulus to speak the sentence,

(2) project in their sequence the directions for the primary control which I had reasoned out as being best for the purpose of bringing about the new and improved use of myself in speaking,

[10]This plan, though simple in theory, has proved difficult for most pupils to put into practice.

and

(3) continue to project these directions until I believed I was sufficiently *au fait* with them to employ them for the purpose of gaining my end and speaking the sentence.

At this moment, the moment that had always proved critical for me because it was then that I tended to revert to my wrong habitual use, I would change my usual procedure and

(4) *while still continuing to project the directions for the new use* I would stop and consciously reconsider my first decision, and ask myself "Shall I after all go on to gain the end I have decided upon and speak the sentence? Or shall I not? Or shall I go on to gain some other end altogether?"—*and then and there make a fresh decision,*

(5) either

not to gain my original end, in which case *I would continue to project the directions for maintaining the new use* and not go on to speak the sentence;

or

to change my end and do something different, say, lift my hand instead of speaking the sentence, in which case *I would continue to project the directions for maintaining the new use* to carry out this last decision and lift my hand;

or

to go on after all and gain my original end, in which case *I would continue to project the directions for maintaining the new use* to speak the sentence.

It will be seen that under this new plan the change in procedure came at the critical moment when hitherto, in going on to gain my end, I had so often reverted to instinctive misdirection and my wrong habitual use. I reasoned that if I stopped at that moment and then, *without ceasing to project the directions for the new use,* decided afresh to what end the new use should be employed, I should by this procedure be subjecting my instinctive processes of direction to an experience contrary to any experience in which they had hitherto been drilled. Up to that time the stimulus of a decision to gain a certain end had always resulted in the same habitual activity, involving the projection of the instinctive directions for the use which I habitually employed for the gaining of that end. By this new procedure, *as long as the reasoned directions for the bringing about of new conditions of use were consciously maintained,* the stimulus of a decision to gain a certain end would result in an activity differing from the old habitual activity, in that the old activity could not be controlled outside the gaining of a given end, whereas the new activity could be controlled for the gaining of any end that was consciously desired.

> *I would point out that this procedure is contrary, not only to any procedure in which our individual instinctive direction has been drilled, but contrary also to that in which man's instinctive processes have been drilled continuously all through his evolutionary experience.*

When I came to work on this plan, I found that this reasoning was borne out by experience. For by actually deciding, in the majority of cases, to maintain my new conditions of use either to gain some end other than the one originally decided upon, or simply to refuse to gain the original end, I obtained at last the concrete proof I was looking for, namely, that my instinctive response to the stimulus to gain my original end was not only inhibited at the start, *but remained inhibited right through, whilst my directions for the new use were being projected.* And the experience I gained in maintaining the new manner of use while going on to gain some other end or refusing to gain my original end, helped me to maintain the new use on those occasions when I decided at the critical moment to go on after all and gain my original end and speak the sentence. This was further proof that I was becoming able to defeat any influence of that habitual wrong use in speaking to which my original decision to "speak the sentence" had been the stimulus, and that my conscious, reasoning direction was at last dominating the unreasoning, instinctive direction associated with my unsatisfactory habitual use of myself.

After I had worked on this plan for a considerable time, I became free from my tendency to revert to my wrong habitual use in reciting, and the marked effect of this upon my functioning convinced me that I was at last on the right track, for once free from this tendency, I also became free from the throat and vocal trouble and from the respiratory and nasal difficulties with which I had been beset from birth.

CHAPTER II

USE AND FUNCTIONING IN RELATION TO REACTION

THE reader who reviews the experiences that I have tried to set down in the previous chapter will notice that at a certain point in my investigation I came to realize that my reaction to a particular stimulus was constantly the opposite of that which I desired, and that in my search for the cause of this, I discovered that my sensory appreciation (feeling) of the use of my mechanisms was so untrustworthy that it led me to react by means of a use of myself which *felt* right, but was, in fact, too often wrong for my purpose.

I draw attention to this point, because over the long period of years in which I have been engaged in teaching pupils to improve and control the manner of their use of themselves, I have found that untrustworthiness of sensory appreciation is present in varying degrees in all of them, exerting, as in my own case, a harmful influence upon their use and functioning, and consequently upon their manner of reacting to stimuli. The whole experience, indeed, convinces me that the prevalence of sensory untrustworthiness is of the utmost significance in relation to the problem of the control of human reaction.

Another point of importance in relation to the control of human reaction is that it was through my discovery of the primary control that I was able to bring about the improvement in the sensory appreciation of the use of my mechanisms which was associated with the improvement in functioning throughout my organism. By the time I had reached the stage when a new manner of use had become established through my conscious employment of this primary control, I was able, when the stimulus came to me to use my voice to recite, to inhibit my instinctive misdirection leading to the old harmful use of my head and neck and vocal organs, and so to my hoarseness, and to substitute for it a conscious direction leading to a new use of my head, neck and vocal organs which was not associated with hoarseness.

This meant that the stimulus to use my voice no longer brought into play the old reflex activity which included the pulling of my head back and down, leading to a shortening of my stature, and which constituted my harmful habitual reaction to that stimulus, but instead, a new reflex activity which included putting my head forward and up to lengthen the stature and which, by its results, proved to be a satisfactory reaction to that stimulus.

The fact that I was able, through my employment of the primary control, to bring about such an improvement in my reaction to the stimulus to use my voice that vocal activity did not result in hoarseness, is proof that quite early in my experiences a practical means had been found, whereby my habitual reflex activity was "conditioned" as a natural consequence of the procedure adopted, since the new reflex activity to which it was changed *in the process* was associated with new and improved general conditions of use and functioning.[11]

Indeed, the results that have been obtained by adopting the procedure described on pages 427-429 furnish evidence of how harmful reflex activity brought about by misdirection of use can be consciously held in check, even in face of the excitation involved in carrying out the procedure.[12]

More than this, my experience has shewn that in cases where the knowledge of how to direct the primary control has led to a change for the better in the manner of the use of the mechanisms throughout the organism, the results of this "conditioning" can safely be left to take their own form. As Professor John Dewey writes, "Science is, after all, a matter of perfected skill in conducting enquiry . . . not 'something finished, absolute in itself,' but the result of a certain technique."[13]

Seeing, therefore, that it proved possible to bring about a conscious control of my reaction through a change in the direction of my use, the reader will understand why, in my opinion, *the substitution of conscious for instinctive direction in the changing of use* is of primary importance, and why I believe a knowledge of the means whereby this change can be brought about would be of inestimable value in all educational work.

---

[11]In this connexion the following quotation from a paper read by Dr. A. Murdoch, of Bexhill-on-Sea, at the St. Andrews (James Mackenzie) Institute on March 6, 1928, may be of interest: "Mr. Alexander has built up the theory on which he has based his practice from the observation of the movements of the body as a whole, and he has made use of lost or unused associated involuntary reflexes with a rare insight, and by recreating them into new conditioned reflexes he has laid the foundation for a new outlook on disease and its diagnosis and treatment."

[12]According to this procedure the subject starts by consciously projecting the directions for the means whereby he will gain a certain end, and, at the critical moment of going on to gain this end, makes a fresh decision as to whether he will employ these "means-whereby" to gain the original end or some other.

[13]*Experience and Nature* (Open Court Publishing Co., 1926).

The experiences I gained in dealing with my own difficulties have proved of the greatest value to me in dealing practically with the difficulties and requirements of my pupils. First and foremost, I learned from these experiences that I could not enable my pupils to control the functioning of their organs, systems or reflexes *directly*, but that by teaching them to employ consciously the primary control of their use I could put them in command of the means whereby their functioning generally can be *indirectly* controlled. My adoption of this principle in the employment of my technique has been fully justified by experience, and I have had no reason up till now for departing from it. Indeed, my continued experience convinces me that unless the building up of a conscious direction of use, in association with an improving standard of sensory appreciation of that use, is made the primary consideration of all those who, in different spheres, are dealing with the problem of the control of human reaction, we are not likely to develop a method for meeting the problem of the control of conscious, or, as it is sometimes called, "conditioned" behaviour.

In any discussion of human reaction certain well-known facts about the nature of human activity may be taken as premises.

Human activity is primarily a process of reacting unceasingly to stimuli received from within or without the self. The first breath taken by a newly born child is a reaction to a stimulus to the respiratory centre, and the child remains a living organism only so long as it is capable of receiving stimuli and of reacting to them. No human being can receive a stimulus except through the sensory mechanisms, and supposing one could prevent the sensory mechanisms from receiving a stimulus, no reaction would be possible and therefore no further activity. Life itself would then cease.

When once it is recognized that every act is a reaction to a stimulus received through the sensory mechanisms, no act can be described as wholly "mental" or wholly "physical." The most that can be said is that in some acts the "mental" side predominates and in others the "physical." For instance, let us take the act of lifting the arm, which would be described offhand by many people as a "physical" act. If we consider what happens between the receipt of a stimulus to lift the arm and the performance of the act, we shall see that a concerted activity takes place which brings into play not only the processes which most people are accustomed to regard as "physical," but also the processes which they regard as "mental." The result of the receipt of a stimulus to lift the arm is, as we all know, a "mental" conception of the act of lifting the arm, this conception being followed by another so-called "mental" process, that of giving or withholding consent to react to the stimulus to lift the arm. If this consent is withheld, the reaction which would result in a lifting of the arm is inhibited, and the arm is not lifted. If consent is given, the direction of the mechanisms required for the act of lifting the arm becomes operative, and messages are sent out which bring about the contraction of certain groups of muscles and the relaxation of others, and the arm is lifted.

But in this connexion it is of the utmost importance to remember that in most people their direction of the use of themselves is habitual and instinctive, so that once consent has been given to react to the stimulus to perform a certain act, they will perform that act, as we say, "instinctively," that is without any reasoned conception of what direction of the use of the mechanisms is required for its satisfactory performance.

Unfortunately, with the increasing prevalence of untrustworthy sensory appreciation,[14] this instinctive direction of use tends, as time goes on, to become more and more a misdirection, having a harmful effect, as was proved in my own case, upon functioning and, consequently, upon the reactions which result.

These unsatisfactory reactions manifest themselves as symptoms of defect, of so-called "mental" or "moral" failing, disorder and disease, and their presence may therefore be taken as an indication of the presence also of wrong use and functioning[15] throughout the organism. My experience with cases manifesting any such "symptoms" has shewn me that where a new and satisfactory direction of the use of the mechanisms has been brought about, leading to an improvement in the associated functioning, these symptoms tend gradually to disappear in the process, and to be replaced by symptoms of health and well-being, or satisfactory reactions. For this reason I claim that the primary requirement in dealing with all specific symptoms is to prevent the misdirection which leads to wrong use and functioning, and to establish in its place a new and satisfactory direction as a means of bringing about an improvement in use and functioning throughout the organism.

This indirect procedure is true to the principle that the unity of the human organism is indivisible, and where there is an understanding of the means whereby the use of the mechanisms can be directed in prac-

---

[14]This is a fact which came to light in my investigations (see Chapter I, pp. 419 and 420) and is one that can be demonstrated.

[15]I wish to make it plain that whenever I use the phrase "use and functioning" in relation to the human organism, I do not indicate by it mechanical activity as such, but include in the phrase all manifestations of human activity involved in what we designate as conception or understanding, withholding or giving consent, thinking, reasoning, directing, etc. For the manifestation of such activities cannot be dissociated from the use of the mechanisms and the associated functioning of the organism.

tice as a concerted activity, in the sense I have tried to define, the principle of unity works for good. But there is a reverse side to the picture. It is in the nature of unity that any change in a part means a change in the whole, and the parts of the human organism are knit so closely into a unity that any attempt to make a fundamental change in the working of a part is bound to alter the use and adjustment of the whole. This means that where the concerted use of the mechanisms of the organism is faulty, any attempt to eradicate a defect otherwise than by changing and improving this faulty concerted use is bound to throw out the balance somewhere else.[16]

This danger is seldom recognized by those who have to diagnose and deal with cases of ailment or disability, but I am prepared to demonstrate that *in the process* of "curing" a wrong symptom by specific treatment, even though this treatment may be outwardly successful, other less easily recognized but often more harmful defects are brought about in other parts of the organism. It is the old story of the seven devils.[17]

The results of my teaching work have shewn me that no diagnosis can be complete which is not based on that principle of the unity in working of the mechanisms of the organism which involves a close connexion between the manner of use of the mechanisms and the standard of functioning throughout the organism.

In what follows I shall bring forward several illustrations to shew how experts in widely differing spheres of activity fail to recognize this principle in their practical dealings with those who consult them with a view to correcting some defect or disability, and how this leads to an incomplete diagnosis and seriously limits the scope of the adviser, whatever his line.

A fair judgment of any procedure can only be reached by an examination of the principle on which it is founded. Where the principle is unsound, the procedure must fail in the long run. I therefore wish the practical procedures which I am now putting forward to be judged by the principle which underlies them.

---

[16]See Chapter IV, pp. 451 and 452.

[17]In this connexion it is very interesting to compare what Sir E. Holderness, the well-known authority on golf, wrote in the *Evening Standard* of March 17, 1928.

> "Here is a true tale of a friend. He suffered from a chronic slice, and in despair went to a professional who offered him an easy cure by making him put his left hand on the top of the club and his right hand underneath. Then he told him to bang away with confidence. Wonderful to relate, the slice disappeared and for one afternoon he drove divinely. But where there had been one devil, seven worse ones came in its place; and for weeks and months he endured the agony of pulls and smothers. His last state was more pitiful than his first."

CHAPTER III

THE GOLFER WHO CANNOT KEEP HIS EYES ON THE BALL

LET us suppose that a golfer who does not make a success of his golf consults a professional with a view to improving his play. After watching him play, the professional tells him among other things that he is taking his eyes off the ball, and impresses on him that if he wishes to improve his stroke, he *must* keep his eyes on the ball. The golfer starts to play with every intention of following out his teacher's instructions, but finds that in spite of all his efforts, he still takes his eyes off the ball.

There are several points in this situation that could be discussed, but I wish, in this chapter, to confine my consideration to the principle which underlies not only the teacher's diagnosis and instructions, but also the procedure of the pupil when he decides to carry the instructions out.

Certain questions at once suggest themselves.

Why does the golfer take his eyes off the ball in the first place, when according to the experts he should not do so?

Why does he *continue* to take his eyes off the ball after he has decided to keep them *on* the ball? Why does his "will to do" fail him at the critical moment?

What is the stimulus that constitutes an apparently irresistible temptation to him to take his eyes off the ball, in spite of his desire to follow his teacher's instructions and in spite of his "will to do"?

To answer these questions we shall have to take them in their connexion with each other, for the answers are as closely related to one another as the questions are themselves.

To take the first question.

When the golfer starts to make his stroke, he brings to the act the same habitual use of his mechanisms that he brings to all his activities, and since for such an essential part of the recognized golfing technique as "keeping his eyes on the ball" the mechanisms concerned with the control of his eyes fail to function as he desires, we are justified in concluding that this habitual use is misdirected.This fact is practically admitted by the instructor when he attributes his pupil's failure to make a good stroke to his failure to keep his eyes on the ball.[18]

To the question why he continues to take his eyes off the ball, in spite of his intention to follow his teacher's instructions and in spite of his "will to do," the answer is that in everything he does he is a confirmed "endgainer." His habit is to work directly for his ends on the "trial and error" plan without giving due consideration to the means whereby those ends should be gained. In the present instance there can be no doubt that the particular end he has in view is to make a good stroke, which means that the moment he begins to play he starts to work for that end directly, without considering what manner of use of his mechanisms generally would be the best for the making of a good stroke. The result is that he makes the stroke according to his habitual use, and as this habitual use is misdirected and includes the wrong use of his eyes, he takes his eyes off the ball and makes a bad stroke. It is clear that as long as he is dominated by his habit of end-gaining, he will react to the stimulus to "make a good stroke" by the same misdirected use of himself, and will continue to take his eyes off the ball.

This process is repeated every time he tries to make a good stroke, with the result that his failures far outnumber his successes, and he becomes more or less disturbed emotionally,[19] as always happens when people find themselves more often wrong than not, without knowing the reason why. And the more he finds himself unable to carry out his teacher's instructions with anything like the necessary degree of certainty for him to get any pleasure out of the game, the worse this emotional condition becomes. The immediate effect is that he tries harder than ever to make a good stroke, falls into the old wrong way of using his mechanisms, and again takes his eyes off the ball.

Now one would suppose that repeated experience of failure would of itself lead him to set to work on a different principle, but my teaching experience goes to shew that in this respect the golfer's method of procedure is in no way different from that of other people who use themselves wrongly, and who are trying, without success, to correct a defect. Strange as it may seem, I have always found that a pupil who uses him-

[18]I admit, of course, that a wrong use of other parts might have a more direct bearing upon the golfer's problem, but for the purpose of illustration I have chosen the wrong use of the eyes, because the experts are unanimously agreed (as unanimously as experts ever are) that failure to keep the eyes on the ball is one of the most common and persistent hindrances to the making of a good stroke.

[19]Unsuccessful effort in any sphere of activity tends to produce emotional disturbance which is not conducive to healthy recreation. For this reason alone the golfer whose efforts to carry out his teacher's instructions are mostly unsuccessful should reconsider his plan of campaign.

self wrongly will continue to do so in all his activities, even after the wrong use has been pointed out to him, and he has learned by experience that persistence in this wrong use is the cause of his failure.

This apparent anomaly can be explained, and in explaining it I hope to shew not only what is at the bottom of the golfer's difficulty, but also of the difficulty which so many people experience when, with the best "will" in the world, they find themselves unable to put right something which they know to be wrong with themselves.

The habitual use of his mechanisms which the golfer brings to all his activities, including golf, has always been accompanied by certain sensory experiences (feelings) which, from their lifelong association with this habitual use, have become familiar to him. Further, from their very familiarity, they have come to *"feel right,"* and so he derives considerable satisfaction from repeating them. When, therefore, he attempts to "make a good stroke," he brings to the act of swinging his club his faulty habitual use, including the taking of his eyes off the ball, because the sensory experiences associated with this use are familiar and "feel right."

On the other hand, the use of his mechanisms which would involve his keeping his eyes *on* the ball during the act of making a stroke would be a use entirely contrary to his habitual use and associated with *sensory experiences which, being unfamiliar, would "feel wrong" to him*; it may therefore be said that he receives no sensory stimulus in that direction. Any sensory stimulus he receives is in the direction of repeating the familiar sensory experiences which accompany his faulty use, and this carries the day over any so-called "mental" stimulus arising from his "will to do." In other words, the lure of the familiar proves too strong for him and keeps him tied down to the habitual use of himself which *feels right.*

This is not surprising, seeing that the golfer's desire to employ his habitual use at all costs in gaining his end, on account of the familiar sensory experiences that go with it, is an instinctive desire which mankind has inherited and continued to develop all through the ages. *The desire to feel right in the gaining of his end* is therefore his primary desire, in comparison with which his desire to make a good stroke is new and undeveloped, and exerts only a secondary influence. This is proved by the fact that although he starts out with the desire to make a good stroke, his desire to repeat sensory experiences that "feel right" acts as a stimulus to him to use himself in the habitual way which is associated with these experiences, although it is this very manner of use that prevents him from satisfying his newer desire to make a good stroke.

The desire to carry out his teacher's instructions to keep his eyes on the ball is a still newer desire, and consequently suffers in intensity as compared with the other two. Moreover, it stands even less chance of being carried out, firstly, because the stimulus which gives rise to it does not come from within, like the others, but from without, i.e., from the teacher, and secondly, because the instruction is framed with the purpose of correcting something wrong with the pupil's use, i.e., the use of the eyes, and so is bound to come at once into conflict with the pupil's desire to employ his faulty habitual use which, as we have just explained, is the dominating influence in whatever he tries to do. The conflict between these two desires is therefore bound to be an unequal one, and his desire to carry out his teacher's instructions goes by the board.[20]

It is the dominating influence of his desire to gain his end by means of a use of his mechanisms which *feels* right, but is in fact wrong for the purpose, that explains not only why he *continues* to take his eyes off the ball and so to fail in his stroke, but also why, in spite of this repeated experience of failure, he does not give up "end-gaining" and set to work in a different way.

Now that we have seen the faulty principle which underlies the golfer's efforts to obey his teacher's instructions, we will go on to examine the principle on which these instructions are based.

The instruction to the pupil to "keep his eyes on the ball" shews that the teacher recognizes that the mechanisms concerned with the control of the pupil's eyes do not function as they should, but when, in order to meet this difficulty, he simply tells his pupil to "keep his eyes on the ball," he also shews that he does not connect the faulty functioning of the eyes with misdirection of the use of the mechanisms throughout the organism. This means that in his diagnosis and treatment he is not considering his pupil's organism as a working unity in which the working of any of the parts is affected by the working of the whole. To this extent, therefore, his diagnosis may be said to be incomplete and his scope of usefulness as adviser to his pupil limited.

Evidence of misdirection of use in human activity is to be found on all sides, and our real interest in the golfer's difficulty is that it is a difficulty not confined to golf, but experienced by all who are trying, without success, to correct defects which hamper them in their various activities, or to perform a certain act satisfactorily.

Misdirection of use is to be found in the person who takes up a pen to

[20]It must be remembered that the greater his desire to obey his teacher, the greater will be his incentive to increase the intensity of his efforts, and it is practically certain that in his attempts to translate this desire into action, he will automatically increase the already undue muscle tension which he habitually employs for the act, thus lessening still further his chances of making a successful stroke.

Cf. Note page 440.

write and proceeds at once to stiffen the fingers unduly, to make movements of the arm which should be made by the fingers, and even to make facial contortions; in the physical culturist whose performance of certain movements of the arms or legs, or of both, is associated with harmful and unnecessary depression of the larynx and with undue tension of the musculature of the thorax; in the person who in reading or singing or talking "sucks" a breath in through the mouth at the beginning of each sentence, though in the ordinary way, in walking or standing, he would breathe through the nostrils; in the athlete, amateur or professional, who, whenever he makes a special effort, employs excessive tension in the muscles of the neck and pulls the head back unduly.

In all these cases, which might be elaborated indefinitely, it will be found that the use of the mechanisms concerned with the movement required is often far removed from that which would best serve the purpose.

This all goes to shew that in every form of activity the use of the mechanisms which comes into operation will be satisfactory or unsatisfactory according to whether our direction of that use is satisfactory or otherwise. Where the direction is satisfactory, satisfactory use of the mechanisms of the organism as a working unity will be ensured, involving a satisfactory use of the different parts, such as the arms, wrists, hands, legs, feet and eyes. It follows that where there is misdirection, this satisfactory use of the mechanisms is not at our command. This is exactly the position of the golfer who cannot keep his eyes on the ball when he desires.

Let us now see how the golfer's difficulty would be dealt with by a teacher who adhered to the idea of the unity of the organism, and so based his teaching practice on what I call the "means-whereby" principle, i.e., the principle of a reasoning consideration of the causes of the conditions present, and an indirect instead of a direct procedure on the part of the person endeavouring to gain the desired end.[21]

First he would diagnose the golfer's failure to make a good stroke as due to misdirection of the habitual use of the mechanisms, and not primarily to any specific defect such as an inability to keep the eyes on the ball. He would recognize that the inability to keep the eyes on the ball was merely a symptom of this misdirection, and could not by any stretch of the imagination be said to be the cause of his failure to make a good stroke. He would observe that immediately his pupil started to make his stroke, he brought into play the same faulty use which he habitually employed for all his activities, and so himself brought about the very thing he wanted to prevent, the taking of his eyes off the ball. He would see that his pupil's difficulty was to a great extent caused by his own "wrong-doing."

[21]Compare *Constructive Conscious Control of the Individual.* P. 230. Note.

A teacher who made a diagnosis on these lines would understand that the difficulty could not be met by any such purely specific instruction as telling his pupil to keep his eyes on the ball, for he would recognize that any "will power" exerted by a pupil whose use of himself was misdirected would be exerted in the wrong direction,[22] so that the harder he tried to carry out such an instruction and the more he "willed" himself to succeed, the more his use would be misdirected and the more likely he would be to take his eyes off the ball. From this he would conclude that he must find some way of teaching his pupil to stop the misdirection of his use, and as he observed that the misdirection began the moment the pupil tried to gain his end and make a good stroke, obviously his first step would be to get the pupil to stop "trying to make a good stroke." He would explain that any immediate reaction to the stimulus to make a good stroke would always be by means of his wrong habitual use, but that if he prevented this immediate reaction, he would at the same time be preventing the misdirection of his use that went with it and was *the* obstacle to the gaining of his end. He would impress upon him that of all the activities that go to the making of a good stroke, *this act of prevention was the primary activity*, since by the inhibition of the misdirected habitual use the way would be left clear for the teacher to build up in his pupil that new direction of the use of his mechanisms, which would constitute the means whereby he would in time be able to keep his eyes on the ball, and thus make a good stroke.

Now if we are to understand the "means-whereby" principle on which the teacher who adheres to the idea of unity in the working of the human organism will base his teaching method, we must recognize that the attainment of any desired end, or the performance of any act such as the making of a golf stroke, involves the direction and performance of a connected series of preliminary acts by means of the mechanisms of the organism, and that therefore, if the use of the mechanisms is to be directed so as to result in the satisfactory attainment of the desired end, the directions for this use must be

[22]Not long ago a professor brought a friend to watch a lesson given to one of his students in whose progress they were both interested on account of her attainments. "You should have no difficulty with this pupil," he said, "because she is so willing and anxious to help you." "Yes," I replied, "that is one of the curses of the 'will to do.'" His companion held up her hands in horror at this, exclaiming, "Surely, even if it's wrong, it's better to exert the 'will to do' than not." This gave me the chance to point out that the "something wrong" meant that there was a wrong direction somewhere, so that what she was really urging was that the addition of the stimulus of the "will to do" would be beneficial, even though it involved an increased projection of energy in the wrong direction. It is not the degree of "willing" or "trying," but the way in which the energy is directed, that is going to make the "willing" or "trying" effective.

projected in a connected series to correspond with the connected series of preliminary acts. If at any point in the series the chain of directions is broken and use misdirected, all the succeeding acts of the series will go wrong, and the end will not be attained in the way desired (for instance, the golfer will not make a good stroke). In most people today the direction of the use of their mechanisms is not reasoned out, but instinctive, and in cases where this instinctive direction leads to faulty use, the connected series of acts preliminary to the gaining of any end will be brought about by a series of instinctive directions operating through faulty use of the mechanisms, so that a series of faulty acts will be the result.[23]

These facts must be taken into account by the teacher who is using the "means-whereby" principle to build up a new direction of the pupil's use. He will recognize in his practice that these preliminary acts, though means, are also ends but not isolated ends, inasmuch as they form a coordinated series of acts to be carried out "all together, one after the other."[24] He will impress upon his pupil that to maintain the unity that is involved in this connected series of acts, he will have to continue to project the directions necessary to the performance of the first act of the series *concurrently* with projecting the directions necessary to the performance of the second, and so on throughout the series until all the preliminary acts have been performed in their connected sequence and the ultimate end in this way secured.

It may be asked what, exactly, is the technique for putting the "means-whereby" principle into practice in building up a new and satisfactory direction of use.

It is impossible to put down here more than a bare outline of this technique, because the sensory experiences which come to the pupil in the process of acquiring a new direction of his use cannot be conveyed by the written or spoken word, any more than the most detailed account that a professional golfer can give of his own sensory experiences when making a drive will enable his pupil to reproduce those experiences. But I would refer my readers back to Chapter I where I described the experiments which led to my discovering that there is a primary control of the use of the self, which governs the working of all the mechanisms and so renders the control of the complex human organism comparatively simple.

This primary control, called by the late Professor Magnus of Utrecht the "central control," depends upon a certain use of the head and neck

[23]See *Constructive Conscious Control of the Individual*, page 368 *et seq.*

[24]This process is analogous to the firing of a machine gun from an aeroplane, where the machinery is so coordinated that each individual shot of the series is timed to pass between the blades of a propeller making 1,500 or more revolutions to the minute.

in relation to the use of the rest of the body, and once the pupil has inhibited the instinctive misdirection leading to his faulty habitual use, the teacher must begin the process of building up the new use by giving the pupil the primary direction towards the establishment of this primary control. The pupil will then project this direction whilst the teacher with his hands brings about the corresponding activity, *the combined procedure securing for the pupil the new experience of use which is desired.* This experience, though unfamiliar at first, will become familiar with repetition.

The teacher then gives the secondary direction to the pupil who *must keep the primary direction going,* whilst he projects the secondary direction and whilst the teacher brings about the corresponding activity. This combined procedure again secures for the pupil the new experience of use that is desired, and again this new experience, though unfamiliar at first, will become familiar with repetition.

By this method of procedure the two directions and their corresponding activities become linked together and will remain linked, and if still further directions are required to bring about the desired change in use, the same combined procedure must apply.

As long as teacher and pupil continue to work together on these lines, never deviating in their procedure from the "means-whereby" principle, they will in time establish in the pupil the desired direction of the use of his mechanisms, and this procedure has only to be repeated until the experiences associated with it have become familiar for the new and satisfactory use to become established in all his activity.

When this stage is reached, it will be found that the improvement in the pupil's manner of use is associated with an improvement in his standard of functioning, and that undesirable specific symptoms, such as unsatisfactory use of the eyes, have disappeared *in the process.* This means that the golfer will be able to keep his eyes on the ball when he wishes to do so, for new and reliable "lines of communication" will have been laid down, which ensures that what he "wills" to do he ultimately does; his "will-to-do," in short, will be effective.

THE END-GAINER'S DIFFICULTIES WITH THE MEANS-WHEREBY

The objection has often been made that this process would prove too lengthy for the ordinary person. I admit, of course, that *if* some way could be found of inducing the golfer who cannot keep his eyes on the ball to inhibit his desire to make a good stroke without going through the process of changing his faulty use of himself, he would then be able to keep his eyes on the ball and make his stroke successfully.[25] But in all

[25]This applies equally to any other difficulties a golfer may experience in his play.

the years that I have been teaching pupils whose use of themselves is wrong, I have never yet found any of them able to inhibit the desire to gain an end directly until this unsatisfactory use has been changed. Even when they have been made aware of the means whereby they can make the change from unsatisfactory to satisfactory use and functioning throughout the organism and by this means overcome indirectly their specific defects, their desire to gain their end directly is so strong that they are very seldom able to profit by these "means-whereby" either to the satisfaction of themselves or of their teachers.

This leads me to the point I wish above all to emphasize, namely, that *when a person has reached a given stage of unsatisfactory use and functioning, his habit of "end-gaining" will prove to be the impeding factor in all his attempts to profit by any teaching method whatsoever.* Ordinary teaching methods, in whatever sphere, cannot deal with this impeding factor, indeed, they tend actually to encourage "end-gaining."[26] The instruction given to the golfer of our illustration to keep his eyes on the ball is typical of the kind of specific instruction given by teachers generally for the purpose of eradicating specific defects in their pupils, and, as we have seen in his case, this instruction was a stimulus to him to try harder than ever to gain his end, and so to misdirect his efforts worse than ever.[27]

This habit of "end-gaining" is so ingrained that it will create a serious difficulty even where the teaching method is based on the "means-whereby" principle, and the difficulty can only be overcome if both teacher and pupil at every step in their combined procedure, even the simplest, adhere strictly to the working principle I have set down, namely, that in a series of acts which have been thought out as the means whereby a given end can be satisfactorily gained, the primary act must not be considered as an end in itself, but must be directed and carried out and *then continued* as the preliminary means of carrying out the secondary act, and so on.

My daily teaching experience has shewn me that the great stumbling-block in the way of the pupil's cooperation in this plan is his idea that as long as he grasps "intellectually" the principle underlying the "means-whereby" procedure and subscribes to it fully in theory, he will

---

26This criticism applies to methods employed by teachers of all sports and games, of physical culture, eurythmics, dancing, singing, etc.

27Even supposing it were possible to restore *at once* to a pupil satisfactory direction of his use and functioning throughout the organism, the pupil's habit of end-gaining would still persist in acts in which he was practised in employing his old familiar use, as, for instance, in making a golf stroke, so that the moment he attempted to make the stroke by his new unfamiliar direction of use, he would bring into play his old habitual misdirection of use, take his eyes off the ball and make a bad stroke.

have little difficulty in working to it practically.[28] It is true that a pupil may start out with an "intellectual" conception of what is required for the "means-whereby" procedure, but in my experience I have found that the moment the idea of performing any act in that procedure comes to him, his habit of "end-gaining" causes him to *try to "do" the act in the habitual way that feels right*, and this in spite of the fact that I have repeatedly demonstrated to him that the sensory appreciation upon which he is depending to "know" whether his means are right or not is deceiving him, so that what he feels is the right use of himself in gaining his end is in fact wrong.

In the case of such a pupil, working on the "means-whereby" principle means working against a habit of life, and difficult as it is to work to a principle against any habit of life (as anyone who tries it will find out), the difficulty is enormously increased when it comes to working contrary to the habit of "end-gaining," for this habit is so closely bound up with faulty habits of use which feel right, that to give it up means giving up the lifelong familiar habits of use that go with it, and employing in its stead a new use which feels wrong.

I therefore claim that if any habit so confirmed as that of "end-gaining" is to be changed and not merely transferred, it is essential that the pupil should be given the experience, at first in the simplest activities,

> (1) *of receiving a stimulus to gain a certain end and refusing to react to it,* thereby inhibiting the unsatisfactory habits of use associated with his habitual reaction;
>
> (2) *of projecting the directions for the new and more satisfactory use* in their proper sequence, primary, secondary, etc., "all together, one after the other," as already explained, *whilst the teacher at the same time with his hands makes him familiar with the new sensory experiences*[29] associated with this new use.

By this procedure a gradual improvement will be brought about in the pupil's sensory appreciation, so that he will become more and more aware of faults in his habitual manner of using himself; correspondingly, as with this increasing awareness the manner of his use of himself improves, his sensory appreciation will further improve and in time constitute a standard *within the self* by means of which he will become

[28]This is a belief that will probably be shared by my readers and is quite understandable, since it is difficult for anyone who has not had the actual experience of working on the "means-whereby" principle to realize what unity of "physical" and "mental" processes means in practice.

[29]I must again impress upon the reader that these new sensory experiences will at first feel wrong.

increasingly aware both of faults and of improvement, not only in the manner of his use but also in the standard of his functioning generally.[30] And since it is by means of the use of the self that he reacts to all stimuli, it is clear that together with the improvement in the manner of the use of his mechanisms and in the adjustment of the different parts of his organism, there will also come about an improvement in his manner of reacting to stimuli in every sphere of activity. This improvement will necessarily include an improvement in his manner of reacting to the stimulus to gain a certain end, shewing that it is possible, by working to the principle involved in the "means-whereby" procedure, to strike at the very roots of the habit of end-gaining which is so deeply embedded in our make-up.

It is obvious that a procedure that makes for the control of the manner of reacting to stimuli must make for the control of habit generally, and for this reason the technique which I have outlined for the building up of a conscious direction of the use of the self should make an appeal to all those who are interested in education in its widest sense.

[30]For instance, with the improvement in his use he will become aware of an increase in the expansion and contraction of the thorax, i.e., of the degree of thoracic mobility. Reliability of the sensory register is essential to all who would make permanent changes from unsatisfactory to satisfactory conditions of functioning.

CHAPTER IV

THE STUTTERER

I WILL take for my second illustration the case of a man with an impediment in his speech who was sent to me for advice and help. He told me that he had taken lessons from specialists who treated speech defects, and had done his best to carry out their instructions and to practise their exercises. He had always had special difficulty with sounds which called for the use of the tongue and lips, particularly with the consonants T and D, but although he had been more or less successful in doing the exercises themselves, his stutter was as bad as ever in ordinary conversation, especially when he was hurried or excited.

As is my custom with a new pupil, I noted specially the way he walked into my room and sat down in a chair, and it was obvious to me that his general use of himself was more than usually harmful. When he spoke, I also noticed a wrong use of his tongue and lips and certain defects in the use of his head and neck, involving undue depression on the larynx and undue tension of the face and neck muscles. I then pointed out to him that his stutter was not an isolated symptom of wrong use confined to the organs of speech, but that it was associated with other symptoms of wrong use and functioning in other parts of his organism.

As he doubted this, I went on to explain that I had been able to demonstrate to every stutterer who had come to me for help that he "stuttered" with many other different parts of his body besides his tongue and lips. "Usually," I said, "these other defects remain unobserved or ignored until they reach the point where the wrong functioning manifests itself in some form of so-called "physical" or "mental" disorder. In your case, your stutter interferes with your work and hinders intercourse with your fellows, and so you have not been able to ignore it, but this may well turn out to be a blessing in disguise if it is the means of making you aware, before too late, of the other more serious defects which I have pointed out to you, and which will tend, as time goes on, to become more and more exaggerated." I assured him that my long years of practical experience in dealing with the difficulties and idiosyncrasies of people who stutter had convinced me that stuttering was one of the most interesting specific symptoms of a general cause, namely, misdirection of the use of the psycho-physical mechanisms, and I did not wish to take him as a pupil, unless he was prepared to work with me on the basis of correcting this misdirection of use generally, as the primary step in remedying his defects in speech. I could promise him, however, that if he decided to come to me and I was successful in making certain changes for the better in his manner of using his mechanisms, a change for the better would also come about in the functioning of his organism, and his stuttering would tend to disappear in the process. He saw the point and decided to take lessons.

Now in my experience stuttering, like the golfer's tendency to take his eyes off the ball, is due to habitual misdirection of the use of the mechanisms, so that the remedying of the defect in both cases presents fundamentally the same problem. Like the golfer, the stutterer needs to have this habitual misdirection of his use changed to a more satisfactory direction, and the new and improved use, associated with this change in direction, has to be built up and sufficiently stabilized in him before he will be able to employ it practically as a means of overcoming his particular difficulties in speaking.

In the case of this pupil, therefore, I began by pointing out to him various outstanding symptoms of his wrong habitual use, one of the most marked of these being the undue amount of muscle tension that he was in the habit of employing throughout his organism whenever he tried to speak. This extreme muscle tension was an impeding factor in the functioning of his mechanisms generally, and rendered impossible a satisfactory use of his tongue and lips, and the more he tried by any special effort of "will" to speak without stuttering, the more certain he was to increase the already undue muscle tension and so to defeat his own end.

The reason for this, I explained to him, was that he did not start to speak until he had brought about the amount of tension which was associated with his habitual use and which caused him to *feel that he could speak*; i.e., he would decide that the moment had come for him to speak only when his *feeling* told him that he was using his mechanisms to the best advantage, and this moment, in the last analysis, was when his sensory appreciation (the only guide he had as to the amount of muscle tension necessary) registered to him as "right" the amount of tension which he habitually employed in speaking and which was therefore familiar to him.

Unfortunately, the familiar amount of tension that "felt right" to him was the unnecessary amount associated with the wrong habitual use of his mechanisms of which his stuttering was a symptom, and I therefore urged him to recognize from the beginning that the "feeling," upon which he was relying to tell him when his use was right for speaking, was untrustworthy as a register of muscle tension, and that he must not depend upon it for guidance in his attempts to speak. How, I asked him, could he expect to judge by his feeling the amount of tension he should employ in speaking, when he was unfamiliar with the sensory experience of speaking with the due amount? Obviously, he could not "know" a sensation he had never experienced, and as sensory experience cannot be conveyed by the spoken work, no amount of telling on my part could convey to him the unfamiliar sensory experience of speaking with less tension and without stuttering. The only way to convince him that he could speak with a less amount of muscle tension would be to give him this unfamiliar experience.

To this end I adopted a procedure based upon the same principle as the procedure employed to the end of giving the golfer the experience of keeping his eyes on the ball, my aim being to give my pupil, first, the experience of employing a conscious direction of a new and improved use of his mechanisms generally, and, secondly, the experience of *continuing to employ this conscious direction whilst using* the mechanisms concerned with the act of speaking in the manner best suited for the purpose.

I began by giving him

(1) the directions for the inhibition of the wrong habitual use of his mechanisms associated with the excessive muscle tension;

(2) the directions for the employment of the primary control leading to a new and improved use which would be associated with a due amount of muscle tension.

I then asked him to project these directions whilst I with my hands gave him the new sensory experiences of use corresponding to these directions, in order that the trustworthiness of his sensory appreciation in relation to the use of his mechanisms might be gradually restored, and that by this means he might in time acquire a register of the due amount of tension required for speaking, as distinct from the undue amount of tension associated with his stuttering.

I continued this procedure, until I had repeated for him the new sensory experiences of use often enough to justify me in allowing him to attempt to employ his new "means-whereby" for speaking and for saying the words and consonants that caused him special difficulty.

It is impossible in the space at my command to put down all the details of the variations of the teacher's art that were employed to bring my pupil to this point, for a teacher's technique naturally varies in detail according to the particular needs and difficulties of each pupil. Those of my readers, however, who have followed the account of the difficulties I encountered when I first attempted to employ the new "means-whereby" in my reciting, will be able to realize the kind of difficulty we were faced with all along, when I say that my pupil was a confirmed "end-gainer."

At the beginning of this new stage in our work together I reminded him how his progress up to this point had been hampered by his habit of end-gaining and of "trying to be right," and I warned him that unless he succeeded in side-stepping it, he would have little chance of applying his new "means-whereby" to his difficulties in speaking, for if, at the critical moment of starting to say a difficult word, he still went directly for his end and tried to say the word in the way that "felt right" to him, he would be bound to revert to his old habitual use in speaking and so stutter.

Events proved how difficult it was for my pupil to take practical heed of this warning. I would repeatedly urge him, whenever I gave him a sound or word to pronounce, always to inhibit his old habitual response to my request by refusing to attempt to pronounce the sound or word until he had taken time to think out and employ the new directions for the use which he had decided upon as best for his purpose. He would agree to do this, but as soon as I asked him to pronounce some sound or word, he would fail to inhibit his response to the stimulus of my voice, and forgetting all about the new directions he had been asked to employ, he would immediately try to repeat the sound, with the result that he was at once dominated by his old habits of use associated with the extreme muscle tension that *felt right* to him, and so stuttered as badly as ever.[31] In short, his very desire to "be right in gaining his end" defeated the end.

In every stutterer of whom I have had experience this habit of reacting too quickly to stimuli is always associated with sensory untrustworthiness, undue muscle tension and misdirection of energy, but in this pupil's case the habit of going directly for his end, and of trying to "feel right" in doing it, had been positively cultivated in him by the methods employed by his previous teachers in trying to "cure" his stutter.[32]

It would appear that the "end-gaining" principle underlies every one of the exercises given by teachers who, whether by orthodox or unorthodox methods, deal with stuttering as a specific defect, and I will take as an example the exercises that had been given to my pupil to meet his special difficulty in pronouncing words beginning with T or D.

His former teachers had recognized that the use of his tongue and lips

[31]In order that the reader should not think this difficulty was peculiar to this pupil, I wish to state that I have had similar experiences with all my pupils. How could it be otherwise when "end-gaining" is a universal habit?

[32]See Chapter III, page 443. Note 1.

was unsatisfactory for the purpose of pronouncing these consonants, and in order to overcome the difficulty had instructed him to practise certain exercises involving the use of these specific parts in saying T or D.

Now this procedure could only aggravate the difficulty, for the idea of trying to say T or D acted as an incentive to the pupil to employ the habitual use of himself associated with the wrong use of his tongue and lips. As long as this wrong habitual use remained unchanged, this association persisted and he had little chance of getting rid of this incentive, so that to ask him under these conditions to practise saying T and D as a remedy for his stuttering was tantamount to giving him an added incentive to stutter.

This was borne out by what I observed when he shewed me how he had been practising these exercises. I watched him closely and saw that as soon as he started to do them, he at once made an undue amount of tension generally, continued to increase the tension of the muscles of the lips, cheeks and tongue, and tried to say T and D before his tongue had taken up the best position for the purpose. This attempt was as bound to result in failure as would be the attempt of a motorist to change gears before the clutch has done its work in getting the cogs into the position in which they will mesh. It was evident that he had been trying in all his practice in the past to gain his end without being in command of the means whereby this end could be successfully gained, and the fact that the majority of these attempts had been unsuccessful had brought him to a state of lack of confidence in himself, which added considerably to the difficulty of breaking his "end-gaining" habit.

As far as I am aware, all methods of "curing" stuttering, however they may differ in detail, are all based on the same "end-gaining" principle. The adviser will select some symptom or symptoms as the cause of his pupil's stuttering and will give him specific instructions or exercises to help him.

I am well aware that it has proved possible by such methods to stop people from stuttering, but I would question the common assumption that because this is so, a genuine "cure" has been effected. For in cases where it is claimed that a stutter has been "cured," there is usually something peculiar or hesitating about the manner of speaking, and those concerned do not seem in the least perturbed that the harmful conditions of undue muscle tension, misdirection of energy and untrustworthiness of sensory appreciation, present in the case when the "cure" was begun, are still in evidence now that what is considered a successful "cure" has been brought about.

No method of "cure" can be accepted as effective or scientific, if, in the process of removing certain selected symptoms, other symptoms have been left untouched and if new, unwished-for symptoms have appeared.[33] *If this test is applied to a stutterer after he has been "cured" by such methods, it will be found too often that the original defects of undue muscular tension, misdirection of energy and untrustworthiness of sensory appreciation have been increased in the process of the "cure."*[34]

I admit that these defects may not bring about a recurrence of the stutter, but even so, they are almost certain to lead to the further development of other undesirable symptoms which constantly remain unrecognized. This invariably happens when defects and diseases are "cured" by specific methods, and explains why, in spite of the immense number of "cures" recorded, the troubles in the human organism would seem to be increasing and calling for more and more "cures."

It is important to remember that there is a working balance in the use of all the parts of the organism, and that for this reason the use of the specific part (or parts) in any activity can influence the use of the other parts, and vice versa. Under instinctive direction this working balance becomes habitual and "feels right," and the point at which the influence of the use of any part will make itself felt will vary and the influence of the particular use be strong or weak according to the nature of the stimulus of the end activity desired. If a defect is recognized in the use of a part, and an attempt is made to correct this defect by changing the use of the part without bringing about at the same time a corresponding change in the use of the other parts, the habitual working balance in the use of the whole will be disturbed.

---

[33]As Dr. Dewey writes in his Introduction to *Constructive Conscious Control of the Individual*, "the essence of scientific method does not consist in taking consequences in gross; it consists precisely in the means by which consequences are followed up in detail. It consists in the processes by which the causes that are used to explain the consequences or effects, can be concretely followed up to shew that they actually produce these consequences and no others."

[34]As an example of this, I will quote a statement made to me by an intending pupil at his preliminary interview. He told me, among other things, that he had cured himself of stammering and I asked him how he had done it. He replied that he had been a very bad stammerer, but that one day he was forced to run to the top of a long flight of stairs to deliver an important message, and found to his surprise that after this experience he was able to speak without stammering, and he had continued to be able to do so. Most people, of course, would look upon this as a "cure," but I could not, because I saw that his use of himself generally was still very bad, and when I said so, he admitted that he suffered from other troubles which, in my opinion, amounted to "stuttering" in other parts of his organism. The fact is, the experience to which he attributed his freedom from stammering had not changed his unsatisfactory conditions of use to those satisfactory conditions which are not found in association with stammering. Consequently, similar experience was just as liable to cause a recurrence at any time of the vocal stammering, and as his unsatisfactory manner of use was still present, he had a predisposition to develop other troubles.

Unless, therefore, the person attempting to make a change in the use of a specific part has an understanding of what is required to bring about at the same time a corresponding change in the use of the other parts which will make for a satisfactory working balance and therefore be complementary to the new use that he is trying to bring about at one point, one of two things is bound to happen:

either, (1) the stimulus of the desire to gain his end, by means of the old use associated with the habitual working balance which "feels right," will be so strong that it will dominate the stimulus to cultivate a new and improved use of a certain part associated with an unfamiliar working balance which "feels wrong";

or, (2) if the change in the use of a part is made in the face of impeding factors in the use of the other parts (as happens in any specific method of treatment employed to correct a defect in a part), the working balance between the use of that part and the use of all the other parts will be so thrown out of gear that the use of the other parts will be adversely affected in their turn, and new defects in the use of these parts developed.

After my pupil had shewn me the exercises he had been told to do, I explained to him that in practising them he had been indulging in his old wrong habits of general use of himself, and thereby actually *cultivating* the wrong habits of use of his tongue and lips which had made him stutter. I impressed upon him once more that if he wished ever to be confident of saying T and D and words in which these consonants occur without stuttering, *he must refuse to respond to any stimulus either from within or without to say T or D*; in other words, whenever the idea of saying T or D came to him, he must inhibit his desire to try and say it correctly, until he had learned what use of his tongue and lips was required in his case for saying T or D without stuttering, and until he could put into practice the necessary directions for this new use of his tongue and lips *whilst continuing to give the directions for the primary control of the new and improved use of himself generally.*

He understood the reason for this, but his attempts at cooperating with me proved more or less unsuccessful for some time. Over and over again I got him to the point where the use of his tongue and lips in association with his general use was such that I knew he could pronounce T and D without the undue muscle tension that made him stutter, but when at this point I asked him to repeat one of the sounds, he would either

(1) forget to inhibit his old response, change back to his old conditions of use and increase the tension to the point when he

felt that he could say T or D, try to say it in this way and stutter, or

(2) on the occasions when he remembered to inhibit his old response and to employ the new "means-whereby" for saying T and D without stuttering, he would make no attempt to repeat the sound.

In both these cases he was actuated by the same motive. He associated the act of speaking, especially the pronunciation of consonants that were difficult for him, with a given amount of muscle tension, and as I have already shewn, he had come to believe that it was impossible for him to speak until he *felt* this undue amount of tension. This explains why he made no attempt to speak until he had deliberately brought about the familiar but excessive tension which caused him to stutter. In this way he simply reinforced the old sensory experiences of undue muscle tension already associated with his habitual use, and with his habit of trying to *feel right* in gaining his end.

To deal with this difficulty I made a point of giving my pupil day after day the experience of receiving a stimulus to gain a certain end and of remembering to refuse to gain that end, since this refusal meant that at one fell swoop he inhibited all the wrong habits of use associated with his habitual way of gaining that end.[35] In proportion as he was successful in inhibiting his immediate response to any stimulus, he became able to defeat his desire to gain his ends in the way that felt right to him, and *as long as he continued this inhibition*, I on my side was able to repeat for him, until they became familiar, the new sensory experiences associated with an improved general use of his mechanisms, including the right use of his tongue and lips. By continuing to cooperate with me on these lines, he gradually acquired sufficient experience in the direction of this new use to be able to employ it successfully as the "means-whereby" of pronouncing the consonants which had caused him special difficulty.

But, more important than this, my pupil in the course of this procedure had learned that if he inhibited his immediate instinctive reaction to any stimulus to "do," he could prevent the misdirection of his use and the associated undue muscle tension which had been the marked feature of all his reactions to stimuli, and which had hampered him not only in his speaking but in all his activities, both "physical" and "mental," and if he chose to apply this principle to his activities in other spheres, he would have at his command a means of controlling the nature of his reaction to stimuli, that is, of acquiring a control of what

[35]Cf. Chapter I, p. 424 foll. Chapter III, p. 444 foll.

is called "conscious behaviour."[36]

> *Certain features of this pupil's case occur with practically every pupil.*
>
> *During the earlier stages of a pupil's lessons when the use of his mechanisms is still unsatisfactory, I have constantly found that he fails to inhibit the old instinctive direction of his use, with the result that his directions for the new use do not become operative. Before I can get a chance to help him, he proceeds to gain his end in accordance with his habitual wrong use, and it is practically impossible under these circumstances to stop him from gaining his end in this way.*
>
> *On the other hand, when he has learned at a later stage in his lessons to inhibit the instinctive direction of his use and the directions for the new use have become operative, so that I am enabled to give him the corresponding sensory experiences, I have found that although he now has at his command the best conditions possible for gaining his end, he will not make any attempt to gain it. He cannot believe that the end can be gained with these improved conditions present; they "feel so wrong," as he puts it, that he instinctively refuses to employ them.*
>
> *When this difficulty arises, it is necessary for me to give him the actual experience of gaining his end by what he feels is a wrong use of his mechanisms, and when I have succeeded in doing this, he invariably remarks how much easier the new way is than the old way, and how much less effort it requires. Yet in spite of this admission, the actual experience of gaining his end in this new way has to be repeated for him again and again before the improved use "feels right" to him, and before he gains the necessary confidence in employing it.*

---

[36]The following is of interest in this connexion. One of my pupils has just told me that before he came to me for lessons he used to have uncontrollable fits of temper, but that since having the work he has no trouble in that way, and that all his family notice the change. He asked me to explain how it was that what he looked upon as a "nervous" or "mental" symptom could be affected by the kind of work I was doing with him. In reply I asked him how other people knew when he had lost his temper, and he answered that they would know by the tone of his voice, the expression of his face, the look in his eyes, or by his gestures and excited manner generally. I then asked him how these reactions could be possible except through the use of what he thought of as his "physical" self. For instance, the voice must be used if we are to judge its tone, there must be use of the eyes if they are to flash, of the muscles of the face for change of expression, and, for excitability to be manifested the whole of the mechanisms of use must be stimulated into undue activity and muscle tension.

Change the manner of use and you change the conditions throughout the organism; the old reaction associated with the old manner of use and the old conditions cannot therefore take place, for the means are no longer there. In other words, the old habitual reflex activity has been changed and will not recur. If loss of control can be manifested only by means of the use of ourselves, it follows that a conscious direction of an improving use will bring us for the first time within striking distance of a conscious control of human reaction or behaviour.

The lesson to be learned from all this is that since our particular way of reacting to stimuli is in accordance with our familiar habits of use, the incentive to try to gain any given end is inextricably bound up with this familiar use. This explains why, if a pupil's familiar use is changed to one that is unfamiliar and therefore unassociated with his habitual way of reacting to stimuli, he has little or no incentive to gain that given end. As long as the conditions of use and the associated feeling are wrong in a person, the incentive to gain a given end by the familiar wrong use appears to be almost irresistible, but when these conditions have been changed to conditions which are best for the purpose of gaining the end, there seems to be practically no incentive to gain it.

This is not surprising, for when a person's sensory appreciation of his use is wrong and his belief as to what he can or cannot do is based on what he feels, gaining an end by a use that is unfamiliar means for him taking a plunge in the dark. Even when I have explained to a pupil why this difficulty has arisen in his case, and he understands the reason for it "intellectually," he will need, more often than not, considerable encouragement and practical assistance in order to be enabled to make the experience of gaining a given end by means of a use that is new and unfamiliar to him. Once this has been done for him, however, he becomes conscious of a new experience that he is desirous to repeat, and repetition of this experience in time convinces him that his previous beliefs and judgments in this connexion were wrong. As a result there gradually develops in him an incentive to employ the new use, and this becomes at last far stronger than the incentive to employ the old use, for its development is the outcome of a reasoned procedure which he finds he can consciously direct and control with a confidence he has never before experienced.

One of the most remarkable of man's characteristics is his capacity for becoming used to conditions of almost any kind, whether good or bad, both in the self and in the environment, and once he has become used to such conditions they seem to him both right and natural. This capacity is a boon when it enables him to adapt himself to conditions which are desirable, but it may prove a great danger when the conditions are undesirable. When his sensory appreciation is untrustworthy, it is possible for him to become so familiar with seriously harmful conditions of misuse of himself that these malconditions will feel right and comfortable.

My teaching experience has shewn me that the worse these conditions are in a pupil and the longer they have been in existence, the more familiar and right they feel to him and the harder it is to teach him how to overcome them, no matter how much he may wish to do so. In other words, his ability to learn a new and more satisfactory use of himself is, as a rule, in inverse ratio to the degree of misuse present in his organism and the duration of these harmful conditions.

This point must be understood and taken into practical consideration by anyone forming a plan of procedure for improving the use and functioning of the mechanisms throughout the organism as a means of eradicating defects, peculiarities and bad habits.

Towards the end of his lessons my pupil asked me why it should be so much more difficult to overcome the habit of stuttering than the habit of over-smoking. He then went on to tell me that at one time he had been an inveterate smoker, but realizing that the habit was getting too much of a hold on him, he had decided he must give it up. He had first tried the plan of reducing the number of cigarettes he smoked per day, but as he found that he could not keep within the prescribed limit, he had decided that the only way for him to succeed in breaking his habit was to give up smoking altogether. He put this decision into practice and had become a non-smoker. He now wanted to know why his efforts to overcome his stuttering had not been equally successful.

I pointed out to him that the two habits presented very different problems.

The smoker can abstain from smoking without interrupting the necessary activities of his daily life, and as the temptation to smoke to excess results, as every chain-smoker knows, from the fact that each pipe, cigar or cigarette smoked acts as a stimulus to the smoking of another, every time he abstains from smoking he is breaking a link in the chain.

The stutterer, on the other hand, cannot abstain from speaking because his daily intercourse with his fellows depends on it. Every time he speaks, therefore, he is thrown into the way of temptation to indulge in his familiar wrong habits of use of his vocal organs, tongue and lips, and so to stutter. The stimulus to speak is one that he cannot evade in the way a smoker can evade the stimulus to smoke if he so wills it, so that the habit of stuttering calls for a much more fundamental form of control.

Satisfactory control of the act of speaking demands a satisfactory standard of the general use of the mechanisms, since the satisfactory use of the tongue and lips and the required standard of control of the respiratory and vocal organs depend upon this satisfactory general use. This being so, the unsatisfactory general use of the mechanisms which, as we have seen, is present in every stutterer, constitutes a formidable obstacle in the way of mastering his habit.

The situation is very different for the smoker, for the act of smoking does not demand any such high standard of use of the mechanisms, and although unsatisfactory conditions of use are frequently present in his case, the influence which they exercise in preventing him from overcoming his particular habit is small in comparison.

Still another element enters into the case. The habit which the smoker is trying to overcome is one which he has himself developed in the process of satisfying a desire. The stutterer, on the other hand, is dealing with a habit which has not been developed in the process of satisfying a desire, but which has gradually grown to become part of the use of the mechanisms which he habitually employs for all the activities of his daily life. This explains why the smoking habit is relatively superficial and in this degree easier to overcome, and why my pupil had been able *by himself* to solve the problem of his over-smoking, but had not been able to deal with his habit of stuttering without the help of a teacher who understood how to give him the means whereby he could *himself* command that satisfactory use of his mechanisms generally which includes the correct use of the tongue, lips and vocal organs for the act of speaking.

I would emphasize here that the process of eradicating any such defect as stuttering by these means makes the greatest demands on the time, patience and skill of both teacher and pupil, since, as we have seen, it calls for

> (1) the inhibition of the instinctive direction of energy associated with familiar sensory experiences of wrong habitual use, and
>
> (2) the building up in its place of a conscious direction of energy through the repetition of unfamiliar sensory experiences associated with new and satisfactory use.

This process of directing energy out of familiar into new and unfamiliar paths, as a means of changing the manner of reacting to stimuli, implies of necessity an ever-increasing ability on the part of both teacher and pupil to "pass from the known to the unknown";[37] it is therefore a process which is true to the principle involved in all human growth and development.

Since this chapter was written, I have received a letter from this pupil, and with his permission I am quoting the following extracts from it, as they are of interest in relation to the development of sensory awareness of an improvement in use:

> "I hope that you have not construed my prolonged silence to mean that I have lost interest in you or in your work. Quite the contrary is the case. I am interested in little else. . . . I feel quite sanguine about the possibili-

[37]The late Mr. Joseph Rowntree after one of his lessons described my work as "reasoning from the known to the unknown, the known being the wrong and the unknown being the right."

ty of making considerable progress again if I can come this year. I am optimistic enough to believe that I am almost ripe for some real new experiences. . . . I have now come to the point that when I feel my back working I also fell my jaws relax. I really believe that I have been using my jaw muscles to keep myself erect! I am really beginning to appreciate how little I have used my tongue and lips in my speech, in fact, I have scarcely used them at all. It is this great improvement in my sensory appreciation that gives me such hope for the future."

CHAPTER V

DIAGNOSIS AND MEDICAL TRAINING

FOR many years medical men have been sending their patients to me, because they know that I am experienced in examining conditions of use and in estimating the influence of these conditions upon functioning. I would say at once that I do not receive these cases as patients, but as pupils, inasmuch as I am not interested in disease or defects apart from their association with harmful conditions of use and functioning.

Some of the cases have been previously diagnosed and treated for such widely differing troubles as angina pectoris, epilepsy, locomotor ataxia, rheumatoid arthritis, sciatica, infantile paralysis, asthma, neuritis, so-called nervous and mental troubles, constipation, voice and throat trouble, flatfoot and stuttering, and on examination of each of these cases I have found present unsatisfactory functioning associated with harmful use of the psycho-physical mechanisms.

In other cases the doctors have been unable to find any cause or explanation of the patient's symptoms, which in some instances have been symptoms of so-called mental trouble such as carelessness, depression, lassitude, unreliable memory, inability to give attention to the job in hand, undue excitability and a low standard of accomplishment generally, and, in other instances, symptoms of a more recognizably "physical" character, such as sleeplessness, indigestion, malnutrition, poor circulation and chilblains. On examination of such cases also I have always found present undesirable conditions of use of the self which have not been recognized, and which have tended to lower the general standard of functioning in the patient.[38]

Further, in all cases where I have found harmful conditions of use and functioning in association, I have also found that the sensory appreciation (that is, the knowledge which comes to us through the sensory

[38]Every medical man has records of cases in which he has been unable to find any specific trouble calling for treatment.

mechanisms as to the manner of our use of ourselves), is not to be depended upon, with the result that the sensory direction of use in all activity is faulty, manifesting itself in bad habits in the everyday acts of walking, sitting, standing, eating, talking, playing games, thinking and reasoning, etc.

My experience in all these cases has brought home to me the close relationship which exists between the manner of use of the mechanisms and the standard of functioning, for where I have found unsatisfactory use of the mechanisms, the functional trouble associated with it has included interference with the respiratory and circulatory systems, dropping of the abdominal viscera, sluggishness of various organs, together with undue and perverted pressures, contractions and rigidities throughout the organism, all of which tend to lower the standard of resistance to disease.

On the other hand, in cases where disease has been previously diagnosed in any of the organs or systems, I have found that the faulty functioning which this implies is always associated with an unsatisfactory manner of use throughout the organism.

This goes to shew that an unsatisfactory manner of use, by interfering with general functioning, constitutes a predisposing cause of disorder and disease, and that anyone who makes a diagnosis and prescribes treatment, without finding out how much of the trouble present has arisen from this interference and how much from other causes, is leaving untouched a predisposing cause of disorder and disease.

For this reason I make the following claim:

> (1) No diagnosis of a case can be said to be complete, unless the medical adviser gives consideration to the influence exerted upon the patient, not only by the immediate cause of the trouble (say, a germ invader), but also by the interference with functioning which is always associated with *habitual* wrong use of the mechanisms and helps to lower the patient's resistance to the point where the germ invader gets its opportunity.
>
> (2) Since the medical curriculum does not include training in the knowledge of how to direct the use of the human mechanisms, the medical man does not bring to his diagnosis an understanding of "use" in the sense I have defined, and so does not recognize the relationship between misdirection of use and that unsatisfactory standard of functioning which is always found in association with disease; any deductions he may make, therefore, will be based on incomplete premises, and the value of his work limited both in the field of prevention and of cure.
>
> (3) A training in the satisfactory direction of the use of his

> own mechanisms is essential to the medical man's personal equipment; for in the course of this training he would be gaining a knowledge which would enable him to judge the manner of use present in the patient, detect any misdirection of use, and, where this exists, determine its relation to any symptoms of unsatisfactory functioning present.

In support of this claim I will take as an illustration the orthodox practice of making tests for the purposes of diagnosis, and I choose "tests" because the result of any test of conditions in a patient is bound to be more or less influenced by the manner of that patient's habitual use of his mechanisms, and if this influence is not taken into consideration, any diagnosis based on the test must to that extent be incomplete.

To prove this we have only to make a test of functioning on a person in whom there are present certain unsatisfactory conditions of use, and make the same test again on that same person after the conditions of use have been changed for the better, and the result of the second test will be found to differ from that of the first; in the majority of cases, indeed, we shall find a marked difference between the two.

An instance in point occurs to me. I was called by a specialist to a case for consultation, and when I went into the room he was testing the patient's chest and lungs with a stethoscope. I realized at once that here was one of the worst cases of wrong use I had ever seen, with the associated contraction and immobility of the thorax, depression of the larynx, tendency to hold the breath in the ordinary acts of life, and harmful stoop. His manner of use was impeding his respiratory processes and circulation and the action of his heart, influencing adversely even his pulse and blood pressure. When the specialist had finished, he asked me to listen so that I could get some idea of the patient's respiratory difficulties from the medical standpoint. I did so, and after noting the result with him, I pointed out the symptoms of wrong use I had observed, and suggested that if he would allow me to make even a slight change in these conditions of use, and then make the same test again while I maintained the changed conditions in the patient, the stethoscope would register an entirely different result. He agreed, I made certain changes,[39] maintained them whilst the second test was made, and the specialist on using the stethoscope found that what I had predicted had taken place. He sent the patient to me with ultimately satisfactory results.

---

[39]I am prepared to demonstrate that, given a reasonable subject, a temporary change to more satisfactory conditions of use can be brought about in a short space of time, although the patient is bound to fall back almost immediately into his wrong habitual use.

I will now go further and try to shew that the medical man is limited, even more in preventive work than in the field of "cure," because he does not recognize the influence of satisfactory use in the maintenance of a desirable standard of general functioning, and so, when he comes to make his diagnosis, he does not possess the knowledge that would enable him to distinguish between satisfactory and unsatisfactory conditions of use in any case he is examining.

Take the case of a child whose parents take him to a doctor purely as a preventive measure. The child shews no symptoms of illness, but the parents want to make sure that there are no harmful tendencies latent which, if allowed to develop unchecked, might lead later on to illness or defect of some kind or another. The doctor examines the child, and finds no symptoms or tendencies which in his opinion call for attention or treatment. He therefore gives the child a clean bill of health.

In appraising the value of this opinion, we must again take into account that the medical curriculum does not include any training that would enable a medical man to employ a satisfactory direction of his own use in the acts of daily life, or to teach his patients to do the same. It is therefore not unreasonable to assume that the doctor of our illustration, when examining the child, does not know what unsatisfactory conditions of use are present, and that if they were present, he would not be likely to recognize them or to estimate their influence upon functioning. He cannot be expected to look out for something, however potent a factor this may be in the development of tendencies to disease and disorder, when he is not even aware of its existence. Consequently, his study of the child's general conditions cannot be said to be complete, for he may give the child a clean bill of health and yet leave unrecognized and unchecked in him conditions of use which, if allowed to develop, may lead in time to the lowering of the child's standard of functioning and resistance to disease.

As an example of a diagnosis based upon a recognition of the close relationship between use and functioning I will cite the following case. On December 12, 1923, a medical man wrote to me as follows:

> "I have just read your book *Man's Supreme Inheritance* as a result of Dr. Peter Macdonald's remarks at the B. M. A. Meeting. I am a medical man and have had to take a rest on account of angina pectoris, and the principles underlying your work appeal to me as being really sound, so much so that I would like to put them into practice in my own case. I am 61, and up to two months ago I was engaged in active practice. . . . If you can help me I should be glad of a reply."

An interview was arranged, and when Dr. X. came to see me, I proceeded in my usual way to make an examination of the conditions of use present. After this examination I told him that I found that his use of himself was most unsatisfactory, shewing a high degree of misuse and maladjustment associated with a dangerous lowering of the standard of functioning of the respiratory, circulatory and digestive systems. This combination of harmful conditions is one which I have always found present in a marked degree in cases of angina pectoris, and would, in my experience, be sufficient in itself to account for the distressing sensations[40] experienced by the patient.

This being my first diagnosis, I explained to Dr. X. that my method of dealing with his case would be to try and change his unsatisfactory conditions of use to those more desirable conditions which are only found present in association with satisfactory functioning. From the first, Dr. X. was particularly interested in my method of diagnosis, and this interest increased as he recognized that during the process of building up a new and more satisfactory use which he employed more or less in his daily life, the symptoms which gave rise to the diagnosis of angina, and which had incapacitated him from work and from playing golf became less and less in evidence in proportion to the change and improvement in the conditions throughout his organism, and so far disappeared that he became free from pain and able once more to work and to play golf.[41] He described the work I was doing as the "first clinical physiology for the human being," and realizing that my method of diagnosis differed fundamentally from that employed in orthodox medical practice, he urged me to write on the subject in order to put my findings before the medical profession.

In what follows I shall make an attempt to carry out his suggestion, and I think I cannot do better than base the comments I have to make on an address that was delivered by Lord Dawson of Penn at the House of Commons on February 24, 1926,[42] because I am assured by my medical friends that the views which Lord Dawson there expressed, as to the efficacy of medical training as a preparation for the successful diagnosis of disease, can be taken to represent current medical opinion on this subject.

My comments will of necessity involve some criticism of medical training, for a lack in the medical curriculum has been brought home to

---

[40]A medical friend tells me that these sensations, as described to a doctor, constitute the only available evidence upon which a case can be diagnosed as one of angina pectoris.

[41]July 10, 1931. I saw this pupil a few days ago and the good work still goes on. F. M. A.

[42]The Report of Lord Dawson's address from which I am quoting will be found in *The Lancet* of March 6, 1926.

me in my capacity as an educator, but in view of Lord Dawson's statement at the opening of his address that "of criticism itself the profession made no complaint whatever," and seeing that I am able to offer a technique which I am convinced from my experience would make good this lack, I have the best reasons for believing that members of the profession will give this criticism their consideration.

On the subject of *Diagnosis and the Medical Curriculum* Lord Dawson said that

> "A necessary preliminary to treatment was a knowledge of disease. . . its causes and its diagnosis. To attempt to treat disease without knowing what is wrong with the body as a whole (not with a part only) was admittedly an act of folly, and to gain such knowledge there must be carefully organized training. . . . There should be no recognition of a man as an independent practitioner until he had had those years of training, and had studied the nature of disease and its diagnosis. . . . And the training should be the same for all. In this matter there could not be the least compromise. . . . Whatever a man's views on navigation might be, whatever his genius, he was not allowed to assume control of a ship until he had passed the tests for navigators. Why should less protection be afforded to the human ship sailing on the sea of life? . . . Everyone was now trying to get control of disease more early, in its more curable stages, and hence *diagnosis was of supreme importance.*"[43]

Let me begin with Lord Dawson's statement that "a necessary preliminary to treatment was a knowledge of disease—its causes and its diagnosis."

It is obvious that once we are aware of the cause of disease, we have some chance of dealing successfully with it, and that there would be less tendency for parts of the organism to become diseased if the functioning of these parts were satisfactory. The connexion between disease and wrong functioning should be generally recognized, and it should also be recognized that where specific symptoms of disease have been diagnosed, *the associated wrong functioning is always associated in its turn with undesirable use of the mechanisms of the organism as a whole.* This association has been borne in upon me by my teaching experience, which has taught me that *in the process* of improving the use and functioning of the organism *as a whole* specific symptoms of disease tend to disappear or to be eradicated.

I therefore fully agree with Lord Dawson that "to attempt to treat disease without knowing what is wrong with the body as a whole (not with

[43]The italics are mine. F. M. A.

a part only)" is "admittedly an act of folly." But when he implies that the "carefully organized" medical training of today does give the student this essential knowledge, I join issue with him on the ground that there is nothing in medical training which would enable a member of the medical profession

(1) to detect and diagnose that wrong *habitual* use of the mechanisms which is associated with wrong functioning and therefore with symptoms of disease, and

(2) to follow up his diagnosis by a process of correcting wrong habitual use and building up in its place a satisfactory use of the mechanisms, a process which, because it is always accompanied by improvement in the standard of functioning, invariably tends to the reestablishing of conditions associated with health.

Now it is clear that such a method of diagnosis and treatment differs fundamentally in principle from orthodox medical methods, whereby definite local symptoms are traced back to specific disorders which are diagnosed as the cause of the trouble and then treated specifically. Suppose, for instance, a general practitioner finds symptoms which he diagnoses as due to trouble in some part, or parts, such as the heart, liver, eye, lung or any other, he will either treat the trouble in the specific part or parts himself, or else send the patient on to a specialist who will proceed to prescribe treatment specially adapted to meet the trouble in that specific part or parts.

I admit, of course, that by this method specific symptoms may be and often are eliminated, but since

(1) specific symptoms are never found apart from wrong functioning,

(2) the wrong functioning associated with such symptoms is always, in my experience, associated with wrong use of the mechanisms of the organism,

(3) by such methods nothing will have been done to improve this wrong use,

conditions will be left within the organism which, if allowed to develop unchecked, will tend to lower the standard of functioning generally, and it will then be only a matter of time before the trouble—either the original disorder, or, as frequently happens, some more serious trouble—will manifest itself.

I submit, therefore, that no person who has not been trained, firstly, to detect the wrong use which is associated with wrong functioning, and secondly, to employ a technique evolved to the end of correcting this wrong use, can diagnose "what is wrong with the body as a whole" or treat the body as a working unity, and that since the study of medicine does not include any such training, and no such technique has been employed in the treatment of disease, the methods of training championed by Lord Dawson cannot give medical students the help they need to enable them to diagnose "what is wrong with the body as a whole."

I cannot accept Lord Dawson's analogy between medical training and the training for navigation. How can it be maintained that medical training includes a knowledge of the "human ship sailing on the sea of life," when the medical student is taught nothing about the use of the mechanisms (either in his own case or in that of his patients) upon which the control of the "human ship" depends? Whatever training a navigator may have received in the management and control of his ship, he would be helpless without a reliable compass to determine his direction. If by chance he took a wrong course and on investigation found that his compass had gone wrong, he would not attempt to proceed until he had seen to it that his compass was put right.

This is where the analogy between the training for medicine and the training for navigation seems to me to break down. For sensory appreciation is to the "human ship sailing on the sea of life" what the compass and other such guides are to the navigator's ship; it is the only guide we have to shew us if in our daily activities we are directing the use of our mechanisms to the best advantage. But the medical man, in his work of navigating the "human ship," does not recognize that sensory appreciation is frequently at fault, and so he proceeds on his course attempting to guide the "human ship" without first seeing to it that his compass is reliable. It has never been recognized in medical practice that sensory appreciation, the human compass, has become more and more unreliable with the advance of civilization, and that in proportion there has come about a growing misdirection of the use of the human organism.

Man has been faced with no greater problem than this. For, as we have seen, the nature of a man's reactions to stimuli in general is in accordance with the manner of the use of his mechanisms, and since use cannot be satisfactory without a reliable sensory direction of that use, his reactions to stimuli will be unsatisfactory in proportion as his sensory appreciation is untrustworthy.

I believe that most of us today are more or less in need of help in cultivating that higher standard of sensory appreciation of use which leads to a more satisfactory control of reaction, and this applies no less to the medical man than to the layman. This is borne out by the practical experience of both, who have constant proof in themselves of unreliability of the sensory mechanisms resulting in such unsatisfactory forms of reaction to stimuli as faulty observation and a low standard of awareness in general. For instance, in cases where it is necessary for several medical men to be consulted, there is too often a wide variance of opinion among them, and we have only to read medical evidence in the law courts to find striking examples of differing diagnoses among men who have all undergone the same "carefully organized" medical training. Many medical men, indeed, deplore the fact that in spite of medical training,[44] members of the profession frequently do not possess the equipment upon which successful diagnosis primarily depends.

Everyone will agree that for accuracy and efficiency in diagnosis the medical man needs to possess not only a high standard of sensory observation and awareness, but also the ability to link phenomena together, to form sound judgments and to take a wide outlook, especially in the presence of unfamiliar conditions. To attain these qualities he needs reliability of the sensory mechanisms concerned with the direction of use of the whole organism in daily activity, and the ability to control instinctive reactions to stimuli, especially reactions to the stimulus of the unfamiliar.

It is my belief that this need can be met by the employment of a technique for the building-up of a conscious direction of the use of the mechanisms, for I have found in my practical experience with pupils that in the process of learning to acquire a conscious in the place of an instinctive direction of their use, there comes about a corresponding improvement in their standard of functioning throughout the organism, and in the nature of their reactions generally.

The explanation of this lies in the nature of the process itself. For the fact that the pupil receives from the hands of the teacher the actual sensory experience of the new use which he is consciously directing, ensures for that pupil a gradual cultivation of sensory trustworthiness and awareness, whilst the second fact that the pupil is not able to employ in his daily activities the new use associated with this unfamiliar sensory experience, until he has consciously inhibited his instinctive desire to employ his familiar habitual use, means that he is gradually developing a reasoning control of his instinctive reactions to stimuli, especially his reactions to the stimulus of the unfamiliar.

[44]It will be remembered that the late Sir James Mackenzie, as a result of researches made by him and his collaborators at the St. Andrews Institute of Clinical Research, found that seventy per cent of human ailments are not yet identified. I have also before me, as I write, an article entitled "Doctors' Vain Guesses," in which the Medical Correspondent of *The Times* discusses the protest made by the Ministry of Health against the institution of record cards "on the ground that our knowledge is as yet insufficient to make general records valuable," and in striking confirmation of this view he cites the findings of the late Sir James Mackenzie to which I have referred.

Although this technique is concerned more with education than with treatment, it is one which, as I have tried to shew, should be incorporated with medical training, for if this were done, and the medical student taught how to consciously direct the use of his own mechanisms, he would be developing within himself a satisfactory standard in his sensory appreciation which would stand him in good stead in diagnosing defects in others. But further, in his treatment of these defects, he would no longer be satisfied to employ purely specific treatment for dealing with specific symptoms, for he would have learned from his personal experience that by a process of restoring and maintaining in activity a reasoning direction of the use of his mechanisms, a satisfactory standard in the functioning of the organs and systems is likewise restored and maintained. For reasons of expediency, of course, he might still be forced in certain circumstances and crises to treat a specific trouble directly, but working on the principle of the indivisible unity of the human organism and equipped with the technique based upon it, he could be both what I will call a "generalist"[45] applying this knowledge practically to the requirements of his patient's case, and also an educator, in that he would be called upon to teach his patient to direct and maintain a satisfactory use of himself in all his activities. Basing his teaching and treatment on the principle of unity, he could hardly fail to recognize the connexion between use and functioning which this implies. He would therefore relate any specific defects or symptoms, which he found present in specific organs or parts, to interference in the interworking of the mechanisms generally, and his method of dealing with such specific trouble would be to correct his patient's wrong habitual use of his mechanisms as the means of correcting the specific wrong functioning associated with particular symptoms or defects; at the same time he would teach his patients how to direct and maintain a new and improved use which, *if employed in all his activities*, would be the means of preventing the recurrence of the old or the development of further defects.

In order to illustrate how this has worked out in my experience I will give three examples, the first of which is particularly pertinent here, since most medical men must have had cases of patients who have experienced in the convalescent stage difficulties similar to those which I describe.

Example I

The first is the case of a lady who had a long and serious illness during which she was ordered to remain in bed for several months, and she

[45]The word "generalist" has been coined for me by my friend Dr. Peter Macdonald of York.

underwent a long course of treatment. The time came when she was told that she could begin to get up and try to walk a few steps at a time, and that as the muscles gradually became stronger, she would in time be able to walk properly. She followed this advice, and after a few months she was able to get about a little with the aid of a stick, but only with great difficulty and fatigue, as acute pain developed in her knees and ankles, which became worse when she walked. The doctor, however, encouraged her to go on trying to walk more, "a little more every day." But this she found she could not do, and as time went on, instead of being able to walk further with less difficulty, the reverse was the case, until her condition became such that if she walked at all on one day, she was obliged to rest upon the next. This condition grew gradually worse, but what caused her real anxiety was that certain symptoms of her original illness gave evidence of returning, and she was then persuaded by a friend who knew my work to consult me.

When she came to see me, I recognized that the manner of her habitual use of herself was most harmful, and that in everything she was doing she was using herself in such a way as to bring about harmful pressures. The results of her work with me proved this to be so, for as I was able to bring about an improvement in her manner of use and to teach her how to direct and maintain it consciously, these pressures gradually decreased. At the time of coming to me she was only able to have six lessons as she was going away to the sea, but after having been away for a short time she wrote to me that she was doing her best to carry on the work, and that she was now able to walk the length of the Parade with only occasional intervals of rest. By the end of the summer she could walk up and down stairs with some degree of ease, and had managed three miles at a stretch. On returning to town in the autumn, she began regular work with me and as an improvement in her use was brought about, the pains gradually disappeared and by the end of that winter she was living a normal life and walking with ease and comfort. In the last four years she has had no return of the original symptoms, in spite of the fact that she now includes gardening among her activities.

Example II

This pupil had been treated for months by a well-known specialist in Boston, because he suffered from severe pains in the lower part of his back, particularly when walking, and his pulse and blood pressure were abnormal. He had been given remedial exercises, and an abdominal belt to wear as a support. As this treatment was not successful, an operation had been suggested, but he had not agreed to this and had come to London to consult another specialist. This specialist after making an examination sent him to me as he believed that the change that I could bring about in his general condition would relieve the pressure and muscular rigidity, which, in his opinion, was the cause of the pain.

When he came to see me, I asked him to perform some of his remedial exercises for me, and as I watched him doing them, it was obvious to me that the wrong manner of use which was present in him had been exaggerated by his practice of these exercises. He was employing an undue amount of tension for the simplest acts, and when he walked, this tension was increased to such an extent that it was not surprising that walking even a short distance caused him intense pain.

I decided that this was a case that could be helped by my work, and I proceeded to shew him how to prevent the wrong manner of using himself which he had been taught in these exercises, and at the same time I gave him directions for the new manner of use which, as I brought it about for him, would relieve the pressure and strain of the lower spinal articulations, which was responsible for his pain and which had been aggravated by his practice of the remedial exercises.

After a few days' lessons the pupil felt relief, and he soon decided that he could dispense with the support he had been wearing. At the end of the second week he was able to take short walks without pain, and after an eight weeks' course of lessons, his medical adviser agreed with me that he was in a fit condition to return to America. Ten months later he returned to England and called to see me. He told me that in the interval he had done his best to keep up what I had taught him and that he had been free from the old pain and discomfort, had not needed to wear any support, and that his doctor, after a recent examination, had said that his pulse and blood pressure were now normal.

Example III

My third example is that of a young woman who wished to be enrolled as a student of an Institution for the Training of Teachers, but on being medically examined, had been told that her condition of health was such that she would not be able to stand the strain involved in the work of training. The doctor who examined her said that he could not diagnose anything definitely wrong that would warrant his prescribing medical treatment; what she needed was outdoor life and freedom from duties which called for effort of any kind. The Principal of the Institution, who was acquainted with my work, brought her to see me, when I found that the manner of her general use of herself would account for the lack of stamina that the medical diagnosis indicated. The upper part of her chest was unduly depressed and her thoracic capacity and mobility reduced to the minimum, seriously affecting her circulation. She also told me that she suffered from chilblains on the hands and feet, and the slightest exertion caused fatigue.

I told her that I could enable her to take the Training Course provided that she came to me for lessons at the same time, and the Principal, understanding the reason for this, made this arrangement possible. She started her training and at the same time a course of lessons with me, and the improvement in her manner of use which gradually resulted so improved her standard of general functioning, that she has been able to meet the demands of her training without interruption, and now, at the completion of her course, is able to take up her work as a teacher.

I have been asked whether the technique I advocate is applicable to cases of people who are anxious, not so much to remedy a so-called physical defect, but to overcome or change what they think of as "mental" or "nervous" troubles, including bad habits of all kinds,[46] as they realize that as long as they cannot control these, they are not getting the best out of themselves. My answer is that the fact that these people are unable to make a change within themselves, which they have reasoned out would be a desirable change, shews that their reaction to the stimulus to gain this end is an unsatisfactory reaction, and that this brings their case at once into line with that of the golfer who cannot keep his eyes on the ball when he wishes to, and of the stutterer who cannot speak as he desires.

I will say at once that of course no one could give a general definition of a satisfactory reaction which would meet the particular circumstances of every case, but we shall surely all agree that in cases where people wish to improve themselves, or to make changes which they consider will be for their good, or to overcome defects and bad habits, their reaction may be considered satisfactory when they succeed in doing what they have reasoned out is the right thing for them to do.

This should make it clear that we are not here concerned with fixed standards of value as to what constitutes right or wrong in any particular case. Such standards are relative and more or less individual, for a man's beliefs and acts are largely the outcome of his upbringing and circumstances, and therefore should not be judged by any fixed standard of right and wrong. Acts which are held to be right by one race and at one period are often condemned by other people or at other periods. Circumstances and conditions play a great part in the question, and each case has to be judged on its own merits.

[46]By these I mean such habits as absent-mindedness, forgetfulness, lack of awareness and observation, undue excitability, twitching, plucking at fingers, inability to sit still, nail-biting, over-sensitiveness, uncontrollable temper, inattention, etc.

But where the use of the self is concerned, there is a standard which can generally be accepted, for it can be demonstrated that a certain manner of use of the mechanisms is found in association with a certain satisfactory standard of functioning and with conditions of health and general well-being. We are surely justified in considering a manner of use that is associated with such desirable conditions to be "natural" or "right" under all circumstances. But this is not a fixed standard of "right" in the accepted meaning of the word, for this manner of use being based upon a primary control of the mechanisms of the organism is one that can be applied and adapted to meet all circumstances, and its "rightness" may therefore be said to be relative to these circumstances. Further, the experiences involved in acquiring a knowledge of such "right" and "natural"[47] use of the self gives a person a criterion of judgment to go by, and also an understanding of relative values, for in this process he is constantly brought up against situations in which, after receiving a stimulus, he has to decide what manner of use is the best to employ in reacting to it, and also to judge which of the directions for this manner of use is primary, which secondary, and so on. The standard of relative values that he thus acquires is one that will stand him in good stead in reacting to the stimuli of modern life, in which conditions change so constantly that they cannot be adequately met by any external standard or fixed code as to what is right or wrong. Seeing that the self is the instrument of all his activities, it follows that a valid criterion relating to the use of this self will be a criterion that is valid in relation to all his activities, both so-called "mental" and "physical."

It is the lack of a valid criterion as to what constitutes right use in the sense of "right for the purpose" that renders people unable to carry out their resolutions and to make certain changes for the better in themselves and in their conduct and attitude towards others. Like the golfer and the stutterer, they want to make a change, but bring into play for the purpose the only use of themselves they know, that use, with its associated habits, which we have called throughout this book the "habitual" use of the self, and the fact that, when using themselves in this habitual way they do not succeed in doing what they have reasoned out is the right thing to do, indicates that their habitual use is misdirected and faulty for the purpose. As long as they have no other criterion to go by but that of the familiar *feeling* of their wrong habitual use, the use they employ will be wrong for the purpose, and their reaction to the stimulus to make the desired change will be their instinctive reaction and

---

[47]By "natural" I do not mean usual; indeed, "natural" in this connexion is, as a rule, the very opposite of usual.

therefore directed along the old wrong channel.

To meet this difficulty I would apply to their case the technique which I advocate for the building up of a conscious direction of use, for its employment demands that instinctive reaction be inhibited and superseded by reasoning processes. I have found that *in this process* of acquiring a conscious direction of use my pupils gradually develop a higher standard of sensory awareness or appreciation of what they are doing in the use of themselves, so that when it comes to carrying out a course of activity that they have decided upon, they possess a criterion *within themselves* which will enable them to judge whether the use they are employing is right or not for the purpose. This will constitute a criterion of self-criticism where impressions conveyed through feeling, and leading to further experience, are concerned.

I wish, however, to emphasize here the importance of inhibition in this process, for on account of the habit of end-gaining which is practically universal, such difficulties as we have indicated cannot be permanently overcome unless inhibition is allied to the process of reasoning out the right "means-whereby" and acquiring a higher standard of sensory direction. The reader will remember how, in my own case, my failure to *continue to inhibit*, due to the habit of end-gaining, was *the* obstacle to my employing the new "means-whereby" in reciting, although I had reached the point where I could command these new "means-whereby" in ordinary speaking and knew by experience that they were "right" for my purpose. I have also shewn how the golfer and stutterer of my illustrations, though constantly warned that the habit of end-gaining would be the greatest difficulty they would have to contend against in making the changes in themselves that they desired, were still unable, when the moment came to gain their particular end, to resist the stimulus to gain that end immediately, which meant that they did not continue to inhibit their habitual reaction whilst projecting the directions for the new use, and so reacted by reverting to the wrong habitual use which "felt right."

In both these cases the habit of end-gaining led them into doing the wrong thing, the golfer with the use of his eyes, the stutterer with the use of his tongue, and this in spite of their desire to make certain changes for the better in the use of these organs, and in spite of their having learned how to direct the use of their mechanisms generally in such a way as to make these particular changes possible.

For this reason, all those who wish to change something in themselves must learn to make it a principle of life to inhibit their immediate reaction to any stimulus to gain a desired end, and, in order to give themselves the opportunity of refusing to fall back upon the familiar sensory experiences of their old habitual use in order to gain it, *they must continue this inhibition* whilst they employ the new direction of their use. By adhering to this principle they will find that this conscious direction of their use will gradually come to be associated with a sensory criterion upon which they can rely as a more accurate register of impressions.

All my experience goes to shew that in cases where untrustworthiness of sensory appreciation has led to a general misdirection of the use of the mechanisms and to unsatisfactory conditions of functioning, a particular stimulus may start up a sensory process which registers a reaction which is quite different from the reaction which has actually taken place.

This is a fact that can be demonstrated, and in view of the admittedly unsatisfactory adjustment of human beings to the demands of modern civilization, the most serious symptom of which is, in my opinion, the growing untrustworthiness of the sensory processes, it is of special interest to me to find that Sir Arthur Eddington, in his Lecture on "Science and Religion"[48] issued the following warning:

> "I have been laying great stress on *experience*; in this I am following the dictates of modern physics. But I do not wish to imply that every experience is to be taken at face value. There is such a thing as illusion and we must try not to be deceived. In any attempt to go deeply into the meaning of religious experience we are confronted by the difficult problem of how to detect and eliminate illusion and self-deception. I recognise that the problem exists, but I must excuse myself from attempting a solution. . . . Reasoning is our great ally in the quest for truth. But reasoning can only start from premises; and at the beginning of the argument we must always come back to innate convictions. There are such convictions at the base even of physical science. We are helpless unless we admit also (as perhaps the strongest conviction of all) that we have within us some power of self-criticism to test the validity of our own convictions. The power is not infallible, that is to say, it is not infallible when associated with human frailty. . . ."

When Sir Arthur Eddington says "we must try not to be deceived," I would venture to submit that in the light of the experiences I have set down in this book, just "trying" not to be deceived will not solve the problem he raises. For all "trying" starts from some personal conviction that in some way we shall be able to do what we are trying to do, and this conviction, like conviction on any other point, is made possible only by virtue of impressions received through the agency of our sensory processes. We must therefore see that the validity of this conviction is dependent upon the nature of the functioning of our sensory make-up.

[48]See Reprint *Science and Religion. A Symposium.* (Gerald Howe Ltd. London.)

If this is satisfactory, our sensory register of impressions of what we are doing and experiencing in response to the stimulus to "try" is likely to be a true register; in other words, the reaction we register is likely to be the reaction that is actually taking place. On the other hand, if the functioning of our sensory make-up is unsatisfactory, our register of what is happening in response to the stimulus to "try" is likely to be deceptive, so that the reaction we register is more than likely to be different from the reaction that has actually taken place.

The reader will remember how in my own case (and this applies equally to the golfer and the stutterer) my "trying" to do the thing which I believed was the right thing to do was based upon the conviction that if I knew what the right thing was, I should, by trying, in time be able to do it, and it was only after a prolonged experience of constant failure that I was driven to the discovery that I was not doing the thing I believed I was doing when I was "trying" to do it. This brought me face to face with the fact that my sensory mechanisms were registering impressions which were not the true impressions of what was really happening.

It is therefore clear that the conviction underlying my "trying," being based upon impressions reaching me through the agency of sensory processes that were untrustworthy, was founded upon a delusion, and to make this conviction, as I did, the premise for reasoning that "trying" would in time bring about the end I desired was only paving the way to further self-deception.

I make no apology for laying such stress upon this personal experience, for the sensory make-up of mankind is admittedly gradually becoming more and more untrustworthy.[49] It seems strange to me that although man has thought it necessary in the course of his development

---

[49]We all of us know of occasions when the impression registered within us of some happening has not been an accurate impression of the nature of that happening; how, for instance, our sensory mechanisms can register "cold" when the thermometer registers otherwise, and how a person will take offence and register a remark as a slight or rebuke, when the speaker intended neither and no one else present registered the remark in that sense. Those who are interested in the subject can find in the newspapers daily proof of the registering of false impressions leading to false judgments in all spheres of life.

See also Introduction to *Constructive Conscious Control of the Individual* where Professor John Dewey writes:

> "In all matters that concern the individual self and the conduct of its life, there is a defective and lowered sensory appreciation and judgment, both of ourselves and of our acts which accompanies our wrongly-adjusted psycho-physical mechanisms. It forms our standard of rightness. It influences our every observation, interpretation and judgment. It is the one factor which enters into our every act and thought."

in civilization to cultivate the potentialities of what he calls "mind," "soul" and "body," he has not so far seen the need for maintaining in satisfactory condition the functioning of the sensory processes through which these potentialities manifest themselves. As a result, the functioning of his sensory processes has become so unsatisfactory that the use of his mechanisms is constantly misdirected in his efforts to "do," and when he "tries" to put right the results of this misdirection, he has no other criterion for self-criticism to guide him in these attempts but that of the untrustworthy sensory processes which originally led him into error.

We must therefore see the danger of continuing to base our efforts to help ourselves or other people upon beliefs, judgments and convictions which have their source in sensory experiences, without ascertaining whether the mechanisms through which these experiences are conveyed are functioning satisfactorily.

I venture to suggest that the experiences described in this book throw light upon the way in which the functioning of the sensory mechanisms can be so improved that they will afford a more valid criterion for self-criticism. Those who have had the experience of putting into practice the technique I have described for the building-up of a conscious direction of their use, have found that the process gives them the opportunity for testing continuously the validity of their sensory observations and impressions of what is taking place, because all the time that they are consciously projecting the directions for the new and improved use, they are obliged to go on *being aware* whether or not they are reverting to the old instinctive misdirection of their use which, associated with sensory untrustworthiness, had led them originally to be deceived in what they were doing with themselves. Further, those who continue to make the principle underlying this procedure their guiding principle in all their activities, find that they are enabled to combine "thinking in activity" with a new sensory observation of the use of themselves in the process. This means that they are not only aware when their reaction is not what they feel it is or what they desire, but, having at the same time a reasoned knowledge of the means to a better reaction, they are also able consciously to keep in check the old instinctive reaction that has been the obstacle to their doing what they desire.

If a technique which can be proved to do this for an individual were to be made the basis of an educational plan, so that the growing generation could acquire a more valid criterion for self-judgment than is now possible with the prevailing condition of sensory misdirection of use, might not this lead in time to the substitution of reasoning reactions for those instinctive reactions which are manifested as prejudice, racial and otherwise, herd instinct, undue "self-determination" and rivalry, etc., which, as we all deplore, have so far brought to nought our efforts to realize goodwill to all men and peace upon earth?

THE END

APPENDIX

In fulfilment of my promise in the Preface to this book, there follows a reprint of the Open Letter to Intending Students relating to the Training Course for Teachers, and also a reference to the work being done in the little school. The reader will have realized ere now that in the matter of gaining the experience of using ourselves in a new and unfamiliar way in the performance of acts both familiar and unfamiliar, time is "the essence of the contract." Experience convinced me that children who came for the ordinary half-hour lesson and attended school outside, or spent the rest of the day without being watched from the point of view of carrying on the work in their daily activities, were not getting a fair chance, and I decided that much better results would accrue if these children could be watched and helped by teachers of my work during their school activities.

The actual simple beginning of the little school at 16 Ashley Place came about in this way. In 1924 a little boy was sent home from India because, although highly intelligent, he was so "nervous" and excitable that his parents realized he would not be able to cope with the conditions of ordinary school life, and so sent him for lessons. When he arrived, I found that his use of himself was so unusually bad that it was decided that in addition to his private lessons he must stay each day and be helped to employ the new use of himself that he was learning for his reading, writing and other lessons. Parents of other children who were taking lessons at the time then asked that their children also might have this help give to them, and in this way the little school started. Since that time children and young people of all ages who have been taking private lessons have entered the class in order to get experience in applying the principles and procedures involved in the technique to other activities, remaining for periods ranging from a few weeks to several terms. Naturally the nature of the school work done by the members of the class differs according to their different ages and requirements, but it is all based upon the principle inherent in the technique, namely, that the end for which they are working is of minor importance as compared with the way they direct the use of themselves for the gaining of that end.

In this development of the work I have been fortunate in having the cooperation of my brother, Mr. Albert Redden Alexander, of Miss Ethel Webb and Miss Irene Tasker, M.A., and, later, of Miss E. A. M. Goldie. Miss Tasker had had a wide and varied experience of teaching, both privately and under the Board of Education, before she became a teacher of my technique. She has arranged and conducted the work of the school, since January 1929 with the assistance of Miss Goldie, and the children have had the advantage of help from the whole staff in their private lessons.

We have now had the experience of five months' work of the Training Course for Teachers, and during this first session we have aimed at correlating the individual work of the students, usually done in private lessons, with the group work necessary to give them the experience required for the making of teachers. To this end the students work for some hours daily under the supervision of a teacher, and they devote the rest of the day to the continuance of this class work, helping one another and aiming always at strict adherence to the principle underlying the technique. The results so far attained in this way justify us in believing that at the end of eighteen months' training these students will be able to help in the little school by working with the children under supervision. This would make it possible to give more individual attention to the children, thus enabling them to make greater progress in a given time.

In the Open Letter which follows the reader will find a reference to a scheme for the development of a larger school in the future, together with details of the Training Course.

OPEN LETTER TO INTENDING STUDENTS OF TRAINING COURSE

16 Ashley Place,
London, S.W.1.

For many years past I have devoted much time and thought to the working out of satisfactory means whereby students can be trained to impart the technique set down in my books "Man's Supreme Inheritance" and "Constructive Conscious Control of the Individual," and in working for this end I have been greatly stimulated by the support given by the members of the medical and other professions who have come to me as pupils. I have hesitated, however, before making definite plans for the practical carrying out of this idea, chiefly,

(1) Because I thought it advisable to be able first to publish the opinion of those most competent to judge whether I am justified in my conviction that I should teach people to carry on in my work.

(2) Because the difficulties which I encountered in my attempts to provide possible students with the material for gaining the necessary practical experience in teaching were for a time insurmountable.

(3) Because I wished to be as certain as possible that at the conclusion of the first course of training there would be a demand for teachers of my work.

With regard to (1) I am now able to quote the following educational and medical authorities who have had the opportunity of observing my work and of testing the value of the principle on which it is based, and whose support has finally decided me to start a course for the training of teachers.

Professor John Dewey (Gifford Lecturer, 1929).
The Earl of Lytton, P.C., G.C.S.I., G.C.I.E.
Sir Lynden Macassey, K.B.E., K.C.
Miss E. E. Lawrence (Principal of The Froebel Institute).
Miss Lucy Silcox, Class. Trip. Camb. (Headmistress of St. Felix School, Southwold, from January, 1909, to July, 1926).
A.G. Pite, M.C., M.A. (Headmaster, Weymouth College, Dorset).
A. J. D. Cameron, M.B.
Mungo Douglas, M.B.
Percy Jakins, M.D., M.R.C.S.
Peter Macdonald, M.D.
R. G. McGowan, M.D., D.P.H.
A. Murdoch, M.B.
A. Rugg-Gunn, M.B., F.R.C.S.

From Professor John Dewey (Gifford Lecturer, 1929). Quotation from Introduction to *Constructive Conscious Control of the Individual*, pp. 224-225.

"After studying over a period of years Mr. Alexander's method in actual operation, I would stake myself upon the fact that he has applied to our ideas and beliefs about ourselves and about our acts exactly the same method of experimentation and production of new sensory observations, as tests and means of developing thought, that have been the source of all progress in the physical sciences; . . . Mr. Alexander has found a method for detecting precisely the correlations between the two members, physical-mental, of the same whole, and for creating a new sensory consciousness of new attitudes and habits. It is a discovery which makes whole all scientific discoveries, and renders them available, not for our undoing, but for human use in promoting our constructive growth and happiness. . . . The discovery could not have been made and the method of procedure perfected except by dealing with adults who were badly coordinated. But the method is not one of remedy; it is one of constructive education. Its proper field of application is with the young, with the growing generation, in order that they may come to possess as early as possible in life a correct standard of sensory appreciation and self-judgment. When once a reasonably adequate part of a new generation has become properly coordinated, we shall have assurance for the first time that men and women in the future will be able to stand on their own feet, equipped with satisfactory psycho-physical equilibrium, to meet with readiness, confidence and happiness instead of with fear, confusion and discontent, the buffetings and contingencies of their surroundings."

Knebworth House,
Knebworth.
March 22nd, 1930.

Dear Mr. Alexander,

I am delighted to hear that the scheme for the training of students in your work has materialised. You know how anxious I have been that your valuable work for the welfare of mankind should be carried on. The experience you have gained and the technique you have evolved are far too valuable to be lost. There must be thousands who like myself have benefited by your help, but we can do no more than tell others of our good fortune; we cannot pass on to them the benefits we have received. If you can train others to practise your technique and thus found a school for the training of teachers of your work it will be a great service to humanity.

I wish your new venture all success.

Yours sincerely,
LYTTON.

27, Abingdon Street,
London, S.W.1.
5th April, 1930.

Dear Mr. Alexander,

It is with the greatest satisfaction that I learn that there is now a definite prospect of arrangements being made for the training of Teachers to acquire and apply your technique and so ensure that your methods will be preserved and perpetuated. It would, in my view, be a calamity if such arrangements were not to be made.

Nothing is required to convince me of the essential value of your work. The beneficial results it has achieved in the cases of the persons known to me, who had exhausted all other advice and remedial treatment, are so outstanding as to carry conviction to the mind of anyone who will take the trouble to investigate what you are doing and see what your methods can accomplish.

I am convinced that it is of the greatest public importance that your methods shall be made known and available to the public as widely as possible.

Yours sincerely,
LYNDEN MACASSEY.

16th April, 1930.

Dear Mr. Alexander,

We are delighted to hear that you have decided to train students in the science and art of your educational work.

From our personal experience of your work and our knowledge of the enormous benefits you have given to both children and adults we think it a matter of supreme importance that an attempt should be made to train students in the handing-on of your own technique.

Simple and fundamental as it is, it is at the same time unlike anything we have come across in our educational experience and we feel it impossible to measure the good that will come from it.

Yours sincerely,
ESTHER E. LAWRENCE,
LUCY SILCOX,
A. G. PITE.

May 8th, 1930.

Dear Mr. Alexander,

May we express how pleased we are to learn that you have decided to undertake the training of pupils in the technique which you have discovered, elaborated, and practised for many years, and in the important principles on which it is based? As medical men we, more than most people, are conscious of the difficulties involved in the undertaking. We realise that the technique you have to impart, being at one and the same time a very advanced craft and a very subtle philosophy, demands special qualities of mind and a certain natural aptitude of body to practise it with success. We rejoice, therefore, that you are now confident that these difficulties can be overcome. As practitioners of medicine we know also how great is the need for its resources at the present time, when the strain of existence exacts such a toll even on the healthy. We believe, from practical acquaintance of its effects on ourselves and our patients, that it is adequate to meet that need, if only because it teaches that satisfactory use of the self which is the basis of physical and mental happiness.

We wish the extension of your valuable work every success and beg to proffer, in so far as we may, our willing cooperation.

Yours sincerely,

A. J. D. CAMERON, M.B.
MUNGO DOUGLAS, M.B.
PERCY JAKINS, M.D., M.R.C.S.
PETER MACDONALD, M.D.
R. G. MCGOWAN, M.D., D.P.H.
A. MURDOCH, M.B.
A. RUGG-GUNN, M.B., F.R.C.S.

With regard to (2) I am now satisfied that I can provide my students with the material for getting practical experience in teaching by combining the work of the Teachers' Training School with that of the little school for children and young people which has gradually been developed in connection with my work. In this school children of all ages are taught how to apply the principles and procedures of my work whilst engaged in the usual school activities, and I am confident that the experience to be gained by combining the work of the students with the work of these children can be of the greatest benefit to all concerned.

With regard to (3) the applications which have come to me from medical men and from those anxious to make use of the work in the field of education and medicine justify me in believing that the demand for teachers is growing rapidly and that it will probably exceed the supply when we reach the end of the three years' training course (1933). To shew how wide a field is opening out for teachers of my work I may mention that during the past 26 years pupils have come to me, not only from all parts of the British Isles and Ireland, but from several European countries, from Australia, New Zealand, Canada, South Africa, South America, Egypt, India, and the United States of America.[50] The enquiries from people who have subsequently taken lessons represent, however, a com-

[50]New York, Massachusetts, Connecticut, New Jersey, Pennsylvania, Ohio, Georgia, Alabama, South Carolina, Illinois, Minnesota, Nebraska, California.

paratively small proportion of those received from people who are unable to come to London and are anxious to find a teacher of my work nearer their home.

For the benefit of those who have not read my books I must point out that would-be teachers of my work must be trained to put the principles and procedures of its technique into practice in the use of themselves in their daily activities before they attempt to teach others to do likewise. Herein lies the difference between the proposed training and all other forms of training. For students may take courses of training in medicine, physiology, theology, law, philosophy or anything else without the matter of the use of themselves being called into question. But in the training for this teaching a considerable amount of work must be done on the students individually so that they may learn to use themselves satisfactorily, and it is only when they have reached a given standard in the use of themselves that they will be given the opportunity for practical teaching experience.

But in addition to this individual work, class work will be necessary, and for this part of the work the classes will be confined to five or six students working together with experienced teachers. When students are working together, however, opportunity will be give to one of the class (a different one each day) to assume the role of guide or adviser during part of the day's work.

Already two substantial donations have been promised towards the formation of a Trust Fund for the establishment in the future of a school in which the teaching posts will be filled by those who are competent to teach in accordance with the technique outlined in my books. The Earl of Lytton, Sir Lynden Macassey and Dr. Peter Macdonald have consented to become Trustees of this Trust Fund, and also Members of a Society which is being formed to extend in every way the scope of the work.

Particulars of fees for the Training Course, and dates of sessions, etc., can be obtained from

THE SECRETARY,
F. MATTHIAS ALEXANDER TRAINING COURSE,
16 Ashley Place,
London, S.W.1.

F. Matthias Alexander
22nd July, 1930.

APPENDIX

Wide Bearing of the Work

The possibilities that open out for the application of the work in widely differing fields will be seen by reference to the following:

In Education

Discussion in *The Times Educational Supplement* (May 12th to July 14th, 1928).

Letters from
The Earl of Lytton,
Miss E. E. Lawrence (Principal of The Froebel Institute),
Miss D. L. Beck, M.A. (Headmistress of the County School for Girls, Ealing).
J. E. R. McDonagh, F.R.C.S. (Author of *The Nature of Disease*).

Introduction by John Dewey to *Constructive Conscious Control of the Individual.*

In Medicine

The Nature of Disease by J. E. R. McDonagh, F.R.C.S. (Heinemann, pp. 44, 54 and 110).

Instinct and Functioning in Health and Disease by Peter Macdonald, M.D., President of the Yorkshire Branch of the British Medical Association (*British Medical Journal,* Dec. 25th, 1926).

Function and Posture (*British Medical Journal,* Oct. and Nov. 1928).

Letters from
Peter Macdonald, M.D.,
R. G. McGowan, M.D., D.P.H.,
Macleod Yearsley, F.R.C.S.,
A. Murdoch, M.B.

In Philosophy

Human Nature and Conduct by John Dewey (Henry Holt, pp. 27-36).

Experience and Nature by John Dewey (Open Court Publishing Co., pp. 296-7).

In Psychology

Survey of Modern Psychology by Arthur J. Busch (*The Brooklyn Citizen*, Jan. 27th. 1929).

Psychology in Vacuo by Capt. C. H. Douglas (*The New Age*, Oct. 4th,1928).

Man: An Indictment by Anthony M. Ludovici (Constable & Co., pp. 309-15, 351-7).

IN PHYSICAL CULTURE

Swedish Gymnastic Teaching by Lucy Silcos, Class. Trip. Camb. (*Journal of School of Hygiene and Physical Education*, March, 1927).

Report on Physical Culture by Alexander Leeper, M.A., LL.D. (Melbourne University), as printed by Teachers and School Registration Board, March 8th, 1909.

IN VOICE CULTURE

See Above Report.

IN SPORT

The Fearful Foozler by Sir E. Holderness, Bt. (*Evening Standard*, March 17th, 1928).

Conscious Control in Golf by John Duncan Dunn, Author of A. B. C. of Golf (*The Golfer's Magazine*, March, 1920).

Copies of extracts from the above will be sent on application to the Secretary.

At the date of going to press the first payments to the Trust Fund have been made by the generous donors and we have the promise of future support from others. I should like to state here that those who are now supporting my work so generously have watched it in actual practice for many years, and have themselves a practical understanding of the principles and procedures involved in the technique. I wish to offer them here my renewed thanks, and also the thanks of my assistants, for their interest and generosity which has opened up possibilities for the development of the educational side of the work in the future that, otherwise, would have been unlikely to occur.

F. M. A.

INDEX

THE UNIVERSAL CONSTANT IN LIVING

With an Appreciation by
PROFESSOR G. E. COGHILL
AUTHOR OF *ANATOMY AND THE PROBLEM OF BEHAVIOUR*

DEDICATED

To the Peoples of the British Empire Whose Understanding of, and Faith in, the Principles of Liberty and Loyalty, and Whose Confidence in Their Own Strength As Defenders of Their Faith, Enabled Them, Alone and Unaided, to Check the Mad Onrush of Mechanized Means of Destruction which, if Unchecked, Would Have Made It Possible for Evil Forces to Overrun the Whole World and to Enslave the Peoples Living in It

A THANKS OFFERING

I WISH to take this opportunity to offer my thanks to the medical men whose names appear under the letter reprinted from the *British Medical Journal* on page 530, and particularly to Drs. Peter Macdonald, Andrew Murdoch and Mungo Douglas for their letters which have appeared from time to time in the *British Medical Journal*; to Drs. J. R. Caldwell, Adam Moss, C. A. Ensor, J. E. R. McDonagh, F.R.C.S., Professors John Dewey and G. E. Coghill, Mr. Aldous Huxley, Dr. Trigant Burrow, Mr. T. G. N. Haldane, and Mr. Eynon Smith for their courteous and valuable appreciations included in these pages; to A. Rugg-Gunn, F.R.C.S. for his article, "F. Matthias Alexander and the Problem of Animal Behaviour" in the *Medical Press and Circular* of April 3, 1940; to President Thos. B. Hall, M.Sc., of the South African Chemical Institute for his appreciative reference to my work in his Presidential Address, "Some Accomplishments of the Chemist"; to Mr. Michael March for his series of illuminating articles in the *Brooklyn Citizen*, one of which drew from Professor G. E. Coghill a eulogy of which he may well be proud; to Professor John Hilton for his broadcasts and for his Address "The New Generation of Workers"; to Miss Lucy Silcox for the excerpts from her paper "Swedish Gymnastic Teaching" in the *Journal of School Hygiene and Physical Education* of March 1927; to Mrs. Alma Frank for her contribution on page 631; to Mr. Aaron Sussman for his help in so many ways; to Dr. Peter Macdonald, Mr. Arthur J. Busch, and Miss Mary Olcott for their suggestions after reading the MS.; to Miss Mary Olcott and Miss Edith Lawson for their help in the correction of proofs; and to Mr. Anthony M. Ludovici, Miss Irene Tasker, Miss Ethel Webb and Mr. Walter Carrington for their help in preparing the subject matter for publication. I must record special thanks to Miss Ethel Webb who has been intimately connected with the work since 1911, consistently rendering most valuable help and encouragement to all engaged in the work at 16 Ashley Place whether as pupils or students. I am particularly indebted to her for the patience and perseverance which has characterized her invaluable help in making the subject matter as clear as possible, in fact, without her help I fear these pages would not be ready for the printers today. I am grateful to Dr. John Dewey for his kind permission to quote from his *Educational Essays*, to Messrs. Harper & Brothers for permission to quote from *Ends and Means* by Aldous Huxley and *Man the Unknown* by Dr. Alexis Carrel, and to Messrs. Macmillan & Co. and The Cambridge University Press for permission to quote from *Man on His Nature* and *The Brain and Its Mechanism* by Sir Charles Sherrington.

I also thank the far-seeing lady—her name is withheld at her request—whose generous gift to the Trust Fund made possible the carrying on of the school at Penhill, Kent, England (now, because of the War, being carried on in this country at The Whitney Homestead, Stow, Mass., through the kindness of the American Unitarian Association); Miss Margaret Goldie who is in charge of the school, for her patient devotion to the arduous task of dealing with the problems set in education by the employment of a new technique, and for the progress made towards the solution of them through her loyalty to the underlying principle of the technique; my assistants Misses Irene Stewart, Marjory Mechin (now Mrs. William Barlow), Erica Webb (now Mrs. Duncan Whittaker), Gurney MacInnes, Richard Walker, Walter Carrington, and Patrick Macdonald (these latter now serving with H. M. Forces) who have helped in the school and given such valuable support on the practical side of the work we are interested in; Miss Lulie Westfeldt for her work in New York and in the South; Miss Marjorie L. Barstow for her work in Boston and in the West; Miss Irene Tasker who has been teaching for some years in Johannesburg, South Africa, and built up a large connexion there; and my brother, Albert Redden Alexander, who has done so much to increase interest in the work in New York and Boston during the last six years, and who will carry on the school and Training Course for Teachers in this country when I return to England after the War.

HOTEL BRAEMORE
COMMONWEALTH AVENUE
BOSTON, MASS.

CONTENTS

Part II Procedures Involved in the Technique —First Principles in the Control of Human Reaction

Definition of Habit—Link between habit and unity of working in human organism—Why the breaking of even simple habits is so difficult—Established habits of use and unreliable feeling—Habitual response and inhibition—Difference between "being right" and "feeling right"—"Feeling wrong" and the "unknown"—Visualizing and self-hypnotic deception—Why real change must be a gradual process—Procedures of new technique analyzed—The vicious circle in "doing"—When trying to be "right" is the direct way to failure—"Doing one's best" and a "dagger of the mind"—Inhibition and reconditioning—Unity of thinking—Sir Charles Sherrington—Indirect method of control—Forgetting to remember—Need for new memory—Why posture visualized as "right" one day will not be the posture associated with future change and improvement—Why the technique is primarily one for the development and control of human reaction.

Part III The Fundamental Approach

Instances to show connexion between use and reaction—Differing manifestations but same processes at work—Postural peculiarities, "mental" and facial expression, etc.—Recapitulation of points dealt with in earlier books—Why new reforming methods have left unsolved the matter of the control of human reaction—Misdirection and the "automatic" working of guidance and control—What decision is required of us before fundamental change can take place—Difficulty in carrying out decisions involving guidance and control of the self during the employment of procedures which is not in line with previous experience in thought and action—Intellectual acceptance of belief and sensory confidence—Unfamiliar means and taking a risk—A unique situation in which man finds himself in carrying out any method of education, training or scheme of living—In what does provision for change consist?—What is implied by the acceptance of a new idea—"Wishing" and "willing" and how to "do" the "doing"—The nature and value of judgment and man's attitude towards dependence upon "physical," "mental" and "spiritual" help—Repression and harmful by-products—Habit and manner of use—The indirect approach in changing habit—New and unfamiliar experiences and unfamiliar procedures—The practical application of concepts and what this involves—A suggestion to those interested in plans for individual and social reform—Specific changes and harmful by-products—Need for providing opportunity to prevent such by-products—Results of man's "willing" and "wishing" and the trial-and-error method—Unreliability of sensory appreciation and judgment as regards judgment of results—Self-suppression and habitual use—Mr. Aldous Huxley—Decision and new experiences of use—Withholding action or non-doing in the fundamental sense.

PHOTOGRAPHS

APPRECIATION

The Educational Methods of F. Matthias Alexander

by

G. E. COGHILL

THE practice of Mr. F. Matthias Alexander in treating the human body is founded, as I understand it, on three well-established biological principles, 1) that of the integration of the whole organism in the performance of particular functions, 2) that of proprioceptive sensitivity as a factor in determining posture, 3) that of the primary importance of posture in determining muscular action. These principles I have established through forty years of anatomical and physiological study of Amblystoma of embryonic and larval stages, and they appear to hold for other vertebrates as well.

In order to make this discussion clear, definitions of certain terms are necessary. Normally, as regards somatic (general bodily) motor function, the organism exists in a condition of mobility or immobility—either as mobilized or as immobilized. The latter condition is illustrated by sleep. In deep sleep the individual is mobilized in regard to its visceral, circular and respiratory functions and the like, but it is immobilized with reference to bodily movement. Reflexes occur, to be sure, to local stimuli, but as an individual the body as a whole does nothing for its own sake. Somnambulism, as a general bodily activity, occurs during periods of imperfect sleep or partial wakefulness. In the condition of immobility the individual may be thought of as in repose. In mobility, on the other hand, the whole individual is mobilized (integrated), or in action as a unit according to a definite pattern. Under these circumstances the organism is in one of two phases of action, posture or movement. Posture is relatively static in so far as the individual as a whole is concerned; movement is transition through space for the organism or its parts. In posture the individual is mobilized for a definite movement in which the energy mobilized in posture is released in a definite pattern of activity. Of course these differences are relative, and one phase passes over imperceptibly into the other, but in their typical manifestations they are clearly differentiated. Likewise the distinction between mobility and immobility is relative, and no absolute distinction can be made between them, but the distinction is useful if not necessary for a clear understanding of physiological principles. It seems reasonable, therefore, to propose that in posture the individual is mobilized (integrated) for movement according to a definite pattern and in movement that pattern is being executed. In posture the individual is as truly active as in movement.

Another term that may need explanation is "proprioceptive," which applies to sensory nerves that serve the muscles, tendons and joints, and the middle ear (vestibular apparatus) and its nerves. The proprioceptive system has nothing to do with local or cutaneous sensation.

Mr. Alexander has found these same principles operative also in man. His work is concerned with the nature of the influence of the working of the psycho-physical mechanisms upon the general functioning of the human organism (posture), and his technique was evolved as an aid in maintaining the general conditions best suited to this working in those in whom they already exist, and in changing and improving them when this working can be shown to be harmful. He has further demonstrated the very important psychological principle that the proprioceptive system can be brought under conscious control, and can be educated to carry to the motor centers the stimulus which is responsible for the muscular activity which brings about the manner of working (use) of the mechanism of correct posture. Of course the time required for this education could be greatly lessened through the assistance of a competent teacher.

To understand the first biological principle mentioned, the relation of the part to the whole, it is necessary to know this relation in the development of behavior, which I have investigated for many years. My studies have been both anatomical and physiological, those of the one method corroborating, supplementing and extending those of the other. For these investigations I used a species of Amblystoma, a type of vertebrate that is well known for its lack of specialization of structure and function and in which movement can be observed under controlled conditions from the first. Like the other Amphibia, it is both terrestrial and aquatic so that the development of locomotion by both swimming and walking can be studied.

In these animals at the time muscular contraction begins the whole functional muscular system is organized as to longitudinal bilateral series of segment, the myotomes. At that time there are no appendages other than relatively homogeneous buds composed of undifferentiated tissue covered with skin. These are not functional organs, and will not be for a relatively long time after the motility of the trunk musculature begins. When the axial muscles begin to contract their contraction proceeds from the head tailward (cephalocaudal). If the stimulus is adequate the whole animal responds as a total reaction. There is never a partial response in the sense of a local reaction except in the anterior end where contraction of a few myotomes may occur in case the stimulus is not adequate to stimulate the entire system, for the organization is such that a stimulus arising anywhere on the trunk or tail must travel headward in the dorsal part of the spinal cord in order to reach the motor centers. Also the motor neurones are integrating neurones of the axial muscles, that is to say, they are at the same time longitudinal conductors in the spinal cord and motor nerves, innervating the muscles simply by means of collaterals (side branches of the axones). These collaterals grow out into the limbs and establish a functional connection with the muscles of the limbs so that the earliest movements of the limbs are performed only as the trunk moves. The limbs are therefore primarily integrated with the trunk, and local reflexes do not occur. These are made possible through another type of neurones, which arise from a different source in the spinal cord from the integrating neurones that give rise to the primary motor fibers. There are, therefore, two possible functions of the limbs: a primary one wholly and always integrated with the trunk, and a secondary one in response to local stimuli. The first gives rise to total reactions and the latter elicits reflexes, and reflexes as partial pattern are normally always subject to the total pattern.

In the course of development of behavior of Amblystoma the earliest partial reactions are postural. If, for example, one can succeed in rolling the animal over from the upright to the supine position by means of a bristle without exciting it to other action, one leg will be elevated and the opposite one depressed in the turning process. The movement has the appearance of a local reaction (partial pattern) but it is not in response to a local stimulus from the skin. It is in response to stimuli arising in the proprioceptive system. There are two possible sources of proprioceptive stimulation. In the first place there are sensory endings in the axial muscles of the earliest reaction stages, and the forced torsion of the axial muscles would stimulate these proprioceptive nerves and they could stimulate the elevation and depression of the limbs. As a second possibility the vestibular system of the ear is sufficiently developed to be functional at this stage of development, and long fibers from the vestibular centers in the brain travel far down the spinal cord and into the motor centers that innervate the limbs. Whether one or both of these sensory systems are responsible for these postural reactions of the limbs it is the animal as a whole that stimulates the response. The earliest postural reactions of the limbs, therefore, is a total reaction, and the sensory factor is in the proprioceptive system. The stimuli arise wholly within the organism.

In the development of Amblystoma I have observed, also, that an appropriate posture is assumed at intervals for an appreciable time before the particular muscular pattern is geared to action. This occurs in the development of swimming, of walking and of feeding. Posture, therefore, is a forerunner of action and must be regarded as basic to it.

These are the simple rudiments of movement which Mr. Alexander calls into play by his methods of reeducation. For he is pre-eminently an educator. He seeks to restore the functions of the body through their natural uses. His methods of doing this are original and unique, based, as they are, on many years of experience and exhaustive study. Yet they can scarcely be adequately described, although the results are marvelous.

One ordinarily considers that rising from a sitting position in a chair to a standing position is a simple process perfectly understood by every adult. But this pattern of behavior is not natural. It was introduced into our behavior very late in our racial development with the invention of the chair, the most atrocious institution hygienically of civilized life. Primitively man sat on the ground or squatted when not standing. Primitive man does so still, and the ease and apparent comfort of the squatting position is witnessed among the less privileged classes, who rest in that position for long periods. This posture requires extreme stretching of the extensor muscles of the legs and abduction of the thighs. Habitual use of the chair, on the other hand, prevents this stretching of the extensor muscles and tends to produce adduction of the thighs, even to the extreme of crossing one leg over the other. This unnatural posture tends to stimulate reflex responses which antagonize the normal total pattern of rising to a standing position.

That this is more than theory Mr. Alexander demonstrated to me in lessons which he kindly gave me. He enabled me to prevent misdirection of the muscles of my neck and back and to bring about a use of these muscles that determined the relative position of my head and neck to my body and so on to my limbs, bringing my thighs into the abducted position. This led to changes in the muscular and other conditions throughout my body and limbs associated with a pattern of behavior more natural (in agreement with the total pattern) for the act of getting on my feet. The whole procedure was calculated to occupy my brain with the projection of directive messages that would enable me to acquire conscious control of the proprioceptive component of the reflex mechanism involved. The projection of the directed messages, Mr. Alexander considers, stimulated nervous and motor activity that was associated with better conditions. This leads to the belief that the motor paths of the spinal cord and the nerve paths through the brain associated with the total pattern were again being used.

In my study of the development of locomotion I have found that in vertebrates the locomotor function involves two patterns: a total pattern which establishes the gait; and partial patterns (reflexes) which act with reference to the surface on which locomotion occurs. The sloth, for instance, has the same total pattern (gait) of walking that the dog has but employs a wholly different partial pattern (reflexes) for he supports himself in suspension with his flexor muscles. Now the reflexes may be, and naturally are, in harmony with the total pattern, in which case they facilitate the mechanism of the total pattern (gait), or they by force of habit become more or less antagonistic to it. In the latter case they make for inefficiency in locomotion. In myself, for example, when I have given attention to details of walking, I have experienced flexion of my toes as if they were trying to grasp the soles of my shoes. This I regard as a reflex brought about by habitual incorrect posture, and antagonistic to the natural gait which my toes, nevertheless, were trying to reinforce.

It is my opinion that habitual use of improper reflex mechanism in sitting, standing, and walking introduces conflict in the nervous system, and that this conflict is the cause of fatigue and nervous strain which bring many ills in their train. Mr. Alexander, by relieving this conflict between the total pattern which is hereditary and innate, and the reflex mechanisms which are individually cultivated, conserves the energies of the nervous system and by so doing corrects not only postural difficulties but also many other pathological conditions that are not ordinarily recognized as postural. This is a corrective principle that the individual learns for himself and is the work of the self as a whole. It is not a system of physical culture which involves only one system of organs for better or for worse of the economy of the whole organism. Mr. Alexander's method lays hold of the individual as a whole, as a self-vitalizing agent. He reconditions and reeducates the reflex mechanisms and brings their habits into normal relation with the functions of organisms as a whole. I regard his methods as thoroughly scientific and educationally sound.

PREFACE

THE reader of the pages of this and my other books will know that I have been consistently concerned with the nature of human reaction in its bearing upon individual and mass activity, for my experience justifies me in asserting that the nature of a person's manner of reacting at a given time determines the nature of his behaviour.

Is it not natural then that at this moment of publishing a new book, I am thinking of the possible reaction of my readers towards the evidence that I have to place before them? In dealing with my subject criticism is unavoidable, but in justification I would point out that in my case it is solely to the end of attempting to help to a better understanding of the constructive plan that I am offering.

A friend of mine once complained that on a particular occasion the remarks of a relative upon the nature of his behaviour was prefaced by a snort, and his attitude interested me because it became evident that his reaction of resentment was a response to the stimulus arising from the snort, rather than from the remarks of disapproval. I desire to preface my subject matter but I have a still greater desire that the manner of this prefacing will not be likely to lead to a snort, or to any accompaniment that would be the forerunner of an impeding reaction on the part of my readers while studying the contents of this book. The subject matter is the outcome of unique experiences during the past eight years in the field of human behaviour, and the book, like Topsy, has "just growed." Should any readers be disappointed that it has not been built to any definite plan, I would remind them that in view of the nature of the subject matter and its source of origin, the limitations that are inherent in a book made to plan have been sidetracked. I am also anxious to address a few words to them on the why and the wherefore of the matter of short and long sentences.

With the help of friends I have given much time to attempts to clarify and simplify what I have written, and, as sidelights on this difficult task, I will quote the remarks of two men after reading my earlier books, one of whom was eminent in the profession of letters and the other in science. The one said he found my sentences involved, but that after further consideration he concluded that this was inherent in the nature of the subject matter. The other pointed out that a particular sentence was too long, but later admitted that he had spent a couple of hours in trying to shorten it or divide it into one or two sentences, but found that when he had succeeded in doing this he was not expressing the full meaning that the sentence conveyed in the original form.

It is comparatively simple to express some idea or experience in a short sentence or in several short sentences if the idea or experience represents something specific, or something that can be done or gained by the *direct method*, for this involves the concept of separation and disconnectedness. But ideas or experiences concerned with unified phenomena and which involve the *indirect method* for general, instead of specific, application can only be fully expressed by a sentence that conveys the meaning of such ideas and experiences so that there can be no doubt that the concept on which they are based is that of a coordinated indivisible whole.

Necessity, we are told, is the mother of invention, and I think my readers may be interested in an experience I had on an occasion when I was brought face to face with the need for solving this problem of reaction. I was officially invited to lecture to the students and teachers of two of the most important Training Schools for Physical Culture in England. In reply to these invitations I made it known that my early experience on the lecture platform had convinced me that lecturing is a waste of time when the lecturer has to advocate procedures with which his listeners are bound to disagree because these are based upon a principle which, if accepted, would demand the giving up of established beliefs. Some of my friends, however, were very anxious that I should give these lectures, so I did not refuse at once but agreed to reconsider the matter and write again later.

On thinking it over it occurred to me that to have any chance of success I must find some way of checking any tendency in my listeners to react too quickly (as we are unfortunately so liable to do) to the stimulus of any statement which happened to be in disagreement with their cherished beliefs and adopted practice. Here I believed that I had come upon means that were worth a trial, and in consequence I wrote to accept both invitations.

The eventful evening arrived. After being introduced to my listeners in the usual way, I told them that I had come there under "false pretences," as it were, because of the reasons I had already given them for hesitating to accept their invitation to speak, but that I believed I was justified in coming, because I was satisfied that I had thought of a means whereby my talk to them could be given, without its leading to any reaction either on their part or mine which would prevent our talk from being beneficial to all concerned.

To this end I began by assuring them that I had not any wish to criticize their beliefs or their methods, and that I assumed their attitude towards my beliefs and work would be the same. I suggested, therefore, that we should join together to apply the test of principle to the beliefs and methods of physical culturists of the past and present, in order to arrive at a sound estimate of their value. There was a pause, my listeners glanced at one another, looked back towards me and eventually there came as a response the word, "Yes."

With a growing confidence in my means, I went on to say my say. There was of course destructive criticism in it, but this was greatly overbalanced by what many of my listeners told me personally they appreciated as being constructive and of great value to them, and at the second lecture I used the same "means-whereby" with the same pleasing result.

I now ask my readers before passing judgment on the experiences described in these pages to apply the test of principle to any evidence emerging from my practice which may chance to conflict with their beliefs in practice or theory, or which runs counter to their individual interests. Then if it is found that this evidence is based upon the same principle as that underlying the practice which it is intended to supersede, judgment should be given against the practice and the evidence discredited. But if the opposite is found to be the case, then the evidence should be put to a practical test by observing the nature of the working of the mechanisms of the psycho-physical organism during the consistent application of the procedures of my practice, and if this working leads to the *raising of the standard of general functioning*, judgment must be given in favour of the practice.

16 Ashley Place,
Westminster, London.
April 1941.

INTRODUCTORY

WHEN my last book *The Use of the Self* was finished, I consoled myself with the thought that I would not need to write another on the subject of my practice and theory, because a detailed description of the evolution of my technique and its application to different fields of activity was then to be found in my books. Obviously such a description was not as full as one could wish, because any change in manner of use of the self, however brought about, is associated with unfamiliar sensory experiences and, as is well known, knowledge concerned with sensory experiences cannot be conveyed by the spoken or written word in such a way as to convey the full meaning to the reader.

This serves to explain why, in spite of the frequency with which I have stressed in my previous books the concept of the indissoluble *unity* of the human organism, some readers still adhere to the concept of *separation* in interpreting what I have written, as if the procedures of my technique and their results in practice could be labelled separately "physical" or "mental." Objective evidence of the dependence of thought and action upon the unified working or interaction of "physical" and "mental" mechanisms and processes is to be found in the first chapter of *The Use of the Self*, and my experience has convinced me that these are manifestations of unified human activity which show at certain stages a preponderance of what is called "physical," and at other stages a preponderance of what is called "mental."[1]

Another source of misunderstanding has arisen through my choice of words for which I have often been criticized. While I do not hold a brief for myself in this regard, I have persistently avoided using words which are labels for ideas and "systems" which I am convinced are fundamentally unsound, and I am able to state that when reasons for such criticism have been given to me, I have always found in my critics a tendency to read into other people's words meanings which fitted in with a particular construction that they were accustomed to put upon them, and I suggest that the habit and the misunderstanding are closely con-

[1] Cf. *Constructive Conscious Control of the Individual*, F. M. Alexander. Page 228.

nected. If the reader will remember that the subject of my study has been, and is, the living psycho-physical organism, which is the sum of a complex of unified processes, he will understand why I refrain as far as is possible from using such terms as "postures," "mental states," "psychological complexes," "body mechanics," "subconscious," or any of the thousand and one labelled concepts, which have, like barnacles, become attached to the complicated idea we have of ourselves owing to the kind of education to which we have been subjected. Instead I prefer to call the psycho-physical organism simply "the self," and to write of it as something "in use," which "functions" and which "reacts." My conception of the human organism or of the self is thus very simple, but can be made difficult by needless complication resulting from the preconceived ideas which readers bring to it.

Since the publication of *The Use of the Self* much water has run under the bridge. There have been happenings of special significance to those interested in the past and future usefulness of my practice, and in the bearing of its underlying principle of unity upon methods and plans of life in general. Biological and physiological findings which have given support to this principle and practice have been published in pamphlet and book form, and appreciative references have been made in books, articles, and in medical, chemical, philosophical, and educational reports.

It is gratifying to have lived to see the principle I have advocated and consistently put into practice for so long, endorsed by authorities in diverse fields of human activity. Unfortunately some of those who in their writings and speeches have given support to the concept of the *organism-as-a-whole* (The Whole Man) do not appear to have understood what is logically implied in putting this into practice, and so are attempting to help others to solve a problem which needs for its solution knowledge in a field in which they have had little or no experience. When making a statement of technique in my books, I have always included a description of the procedures necessary for putting into practice the theoretical conception that was the counterpart of this practice, and I can only regret that some of those who have restated and are now championing the concepts I have arrived at experimentally make no mention of any technique by means of which these concepts can be put into practice.

I have decided therefore that a new book may be of help in clarifying misconceptions, and in emphasizing the oneness of control and guidance of use and reaction, as well as in stressing the importance of gaining the knowledge and experience required for putting the concept of The Whole Man into practice consistently. This knowledge and experience is essential if our acceptance of the concept is not to remain merely an intellectual belief. A great deal of the confusion and perplexity in the world today is due to the acceptance and spreading of theoretical concepts which have not sprung from the personal experience of those who advocate them.

In the educational and medical world especially, writers and speakers have been putting forward the concept of The Whole Man as the one upon which sound methods in all fields of activity should be based, but few among these offer knowledge concerning the means of translating the concept into experience, or give a technique to be employed in applying the principle in practice. Yet as Professor G. E. Coghill writes in regard to the concept of the organism-as-a-whole: "It is a very different thing to state a theory and to demonstrate it as a fact. It is the demonstration that places the concept on a scientific foundation." He continues: "In my own case the concept came through the demonstration. I adopted the concept after I had the demonstration."[2]

Dr. Coghill's statement is especially interesting to me as it is entirely in line with my own experience, and clearly removes a scientific concept from the status of an intellectual belief. When I began the observations which led to the evolution of my technique,[3] I did not hold any hard and fast theory as to the working of the organism, though in common with most people, I conceived of "body" and "mind" as separate parts of the same organism. But the time came when I saw that the defects in my reaction at a given point, which I and my advisers had tried to change by *direct* method and treatment, were not primarily due to defects in the use and associated functioning of the parts of the mechanism seemingly most immediately concerned (in my case the vocal organs), but were the *indirect* result of defects in my general use of myself which were constantly lowering the standard of my general functioning, and harmfully influencing the working of the musculature of the whole organism. The close connexion which I observed to exist between the processes of use and functioning,[4] and which worked as I saw from the

---

[2]See "Psychological Controversy" in the *Brooklyn Citizen*, Brooklyn, N.Y., May 12, 1939.

[3]For those readers who have not read my books, the details of my observation will be found in the chapter headed "Evolution of a Technique" in *The Use of the Self.*

[4]The phrase "use and functioning" is often used by me in my writings; and as it has been suggested to me that the word "and" in the phrase might be misconstrued as implying a separation between the two processes of use and functioning—that, in fact, I might be accused of breaking faith with my well-known advocacy of unity by using the phrase, I think that reference to the experiences outlined in the first chapter of *The Use of the Self* will clear me from any misunderstanding on this score, because the order of the happenings I have recorded there is in accordance with the order of the words in the phrase.

whole to the part, was sound evidence to me of an integrated working of the organism, and when in working to this principle I discovered the existence of a control of this integrated working, which, according as it was employed, influenced for good or ill my general functioning, I realized that I had not only come upon the primary control of the integrated working of the psycho-physical mechanism in the use of the self that I needed to bring about a change in my own reaction, but that, by the objective proof emerging from my observations and the procedures I employed, the concept of the organism-as-a-whole had been placed upon a foundation that could be scientifically established.

The full significance of the foregoing has not been grasped even by those who have written on the practice and theory of my work, but emerging as it does from the practical application of my technique, it is fundamental to the comprehension of its wide implications and the fuller understanding of their nature in respect to man's reaction in living. It has not been realized that the influence of the manner of use is a *constant* one upon the general functioning of the organism in every reaction and during every moment of life, and that this influence can be a harmful or a beneficial one. It is an influence for ill or an influence for good in accordance with the nature of the manner of use of the self in living, and from this there is not any escape. Hence this influence can be said to be *a universal constant in a technique for living.*

I have in daily lessons for nearly fifty years demonstrated to pupils and others the influence for good or ill of this constant upon their general functioning, and the fact that repetition of the demonstration is possible provides that kind of proof of the soundness of concept and principle, and of the technique, plan or method based upon it, which is acceptable to the scientific engineer when he finds that in working to a concept or principle he can build a machine that, as a working mechanism, satisfies the need for which he designed it.

My experience and the course of events have only strengthened my conviction that we cannot hope to understand what is essential to the task of bringing about improvement in the manner of human reaction without first acquiring that knowledge of the integrated working of the self that will enable us either to prevent this working from being interfered with, or to restore it if such interference has already intervened. I would say that it is man's failure to perceive this necessity that has resulted in the tragic events that disfigure and tend to undermine the civilization that he has built up.

As I hope to show fully in what follows, any attempt on man's part to bring about changes in his own reaction or that of others must begin by throwing overboard the conceptions and beliefs that are associated with the feeling upon which he has previously relied for guidance and control in the use of himself in carrying out all his activities. He will need to substitute for these a new conception leading to belief in new procedures, if he is ever to understand what is necessary to the making of fundamental change in reaction. This will call for a change in guidance and control in carrying out the new procedures that have been reasoned out as best for his purpose, but as these lead to changes in the use of the organism which are associated with unfamiliar motor and sensory experiences, sometimes disconcertingly so, much more is needed than a belief arising from intellectual considerations alone, if he is to hold to this belief *during* the employment of these procedures.

I am of the opinion that the presentation of the material that I am now putting forward will make it clear that my technique provides a practical counterpart to the concept of The Whole Man which is stressed in certain of the writings of authorities I shall quote. I have gathered together a variety of significant material from my own experience, to which I am relating the ideas, arguments and conclusions of others in various fields of activity, and while this material may appear at first glance to be discrete, it is in fact linked together by being analyzed and considered in the light of adherence to the principle of the psycho-physical unity in the working of the human organism. To judge from the opinions expressed by authorities in many fields since the publication of *The Use of the Self*, my experience may one day be recognized as a signpost directing the explorer to a country hitherto "undiscovered," and one which offers unlimited opportunity for fruitful research to the patient and observant pioneer.

After working for a lifetime in this new field I am conscious that the knowledge gained is but a beginning, but I think I may confidently predict that those who are sufficiently interested in the findings I have recorded, and who will be guided by them in any further search, will find their outlook and understanding towards the question of the control of human reaction (behaviour) so completely changed that they will see that knowledge of the self is fundamental to all other knowledge, particularly to that which can make for the raising of the standard of human understanding and reaction essential to a sane plan of civilization. I trust that the reader will appreciate that the subject matter of this book is a warrant for this prediction, and suggest that if he will embark on the adventure he will find my prediction fulfilled.

CHAPTER I

THE CONSTANT INFLUENCE OF MANNER OF USE FOR GOOD OR ILL

> "The classic observations of Dr. George E. Coghill on the growth of the nervous system and the earliest development of embryonic behaviour showed that behaviour first appears as a total reaction of the organism, which is integrated from the beginning, and that the smaller patterns of behaviour, or specific reflexes, arise by a process of individuation from the total pattern."
> (Extract from the *Six Year Review*, 1930-1936 of Josiah Macy, Jr. Foundation.)

FEW of us hitherto have given consideration to the question of the extent to which we are individually responsible for the ills that our flesh is heir to; this, because we have not come to a realization of the faulty and often harmful manner in which we use ourselves in our daily activities and even during sleep,[5] or of the misdirection, strain and waste of energy due to this misuse. We have mostly taken it for granted that we are able to make the best use of ourselves at our work and in everything else we do.

In recent years, however, certain harmful effects of factory work (as apart from factory conditions, working hours, ventilation, etc.) have begun to be publicly recognized, an admission that something is wrong, and this has led to efforts being made to deal with the troubles of these workers.[6]

Unfortunately, up to now, only palliative measures have resulted from the efforts of those most concerned to remedy these troubles, because

[5]As far as investigation has been possible, it has been found that people often tend to exaggerate in sleep the harmful manner of use they employ during their waking hours. It is not generally appreciated that although the need of activating the mechanisms responsible for the process of living may perhaps not be so great during sleep as during the waking hours (because of the generally lowered tone and tempo of the functions), it is nevertheless present, and may be interfered with by the same harmful habits of use as prevail in wakeful activity.

[6]See Appendix D for excerpts from an address by Professor John Hilton, M.A.

in their consideration of what is necessary for the solution of their problem, they did not take into account the part played by the psycho-physical mechanisms of the human organism, both in those activities which are labelled physical and manual, and in those which are labelled mental and intellectual. No matter whether the activity is:

> (1) one which calls for the use of the limbs in general movement and locomotion, or for the use of the hands in employing tools and instruments, or
>
> (2) one through which the processes of conceiving, reasoning and understanding are set in motion, and through which the results of these processes are expressed in speaking or writing, as in education, religion, politics, science, etc.,

the part played by the organism in these two fields of psycho-physical activity is common to both.

> With regard to the use of the word *psycho-physical,* I would refer my reader to what I wrote in my book, *Constructive Conscious Control of the Individual* (page 228): "The term *psycho-physical* is used both here and throughout my works to indicate the impossibility of separating 'physical' and 'mental' operations in our conception of the working of the human organism. As I wrote in *Man's Supreme Inheritance,* 'In my opinion the two must be considered entirely interdependent, and even more closely knit than is implied by such a phrase.' Hence I use the term *psycho-physical activity* to indicate all human manifestations, and *psycho-physical mechanism* to indicate the instrument which makes these manifestations possible. Psycho-physical activity must not, however, always be considered as involving equal action and reaction of the processes concerned, for, as I hope to show, the history of the stages of man's development reveals manifestations of human activity which, at certain stages, show a preponderance on what is called the 'physical' side, and at other stages a preponderance on what is called the 'mental' side. I am forced to use the words 'physical' and 'mental' here and throughout my argument because there are no other words at present which adequately express the manifestations of psycho-physical activity present at these various stages, not in any sense because the 'physical' and 'mental' can be separated as such. I wish, therefore, to make it clear that whenever I use the word 'mental,' it is to be understood as representing all processes and manifestations which are generally recognized as not wholly 'physical,' and vice versa, the word 'physical' as representing all processes and manifestations which are generally recognized as not wholly 'mental'." This also applies where I use the words "physical" and "mental" in this book.

Every living human being is a psycho-physical unity, equipped with marvellous mechanisms through which, when set in motion by the stimulus of some desire or need, all reactions take place. Every reaction, therefore, is associated with a particular manner of use of these mechanisms, and it is because of this close association of manner of use and manner of reaction that all manifestations of human activity, whether labelled manual or mental, are constantly influenced by manner of use.

Take first the manual or skilled worker. His manner of use influences for good or ill not only his general functioning, but also the way in which he employs the instruments or tools of his trade. All his activity is his particular reaction to some stimulus. It is the stimulus that sets in motion a certain manner of use of himself, and the way he reacts is determined by this, and in a lesser degree by the comparative strength or weakness of the stimulus in its effect upon his manner of use. In this case there is *one stimulus* to reaction, his desire or need to employ tools or instruments as the means whereby he can gain his end.

The position is not so simple when it comes to workers in intellectual fields such as education, religion, science, politics, etc. They employ theories or plans which they have formulated as the instrument or means whereby they can instruct others or convert them to their ideas. Here, even with the help of the very best possible "means-whereby," success in gaining their end depends upon the manner of their reaction not to one, but to several stimuli of varying intensity. For instance, there is the stimulus of the ideas they wish to put forward; there is the stimulus of the desire to convert other people; in certain cases, there is the stimulus of the presence of an audience and so on, and to each of these stimuli they will react in accordance with their habitual manner of use. In addition to all this, their success in the last resort will depend upon the manner of the reaction of the people to be converted or instructed, since these, in their turn, will react according to the manner of use of themselves which is set in motion by the stimulus of the new idea, and also by the stimulus, potent or weak, resulting from the personality and manner of those who are presenting it.

It is surprising how few people realize that reaction is influenced, just as functioning is, by manner of use, and not many, even of these, are aware how intimately the individual's use of self modifies the functioning and reaction of his whole being.

> We all know from experience that the obvious often escapes our notice, and that we constantly fail to see things of great importance even when they are close to us. When we come into contact with a new and unfamiliar fact or experience, we do not bring the knowledge and experience we already possess to bear upon it, and so, frequently fail to make any

> connexion between the familiar and the unfamiliar. We therefore miss that new knowledge which we might have acquired if we had connected up the new and unfamiliar experience with what we already know. This explains why so few people among those who know my work have yet fully appreciated the truth of what I have just written as to the nature of the influence of use upon functioning and upon reaction, the association of manner of use of the self and manner of reaction and conditions of functioning being so close that control of one depends upon control of the other. Yet surely this association is the fact of all others which should have emerged from knowledge of my work, and study of my books. That it has been overlooked, however, will be apparent to anyone who reads the various appreciations of my work which have been published over a long period in reviews, articles, and references in books. Well-known authorities in their own sphere have expressed their opinions endorsing the value and soundness of my practice and theory, but no reference will be found in their writings to what is implicit in the acceptance of a truth which is fundamental to that practice and theory, and which I am now about to stress.

The question of the nature of use in its relation to functioning and reaction in our daily activities presents a problem requiring solution, and it will be found that the attitude of most people, with very few exceptions, is that Nature makes provision for us in this respect. How often have I been asked, "Why should our use of ourselves go wrong? What is the cause?" and so on.

These questions have been answered very fully in my other books. It is true that Nature has provided us all with the potentiality for the reasoning out of means for preventing wrong use of the self, but we have not developed any preventive measures to this end because we have assumed, quite erroneously, that our manner of use of ourselves cannot go wrong or fail us.

But now that it can be demonstrated that the influence of the manner in which we use ourselves is operating continuously either for or against us every moment of our lives, it is unreasonable to cling to this assumption. A good manner of use of the self exerts an influence for good upon general functioning which is not only continuous, but also grows stronger as time goes on, becoming, that is, a *constant* influence tending always to raise the standard of functioning and improve the manner of reaction. A bad manner of use, on the other hand, continuously exerts an influence for ill tending to lower the standard of general functioning, thus becoming a *constant* influence tending always to interfere with every functional activity arising from our response to stimuli from within and without the self, and harmfully affecting the manner of every reaction.

In estimating the extent of this influence of use upon functioning and reaction, the vital point to consider is whether it is spasmodic or constant. If by chance it is spasmodic, it will have a comparatively slight effect upon the nature of the functioning, but if, as is usually the case, it is constant, its effect upon functioning will tend as time goes on to grow stronger and stronger.

We all know that constant attention to what we are doing in the daily round of life makes for success, that constant energizing in a given direction is the most effective way to produce a given result, that constant application to a given task by a slow dull person can bring success where a quick brilliant person who indulges in spasmodic application will fail, that constant dripping of water will wear away stone, that constant pressure on parts of the human body produces irritation and pain, that constant repetition of a sound at a given interval will drive men mad, indeed, has actually been employed for that purpose, and that constant indulgence in bad habits leads sooner or later to irritation, undue excitement, depression, demoralization and even insanity.

The kind of *constant influence*, therefore, which our manner of use exerts upon functioning, is of the utmost importance. If it is one that tends to raise the standard of general functioning, it will be a constant influence for good, but if it is one that tends to lower this standard, then it will be a constant influence for ill. *Habit, indeed, may be defined as the manifestation of a constant.*

For this reason we should know and be able to employ the means whereby we can establish a good manner of use as a constant. Readers of *The Use of the Self* will remember that when I was experimenting with various ways of using myself in the attempt to improve the functioning of my vocal organs, I discovered that a certain use of the head in relation to the neck, and of the head and neck in relation to the torso and the other parts of the organism, if consciously and continuously employed, ensures, as was shown in my own case, the establishment of a manner of use of the self *as a whole* which provides the best conditions for raising the standard of the functioning of the various mechanisms, organs and systems. I found that in practice this use of the parts, beginning with the use of the head in relation to the neck, constituted a primary control of the mechanisms *as a whole*, involving control *in process* right through the organism, and that when I interfered with the employment of the primary control of my manner of use, this was always associated with a lowering of the standard of my general functioning. This brought me to realize that I had found a way by which we can judge whether the influence of our manner of use is affecting our general functioning adversely or otherwise, the criterion being whether or not this manner of use is interfering with the correct[7] employment of the primary control.

Unfortunately, the great majority of civilized people have come to use themselves in such a way that in everything they are doing they are constantly interfering in a greater or lesser degree with the correct employment of the primary control of their use, and this interference is an influence constantly operating against them, tending always to lower the standard of functioning within themselves and to limit or affect adversely their achievements in the outside world.

This adverse influence will still be operative even in the case of patients who are undergoing medical, surgical, or any other form of treatment for the "cure" or alleviation of some specific trouble, for it will tend constantly to lower the standard of their general functioning, not only *during* treatment but also *after* it is finished. And this will be so, no matter how successful as a specific "cure" the treatment may be. This applies in all fields of man's activity and also to pupils being taught under any educational method. Whether they are being instructed in a school subject such as mathematics, French, etc., being coached for games or athletics, or being taught the specific technique of some art or craft, the adverse influence of any interference with the correct employment of the primary control of their use will tend constantly to lower the standard of their functioning and the quality of their output.

When, on the other hand, a person's manner of use is such that there is no interference with the correct employment of the primary control, it means that an influence is constantly operating in his favour, tending always to raise the standard of functioning within the self, both in outside activity and during sleep.

The full significance of this will be apparent to those of us who have had the experience of applying my technique consistently to the task of changing use by the indirect method of preventing interference with the manner of employment of the primary control, for this experience involves a practical demonstration that *our manner of use is a constant influence for good or ill upon our general functioning.*

When once we have accepted what this implies, we shall appreciate the part played by wrong manner of use in the bringing about of general psycho-physical inefficiency and ill-health, and conversely, the part played by an improving manner of use in the restoration and maintenance of psycho-physical efficiency and conditions of well-being. We

[7]When in my writings the terms "correct," "proper," "good," "bad," "satisfactory" are used in connexion with such phrases as "the employment of the primary control" or "the manner of use" it must be understood that they indicate conditions of psycho-physical functioning which are the best for the working of the organism as a whole.

shall also see how important it is that every one of us should know how to estimate the degree in which our functioning is being influenced in one direction or the other by our manner of use, so that we can with confidence check any trend of this influence in the wrong direction. In short, it will be seen that the ability to assess the influence of manner of use upon general functioning provides a basis that is fundamental for diagnosis.

The acceptance of this basis for diagnosis means a changed outlook for all who are seeking to help themselves out of their difficulties, or to make some change of thought and action. No matter what means they may employ for self-help, whether by orthodox or unorthodox methods of treatment, self-discipline or anything else, the most potent force working with them for the gaining of their ends is the constant influence of an improving manner of use, tending to a gradual raising of the standard of their functioning in all activities and so affecting for good their every reaction.

It is only during the last forty years that this fact has begun to be appreciated, so that comparatively few of us today recognize that our manner of use has anything to do with the nature of our functioning or of our reaction to stimuli, nor the extent to which our physical-mental well-being depends upon the manner in which we use ourselves during our sleeping and waking hours. Unfortunately, we are not conscious of any interference with our well-being in terms connected with the manner of use, although this interference may be lowering our standard of functioning, but we are conscious of interference in terms of having a temperature, harmful tensions, internal pains or disorders, etc., as when we say we "do not feel in good form" or "are not up to the mark," or, sometimes, "feel ill." We know that under these conditions we are not likely to react to a given stimulus in the same way as we should if we were "feeling well" or "in good form." On the contrary, we show symptoms of irritation, peevishness, perversity, loss of temper, but we do not recognize these as manifestations of a lowered standard of our well-being which is associated with an interference with our manner of use and a consequent lowering of our standard of functioning. When once we appreciate that even in the absence of symptoms of "not feeling well," the majority of the people today have developed a manner of use of themselves which is constantly exerting a harmful influence not only upon their functioning but also upon their manner of reaction, we should be able to see that this wrong use can be a source of individual failings, peculiarities, wrong ideas and ills of all kinds, as well as of that inward unrest and unhappiness which is so evident in the social life of today. From my long experience I can now assert with confidence that the underlying cause of our personal and social difficulties will persist until we adopt "means-whereby" which will not only *prevent* the children of our time and of the future from developing a manner of using themselves that is a constant influence for ill in everything they do but, in those cases where harmful conditions are already present, will restore a manner of use which will be a constant influence for good. This remains true no matter what other means for alleviating them are adopted.

For a faulty manner of use, whether inherent or developed, will, as time goes on, become a more and more firmly established habit, and therefore more difficult to change. On the other hand it is easy to picture the beneficial effect of the cultivation and employment of a manner of use of the self that is associated with a gradual raising of that standard of general psycho-physical functioning which is a constant influence for good in the development of the human being.

End-Gaining and "Means-Whereby"

These terms stand for two different, nay opposite conceptions, and for two different procedures. According to the first or end-gaining conception, all that is necessary when an end is desired, is to proceed to employ the different parts of the organism in the manner which our feeling dictates as necessary for the carrying out of the movements required for gaining the end, irrespective of any harmful effects due to misuse of the self during the process; a conception which implies the subordination of the thinking and reasoning self to the vagaries of the instinctive guidance and control of the self in carrying out the activities necessary to achieve the end.

It will be seen therefore that end-gaining involves the conception and procedure of going *direct for an end* without consideration as to whether the "means-whereby" to be employed are the best for the purpose, or as to whether there should be substituted for these, new and improved "means-whereby" which, in their employment, would necessarily involve change in the manner of use of the self. This end-gaining plan is one of trial and error, and it proved more or less successful when man's manner of using himself was satisfactory, but during his experiences in civilization this use of himself has become more or less harmful (a fact that can be demonstrated), so that the end-gaining procedure no longer meets individual needs.

According to the second term, the "means-whereby" conception, this fact is recognized. Consequently, when an end is desired, the procedure is based on the conception that the manner of use of the self is no longer satisfactory, and that the associated mechanisms, being misdirected, are responsible for activity which does not meet the requirements for the gaining of desired ends; that this, therefore, necessitates the thinking out of new and improved "means-whereby" which will ensure that the manner of use of the self will not be associated with misdirection of the associated mechanisms, and so prove a stumbling block in achieving the end.

This is an *indirect* procedure, and, as has already been shown, it involves the inhibition of familiar messages responsible for habitual familiar activity, and the substituting for these of unfamiliar messages responsible for new and unfamiliar activity.

I wish it to be understood that throughout my writings I use the term "conscious guidance and control" to indicate primarily a plane to be reached rather than a method of reaching it. (Cf. *Constructive Conscious Control of the Individual.* Page 227, note.)

CHAPTER II

THE CONSTANT INFLUENCE OF MANNER OF USE IN RELATION TO DIAGNOSIS AND DISEASE

EVER since I first started taking pupils, medical men have been sending me their patients because they believed that I had evolved a sound technique. I am deeply indebted to them for their encouragement and support, and especially for the effort they are now making to bring a knowledge of my technique to the notice of those who are responsible for determining the range and nature of the medical curriculum with the aim of its being included in medical training. This is evidenced by the following letter signed by nineteen medical men and published in the *British Medical Journal* on May 29, 1937, vol. 1, p. 1137:

"Constructive Conscious Control"

To the Editor of the *British Medical Journal*

Sir,—In a review of Mr. F. Matthias Alexander's book *Constructive Conscious Control of the Individual*, which appeared in your columns on May 24, 1924, your reviewer wrote: "He (Alexander) would certainly appear to have something of value to communicate to the medical profession."

We, the signatories to this letter, are at one with your reviewer in this belief. As the medical men concerned we have observed the beneficial changes in use and functioning which have been brought about by the employment of Alexander's technique in the patients we have sent to him for help—even in cases of so-called "chronic disease"—whilst those of us who have been his pupils have personally experienced equally beneficial results. We are convinced that Alexander is justified in contending that "an unsatisfactory manner of use, by interfering with general functioning, constitutes a predisposing cause of disorder and disease," and that diagnosis of a patient's troubles must remain incomplete unless the medical man when making the diagnosis takes into consideration the influence of use upon functioning.

Unfortunately those responsible for the selection of subjects to be studied by medical students have not yet investigated the new field of knowledge and experience which has been opened up through Alexander's work, otherwise we believe that ere now the training necessary for acquiring this knowledge would have been included in the medical curriculum. To this end we beg to urge that as soon as possible steps should be taken for an investigation of Alexander's work and technique, he on his side having given us an assurance that he is ready and willing to give us the benefit of his experience for the carrying out of any plan which those concerned may suggest, provided that in his opinion the plan is one that would make it possible for him to help us to the desired end. We are, etc.,

Bruce Bruce Porter
J. R. Caldwell
J. H. Dick
Mungo Douglas
H. Duffett
C. A. Ensor
W. J. Graham
A. Rugg-Gunn
Percy Jakins
J. Kerr
D. Ligat
J. E. R. McDonagh
Peter Macdonald
R. G. McGowan
Adam Moss
A. Murdoch
F. J. Thorne
Harold Webb
A. H. Winchester

This endorsement of what I wrote in my chapter on "Diagnosis" in *The Use of the Self* comes from medical men who have been associated with my work for many years, and I am particularly anxious that my readers should grasp the full significance of their support of my contention that diagnosis of a patient's condition cannot be complete, unless in making it, the medical man can assess the influence for good or ill of the patient's manner of use upon his general functioning. It means that medical men are beginning to appreciate that a fundamental need in medical training and diagnosis has remained unrecognized until now, to the detriment of the medical man's usefulness and the best interests of his patients.

This should appeal especially to the layman, because prevention and alleviation of his ill-health depends upon treatment which is the outcome of his doctor's diagnosis, and if the diagnosis is not a complete one, any treatment prescribed as a result of that diagnosis can be assumed to be equally incomplete.

Apropos of diagnosis, it has often been tactfully suggested to me in the past that the medical man, by virtue of his training, has made the field of diagnosis entirely his own. The time came, however, when my experience enabled me to suggest, with equal tact I hope, that this attitude was not justified, since medical investigation and training had only covered a part of the field, indeed, in my opinion had left the most fertile part unexplored, particularly where full diagnosis was required for the purpose of prevention. This reasoning has had effect with a number of medical men and women who have written to me admitting that they have not been able to diagnose what was wrong in certain cases, asking me to try to do so and, if successful, to help them in any way that would be to the benefit of their patients.

This has been a source of much gratification to me and has afforded me some consolation for the opposition which I have met with in the past when trying to make known what is now recognized as being demonstrably true by many leading authorities, both in the medical and other professions.

For many reasons I have refused up to the present to publish particulars of cases, but I am now tempted to quote from some of the medical evidence at my disposal, because it supports my contention that interference with the correct employment of the primary control of our manner of use is a potent factor in inducing and maintaining the harmful functioning accompanying conditions of ill-health. For many years I have demonstrated in my daily work with pupils that wrong employment of the primary control of use can be checked, and the evidence of my medical friends and supporters encourages me to believe that a fuller understanding of the nature of the working of the primary control, and of the influence of this upon the general working of the organism, will help us to understand more fully the nature of the interference with manner of use and standard of general functioning which is becoming an ever more determining factor in the growing incidence of defects and disease.

In the particulars of the cases which are to follow it will be seen that underlying the diversity of symptoms, there is a factor common to them all which is the fundamental cause of interference with conditions of well-being. All that is written about these cases might be applied to many others, and this would show how wide is the range of human ills and ailments to which the technique has been successfully applied. Among cases sent to me by medical men I can mention those diagnosed as neurasthenia, visceroptosis, angina pectoris, epilepsy, locomotor ataxia, *tic douloureux*, migraine, short sight, stuttering, nasal and throat troubles, loss of voice, respiratory and heart troubles, severe damage from accidents. Children and young people have been sent to me because they were considered backward or defective, some of them actually diagnosed as mentally defective.

From these I have chosen for illustration examples which I think will best serve my purpose. They were sent to me for help by their medical advisers because the medical or other remedial measures prescribed had not met with the success hoped for. The striking characteristic which I observed to be common to all these cases was a misdirection and misuse of parts which was associated with an extreme interference with the subject's employment of the primary control of use, leading to such harmful conditions as undue lumbar curve of the spine, undue tension of the neck, arms and legs, and overaction of muscle groups of the organism. All these conditions I found to be unduly affecting the extensors at one time and the flexors at another, thus tending to bring about maladjustment, misplacement of viscera, harmful pressure on the joints, ribs and vertebrae. The use of the anti-gravity muscles was so misdirected that the working of these muscles tended to lessen the anti-gravity influence which is of vital importance in maintaining equilibrium. Any attempt to move the head involved movements of other parts of the organism which should have remained passive. This meant a misdirection of energy and a spasm or overaction of muscle groups, and the greater the desire to turn the head, the more energy was expended in misdirection and consequent overaction of the muscle groups.

To take first the case of osteo-arthritis. Mr. B. was a patient of Dr. Caldwell, of Milnthorpe, Westmoreland, and the most striking characteristic I observed in his use of himself was the way his head was tilted backward and downward, and that the degree of tension he employed in activity was such that the head and neck had become practically fixed. There was also an extreme lumbar curve, and in standing and walking the pelvis was brought relatively too far forward. When an attempt was made to move the head from side to side, the movement was infinitesimal, but because of the overaction of muscles and spasm which ensued, even that movement caused acute pain.

The following gives a fair description of the nature of the disease diagnosed in this case from the orthodox point of view. There were definite organic defects and growths (nodules) which played their part in the fixation, deformity and wrong axis of the head, and also other manifestations which, collectively, had led to the conclusion that the case was one for orthopaedic treatment. As a result a collar two and a half inches high was prescribed by an orthopaedic surgeon to check any further increase in the pulling down of the head. The patient was wearing this collar when he came to see me.

Mr. B. started his lessons with me on October 13, 1936, and the collar was removed within a fortnight or three weeks after the first lesson.

About two months after his lessons started Dr. Caldwell wrote to his patient:

December 19, 1936

Dear Mr. B.:

I have been so convinced from the very first of the essential rightness of Alexander's technique that I have read his book through four times, and if proof were required that his teaching is fundamentally correct, you provide the living proof.

It is true, that by wearing a collar, the disease might be arrested, but without removing the deformity and without correcting the wrong axis of the head. So that in due course a relapse would be almost certain and recourse would have to be made to the collar.

Arthritis of the cervical spine at your age is a "postural" disease. . . . With the onset of arthritis in the spine, or indeed anywhere, there occurs reflex spasm or overaction of muscle groups which is a vicious circle as this very reflex spasm further menaces the deformity and increases the pain.

Alexander teaches how to inhibit the reflex spasm, that is the real secret and what I have longed to do for years. . . .

Yours sincerely,

(signed) J. R. CALDWELL.

Shortly afterwards, Mr. B. sent me a copy of a letter he had just received (December 22, 1936) from the orthopaedic surgeon on whose advice he had worn the collar referred to in Dr. Caldwell's letter.

Dear Mr. B.:

Thank you very much indeed for your extremely interesting letter which I am delighted to have and to hear all you say is being done for you by Mr. Alexander. There is no doubt he has done you good, not only physically but mentally, and you now have an aim and an object which unfortunately surgery could not give you and in that way, if in no other, Mr. Alexander has done you good.

In regard to the exercises, I probably am a sceptic, and I know that as long as the muscles are developed temporarily *by any system of exercise*,[8] you will undoubtedly feel better until ordinary times come and these muscles return to the condition in which nature meant them to be to accommodate with the conditions of your cervical spine. I shall be very interested to hear what your condition is in three or six months' time, if you will let me have another report.

As you know, medical men are frequently blamed for being reactionaries but it is really not so. We are delighted to know anything new, anything that can improve a patient because naturally that is all to our

[8]I have italicized the points in this letter which I am taking up in my argument to follow.—F. M. A.

credit and to our own benefit, but *occasionally we find systems of treatment which temporarily relieve*, but unfortunately in at least some cases, the relief is not permanent. *I only hope your relief is permanent* and you do improve because you have tried hard, and you deserve improvement if any man does.

(*signed*) M.

By the date of this letter, it is clear that Mr. B's condition had continued to improve, and this is corroborated by the following letter:

December 15, 1936

Dear Mr. Alexander:

I saw Dr. Caldwell yesterday and he was extraordinarily pleased and interested.

He said, that when he had read your book, he was convinced that your lines were the right ones.

Caldwell says, of course, the bones in the spine have got on a cant, and the cartilage is probably worn away on the side where the pressure comes.

He said, that with the relief I have now got, this cartilage will grow again, but he expects it will take about two years before that has entirely taken place.

The arthritic nodules which have formed, he agrees will disappear. . . .

He thinks it a very wonderful result.

With kindest regards,

Yours sincerely,

(signed) G. E. B.

These letters are of special interest to me as in them Dr. Caldwell has linked up his medical knowledge with that which came to him through observation of his patient's improvement from the time that he came to me and analyzing the nature of the changes he noted. This is shown by the statements in his first letter where he connects what he has read about my work in *The Use of the Self*, with the changes brought about in his patient's general condition by the application of my technique. In this book I am trying to show that the field in which I have worked is one in which those who are interested in therapeutics must also work, if they are to gain the knowledge and experience required for that full diagnosis upon which sound methods of prevention, and the restoration and maintenance of conditions of health depend. But beyond this I am hopeful that workers in other fields of activity will be stimulated to follow Dr. Caldwell's example, and link up the knowledge they possess in their own sphere with the new knowledge which is now available of the use of the self.

Dr. Caldwell in his letter clearly shows that after reading my book, he had no doubt that my technique was based upon a sound principle, and that for a patient suffering from the effects of a "postural disease" called osteo-arthritis of the cervical spine, the means I used for making structural and other changes would prove to be the right means. As the work progressed, what he saw happening in his patient confirmed him in his belief. For not only was the deformity being removed and the wrong axis of the head prevented, but, most significant of all, the reflex spasm which Dr. Caldwell states "occurs with the onset of arthritis of the spine" was being consistently inhibited, and the associated pain grew less and less until there was permanent relief.

Now if we look at the letter Mr. B. received from the orthopaedic surgeon, we shall see that he doubted whether the changes brought about would afford "permanent relief," because being unacquainted with the nature of my work, he assumed that my technique was some "system of exercise." If he had read my books he would have known that his contention that "systems of exercise" give only temporary relief in most cases corroborates what I have written on this subject, and that in employing my technique, no attempt is made to gain specific results by *direct* means. This is indeed where it differs from all "systems of exercise." The changes in Mr. B.'s condition were brought about *indirectly* by improvement in his manner of use of himself, and it was the influence of this improvement upon his general functioning that was also responsible for the other changes noticed by Dr. Caldwell. The abnormalities,[9] so evident in his case, would not have been likely to develop if his use of himself had not been harmful, the fundamental influence constantly operating towards the development of these abnormalities being his habitual interference with the employment of his primary control in all the acts of life. Therefore only by changing his habitual manner of employing the primary control of his use of himself could a permanent improvement in these abnormalities be expected. But as this improvement occurred in the course of applying the technique the actual changes that Dr. Caldwell described were gradually brought about even in the structural condition.

For instance, the nodules were disappearing, the worn vertebrae were gradually growing back to normal, and the deformity of the cervical spine was corrected. This meant that distinct and permanent changes were also brought about in the bony structure of the thorax

[9]As there is much confusion in the general use of the words "abnormal" and "abnormality," I wish to state that I use these words to indicate conditions which are associated with a manner of use that is tending to lower the standard of general functioning of the organism, and not in relation to conditions which may be variations only.

(chest) and of the spine, and with these changes came changes in the functioning of the abdominal viscera, with an increase in the mobility and capacity of the thorax.

Since these structural changes came about through changes made in the manner of use, it follows that the muscle groups throughout the organism had to play their part both in making the changes and in accommodating themselves immediately and continuously to the changes they were bringing about.

For instance, during the making of changes in manner of use which accompanied the modification of the deformity of the curved spine, the muscle groups were accommodating themselves to the new and better structural conditions which they were bringing about, and *as long as the improvement in the manner of use was maintained*, there could be no question of the muscles reverting to the original conditions to which they had formerly accommodated themselves, for these conditions, including the deformity of the cervical spine, no longer existed. This, as the surgeon points out in his letter, is not the case where exercises, remedial or otherwise, are employed.

Dr. Caldwell throws light upon the bringing about of structural and other changes through action of muscle groups when he states in his letter: "With the onset of arthritis of the spine, or, indeed, anywhere, there occurs reflex spasm or overaction of muscle groups which is a vicious circle as this very reflex spasm further menaces the deformity and increases the pain." This condition of overaction of muscle groups is not present in cases where there is correct employment of the primary control, but this is not taken into account by those who diagnose postural defects without consideration of the influence of use upon general functioning, and who prescribe the practice of exercises, remedial or otherwise. They do not recognize that the overaction of muscle groups associated with wrong employment of the primary control is constantly exerting an influence towards the formation of bad "postural" and other habits, and that the performance of exercises could only exaggerate this bad influence.

Dr. Caldwell's next statement, therefore, that "Alexander teaches how to inhibit the reflex spasm, that is the real secret" is most significant, for it shows that he understands *why* the particular means employed in my technique in Mr. B.'s case came about as an *indirect* result of the pupil's learning to inhibit the wrong employment of the primary control of his use. When he became experienced in inhibiting the misdirection which led to the wrong employment of the primary control, and *could maintain the resultant new manner of use when responding to any stimulus to activity* in his daily life, his reaction no longer resulted in overaction of the muscle group or reflex spasm.

Such a change could not have been brought about without the inhibition of his habitual manner of use, for this was associated with misdirection and the high degree of muscle tension throughout the organism, and was *indirectly* responsible for much of the overaction of the muscle groups resulting in the spasm.[10] The change made in his use through the inhibition of this misdirection brought about many changes in conditions, including a lowering of the standard of muscle tension throughout the organism generally, and, with it, a reduction of the undue tension involved in the spasm.

Dr. Caldwell's generous admission encourages me to believe that others will also wish to analyze the principle underlying my technique, which, although it has been evolved out of experiences gained in a field which is new to them, has a distinct bearing upon the whole question of diagnosis and prevention in all fields of man's activity in living. It is true that my technique, when compared with medical practice, is based upon a new and unorthodox principle, but this is equally true if it is compared with osteopathy, remedial exercises, physical culture, and teaching methods in general.

I have described in my last book how and why I came upon this new principle. It was not merely the outcome of an idea, a vision, a theoretical conception without a practical counterpart; it was the outcome of practical experience, the at first tantalizing experience of discovering that IT WAS WHAT I WAS DOING MYSELF that was causing the throat trouble which had defied all previous treatment. While I was evolving a technique to meet the needs of my own case, I gained experience which convinced me that the orthodox method of treatment which I had tried for my throat trouble and which had failed, was based upon a wrong principle.

I had worked patiently at the breathing, vocal and other exercises suggested by my teachers, and had carried out to the letter the treatment prescribed by my medical advisers, but all to no purpose. But when I came to appreciate fully that it was WHAT I WAS DOING in following out instructions that was leading me into the wrong use of myself that was causing my throat trouble, I realized that self-accusation must replace self-pity, and that, in fact, I had to accuse myself of "doing" the undue depression of my larynx, the contraction of my chest, as well as the

[10]Hence the futility in such cases of exercises which tend rather to raise the degree of muscle tension than lower it. This applies equally to methods of "relaxation" which in my experience bring about under certain conditions a form of collapse, while in others there occurs with the collapse of certain muscular groups a compensatory overaction of others, tending to increase the irritation and pressure already present.

wrong axis of my head, which were some of the most serious symptoms in my throat trouble, and I saw that what I had needed at the outset was someone who could have explained to me, first, what it was that I was *doing* in the use of myself that was wrong, and then, as a *primary procedure*, show me how to prevent this. Obviously, for me to be told by a teacher TO DO something new as a remedy for my trouble, practically amounted to my being told to continue using myself in the old wrong way in order to do the new thing he suggested.

For this reason, the idea of going to a teacher working on the old lines was out of the question, and as my medical advisers by their own admission could not help me here, I saw that I must find out for myself WHAT I WAS DOING that constituted a wrong use of myself, and then learn how to prevent myself from continuing in this "wrong-doing."

At the time I thought this would be a simple matter and on the face of it it would seem to be so, at any rate, theoretically. But when I came to work out the problem practically I found I was mistaken. Later on, when I had learned through experience what a harmful influence wrong employment of the primary control of use, associated as it is with perverted sensory appreciation (feeling), can exert upon functioning, I came to understand why I had miscalculated the difficulty of my problem.

Obviously, in all "doing" there is a conception of what is to be done and how to do it. Whether we react to this conception by giving consent to do the act, or by withholding that consent, the nature of our reaction is determined by our habitual manner of use of ourselves in which we depend upon feeling for guidance.

It is well known that different people will get a different conception from the same word, spoken or written, and from the same gesture, showing that conception is dependent upon the nature of the impressions taken through the sensory mechanisms which control the functioning of the cells (receptors and conductors) of the eyes and ears, etc. The conception likewise of what is happening within ourselves is dependent upon impressions which come to us through the sense of feeling (sensory appreciation) upon which we mostly rely for guidance in carrying out our daily activities. When our sensory appreciation is deceptive, as is the case more or less with every one today, the impressions we get through it are deceptive also. The extent of this deception depends largely upon the extent to which our manner of use has been put wrong and the nature and degree of the faulty guidance of deceptive feeling. When a certain degree of misuse has been reached, the deceptiveness of these impressions reaches a point where they can mislead us into believing that WE ARE DOING SOMETHING WITH SOME PART OF OURSELVES WHEN ACTUALLY WE CAN BE PROVED TO BE DOING

SOMETHING QUITE DIFFERENT. This is equally true of things we believe we think, which more often than not are things we feel.

Here then we have a vicious circle. Directly we get a conception of doing something, we react according to our habitual misuse of ourselves, the functioning of some one part or other is thereby impaired and, as the organism works as a whole, this means that all parts will be more or less affected.

In working out my own problem, I was immediately caught in this vicious circle, for my habitual reaction to any conception of "doing" fitted in with my own peculiarities of misuse and faulty functioning, and with the deceptiveness of sensory appreciation that went with these. As soon, therefore, as I tried to change my reaction *directly*, I found that these impeding influences stood in my way, and there was no escape from the vicious circle. Repeated experiences of this kind made me see that if I were to succeed in solving my problem, any technique I might be able to evolve must be one which would enable me to eliminate the impeding influences which were baulking my effort, and so *indirectly* bring about a real psycho-physical change in my habitual reaction, for when once we admit that change of some kind must be made in order to bring about improvement in reaction, it is evident that change of habitual use is fundamental to success.

As long as we continue to react in "doing" according to our familiar habit of use, we, *by our own doing*, make change of use and reaction impossible. My experiences, therefore, convinced me that in any attempt to control habitual reaction, the need to work to a new principle asserts itself, the principle, namely, of inhibiting our habitual desire to go straight to our end trusting to feeling for guidance, and then of employing only those "means-whereby" which indirectly bring about the desired change in our habitual reaction—the end.

The task of reasoning out and selecting the effective means of bringing about psycho-physical change according to this new principle is not an easy one, but the real task begins when we start to put into practice the procedures which we have decided upon, for this, as Dewey puts it, presupposes a "revolution in thought and action." It means that on the receipt of a given stimulus to perform some act which we have decided is necessary for the change of our habitual reaction, CONSENT TO PERFORM THE ACT MUST BE WITHHELD NOT GIVEN, in order that our habitual reaction may be held in check, and the usual messages to the motor nerve and muscle mechanisms which determine our manner of employing the primary control of our use in our habitual reaction, not projected. This clears the way for us to project new messages which in time will be associated with new and unfamiliar use of the mechanisms in activity, thus bringing about a change in the employment of the primary control, and thereby indirectly a change in the manner of our habitual reaction.

Here we have two procedures fundamental to our new technique, which, if repeated, will (1) cause the habitual means whereby we have energized our old reaction to fall into disuse, and (2) cultivate new means whereby we shall energize new and desired reaction. This new reaction comes in time to take the place of the former habitual reaction, to be equally part of ourselves and therefore to "feel right."

This change, brought about by means which determine the manner of employment of the primary control, goes on throughout the organism, and brings about improvement in the use of the self in general. In my own case, it was not until I could work to this principle that I was able, at the moment when I decided to use my voice, TO INHIBIT THE MESSAGES BEING SENT which had been responsible for my habit of bringing about misuse of my vocal organs by overaction of muscle groups and misuse of myself in general.

In this process we have a connecting link between what happened in my own case and in that of the case of osteo-arthritis which we have been discussing. In both there was evidence of overaction of muscle groups due to misuse, the influence of which had been constantly operating against any form of treatment. It was the inhibition of the misdirection of my use which finally enabled me to regain the proper functioning of my voice, and it was this same inhibitory process at work, which, in the case of osteo-arthritis, led in time to what Dr. Caldwell described as the "inhibition of the reflex spasm."

There was similar evidence of misuse and overaction of muscle groups in the case of spasmodic torticollis and in the other cases sent to me by the medical men referred to later in this chapter. Moreover, this misuse and overaction is happening in all cases where there are symptoms of disease or any of those peculiarities or conditions which are considered to require medical treatment, remedial or other exercises, or physical culture. If there is deformity, pain, wrong axis of the head or all of these conditions present together, there will also be present harmful psycho-physical tension which tends constantly to increase, and to add to the degree of overaction in muscle groups which are already overactive.

To illustrate this point, I will refer again to the conditions I noted in the case of osteo-arthritis from the point of view of what *he was doing himself* in bringing these conditions about. To me, they revealed a man unknowingly indulging in the most harmful use of himself in every activity. This was particularly noticeable in his breathing, when he was trying to rest in a chair, when he was moving an arm or leg, or taking part in ordinary conversation. The relative position of the head to the neck, and of the head, neck and torso to the limbs, was habitually being interfered with. This afforded proof that as soon as he gave consent to perform any act, messages were projected which resulted in an interference with his direction of the primary control, causing overactivity and a gradually increasing tension not only in the groups of muscles concerned, but also in others which were taking a too prominent part in the performance of the act. As soon, therefore, as he gave consent to doing anything in an endeavour to help himself, these impeding influences at once came into play, operating against him in his "doing" as they would operate against him in any "doing" in physical culture, remedial exercises, or any other method. The deformity of the neck, the fixation of the cervical spine and head, the round humped back, the uneven position of the shoulders, the undue lordosis and slight lumbar curve of the spine, the extreme anterior position of the pelvis in standing, the unduly protruded abdomen, the contracted chest, and the undue tension of the arms and legs even when he was in a sitting position, his habitual tendency to slump when seated—all these were evidence of the vicious circle involving reflex spasm in overaction of muscle groups, which Dr. Caldwell wrote was "further menacing the deformity and increasing the pain." To put it simply, a person manifesting these conditions is being gradually pulled down and bent forward, the forward bend being chiefly from the pelvis, in much the same way as if his feet were fastened to the floor and he were being, day by day, more and more pulled forward and down by means of a rope fixed round the neck.

It is not possible to set down full details of the stages this pupil passed through before he learned to inhibit his end-gaining habit, and to modify the undue and harmful tension which he exerted throughout his organism, and which impeded me in my attempts to give him with my hands the experience he needed for improving the employment of his primary control. The time came when the changes made in the relativity of the head to the neck, and the head and neck to the torso and limbs and therefore in the manner of use generally, tended to reduce the pressure exercised by the old use upon the cervical spine. These changes in relativity were the indirect means of correcting the wrong axis of the head, of modifying the reflex spasm or overaction of the muscle groups, and the comparative fixation of the neck and the accompanying deformity, and last but not least, of diminishing little by little the headache and the pain. As this improvement in use continued, the range of movement of the head from side to side gradually widened, the pain decreased and the headache ceased. There was also a continuous lessening of the tension of the legs and arms, and of the tendency to slump when sitting.

I have gone into this case at some length in order to show that the field of experience with which I am dealing is one that is quite outside any which comes within the survey of the practitioner and patient when such a case is dealt with by orthodox methods. The set of conditions such as "wrong axis of the head," deformity, reflex spasm, which, as we have seen, Dr. Caldwell describes and diagnosed as symptoms of a "postural disease" called osteo-arthritis, were conditions which, according to the orthodox outlook, would be recommended for medical or orthopaedic treatment or remedial exercises, or in many cases indeed, there might be recourse to methods such as those of the osteopath, chiropractor, or bonesetter. But the point I wish to make clear is that the treatment given in the case we are interested in had not been successful, and as Dr. Caldwell testifies that his patient is now a "living proof" that the "means-whereby" which were employed in teaching him were fundamentally correct, I trust I may be pardoned if I emphasize here that these means were not part of a new method of treatment for the condition which Dr. Caldwell described as a "postural disease," but were the outcome of a new outlook towards a fundamental cause of these conditions, and that, on Dr. Caldwell's showing, help is to be found for such cases in a new field, which is not one of treatment orthodox or unorthodox, but of education in the widest sense of the word in that it deals with the control of human reaction.

* * * * *

Having dealt with one case very fully, I shall now give in brief outline the special characteristics which I observed in other cases to which my technique has been successfully applied.

A. *Spasmodic Torticollis*

Associated with an overaction of muscles of the neck so extreme as to be apparent to the casual observer, there was in this case a constant spasmodic movement of the head, undue and harmful lordosis and lumbar curve of the spine, extreme protrusion of the abdomen, and extreme anterior position of the pelvis in standing and walking, which increased the strain and stress in attempts to preserve equilibrium. There was definite injury to the vertebrae resulting from pressure, lordosis and lumbar curve, harmful displacement of the viscera, together with the reflex spasm of the neck muscles. These conditions were so acute that I would not give the doctor any assurance of what I could do, until I had given the pupil a fortnight's lessons. In this case, aid had been sought from physicians, surgeons and psychologists all of whom pronounced the case hopeless.[11]

[11]This is the case to which Dr. Adam Moss refers in his letter reproduced on p. 546.

B. *Stuttering*

The tendency to fixation of the head and neck, which was so noticeable in the cases of osteo-arthritis and torticollis, characterized this case also. In any attempt to move the head there was a spasmodic movement associated with overaction of neck muscles similar to that of the spasmodic torticollis case. Special to this case was the undue excitement of the fear reflexes in response to any stimulus to move or speak. The orthodox view of this case had led to treatment and teaching for the specific improvement of the use of the organs of speech. The lessons given by teachers were based on the orthodox principle of telling and showing the pupil *what to do* with the tongue and the lips, and how "to take breath" to the best advantage and so on. No attempt was made to change the manner of the pupil's general use of the self, and as a result the attempt to "cure" the stuttering had not only failed but was actually responsible for the cultivation of new bad habits of use and the exaggeration of those already present. The lessons I gave were based upon the principle that the pupil's manner of general use was responsible for the trouble. This being so, the first thing to be done was to prevent the projection of the messages which brought about this wrong manner of use, and so to effect a change in the pupil's habitual reaction to any form of "doing" in daily life, including the act of speaking. Thus, the change brought about in the manner of use of the vocal organs was an *indirect* result of the change in the pupil's manner of general use of the self.

C. *Asthma*

I shall now refer to a typical case of asthma in which the manner of use was what may be described as particularly harmful. One of its results was the misdirection of the musculature of the chest and throat so that the ordinary breathing act was more or less impeded, particularly in expiration; and during an attack of asthma, the ill effect of this misdirection was noticeably increased. Misdirection of this kind, no matter in what type of case, always has its source in interference with the working of the primary control, and in the case under consideration this was manifested in an undue and harmful pulling back and down of the head, and in the fixation of the bony structure of the neck in the region of the occipital muscles, while the lower part of the back of the head was pulled down on to the ordinary collar worn by the sufferer. There was an extreme lordosis curve, the chest was raised unduly (pigeon chest) and the pelvis thrown too far forward—all of which conditions tended to decrease the stature and unduly widen the front of the chest, resulting in harmful tension and the minimum of mobility. The act of breathing even during the slightest attack led to an exaggeration of the harmful manner of use with increased tension and, as a consequence, the severity of the attack was accentuated. The effect of undue tension can readily be understood when it is remembered that muscular tension tends to induce chest rigidity and breathlessness.

D. *Seriously Damaged Neck, Owing to Riding Accident*

This pupil was thrown from his horse and the spine was severely damaged in the region of the neck. After eight months of medical treatment he was still unable to walk and came to me for help. He was wheeled into my teaching room in an invalid chair, accompanied by his nurse, and I needed the help of assistant teachers to get him out of it. He was wearing a support to prevent the head from falling so far backward that it became completely out of his control. In a few days he was able with a little assistance to walk from his invalid chair into the house, and shortly afterwards found that the support to the head was not needed and that he could walk without assistance. His improvement has been gradual but continuous and some time ago he resumed riding.

E. *Tic Douloureux*

In this case there was extreme mal-coordination and maladjustment associated with undue and harmful interference with the employment of the primary control of the manner of use of the different parts of the organism. The right eye was almost closed, the skin was very dark under the eyes and red and inflamed on the forehead. The abdominal viscera were harmfully dropped, the spine unduly curved in the lumbar region, the head thrown too far back, and the general use was such that even attempts to move the jaw in the act of speaking caused pain which was often intense, and this obtained when attempts were made to wash the face or comb the hair.

Five members of the medical profession who had been consulted decided that the only thing to do was to operate and inject alcohol.

The sufferer came to me three weeks before I left for my holiday at the end of July, and by the time I went away there was a distinct improvement in the manner of her general use and a corresponding diminution of the symptoms including the pain. Lessons were begun again on September 6 and ended on September 23 when the pain had practically disappeared, the eye was normal and the general condition much improved.[12]

[12]For further reference to this case see Appendix E.

I will now give further extracts from letters which I have received from medical men with reference to patients they have sent to me.

F. *Sciatica*

From C. A. Ensor, Esq., M.R.C.P., L.R.C.P., dated April 27, 1937:

> My daughter's improvement which began so soon after coming under your care, continued until her complete recovery. Her left sacro-iliac pain was of such long standing and the treatment hitherto given of so little help that I began to fear that the condition would become permanent. Both she and I are very grateful to you for all you have done for her.
>
> June 30, 1939
>
> My daughter whom I saw today is very well indeed and has had no recurrence of her sciatica.

G. *Legs Damaged in Flying Accident*

Extract from letter from S. B., received January 22, 1940:

> My legs were broken in August, 1914.
>
> *Right leg*: Tibia and Fibula and Femur; not compound. Lost 2 inches of length.
>
> *Left leg*: Knee cap in several bits. This was wired. The right leg was badly set with the toe rather turned in. The left leg was admirably done. Only slight muscle wastage and can bend well past the right angle.
>
> You completely did away with all lameness.

After examination of this patient J. E. R. McDonagh, Esq., F.R.C.S., wrote to me on September 17, 1937, as follows:

I have seen S. B. and must congratulate you on the work you have done on him. I consider this to be the best example of your work.

H. *From Adam Moss, Esq., M.D.*

> June 8, 1939
>
> Dear Mr. Alexander:
>
> I feel that I ought to place on record the remarkable results of your work upon a number of my patients who had been regarded as derelicts.
>
> Ten years ago I sent to you Mr. D. C. a bad spasmodic torticollis case about whom a London nerve specialist had written, to say that "he had never known such cases to get better."
>
> His stay in London, under your care, was interrupted, but the improvement in the short time was extraordinary.

The next was Mrs. D., spasmodic torticollis,[13] in a pitiable condition, having to be fed. She had been seen by consulting physicians, surgeons, and orthopaedic surgeons; and just before I saw her she had been for ten weeks in a psychologist's nursing home. I advised that she should see you. She is now perfectly well, living a full life and driving her own motor car.

Next Mrs. B., scoliosis, head almost in the axilla, and torticollis on top of that; she had had osteopathic treatment and was wearing a collar prescribed by an eminent orthopaedic surgeon, she was partially bedridden. Six weeks after she came to you I was in London and watched you give her her lesson; she was then quite erect—lateral curvature gone. Her brother told me a few days ago how much better she was, and that she was going to you for another fortnight's treatment.

Then Mrs. R. who might be described as a hopeless neurasthenic bordering on melancholia, she had been in and out of nursing homes for four years and had seen many physicians, the last one told her that nothing could be done. She is now well and radiantly happy. There is much more that I should like to say. Your books have been most instructive and thought provocative.

Your personality, your strict honesty of purpose, and the generous way in which you explain your methods and technique has earned you the esteem and regard of your many medical friends, from all over the country, who know of your splendid work.

Yours sincerely,

(signed) ADAM MOSS.

OLD AGE

The following letter from Dr. Millard Smith of Boston, Mass., was addressed to my brother, Mr. A. R. Alexander, who has been teaching my technique in Boston for the last six years:

January 20, 1941

Dear Mr. Alexander:

I want to tell you that the sudden death by cerebral accident of your pupil and my patient Mr. A., at the age of 81, does not alter in my mind the appreciation of the remarkable rehabilitation that you had been able to give him. When I first saw him in 1931, shortly before he became your pupil, he showed a very disabling degree of hypertrophic arthritis of the spine. While it is my belief that most arthritic joints chronically affected should be mobilized, I felt very dubious about carrying out mobilization measures in his case after seeing the marked hypertrophic changes in the x-ray of his spine. The usual course of such a situation at that age is

[13]See note p. 543.

> increasing disability, and comfort can be given only by the use of orthopaedic appliances that lead to further fixation. There is no question but that he had reached a turning point in his life's physical activities and I am sure that there is no known medical procedure that would have resulted in the remarkable rehabilitation that he had shown progressively during the past seven or eight years. He has had a steadily increasing well being and interest in living, especially during the past two years when he has probably had harder burdens to bear than at any time in his life. From the medical standpoint he has really shown a reversal of the aging process and his performance has been quite contrary to what one would have predicted for him nine years ago. His blood pressure has been lower, and he has lost angina symptoms that he had nine years ago. X-rays of his spine have been taken periodically and they showed a slight diminution, rather than an increase as would be expected, in the hypertrophic process. During the past two years his zest for living has been such that he has taken regular vocal lessons. He has been able to play regularly a very good game of 18 holes of golf. This fall he skated regularly two or three times weekly and I have it on good authority that he did very difficult figure skating and was excelled by very few of the best amateur skaters. In fact his sudden death occurred just after he had completed a difficult figure. I consider his death a mere incident to the fact that his work with you had made it possible for him to live a very active, normal and happy life as compared with the probability of increasing marked disability when he first became your pupil.
>
> Sincerely,
>
> *(signed)* MILLARD SMITH.

Many of my medical supporters are anxious that I should refer to the influence of use in its relation to functioning during childbirth and the preceding period, and by way of introduction I do not think I can do better than quote the remarks made on the subject of faulty bodily coordination and its evil effects on childbirth by Mr. A. M. Ludovici.[14] This will at least draw attention once more to a fact which cannot be too often emphasized, namely that it is the whole psycho-physical self, the whole human organism with all its manifold functions, which gains in efficiency and well-being from the correct employment of the primary control of use in every activity of life.

Mr. Ludovici writes:

> This faulty bodily coordination affects health and efficiency in men just

[14]In *The Truth about Childbirth* (London & New York, 1937).

as much as in women, but whereas the former, I repeat, are not in peace-time called upon to perform any feat which reveals on a large national scale the extent of their deterioration, the latter have their lack of efficiency constantly brought into the limelight by childbearing and childbirth.

Twenty-five years ago Mr. F. Matthias Alexander was probably the only man in the civilized world who was insistently calling attention to this evil and showing us how to correct it. And in two books published respectively ten and four years ago I tried to convey to the English and American reader the fact that in this vicious use of the body as a mechanism we had a veritable modern plague, which was all the more alarming seeing that there was no escape from it along the ordinary lines of disinfection, medicinal pills, squills and tabloids, or even serological therapy—hence the great importance of Alexander's work.

Again let me avoid Alexander and quote from the much belated orthodox reformers in this field. In *Body Mechanics* we read:

"Much of the gynaecological disability and long periods of weakness following some pregnancies can be explained on the basis that the compensation for long-standing faulty body mechanics has been broken by the burden of pregnancy and parturition, and when once broken, the badly used body is unable to regain its compensation and strength."

Suppose that, through faulty coordination and wrong use of self—and Alexander leaves us in no doubt about this—we get a general shortening of the trunk so that cavities are distorted, organs dropped, respiratory function hampered, and the abdomen made to bulge and sag. Can a gravid uterus in such a body fail to suffer from the abnormal conditions?

Is it not fantastic to expect normal functioning, or anything approaching easy and pleasant functioning where such a state exists? And yet Alexander tells us, and has been telling us for over thirty years, that such conditions are almost universal in modern urban people![15]

Since then, however, orthodox orthopaedic surgeons seem everywhere to have appreciated that vicious bodily coordination is a grave danger to modern man, even if they have not always recommended the best means of correcting or preventing it, and such enlightened books as *Body Mechanics*[16] and such recent articles as that by Mr. Philip Whiles in the *Lancet*[17] show, although strangely incredible as it may seem, neither mentions Alexander's work, that scientific medical interest is beginning to be directed to this fundamental problem.

Now all that Alexander used to say, when he was alone in saying it, is

[15] *The Truth about Childbirth*, pp. 234-238.

[16] By Drs. J. E. Goldthwaite, Lloyd T. Brown, Loring J. Swain, and J. G. Kuhns. (London, 1932).

[17] Issue of 7.4.37.

being emphatically restated by modern orthodox orthopaedic surgeons. And nobody can read the latest scientific contributions to this subject without appreciating the accuracy of Alexander's original criticism of modern man.

Take, for instance, the following:

"Poor health may be found with no disease of the organs, but it is always associated with faulty adjustment of the body or what is better called faulty body mechanics."

This may strike many as a passage from one of Alexander's books. But, as a matter of fact, it is taken from the book above quoted, by four orthopaedic surgeons, and published in 1934.

There is hardly a bodily function, from digestion to respiration, which cannot be gravely interfered with by faulty bodily coordination. And, in view of the wide range of its evil effects, it is impossible to take too serious a view of this question. Nor need I quote from Alexander to show any of the specific effects of this evil; but again turn to the four orthopaedic surgeons already mentioned. They say:

"Is it not possible that much of that which concerns chronic medicine has to do with the imperfect functioning of sagged or misplaced organs? Is it not possible that such sagging results in imperfect general secretions, or mixtures that at first are purely functional but which, long continued, may produce actual pathology?"

THE EFFECT OF FAULTY USE OF SELF ON CHILDBIRTH

There is neither the space nor the need to deal with the general aspects of this question. And even its immense importance in obstetrics and gynaecology should be fairly obvious. For if it be admitted that, by faulty coordination, the normal and natural relations of the organs, their condition and their tone may be adversely modified, if it be acknowledged that by the wrong use of self an abdominal wall may sag, abdominal viscera may be displaced, and a thorax may expand so inadequately as to restrict the respiratory function, then here alone we have a sufficient amount of mischief to impair not only the course of pregnancy but also and above all that of childbirth.

It is with great pleasure that I am able to reproduce the following extracts from a letter from Mr. Gaston M. Martineau after his wife had given birth to her second child. Mr. Martineau writes:

A son was born to us early this morning; he is thriving nicely and my wife is wonderfully well. I am writing to you personally because I want you to know that both my wife and myself will be eternally thankful to you for what you have done for her, because we know that her extremely robust health right through pregnancy and now that all is over to be due to your work.

We think it due to tell you now that the supreme test of birth has been put upon the worth of your work on her successfully that she carried the child right through pregnancy and required no support for the abdomen the whole time through.

When we remember the acute trouble Catherine (the first child) caused and the deplorable way in which the abdomen sagged in the later time of gestation we are both gratefully amazed.

It must be remembered too that a solid five years have elapsed since your training was received, during which time she has enjoyed perfectly robust health, vastly different from anything she experienced before, being entirely without corsets of any kind, so that it cannot in any way be said that the benefit is a "flash in the pan."

Will you accept this short description of her well-being as a small token of our great thanks to you, please Mr. Alexander, for all your share in our possessing it. You will live with us for the rest of our lives even though we never saw you again, because of what you have given us, and because your training is progressive daily through a lifetime.

If this description should be of any help in your work as evidence of long distance results please use it in whatever way you may desire.

Ever yours, etc.,

(signed) GASTON M MARTINEAU.

My justification for deciding to take Mr. B. and the other pupils I have mentioned was this:

Experience had taught me that by employing the procedures of the technique which I have outlined one can help a person afflicted with osteo-arthritis, spasmodic torticollis or any other trouble to gradually overcome his habit of interfering with the employment of the primary control of the use of himself, and so indirectly bring about a constant improvement in the manner of his general use. The pupil who, with the aid of his teacher, learns to employ these procedures as the means of gaining the end he desires, begins a process of change by starting with the inhibition of the misdirection of his habitual employment of the primary control associated with his harmful functioning. In this way, he influences for good his manner of use and indirectly raises his standard of general functioning, and in the process, he gradually modifies the deformity, the wrong axis of the head and the overaction of the muscle groups (reflex spasm), and with this the irritation and pressure, headache and pain associated with the condition disappears. At a certain stage of his work, the pupil becomes able to project with confidence the new messages necessary to an improving employment of his primary control, and continues this reconditioning process in his daily life. This means a constant influence in the right direction leading to change which will prove permanent, for it will become associated with a tendency for the defect or disease to be diminished, and when a given point of change is reached, the undesirable symptoms will disappear. The reconditioning process will include a continuous raising of the standard of reliability of his sense of feeling, so that in time he will find it almost as difficult to revert to the old habitual manner of use which once *felt right*, as it was at the beginning of his lessons to employ the new and better manner of use which, at that time, despite all the help given him by his teacher, still *felt wrong*.

I ask the reader to be patient with me for wishing to re-emphasize here that in the cases we have been considering, I was not concerned with the *curing* of osteo-arthritis, spasmodic torticollis, deformity, wrong axis of the head, reflex spasms, headache or pain *as such*; and this is true of my attitude whenever a case is sent to me by a doctor, no matter what the trouble may be, and is in keeping with the facts which I have accumulated and noted during the varied experiences of a long teaching career. My concern is always to try to reestablish as a *constant* that employment of the primary control of use with its associated standard of functioning, which is found present in people who are not in need of "cure," but are instead in what can be described as good health.

I have yet to see a person afflicted with the conditions in need of "cure" which were present in such cases as those we have been discussing, whose employment of the primary control is not having a *constant* harmful effect upon his manner of general use, and therefore upon the standard of his general functioning.

Should I chance to find such a case, I should at once admit that the contentions I have been making almost all my life were wrong, and I should seek some other outlet for my energies.

CHAPTER III

A REVIEW OF THE REPORT OF THE PHYSICAL EDUCATION COMMITTEE OF THE BRITISH MEDICAL ASSOCIATION

Part I

Fallacies and Limitations in Physical Culture

In November, 1937, a committee with Dr. (now Sir) E. Kaye Le Fleming as chairman, reported on methods of physical culture for the purpose of offering suggestions for improvement. The opportunity offered them was an exceptional one. It was sponsored by the British Medical Association at a time when, for special reasons, it was considered necessary by the authorities to encourage a national movement in the direction of improved physical development, and to ensure that the very best possible means be employed for putting this idea into practice. The members of the committee were entrusted with the task of examining methods of physical culture in vogue, both today and in the past, together with all available knowledge bearing upon this subject up to date. If they decided that any of these methods were unsatisfactory, and they could by availing themselves of recent advances in knowledge offer something better, they were pledged to do so.

When the report was published several copies reached me within a week, some sent by medical men who did not hesitate to condemn it, and others by laymen who urged me to reply to it in the press or in my next book.

I am about to carry out this last request and shall begin by giving a quotation from the report:

> Each of these exercises is designed for the purpose of producing specific effects which taken together, bring about the desired physical development.

Just so! But the question is, when the members of the committee wrote this, what was the picture of "desired physical development" which they had before their eyes and wherein does this differ from the conception of those whose methods they set out to examine? By what scientific findings were they guided when they arrived at the conclusion that the performance of exercises designed for the purpose of producing a given number of specific effects could, "taken together, bring about the desired physical development"?

Anyone who reads the report will see that the conception of the members of the committee does not differ from that of the traditional physical culture experts and teachers past or present. There is nothing new or original—just the same old idea of muscle development of specific parts by direct means. There is nothing in their suggestions to show that they recognize that all physical effort tends to increase thoracic rigidity and to cause breathlessness, and that consequently the performance of exercises for the development of muscle tension in specific parts tends to develop undue contraction and raising of the chest and to increase any lordosis curve of the back which may be present.

Those who designed the exercises provide no means for countering or minimizing tendencies such as these, which should surely be countered in people who are in a condition requiring help. I admit that the performance of exercises can and does build up the muscles on the outside of the chest, but the tendency to increased rigidity is not thereby diminished; indeed such structural defects as may be present are merely exaggerated. As a good instance of this I will cite that of a famous athlete who advertised that he had a ten-inch chest expansion, his claim being supported by doctors who measured him. One doctor, however, was not satisfied with the methods of taking the measurements and, after making an extensive examination, was able to prove that the man had only a two-inch thoracic expansion, the other eight being due to muscle expansion on the outside of the bony structure of the chest.

Further, anyone who examines the practice approved by the committee will see that the means they advocate for putting their theories into practice do not differ *in principle* from the means which have been employed ever since physical exercises were first devised by man. It is just this: The members of the committee realize that something is wrong with the physical development of many of our people; they therefore advocate physical exercises and recommend people to practise them. This is evidence of a complete misunderstanding of cause and effect. In my previous books, as in this one, I have dealt fully with the defect in diagnosis which has led to this misunderstanding, and so to the adoption of the wrong principle underlying all physical culture methods. I have shown that if there is something wrong with a person's physical development, it can be demonstrated that this wrongness is caused chiefly by his wrong manner of use of himself, and that this wrong manner of use is really *what he is doing himself* as a result of depending upon unreliable sensory guidance in carrying out his daily activities, including of course any exercises he may perform. The reliability or otherwise of sensory guidance is a matter of immediate concern and importance in the carrying out of any instructions which are given for physical exercises. Those in need of physical development will always be people whose manner of use of themselves is tending to lower their standard of general functioning, and this will be associated with misdirection of energy to the musculature through unreliable and deceptive sensory guidance (feeling).

Today the unreliability of our sensory mechanisms is widely recognized, as, for instance, in a deterioration in our sensory observation and awareness. A medical man at a meeting of the British Medical Association at Bath in 1925 was reported to have expressed the wish that something might be done to raise the standard of the medical student's observation and awareness. But in the B. M. A. report the reliability of the sensory guidance of those they wish to help through physical culture is taken for granted. The committee ignores the fact that those who practise the exercises they advocate will be guided in the performance of them by the same unreliable sense of feeling which has guided them hitherto in all their activities, and has brought them to the pass where they are in need of the help which physical exercises are supposed to give. Hence it follows that the unfortunate victim of faulty sensory guidance and deceptive appreciation of what he is doing will do *what he feels is right* as soon as he starts to do the exercises, and since in this he will be relying upon the same old sensory guidance and appreciation which led him into wrongness, his "right," while he is still so guided, will be wrong. Most important of all, his unreliable sensory guidance will lead him to a wrong employment of the primary control of his use of himself which will be a constant influence working against him during the performance of his exercises, while in most cases the harmful effect of this influence upon his general functioning will be increased by any effort he makes TO DO the exercise "right" because, as already explained, his "right" is wrong in the use of himself.

I admit that it is possible for such an individual to get an exercise "right" as such, but it is hardly possible for him to put his use of himself right in doing so, since this would mean doing what he *feels to be wrong*. For a person to do what he feels to be wrong in order to be right is as unlikely as it would be for him to take what he believes to be the wrong road to a place and expect to arrive there. In fact one can guarantee that the one thing a person in need of help will not do is what is *right in the use of himself* in performing exercises, no matter by whom they are designed. *All exercises are fundamentally the same in the sense that the activity which goes to their performance is inseparable from the habitual manner of general use of the performer.*

This being so, the reasoning should be: Here are people whose physical development is unsatisfactory, and this is associated with their sensory misdirection of their habitual use of themselves. Surely then, before they are given anything TO DO in the form of exercises, we should point out to them wherein this misdirection lies and give them the means of preventing it.

I ask any readers who doubt what I have written on the subject to watch the performance of exercises such as I am condemning, and, if they will take the time necessary for such observation, they will confirm me in maintaining that the performance of any exercise by those in need of physical development for health not only tends to exaggerate the bad habits of use always present in such people, but cultivates new bad habits.

John Dewey, long before he had lessons with me, had seen that in methods of general education new defects are cultivated during attempts to eradicate old ones, and wrote in his *Educational Essays*:

> It is through a partial and defective psychology that the teacher, in his reaction from dead routine and arbitrary moral and intellectual discipline, has substituted an appeal to the satisfaction of momentary impulses. It is not because the teacher has a knowledge of psycho-physical mechanism, but because he has a *partial* knowledge of it. He has come to consciousness of certain sensations and certain impulses, and of the ways in which these may be stimulated and directed, but he is in ignorance of the larger mechanism (just as a mechanism), and of the causal relation which subsists between the unknown part and the elements upon which he is playing. What is needed to correct his errors is not to inform him that he is only misled by taking the psychical point of view, but to reveal to him the scope and intricate interactions of the mechanism as a whole. Then he will realize that, while he is gaining apparent efficacy in some superficial part of the mechanism, he is disarranging, dislocating, and disintegrating much more fundamental factors in it. (*Educational Essays*, p. 151.)

Yet I have never heard of a teacher of physical culture who had awakened to this fact in connexion with the performance of exercises designed to eradicate specific defects. Many years ago, when speaking before a child study group, I offered to visit any class of physical culture with some of the members, and said that if I could not point out that the pupils during the lessons given for the purpose of remedying some specific defect were cultivating new defects which sooner or later would prove more harmful than those they were trying to eradicate, I would then and there give up my work and seek some other occupation. No advantage was taken of this, but some time afterwards I was lecturing to the students of a College for Physical Training and was asked to demonstrate my technique on a few students chosen because they were considered especially good at their work. I shall never forget how sorry I was for those selected, because from my point of view, in whatever they did for me, their use of themselves could not have been worse.

After the lecture I was asked to look at the back of one of their best teachers, because of a trouble it had been found impossible to remove. It was obvious to me that the trouble was brought about by her bad manner of use of herself generally, which also accounted for other specific defects which I noticed, such as her habit of over-stiffening the muscles of her legs and throwing them unduly backward at the knees in her attempts to keep her equilibrium. I pointed this out and another teacher then said: "We teach them to do that in order to improve the condition of the abdominal muscles." Could one have a better example of a harmful by-product being cultivated through the practice of exercises "designed for the purpose" of producing a "specific effect"?

I challenge any or all of the members of the B. M. A. committee to demonstrate to me that the person engaged in the performance of "each of these exercises" will not, in producing a specific effect (obviously the effect believed to be the right means for producing the "desired physical development"), also produce what I call by-products in the way of new bad habits of use, with harmful effect upon the general psycho-physical functioning, making normal physical development impossible. Obviously the greater the number of "specific effects" aimed at, the greater will be the opportunity for the further misuse of the mechanisms, and the production of harmful by-products.

One more point. The committee, in telling us that each of the exercises is "designed for the purpose of producing specific effects," is assuming that the designers know exactly how many specific effects will be required for bringing about the "desired physical development" in people who practise them. Otherwise, how could they have arrived at a calculation of the number of exercises they would have to design for this purpose? Such a task would call for a complete diagnosis of the conditions present in every person whose needs the exercises are designed to meet, for it is a matter of common observation that people's defects in "physical development" differ as much as defects in their handwriting.

Those who practise the exercises will almost certainly not be able to diagnose their own physical shortcomings, let alone the defects in their manner of use responsible for these.[18] This means that they will be forced to practise indiscriminately a set of ill-assorted exercises, the effect of which they no more foresee than they can check, and therefore, have little chance to avert the harmful effects the practice must have upon their general use and, in the long run, upon their functioning.

In Australia over forty years ago, in the rooms of one of the best teachers of physical culture I have ever known, I had my first experience of observing the results of exercises designed to bring about "specific effects." Although I disagreed then, as I still do, with the principle underlying his and all such teaching, we were both impressed by the fact that *the same set of exercises was responsible for quite different effects in different people.* How could it be otherwise?

We all notice differences in people's manner of walking and speaking, and this same difference in use they bring to the performance of the exercises. The specific effect desired, as well as the by-products of one exercise or more, will not be exactly the same in any two people, and if this be so, who is to decide which of the exercises—whether all or only a selected few—are to be used, and in what order they are to be practised if they are to meet the variations in kind of the various mal-conditions which in most people create the need for the "desired physical development"?

Who is to decide what is "cause" and what "effect"? Or which are the particular parts affected and needing attention? Anyone who by training and experience is equipped with the sensory observation required for detecting these differences can satisfy himself, by examining a number of people performing the same set of exercises, that the result will differ according to the difference in conditions present in each.

Suppose, for instance, that two people, one with round shoulders and an unduly contracted chest and the other with an unduly protruded chest and lordosis curve, take up the practice of the same set of exercises selected from among those recommended by the B. M. A. committee. In these two people the habitual manner of use will be so different that the process of gaining the specific effects desired from the

[18]In his *Human Nature and Conduct* (pp. 27-29), Professor John Dewey discusses what happens when the ordinary man, slouching along with a stoop, is told to stand up straight. He immediately pulls himself up, and imagines that, by conforming to the idea suggested by the command, he is, for the time being, improving himself, and Professor Dewey proceeds: "Of course, something happens when a man acts upon his idea of standing straight. For a little while, he stands differently, but only a different kind of badly." That is to say, unless he has been taught the correct use of his primary control, his "standing-up" will only be another form of the wrongness associated with his slouching.

practice of any one exercise will make on the muscles immediately concerned a much greater demand in one of them than in the other, and this will be found to be the case in respect of the demand made upon other muscles throughout their organisms.

If the committee should argue that it is not concerned with the effect of the exercises upon muscles, or with muscle development as such, but with the "physical development" generally found in association with health, then their case becomes worse still. The idea of health cannot be disassociated from that of an optimum standard of functioning, and no person can enjoy an optimum standard of functioning when, in all his activities, there is such interference with the employment of the primary control that his manner of use of himself is constantly lowering the standard of his general functioning. It is certain that the practice of the exercises advocated will tend to exaggerate any such interference with the primary control of use, and so lower still further the standard of general functioning.

With these considerations before us, I repeat the question with which I opened this chapter: By what scientific findings were the members of the committee guided when they arrived at the conclusion that the performance of exercises designed for the purpose of producing a given number of specific effects could, "taken together, bring about the desired physical development"?

To this question there can be but one reply: They could not have been guided by any scientific findings. Only by ignoring a whole field of essential data could the committee have come to the conclusion formulated in the report.

The members of the committee must surely see that if the procedures they advocate for the purpose of producing a "desired physical development" can be shown to make for the development of harmful by-products, these procedures cannot be in accordance with scientific method which demands that in an experiment, the means employed shall produce just the results they are supposed to produce *and no other*, and that the relationship of the results to the means employed shall be subject to sensory observation.

In teaching people who are in need of physical development, some of whom manifest symptoms of chronic disease, my daily experience proves to me that if specific effects are to be secured in accordance with scientific method and in such a way as to be lasting, they must be gained not by direct but by *indirect* means[19] which involve a knowledge of the

[19]It is interesting to remember the number of valuable discoveries that have been made *indirectly*. For instance, Faraday was interested in the effect of a magnet on a piece of steel, Pasteur in crystals. Watt was first interested in the lifting of a pot-lid by the steam, and so on.

use of the primary control. Anyone who employs the technique described in my books can demonstrate this for himself, for the technique is based on the indivisibility of individual human potentialities in activity, of which the primary control is the governor. But the committee makes no mention of such a control, despite the fact that the findings of the late Rudolph Magnus established its existence, and also that a detailed description of my discovery and use of this control in a technique is to be found in *The Use of the Self.* A medical friend of mine who realized the importance of this in the field of "physical development" assures me that he urged influential members of the committee to take my work into their survey, but they refused to do so. It is inconceivable that the members should have consented to serve on such a committee unless they were dissatisfied with methods of physical development in vogue, and were determined to examine and make use of any available new knowledge on the subject in an endeavour to improve these methods. Yet there is no reference in their report to the contributions made in recent years to a field in which experience has been gained which has an all-important bearing upon scientific physical development. I cannot find anything in the report which has not been in use since I was a young man, and the principle underlying the practice involved in their suggestions can be demonstrated to be unscientific. When arriving at their conclusions they placed themselves at great disadvantage by ignoring:

> (1) the discovery of a primary control of use[20];
>
> (2) that the sensory guidance of all people needing physical development is unreliable;
>
> (3) that such people will employ their primary control wrongly in their activities, and that this is a *constant* influence for ill working against them both before and after the practice of their exercises; and,
>
> (4) that no method of help can meet their needs unless in carrying it out they are taught to employ the primary control in such a way that their manner of use becomes a constant influence for good, tending always to raise the standard of their functioning.

These are the points they could and should have brought forward, not only to prove the shortcomings of present methods but also to bring before the public, now so deeply interested in "physical fitness," new knowledge which would set them thinking along new lines, and so help

[20]See Anthony M. Ludovici, *Health and Education Through Self-Mastery*. Chap. I. "Use of Ourselves," pp. 23-30.

them to avoid the pitfalls which exist in the practice of physical culture exercises. *This could have been a beginning of a practical campaign in prevention.*

The substitution however of preventive for curative measures was not even recommended in the report of the British Medical Association, nor were any "means-whereby" offered which would have made the carrying-out of this recommendation possible.

In ordinary mechanics, if we knew that the control or controls of a machine were out of order, we should at once decide to have them put right before expecting the machine to show the mechanical stability and usefulness of which it is capable. But this common-sense point of view must have escaped the committee, for the suggested plan implies that we should take an already ill-controlled piece of human machinery and proceed to increase the work done by it. If their advice is followed, the working of the controls will only be further interfered with and the general misuse of the mechanism increased, with the result that new defects will be produced by the practice of exercises designed to eradicate other defects.

It can be demonstrated by means of my technique that interference with the working of the primary control of the psycho-physical machine cannot only be prevented but also be remedied in those in whom the working of this control has already been interfered with. Anyone who has learned this technique of the correction of interference with the working of the primary control will be able to put it into practice in daily life in any sphere, and in any form of activity, including games and all forms of outdoor exercise. All that is necessary is to see to it that during games and all forms of outdoor exercise there is no interference with the working of the primary control.[21] In this way any reasonable standard of physical development can be attained without fear of producing harmful by-products, and the act of living itself will become a constant means whereby changes in the direction of more and more desirable physical development can be brought about.

---

[21] In discussing this matter recently with a public official, I asked him why the people concerned with health movements were making such a definite stand for physical culture. He said it was because they had not found the development gained through the agency of games satisfactory. I then explained to him that a different result could not be expected, because it is highly probable that those for whom the games were planned were already interfering with the proper use of the primary control, and that they would exaggerate this misuse in playing games. For the same reason, I pointed out, physical culture schemes would prove equally unsatisfactory. If it could be arranged, I should like to take a group of adults or young people who have learned to prevent interference with their use of themselves while playing games or performing exercises, and compare the results in physical development with those obtained by a similar group practising any physical exercises and games in accordance with orthodox principles. *(continued on next page)*

Under the committee's plan, this "desirable physical development" is to be produced in people by the performance of exercises for a certain time during the day, and we are actually asked to believe that muscular tension, exerted for a comparatively short space daily by people whose habitual use is so defective that they are in need of help, will counter the general wrong functioning which is due to a misuse that is operating against them all day long. To believe this is to carry credulity very far. If the people who are in need of physical exercises are habitually interfering with the working of their primary control to the extent of upsetting their functioning, it stands to reason that any extra muscular tension they exert in the practice of exercises will increase this habitual interference, so that their daily exercises will simply afford yet another opportunity of exaggerating their bad habitual use of themselves, and of repeating and therefore establishing more and more firmly wrong sensory experiences.

In the practice of my technique, the boredom of performing exercises for a given time daily is avoided, and the opportunities for wrong experiences in practice minimized. As long as we adhere in everything we do to the principle of consciously inhibiting interference with the employment of the primary control, then our ordinary daily activities can be made a constant means of psycho-physical development in its fullest sense. The instinctive misdirection which led to interference with the employment of the primary control will be changed to a conscious guidance of the use of the self, associated with reliability of sensory appreciation.

This means that it may be possible for us to live a full life in civilization, in which the activities necessary for the support of life can be made

---

In a lecture given by her to the Ling Society, Miss Lucy Silcox, Class. Trip. Camb., formerly Head Mistress of St. Felix School, Southwold, said: "I have to judge your system . . . as an onlooker, by the eye, and in doing so I take the simple and obvious tests that meet the eye, tests of sitting down and standing up, of running and walking, of speaking and listening. Not in the gymnasium, but in the house and in the field and in the street, I have put these tests; and it is only the rare exception that has, in the simple ways of life, aroused in me the emotion of living, moving beauty, that beauty of movement which, though often found with beauty of form and face, is independent and can and does exist apart. Everywhere that I have gone out and about, I have shamelessly made notes, asking myself *quid deficit?* What is lacking? Why is it that of specially selected and specially trained persons, A is unable to stand in quiet repose, B moves across the room with a lurch, and C nods her head whenever she speaks? Why is the heavy step so frequent among teachers and taught? (not, of course, in the drill class). A Head Mistress friend of mine, whose sitting room was under her large hall, said to me: 'During the dancing class, the movements were almost noiseless; the lesson over, you would say the room was full of rhinoceroses.' What had become of the lightness they had shown? What good was it if it ended with the lesson?"

These questions lead to the core of the whole matter.

as effective in securing and maintaining a satisfactory standard of physical development, as were the activities of man in uncivilized life when he was a hunter and his very existence depended upon the standard of development required for survival.

* * * * *

It has struck me that I could not conclude this chapter on Physical Culture more appropriately than by reproducing two photographs with the comment they received which have caught my eye in the English press. Each is profoundly interesting in its own way, as revealing how consistently both by precept and example, wrong values in matters of physical culture are now being inculcated upon the general public.

The first photograph entitled "THE ROWERS" appeared in the *Evening Standard*, March 1, 1939, with the following words:

> This remarkable study of the Oxford Boat Race crew rowing a sharp burst in their training at Henley was taken by long-focus camera. The tenseness of the various facial expressions reveals the effort put into the work.

The caption read:

DETERMINATION MIRRORED IN THEIR FACES

I have carefully studied the expression on the faces of the young men in the picture, but have failed to find any justification for the above caption. Four of them look as if they were being tortured on the rack, three as if in a trance, and just one, the third from the left, as if he had taken part in a rowing race and had the right attitude towards a rowing contest. Surely a university boat race should be a friendly contest between men animated by the sporting instinct. Every one of them should wish the victory to go to the best crew. It should be an experience of pleasure, happiness and healthy recreation to all concerned, not an unnatural struggle involving distortion and loss of consciousness through the "determination" to gain an end even at the cost of personal exhaustion and damage. What difference does it really make in the long run whether or not an Oxford or Cambridge crew wins the boat race in a particular year? None whatever—particularly when we remember that over a period of 111 years Oxford has won forty-two contests and Cambridge forty-eight.[22] People indulging in sport today whether it be rowing, football, cricket or what-not, seem to be losing all sense of pro-

[22]There were no contests in the years 1830 to 1835 inclusive, none in 1837, 1838, 1843, 1844, 1847, 1848, 1850, 1851, 1853, 1855, 1857, and 1915 to 1919 inclusive. There were two contests in the same year in 1849 and one dead heat in 1877(?). This accounts for the apparent discrepancy in the figures.

portion, all idea of relative values. In the interest of all concerned, it were far better if we engaged in sport for sport's sake. End-gaining in sport, as in every sphere of life, is in the long view a delusion and a snare.

The second photograph entitled "THE SERGEANT MAJOR" appeared in the *Sporting and Dramatic News*, November 26, 1937, with the following caption:

THE FINISHED OBJECT! HOW THE SERGEANT MAJOR STANDS.

This is an example of the harmful result of building posture on the "plumb line" theory and practice.

When shown this photograph, a medical man I know uttered the one word: "Monstrosity!" It is just another proof of the ignorance and stupidity that prevails today in spheres where experts rule supreme. Study this photograph and use your own common sense in judging the contorted form before you, then look up your manuals of physiology and anatomy, and see if you can discover anything in favour of the posture assumed, thanks to the misguided people who advocate this degradation of the human self. You will not succeed in finding anything to justify it, but you will certainly find that in this picture physiological, anatomical, and biological laws have been outraged. The passing of new laws is in vogue nowadays, and as many people are likely in their ignorance to be led into serious error by attempting to imitate the posture of the unfortunate man in the picture and much value is now being attached to health and well-being, I suggest that probably the most important law to be passed at the moment would be one to prevent human forms from being harmed and degraded by physical culturists whose work and ideals lead to the posture shown in our picture. It would have seemed incredible to me before seeing it that anyone should find it in him to wish to distort the body of a human being in this way, and still more incredible that anyone could be found who would submit to the indignity and folly of procedures that can bring it about.

Large sums of money are being spent in a campaign for physical fitness and well-being, and thousands of people are being placed in the hands of physical culture teachers to be subjected to the carrying-out of special exercises to gain certain ends. It is in the interest of my readers that I am including in these pages this photograph of a man trained in accordance with this plan.

*　　*　　*　　*　　*

It has been shown that man, by using exercises as a means of improving his physical condition, becomes a specialist in the production of harmful by-products, and that, by doing this, he not only nulli-

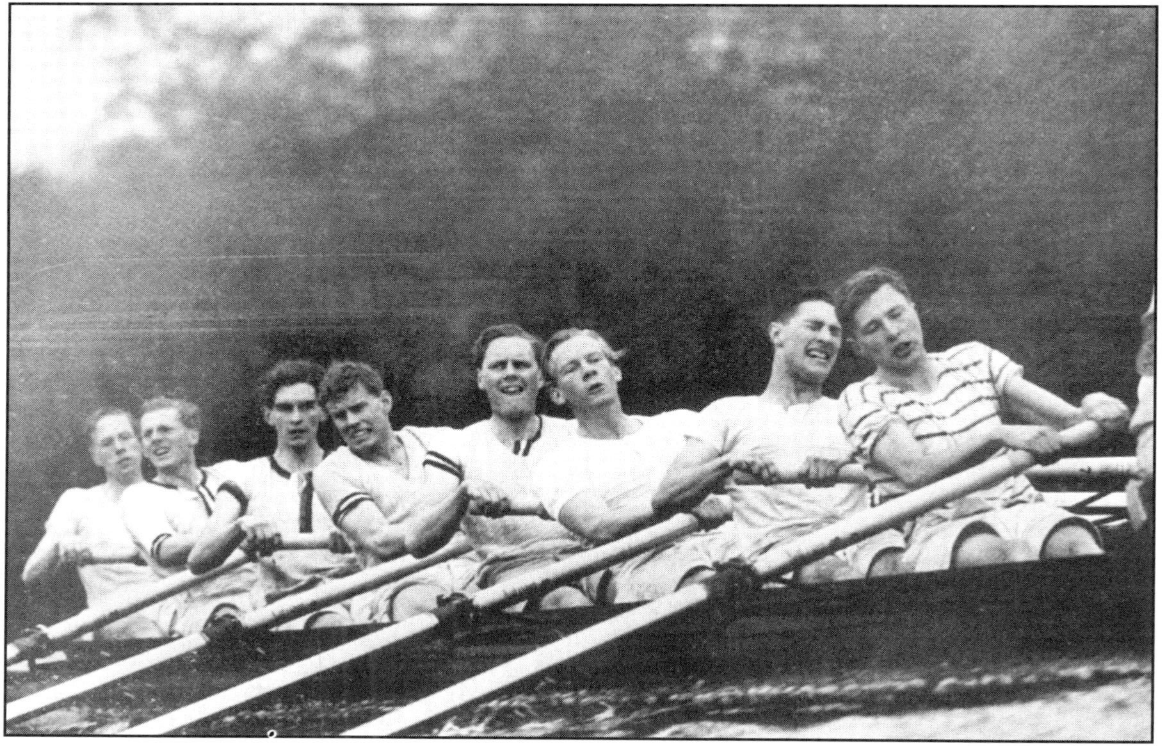

THE ROWERS

And they call it sport! The Oxford Boat Crew showing what *The Evening Standard* called "Determination mirrored on their faces."

See page 563

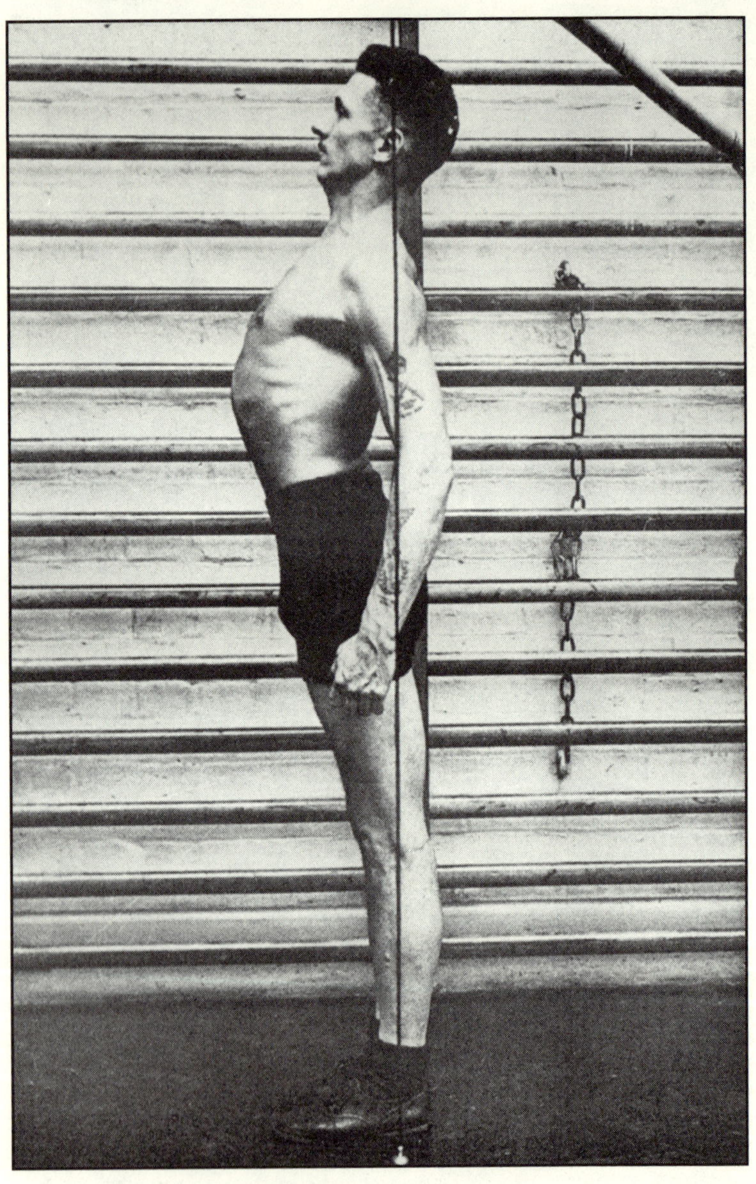

THE SERGEANT MAJOR
Building posture on the plumb line

See page 564

fies anything he may gain at one point, but, in the long run, tends to lose rather than gain in the aggregate.[23] In a large majority of cases, the practice of exercises leads to the cultivation of harmful psycho-physical habits associated with a lowering of the standard of general functioning. In this way man, in the fundamental sphere of activity within the self, defeats his own ends, and his habit of end-gaining is so deeply ingrained, that it persists as a menace to him in his relations with the body politic and the outside world.

We have proof of this in every field of his activity, scientific and otherwise. It matters not whether he considers it necessary to do something to improve his personal well-being or that of others, to "cure" some defect or disease, or to make some social, political, financial, business, religious or educational reform; in the long run he will defeat himself by his habit of concentrating on his end, without having first thought out the means whereby harmful by-products will not be created in the process of gaining it.

Part II

My indebtedness to Mr. Aldous Huxley for the article that follows calls for my best thanks. I have included it in this chapter, because of its bearing upon the subject matter, and because I believe that the reader will be interested in the happenings which Mr. Huxley has presented in the unique manner that is so characteristic of his writing.

A NEW TECHNIQUE FOR NEW SOLDIERS
by Aldous Huxley

"Good news is always less sensational than bad, and therefore, even at the best of times, gets less attention. In a world at war there are so many, such horribly absorbing stories of destruction and sudden death that neither journalists nor their readers have much time for anything else. But even in a world at war human decency and reason still survive and actually succeed in scoring their small successes. The record of one of these inconspicuous triumphs may be found, well buried, so far as the general public is concerned, in the correspondence columns of some recent issues of the *British Medical Journal.* Here, from an exchange of letters between Dr. Andrew Murdoch and Colonel Wand-Tetley, Inspector of Physical Training for the British Army, we learn that, in recent months, the physical training of English soldiers has undergone

[23]In this connexion I would refer the reader to Appendix F in which are disclosed the harmful by-products produced by the methods in force in the German Army.

a radical change for the better. The nature of this change is such, and its implications are so important, that it seems worth while to give a brief account of it.

"Physical training for soldiers has its origin in parade-ground drill. Now, parade-ground drill had a twofold object: it was intended, first, to teach the use of arms and the performance of certain maneuvres; and second, to provide an agreeable spectacle for the important personages in the reviewing stand. Among these important personages a convention grew up during the eighteenth and nineteenth centuries that the most agreeable of all military spectacles was that of large bodies of men standing in positions of extreme tension and rigidity, moving with the stiff precision of automata, and doing difficult and unnatural tricks like trained animals. Hence those blown-up pigeon chests, those shoulders stiffly thrown back, those concave spines, those taut necks and raised chins. Hence, too, such horrible monstrosities as the Prussian goose step and its recent fascist imitation, the *passo ginnastico*.

"Some fifty or sixty years ago the first signs of a change began to manifest themselves. Physical culture came to be taught in schools and as an adjunct to medicine, and it was found that the traditional military methods were far from giving satisfactory results. Even in the armies, enlightened officers began to talk about physical training for health and general well-being, not merely for smart appearance on the parade ground. But just what sort of physical training would give men health and general well-being? That was the question; and while the experts argued back and forth about the proper answer, soldiers, and to a lesser extent, school children went on being taught in the old bad way. Chests were still thrown out, spines bent backwards and neck muscles strained, just as they had been in the days of Frederick the Great.

"Meanwhile, many new systems of physical culture were tried out. Most of them were better than the traditional parade-ground drill; but none was wholly satisfactory. For in all of them the organism was conceived, not as a whole, but as a collection of parts, each of which was to be exercised and strengthened in turn; and corrective treatment was aimed at palliating the manifest symptoms of weakness and deformity, not at removing the underlying causes. The trouble was that nobody knew what those underlying causes might be. All that the physical culturists could be sure about was the obvious fact that some people seemed to be naturally gifted with the power to use their bodies well, while others (an actual majority in urban, industrial communities) could only use their bodies badly. Why this should be so, nobody understood. Then, in the early years of the present century, an obscure young Australian, F. Matthias Alexander, completely revolutionized the situation. By long and patient experiment first on himself and then on others, Mr. Alexander became convinced that the underlying cause of most physical maladjustment was to be found in the faulty carriage of the head in relation to the spinal column. We can summarize his conclusions by saying that, in man as in other animals, there is a certain natural and correct relation between head and spine—a relationship which, when it is preserved, guarantees that all the organs shall be in their proper position and functioning harmoniously. Animals in a state of nature tend to retain this correct adjustment instinctively. It is only when human beings interfere with them that they go wrong. Thus, the bearing rein was introduced to 'improve the appearance' of carriage horses, by drawing back the head in relation to the neck. The result of its use was that the poor beasts so harnessed suffered great discomfort, lost half their pulling power and were rapidly exhausted. What men did to their horses by means of the bearing rein they have done to themselves by means of the bad postural habits acquired under the stresses of urban and industrial civilization. How or why these habits are acquired, we do not know; but that they are acquired is certain. And what is equally certain to anyone who has followed the work of F. Matthias Alexander and his pupils is that the correction of these bad habits produces far-reaching results, of benefit to the entire psychophysical organism. It is, of course, impossible in a short article to describe Mr. Alexander's discovery in any detail. Nor is it necessary; for he has done the work himself in a series of books, of which the most recent and the most explicit is *The Use of the Self*. Let it suffice to say that the correct relation of head to spine can be obtained, when the head continuously and progressively obeys the injunction, 'Forward and up.'

"The importance of Alexander's discovery was early recognized by that eminently practical philosopher and educationist, John Dewey, who contributed prefaces to his first two books. But in spite of this and of his great success as a teacher, both in London and New York, where he is now teaching, Alexander received, during many years, little or no recognition from official quarters in the fields of medicine and physical education. Recently, however, a change has set in. Biologists and physiologists are coming more and more to think in terms of the organism as a whole. Moreover, studies of animals in motion have revealed the significant part played by the head and neck in the co-ordination of the body. In consequence of all this, official medicine and official physical culture have become increasingly receptive to the hypothesis which Alexander has been so clearly verifying during his forty years of teaching. For the last few years Alexander has been enjoying that curious kind of triumph which comes to unorthodox and professionally unqualified men of genius, who live long enough to see their ideas appropriated (without acknowledgment) by the orthodox and the qualified.

"The latest and most striking tribute paid to Mr. Alexander's ideas is the fact that physical training in the British Army is henceforward to be based upon the principle which he was the first to formulate: that the secret of proper physical co-ordination must be sought in the correct relation of the head to the spinal column. If this principle is properly taught, it means that hundreds of thousands of young Englishmen will be shown how to unlearn the bad habits forced upon them by urban and industrial life and will acquire one of the indispensable conditions of health and well-being, a correct and natural carriage of the body. Because it is not dramatic, because it refers to an event which can produce results only slowly and at long range, this piece of information is likely to go unrecorded. That is why I have drawn attention to it. Good news is too scarce nowadays for us to be able to afford to ignore it."

CHAPTER IV

A TECHNIQUE FOR PREVENTION

WE are all familiar with the saying, "Prevention is better than Cure," and as far as I can gather, the general interpretation of the word prevention is that accepted in medicine, where it is understood to mean the doing or taking of something either to make the subject temporarily immune to germ infection, or to slow down, if not to arrest, the progressive aggravation of a functional disorder already present so that it may not become acute or organic, or to forestall and remove the more obvious conditions making for dysfunction or distress at a particular crisis.

People may argue with some justice that this is to narrow unduly the scope of prevention, and that if the word is used in its full sense, its primary object must surely be to promote such conditions of well-being in the individual as a whole as will prevent the possible development of specific functional or organic trouble.[24]

In the course of my experience I have found that in cases where such changes for ill have developed, the employment of the primary control is being interfered with in all activity, and there is a constant tendency towards wrong conditions, whereas, and equally beyond dispute, where this control is not interfered with, the tendency towards wrong conditions is changed to a tendency towards good conditions. From this we can postulate that the human being who would be a good subject for the application of the principle of prevention in the wider sense, would be one in whom the employment of the primary control of use ensures the best possible standard of functioning of all parts and processes, as well as the healthiest chemical composition of the tissues.

Unfortunately, the medical man's training, through no fault of his own, does not equip him to work to the principle of prevention in this

[24]These contentions are supported by the subject matter of the letter signed by nineteen medical men quoted in Chapter II. The reader who is not familiar with my books, and is anxious to become better acquainted with the means employed in making changes from unsatisfactory to satisfactory conditions of use, should read *The Use of the Self*, as there is not space in this work for a restatement of the evidence there adduced.

wider sense, because, as has been pointed out, it does not provide him with the knowledge that would enable him, in making his diagnosis, to take into consideration the influence of use upon his patient's general functioning. Therefore, even if he chances (though this is most unlikely) to be asked to give advice to a patient whose employment of the primary control has not been interfered with, he cannot pass on to him the knowledge which would enable him to prevent himself from doing anything that would interfere with this employment in carrying out his future activities, much less give to a patient who is found to be interfering with the employment of his primary control, the means whereby the correct employment of this primary control could be restored. If in this latter case the doctor should attempt to improve the patient's health and well-being by means that do not include the bringing about of an associated improvement in the employment of the primary control of the use of himself, he will be leaving the constant harmful influence of this use upon the patient's general functioning as a legacy for future trouble.

In the same way if the doctor is to practise prevention in this wider sense with his baby patients, he would need to provide mothers and nurses with the knowledge that will enable them to avoid inducing bad habits in the baby's use by their manner of handling it, or allowing bad habits in its use to be cultivated during its rest and sleep, and particularly whilst it is getting its first experiences in sitting up and in learning to crawl and walk. It is equally essential that when changes for ill have already been allowed to develop in the growing child, the doctor should be able to provide the means whereby right conditions can be restored, and a recurrence of the trouble be prevented in the future. This, for want of a better name, I will call "comparative prevention," and the technique we employ has been found to meet the demands of this form of prevention as well as of prevention in the wider sense.

When a baby is born with a correct working of the primary control, the application of prevention will resolve itself into providing the means whereby this state of use and functioning could be maintained in living. This would be equally true of the adult in whom conditions had been right from the beginning and had been maintained. But such an adult would be hard to find, for the history of man shows that under the demands of civilized life certain undesirable changes are brought about in the working of the human organism, and the human being of today manifests the harmful effects of these changes in his use of himself not only during his working hours but also during sleep. One has only to watch a child or adult *begin to learn* to dance, skate, play some game, write, read or take up some kind of work for the first time, to note the beginning of new bad ways of using themselves which, if repeated, will become new bad habits of use and tend in due course to lower the standard of their general functioning.

In support of this I will quote Mr. (now the Rt. Hon.) Ernest Bevin's Presidential Address at the Trade Union Congress in 1937[25]:

> "The nation has awakened," Mr. Bevin said, "to the fact that too great a price can be paid for the mad rush to increase production. Notwithstanding all the money which has been spent to cure known diseases, industry is constantly creating others."

One can assure Mr. Bevin with the utmost confidence that not only will industry continue to create new diseases, but that, as time goes on, the victory will remain on the side of industry until the worker knows enough about the principles on which the technique of the use of the self is based to enable him to avoid cultivating bad habits of use in meeting any unfamiliar demands made upon him either in prosecuting his particular task, or by unfamiliar environmental conditions.

Any interference with the right working of the primary control of our manner of use during our daily activities is certain to become exaggerated in learning to carry out new industrial work, or in practising physical or other exercises. Witness the extent to which people misdirect their energy in their daily activities, in order to appreciate the opportunity such misdirected activity affords for the development of new harmful habits of use. Hence the fundamental importance of *preventing* the cultivation of these bad habits in learning and learning to do.

Similarly, bad habits are being cultivated by children at school, not only in the sitting or standing positions they assume when learning from a book, or in carrying out their other school duties, but also in playing games and in all other activities which call for the use of the hands or legs or both.

Bad habits are also being cultivated in every hospital and sickroom, particularly when the patient has recovered sufficiently to be allowed to sit up or to begin to walk. I yield to nobody in my respect for the doctors, surgeons and nurses of our hospitals, but this does not prevent me from maintaining that they have not the requisite knowledge to recognize whether the manner of use which the patient adopts in his early attempts to sit up or move about are impeding him. Hence, whatever the patient's difficulties may be, they are made greater than they need be, and what is more serious still, each successive attempt he makes to carry out instructions only exaggerates the impeding or obstructive manner of use which, sooner or later, becomes habitual. This applies of

[25]Reported in *The Daily Herald*, London, December 7, 1937.

course equally to the effort of all who are responsible for the welfare of invalids in the home.

The letter quoted from the *British Medical Journal* in Chapter II is evidence that there is a growing body of medical opinion in favour of including the subject of the use of the self in the medical curriculum. "Diagnosis of a patient's troubles," write the signatories, "must remain incomplete unless the medical man, when making the diagnosis, takes into consideration the influence of use upon functioning." A few months after the publication of this letter, Lord Horder, writing in *The Daily Telegraph* on "The Future Role of the Family Doctor," said:

> And if it be advanced that the doctor's training has not up till now fitted him for work of this sort, then the sooner it does so fit him the better. Inevitably the doctor's work in the future will be more and more educational and less curative. More and more will he deal with physiology and psychology, less and less with pathology. He will spend his time keeping the fit fit rather than trying to make the unfit fit. . . . It is a duty we owe to the panel doctor to enable him to get back now and again to the stimulating and enthralling atmosphere of the wards and laboratories, and—no less helpful—to the atmosphere of his colleagues and teachers.

In this passage, as in his other writings, Lord Horder shows himself to be on the track of prevention. He sees that the successful and useful medical man of the future will be one who can help people to *prevent* unfitness and illness. Unfortunately the plan recommended of sending the medical man back to the wards, laboratories and medical schools, will not give him the help he needs to make his methods "less curative" and "more educational." For up till now medical investigation and experimentation have been devoted to the acquisition of knowledge for the purpose of finding methods of "cure" for disease, rather than knowledge which would enable the doctor to diagnose conditions for the purpose of the *prevention* of disease, the preservation of well-being and a full understanding of the nature of health. The clue to what is wanted in medical training, if the medical man's usefulness in the field of prevention is not to be limited, is to be found in the acquisition of that knowledge of the influence of use upon functioning which the group of medical men in the letter to the B. M. J. state "should be included in the medical curriculum."

If a knowledge of the influence of use upon functioning, and the experience of applying such knowledge in practice is essential to medical men in general, how much more essential must it be to the doctor working according to a plan of prevention in its full sense for, when making his diagnosis of conditions in the child at an early age, he should be able to detect those incipient errors in use which are found associated with a lowered standard of functioning and which, if left unchecked, lead in time to the development of disorders, and are the forerunners of disease.

By means of the knowledge which my technique makes available, the medical man would be able, when diagnosing conditions in a child, to detect from the very start any interference with use and functioning, and would then be equipped for the work of prevention in its full sense; that is to say, with his help, the standard of the child's functioning would be maintained from its earliest days up to adolescence at a level so much higher than at present, that the ills which beset the adult would be lessened and their effect greatly minimized. Moreover, the idea of a "palliative method of cure" which still narrows the practice of medicine, would pass and make way for a new outlook leading to a plan of procedure in which preventive medicine in the widest sense would be a practical possibility.

As matters stand today, the outlook of the patient is as much at fault as that of the doctor and of those responsible for the curriculum of medical training. There is a vicious circle in the attitude of all three. The patient does not consult the doctor until he is ill. We all know that most people keep away from their doctor until they are forced to go to him. Probably this is because of the layman's belief that the doctor is a person trained to treat disease. In any case he goes to a consultation with a fear that there may be something seriously wrong. How different it would all be if he looked upon the doctor as a person trained to *prevent* the development of disorder and disease!

But prevention, in the sense I mean, cannot become a practical possibility until the attitude of people generally changes in favour of preventive methods, and medical men, in making their diagnosis, are mainly concerned with the influence of use upon functioning. In order to succeed in this field of prevention they will need to subject themselves to a form of training which, to those who undertake it, means the "revolution in thought and action" of which Dewey speaks. The experience they will gain however should lead them to see that the art and science of assessing the influence of use upon functioning comes first in the practice and theory of any scheme of preventive medicine, and that any other knowledge required for their medical training can be best applied, not as a principle, but as an auxiliary measure.

Life is the manifestation of use in association with the functioning of the organism, and it is this combination, working as a unity, that makes reaction to stimuli possible. Health in living, therefore, may be defined as the best possible reaction of the organism to the stimuli of living as manifested in its use and functioning. To ensure this we require as a *con-*

stant the best possible manner of use and the highest possible standard of functioning at a given time, in a given environment and under given circumstances; and this I submit constitutes the ideal of human attainment in the field in which we are interested.

It may be argued that this ideal is unattainable, but those who argue in this way are influenced by past experience of failure in making the changes necessitated by the acceptance of new knowledge, and they fail to realize that they owe their failure to the fact that their end-gaining outlook led them to try to make those changes *directly*. Such changes cannot be made by direct procedures, and should not be attempted with undue speed. The end-gaining outlook, which has been and still is almost universal, must therefore pass and give way to a new outlook, in which allowance is made for the time required for the consideration and for the working out of the means whereby any particular change can be made.

In many instances this is a difficult problem to solve, but it is not unduly difficult. The first step is to make the necessary training in the subject of the use of the self a feature of the curriculum at as many medical schools as the number of teachers of my technique now available will permit. Qualified men with this training should be engaged exclusively in making diagnoses of conditions of use for their own patients and for the young patients who are sent to their colleagues, in cases where conditions of use are exerting a harmful influence upon the functioning. If required, they could take advantage of the assistance of teachers trained in my work, the number of whom is steadily increasing. Meanwhile medical men generally could avail themselves of the help we can give them now in the diagnosis and improvement of the manner of use of their child patients; for with the best intentions in the world, medical men class children as satisfactory specimens of well-being when they can be shown to be unsatisfactory specimens of use and functioning. The result is that in many cases a bad manner of use, which should have been diagnosed early, continues to grow worse and to lower the standard of general functioning, until sooner or later functional disorders arise, serious enough to be recognized by the parents. The child is then taken back to the doctor who, from what he finds, diagnoses actual functional disorders, and in consequence begins a course of treatment the need for which could have been *prevented*.

The opposite condition would have come about if in the beginning the doctor had diagnosed the bad manner of use present, and had taken measures to correct it. Then, instead of a gradual lowering, there would have been a gradual raising of the standard of general functioning, with the result that the child in question would be enjoying a state of comparative well-being, instead of being beset with conditions which are undermining his constitution and retarding his psycho-physical growth and development. I have recently seen a girl of twelve with the body frame and general characteristics of a potentially fine type of human being, who had been passed by her doctor the week before as perfectly healthy. It is true that the doctor had suggested that it might be advisable to have her tonsils taken out, but to this the parents would not consent. The mother, however, was not satisfied with the condition of her daughter's back, and for that reason brought her to me for examination. Now in all my long experience I have seldom seen a worse manner of use associated with unsatisfactory conditions than was present in this girl. There was an extreme lordosis curve of the back, a protruding abdomen, fallen arches, and the pelvis was held too far forward.

I particularly noticed a bad curve of the cervical spine, and undue tension of the muscles in the left side of the neck due to her wrong employment of the primary control, and the resultant misdirection was apparent in everything she did. The diagnosis of good health given in this case was a clear example of the failure to detect seeds of future trouble which would in time germinate and lead to acute functional disorder.

The following is another example of what can happen if the influence of the manner of use upon functioning is not taken into account in diagnosing conditions. A school-boy was sent to me because of an impediment in his speech. Various treatments had been tried to rid him of his trouble but without success. When I pointed out to his parents that his stuttering was due to his harmful manner of use, I was told that he was quite successful at games and was the best boxer in the school. This did not impress me as much as they thought it would, and I went on to explain that they evidently had no idea of the harm that such strenuous exercise was doing to the boy, affecting not only his general well-being but also adding to his difficulty in speaking. I agreed to take him as a pupil, but only on the understanding that he should give up strenuous games and discontinue boxing, at any rate for the time being. This was agreed to and good progress was made, until at length he reached the stage when a lesson at intervals was all that he needed.

After one of these intervals he came back for a lesson, and I was alarmed by the rapidity of his heartbeat. I questioned him and found that he had been sprinting regularly. I reminded him that I had warned him against strenuous exercise, and arranged for him to consult a relative of his, a medical man in whom the family had confidence; and there for the time being the matter rested as far as I was concerned.

After a much longer interval than usual, another appointment was made for a lesson, but on the day on which he should have kept his appointment, I heard from his headmaster that he would not be able to come for the lesson as he had broken his arm at football. I wrote at once to say that I was greatly disturbed to hear that he had been allowed to play football because of his heart trouble, but received the reply that the school doctor had given permission for him to play, as he was of the opinion that there was nothing *organically* wrong with his heart. I wrote to say that I was well aware of this, but pointed out that there was serious *functional* trouble which would soon develop into organic disorder if he continued to indulge in strenuous exercises. Meanwhile, I heard from the doctor whom I had advised the boy to consult, that he fully agreed with my view of the case, and that he disagreed with the school doctor with whom he took the matter up.

It is the school doctor who is especially hampered in his work because his training does not equip him as it should for his important job. To undertake to diagnose the condition of children in a school, and to advise whether or not they should take part in strenuous games or exercises is a grave responsibility, and not less grave is the responsibility of having to suggest preventive methods to help those children who have already developed functional trouble which, if left unchecked, can lead to serious disorders. As far as my experience goes, the school doctor seems to diagnose chiefly for organic, not functional trouble. But if he cannot diagnose those incipient functional troubles of which wrong employment of the primary control of use is the forerunner, it is not his own fault but that of his training. Yet it is just in this field that the real usefulness of guidance on preventive lines is needed. The fact that such advice and guidance are not vouchsafed to the child during school life means that its potentialities for health and well-being are not being fully developed, that in most cases trouble is being laid up for the future, and that the child's efforts in the actual school work are being seriously impeded.

When it is pointed out to the headmaster or to the parents that a pupil should not play strenuous games or be made to drill and perform exercises, it is disappointing to find that the school doctor, when appealed to by the headmaster, almost invariably proves to be the stumbling block. Yet in all such instances, I am able and willing to demonstrate that the manner of use of the pupil is not only leading to functional trouble, but is also associated with it, and that in consequence, any strenuous exercise or drill must tend to exaggerate the pupil's habitual manner of use, and so tend to lower gradually the standard of his functioning—the sure and certain way to disorder and ultimately to disease.

I number amongst my pupils headmasters and teachers who are only too well aware of all this. But they sometimes encounter difficulties, because parents through force of habit, are inclined to rely upon the school doctor's opinion regarding the condition of their child and its well-being, irrespective of any evidence that may be put forward to confute it. Nor, seeing how little is done to enlighten them in this matter, is this to be wondered at.

Few of them have either the time or the inclination to seek for such new knowledge as would help them to check the school doctor's opinions, or to adopt a new outlook towards the subject of use and functioning in its relation to child welfare.[26]

I can hardly leave the question of the child's school life without referring to another aspect of it which is of paramount importance. I mean the influence of imitation on the child and the way the average parent approaches this problem.

Example and imitation are potent influences in education. There can be little doubt that most of us, particularly in childhood, are influenced by good or bad example, and whether for good or ill, are certainly prone to imitation. It may therefore be interesting here to relate the experience I have had of the parental attitude towards this matter since I began interviewing parents intending to send their children to our school, first at 16 Ashley Place, and later at Penhill. These parents had heard of our successes in the field of prevention with children considered normal, with backward children, and with those who, owing to some disability or other, could not be helped in ordinary school.

Now the parents of children who, from the ordinary standpoint, would not be considered normal invariably point out that they would not like their child to attend the school if there were children there with peculiarities which their child might imitate. It never seems to occur to these parents that their own child, whose defects they are prone to overlook, might be a bad example to the children already at the school, and that the parents of the latter might justly raise the same objections to the new recruit as they themselves are raising to the existing scholars.

In order to begin to bring such parents to a more reasonable point of view, I try to demonstrate to them that the habits which are the objects of their dread are the particular reaction of a given child manifested in its wrong use of itself in all the acts of daily life, and that although they

[26]Similarly, as far as I can gather, a new outlook is required towards the food eaten, towards the way it is cooked and towards many other matters on the domestic side of the child's life. It is during this period that the best quality of suitable food should be supplied, such as will provide the nourishment required for the development of health and strength in the growing young. Admittedly, however, more has been and is being done in this matter than in regard to the question of the manner of use.

may consider their child normal, I could show them that he displays bad habits of use which other children might imitate. When I succeed in making this clear, I draw their attention to the very bad use present in the great majority of teachers today, and they quickly appreciate the bad example these teachers set to their pupils. For in such cases the greater the teacher's influence over the pupil, the greater the danger of imitation affecting the child adversely during school hours.

I have always recognized this, and that is why all teachers at Penhill School have to become more or less proficient in employing the technique of conscious control in their own use of themselves before taking up their teaching work, and most of them have been through my three years' Training Course for Teachers. Their first aim is to be good examples of use to their pupils, and the experience of having to apply the technique gives them the standard by which to judge.

Having explained all this to parents, I then answer their original query, and assure them that in our experience children do not copy one another's bad habits of use when working to principle in applying the technique employed in the school to their activities in learning and "learning to do." As a matter of fact, instead of imitating such habits, even the youngest child will, after being at the school for a few weeks, often begin to notice faults and find out how and when they occur, the cause being invariably failure to apply the technique in some activity. The manner of use of both teachers and pupils resulting from the application of the technique is of first importance in our school, because the employment of a correct manner of use of the self ensures that the best conditions possible at a given time will be present in the organism while it is being employed in learning and "learning to do."

CHAPTER V

THE CONSTANT INFLUENCE OF MANNER OF USE IN RELATION TO CHANGE

Part I

The Human Element

WE all know how difficult it is to change habit and to keep newly made resolutions which involve our reacting in a different way from that which is habitual to us. Many people will tell you that they have succeeded in doing so by exercising self-control, but as a friend once said to me: "I am coming to the conclusion that what most people call exercising self-control against a bad habit is merely a process of elimination," and I agree with him. My friend was thinking of all those cases of immoderate indulgence in drinking, smoking, etc., in which the persons concerned were forced to give up smoking and drinking entirely, because they found that if they drank and smoked at all they did it to excess.

An attitude of dependence upon instinct (nature) is revealed in the ordinary attitude towards self-control. If a person habitually manifests undesirable emotional or other reactions, such as outbursts of temper, irritability, lying, drunkenness, stealing, etc., it is assumed that, except in special circumstances, these reactions can be controlled by that person, and he is advised or urged to exercise control, or he may decide to do this independently. The same is true of the general attitude towards functional troubles, defects and peculiarities.

Strange it is that this belief in control, as such, still exists, seeing that few people are intentionally uncontrolled, and that throughout man's experience in civilization the need and value of self-control has been advocated by all moral, educational, and religious teaching. Those who accepted the teaching have met with small success however and this must be evident to any unbiased observer of individual or mass reaction today.

The truth is that so far man has failed to understand fully what is required for changing habit if the change is to be a fundamental one, because he has not realized that the establishment of a particular habit in a person is associated in that person with a certain habitual manner of using the self, and that because the organism works as an integrated whole, change of a particular habit in the fundamental sense is impossible as long as this habitual manner of use persists.

True, we have all heard of people who claim to have succeeded in "curing" habits by following the precepts of some teaching method, just as others will claim that they have made changes in themselves by "willing" themselves to do, or not to do, on the trial and error plan.

Yet it is a demonstrable fact that control of the use of ourselves and control of emotional and other reactions is as closely associated as control of manner of use and control of all that prevents interference with the raising of the standard of functioning. Therefore, if people beset with defects and bad habits try to make changes in themselves without first making that change in their use which raises the standard of their general functioning, the constant influence for ill associated with their wrong habitual manner of use remains, and any change claimed to have been made may justly be deemed merely a matter of transfer.

Understanding of this whole problem has been retarded by mistaking "cure by transfer" for permanent change. It is true that the activity, which up to a certain time has habitually manifested itself in one form of reaction, may in response to some new stimulus manifest itself in another form, and one which, when taken by itself, may be considered according to individual outlook to be a great improvement on the old reaction (habit). But unless our aim is merely that of suppressing one specific symptom, or of dropping some specific form of indulgence without reference to the effect upon the organism *as a whole*, the value of the improvement brought about by any method of change must be judged entirely according to whether or not the standard of general functioning is being raised or lowered in the process, and in the latter case, whether by-products harmful to the general functioning have been brought about.

To change habitual reaction permanently without the accompaniment of harmful by-products it is necessary to change the manner of use of the self that is associated with it. This reconditions the reflex activity of which this manner of use is a manifestation, and means that for the old reaction associated with the old reflex activity, there is substituted a new reflex activity resulting in a new changed reaction, and a consequent disappearance of the old reaction.

The possibility of reconditioning opens up the way to an unlimited development of control, but not simply a control which results from a fixed conditioning, as in the case of the dog reacting to a prearranged and regularly repeated stimulus along the lines contrived by Pavlov. For, as John Dewey puts it, "The latter, as usually understood, renders an individual a passive puppet to be played upon by external manipulations." The control that is meant by reconditioning in my sense is made possible by that employment of the primary control which—again as Dewey puts it—"conditions all other reactions, brings the conditioning factor under conscious direction and enables the individual to take possession of his own potentialities. It converts the fact of conditioned reflexes from a principle of external enslavement into a means of vital freedom."[27]

Thus the person who by some direct means has conditioned himself to exercise control which depends upon the elimination of specific stimuli, such as alcohol or tobacco, or those arising from emotional disturbance, some distressing environment or the like, does not constitute a case of control of reaction by reconditioning in my sense. This calls for that "vital freedom" in reaction (freedom IN thought and action), which enables us to give effect to a decision previously reasoned out, such, for instance, as the decision to take or not to take alcohol, to smoke or not to smoke tobacco, or to use either in moderation whenever it is decided to do so and to be able to stop at any time.

In the case of the addict such a decision is difficult to carry out, because of the nature of the sensory experiences which have been habitually associated with his attempts to satisfy his need. As long as this need persists, these experiences are a continuous stimulus to indulgence in his bad habit, and hence the carrying-out of a decision not to indulge implies inhibiting his habitual reaction to the stimulus arising from the sensory experiences which are the background of his craving. These sensory experiences are as much a part of such addicts, and exercise as harmful an influence towards indulgence, as the habitual sensory experiences which influence people towards indulgence in certain harmful ways of using themselves in keeping their equilibrium, in standing, sitting, walking and other activities. The sense of satisfaction which comes from the indulgence in both these cases is associated with "feeling right" and comfortable, although associated with a particular manner of use which is lowering the standard of general functioning and bringing about ill-health and disease.

Bad habits of use are fundamental conditions of abnormality, and it

---

[27]See Introduction by Prof. John Dewey to *The Use of the Self.*

is reasonable to expect them to be associated with such other abnormalities as an excessive craving for alcohol or tobacco, and even more reasonable to conclude that when we begin to eradicate the fundamental conditions of abnormality throughout the organism by changing the manner of use, we are taking the first step to the gradual eradication of other forms of abnormality within the self. In the ordinary way a person who is an addict whether to tobacco, drink or drugs, is considered to be "cured" if he ceases to indulge his particular habit or craving, without due attention being paid to other bad habits which are certain to be present, or to new bad habits which are likely to be cultivated during or after the "cure." Too often the alleged cure leaves him depressed, unhappy, and discontented, and I have known cases in which these after effects have been so distressing and deleterious that I was forced to the conclusion that the "cure" was worse than the disease.

The close connexion between habit and an associated manner of use has been missed in all schemes of reform, and when we add to this that, concurrently with the training man has derived from past and present methods of education and development, harmful changes in the use and functioning of his organism have been allowed to develop unchecked, we cannot wonder that man's reactions in general seldom correspond to the ideals he professes, but approximate too often to those of the caveman, especially now that the fruits of his invention on the material side are gradually becoming an ever-increasing danger to himself and those around him.

He has forgotten that in the last resort it is the human element that counts, and my work has always been a practical plea for this truth. The forces of mechanization are being used in a way that prevents the full development of human potentialities. This is the price we are paying for so-called progress and improvement, scientific and otherwise, achieved by changing conditions in the outside world regardless of the cost in human sacrifice and of the means employed to gain our end. Unfortunately this so-called "progress" is associated with a lowering of the standard of man's sensory awareness of harmful changes that are taking place within his organism, changes which are recognized only when their harmful effects are manifested as bad habits, defects and disease.

Hence the importance of understanding the means whereby such harmful conditions may be prevented from developing unknowingly within the human organism, or, if they have been allowed to develop, may be changed back to those which were present before undesirable reactions manifested themselves.

Part II

Procedures Involved in the Technique

First Principles in the Control of Human Reaction

Before going on to consider what is fundamentally involved in the changing of habit by the employment of my technique, I wish my reader to understand that I use the word "habit" in its widest sense, as the embodiment of all instinctive and other human reactions, observable through and determined by the manner of use of the self as a constant influence operating for or against us under given circumstances and at a given time.

If we view habit from this wider angle which shows the link between the manifestation of any single reaction with the working of the whole organism, it will be easier to understand the difficulty we all experience in breaking even simple habits, and that this difficulty increases in proportion to the intensity of the stimulus to indulge in the habit. In the employment of my technique this added difficulty is taken into account from the start of the lessons, and hence, in any attempt to help a pupil to change habitual reaction, I begin with procedures that involve only simple activities on the pupil's part, such as sitting and rising from a chair, in order to give him in the easiest way the opportunity to inhibit his habitual response when any stimulus to activity comes to him.

Unfortunately even when the work is limited to the simplest activities, there are difficulties to be overcome which are almost incomprehensible to people inexperienced in trying to bring about such psycho-physical changes as we are concerned with, and I shall try therefore to show the why and the wherefore of this.

The attitude of most people towards learning to do things which they hope will bring about the changes they desire, is one leading to more or less anxiety and tension which in many reaches a stage of emotional disturbance, particularly if they are being assisted by a teacher. This is not to be wondered at when we remember that under orthodox teaching methods, the teacher expects his pupil to try to be "right" from the very start in carrying out whatever he is asked to do, and the pupil also believes in this idea and acts accordingly. In expecting this of his pupil, the teacher is not only asking him to overcome at one stroke the influence of long established habits of use, but also to accomplish this feat while being guided by the unreliable feeling which had led him into his wrongness.

To make this point clear, let us consider the case of a person in whom posture and structural conditions and standard of functioning are unsatisfactory, and for whom a course of lessons in physical culture, remedial exercises, dancing or other methods has been decided upon as a remedy. Here let me re-emphasize the fact that as such a person has been guided hitherto by what he has felt to be right in all he has done in daily life, and as this "doing" has led to the unsatisfactory structural conditions of posture and functioning present in his case, it is obvious that what in the past had felt right to that person must have been wrong. In other words, his "right" is wrong. If then he goes to his teacher convinced that he must try to be right in all that he does, and so attempts to conform to the teacher's and his own conception of what is right in performing exercises or anything else he may be asked to do, he will continue to do what he feels is right (the known), and so will unknowingly tend to exaggerate the wrongness which is, and has been, the background of his trouble.

The only way in which such a pupil could perform exercises or any other activity so that his practice of them would not have this result, would be by doing what he feels is wrong; and he is not likely to do that *for it would be the unknown to him*. It is difficult enough as experience shows, for a pupil, in carrying out any ordinary activity, to allow one to do something for him that feels to him wrong, but it is still more difficult to get him to carry out an unfamiliar activity himself by means which feel wrong to him. All of which goes to show that a pupil who believes he must try to be right and when he comes to a lesson worries about whether he is going to be right or wrong, adds to the difficulties he is faced with in any case when making changes in his way of doing things. It is almost certain, too, that this same pupil will be convinced that the teacher can and should tell him what is the "right" standing, sitting or other position, and enable him to acquire and maintain this position in each instance, and that to be a good pupil he must concentrate on trying to be right, and must visualize how he is to carry out his teacher's instructions in the course of his work.

It can be demonstrated that the attempt to concentrate in such cases resolves itself into a condition of increased muscle tension and self-hypnotism, and therefore tends to lessen rather than increase the chance of success. This can also be said of the beginner's attempts to visualize what is to be done and how to do it, seeing that in taking impressions he depends for guidance and judgment upon the same feeling that he has always depended upon in the past, and which has led him into the wrongness he wishes to change into rightness.

Then as to the idea that it is helpful to know and to be able to acquire the "right" position in, say, standing, sitting or in any other activity, let us for a moment consider the facts. To pass from wrong to right conditions associated with posture and functioning means change, and if a person is to make this change successfully, it must be by a gradual process of change from day to day so that the effect of the readjustment of the bony structure, the abdominal viscera, the vital organs, the interference with the habitual sense of equilibrium and the disturbing influence of experience in doing what feels wrong, may not retard the process.

Hence common sense dictates that changes such as these can not be made in a single lesson or in a month of lessons. If therefore at the first lesson, or indeed at any lesson, a pupil visualizes the position of standing or sitting which is advocated on that day as the right one, and henceforward continues to adopt it as right for good and all, he cannot make further improvement. He will be adopting for all time a posture and conditions of functioning which were advocated as right at a certain stage of his progress, and which he has visualized and worked for at that stage, but he will not get past that point. Whereas if he is to make further change and improvement of conditions from day to day, what he visualized yesterday as the "right" posture will not be the posture associated with future change and improvement.

Hence ideas or methods which lead to fixed right postures do not meet the needs of those who desire to change conditions which are associated with unsatisfactory use, functioning and postural effects. A satisfactory technique for making the changes we are considering must be one in which the nature of the procedures provides for a continuous change towards improving conditions, by a method of *indirect approach* under which opportunity is given for the pupil to come into contact with the unfamiliar and *unknown* without fear or anxiety.

To this end from the beginning of the first lesson the teacher does his best to reassure the pupil and allay any anxiety on his part as to whether or not he will be able to carry out instructions rightly. He explains to him that he does not want him to try and be "right" in carrying out any instructions, because this would only mean projecting messages which would result in his reacting to the instructions by the habitual use of himself which "feels right," but that he can prevent this if, on receipt of any stimulus to activity (such, for instance, as a request from his teacher to sit down or to perform some other simple act), he will make the decision to refuse to give consent to carry out the activity by that habitual use of himself which is in accord with his conception of HOW the act should be performed. By adhering to this decision the pupil inhibits his immediate response, and therefore cuts off at its source his habitual reaction to the stimulus of the teacher's request, and the way is thus cleared for the teacher to help him to employ new means whereby he can gain his end by a new and improved manner of use, the responsibility for the pupil's being wrong or right in the employment of these means being the teacher's responsibility alone. It is pointed out to him that under the changed conditions the new use of himself may, and probably will, feel wrong to him at first, but that through the experience he will gain in his lessons, the new use will in time come to feel right, and he will come to see that the conception which underlies this new way of using himself is not based on any arbitrary theory of what is "right" in the circumstances, but on a practical knowledge of what change in his habitual use and functioning is required if he is to gain a new control of his reaction, with all that this connotes, in performing the act.

When these points have been explained and demonstrated as far as possible, the pupil will as a rule find little difficulty in accepting them theoretically. Indeed, like some others, he is inclined to accept them too quickly, in the sense that he appears to have no doubt that when he receives a request from his teacher to carry out some simple act, he will be able to adhere to his decision to inhibit his immediate response to the stimulus of this request, and will be able to put into practice the new "means-whereby."

In spite of this optimistic outlook however it is practically certain that the first time the teacher asks him, for instance, to sit down, the pupil will fail to adhere to his decision to inhibit the immediate response to the stimulus of this request, but will instead give consent to the request and sit down in his usual way because it "feels right" to him, with the result that, as his teacher has warned him, he will merely repeat and probably exaggerate his habitual wrong manner of use of himself in sitting down. As a pupil wishing to be helped this is not what he desires; on the contrary he wants to change and improve his manner of using himself. My observations as a teacher however have shown me that a pupil with the best possible intentions is at first incapable of carrying out a decision which runs counter to all his earlier experiences in the use of himself, because the carrying out of the decision would cut him off from ways of reacting which are familiar to him (habit). To begin with, the methods of training and education in which he is versed, have developed in him a habit of end-gaining through a too quick and unthinking response to stimuli, and hence at the moment when in order to carry out his considered decision, he is obliged to depend upon procedures which are unfamiliar to him, his habit of responding too quickly overrides his new decision, and he relapses once again into doing what he has habitually done to gain his end, repeating experiences known to him.

Another incentive to end-gaining on the pupil's part is his desire to gain in a given time the maximum benefit from his lessons irrespective of the conditions to be changed. Unfortunately for him, in view of the nature of his educational training, this very commendable desire causes him to make a special will-to-do effort in his desire at all costs to be "right." But as his "right" is wrong, this merely means a stronger effort in the wrong direction,[28] and an exaggeration of his habitual way of "doing" the very things he must get rid of if he is to gain the improvement he desires. Only time and experience in the working out of the technique will convince him that where the "means-whereby" are right for the purpose, desired ends will come. They are inevitable. Why then be concerned as to the manner or speed of their coming? We should reserve all thought, energy and concern for the means whereby we may command the manner of their coming.

According to my experience, although a pupil may believe or assert that he has reasoned out why he should not give consent to a certain act and consequently desires to inhibit his habitual reaction, he is clearly more concerned at the moment with gaining his end (i.e., carrying out his teacher's instructions, hoping to be right and fearing to be wrong), than with the inhibition of his habitual reaction to the teacher's request. He has yet to learn by experience that *trying* to gain his end, *trying* to be right, is the surest way to failure in carrying out his newly made and reasoned decision. He must become convinced by his own experiences that what he feels is right is wrong, and that the idea involved in trying to do better at one time than another is merely a myth, "a dagger of the mind."[29] Time will be required to help him to stop trying to be right and afraid of being wrong; but, given time, he will learn to withhold consent to the giving of the messages which would be his instinctive response to the stimulus to accede to his teacher's request, and so will be able to inhibit his habitual reaction while giving consent to the new messages necessary for bringing about that change in the manner of his general use which will be present as he moves—say, from standing, to sitting in a chair.

---

[28]See *The Use of the Self* p. 440.

[29]To make my point clear I ask the reader to think over the following: Suppose a friend tells you he is going to do his best today. Just ask him to tell you in concrete terms what he intends to do that will be different from what he does at any other time, the times when he is not especially intending to do his best. I have tried this for years and the response has always been—first a blank look, then a recovery and some rather weak explanation. Although I have pressed for a plain straightforward explanation, up till now I have not been given one. How could it be otherwise? People do not know what they do in the use of themselves in their activities. Apropos of this, I recall the account I read in the *Evening Standard* of the taking of slow-motion pictures of four famous golfers making a stroke. According to the account, they were asked if they knew what they did to make a particular stroke. *(continued on next page)*

The length of time needed for bringing the pupil to this point varies in different people, but as soon as the teacher is satisfied that up to this point his pupil has a satisfactory understanding of the theoretical side of his work, he can take him on to further stages. He will continue as before to employ the variations of his teaching art to prevent the pupil from becoming emotionally disturbed, assuring him again that as he reaches further stages in the procedure of the technique he does not want him, any more than in the earlier stages of his work, to be concerned as to whether he is right or wrong, but merely to go on as before seeing to it that he inhibits his habitual reaction to any request from his teacher during the lesson.

This accomplished the teacher will ask the pupil to give the new messages necessary to carrying out the new "means-whereby" required for bringing about that employment of the primary control of the use of himself which is fundamental in reconditioning reflexes. At the same time the teacher will with his hands give the pupil the actual sensory experience of this new employment of the primary control, and thus will be able to help him to maintain the improving manner of use which results from this new experience in making any movement that may be required in the course of the lesson such as that of moving from standing to sitting in a chair. By this means a real change, however small, will have been made, and it will be found that this is the beginning of a process of reconditioning leading in time to permanent change in use, functioning and structural conditions. This is necessarily attended by a variety of unexpected experiences, such as a slight and momentary disturbance of equilibrium and some doubt and uncertainty about the success to be gained by unfamiliar means (although from the start of the lessons it is made clear that the responsibility for being "right" is not placed upon the pupil), together with other misgivings arising from a situation in which doing what feels wrong is paradoxically associated with a gradual improvement in the pupil's general use and functioning. In

"Yes," came the reply. "Very well, tell me what you do!"They each did so, and notes were made of their statements. When the pictures were taken, it was found that not one of them had done a single thing they claimed they did in making their stroke. In the same journal I once read an account given by one of Mr. W. H. (Bunny) Austin's friends about an experience Austin had had at Wimbledon. Austin had told him that at one stage in the game, he was playing so badly he decided not to try to win the set but that as soon as he had made that decision, he began to play up to his usual form. In consequence, he decided that now he would try to win the set after all, and immediately reverted to the indifferent play that had caused him "not to try." It does seem sometimes as if human beings not only like to be fooled by others but are keen on fooling themselves.

time, however, these difficulties are overcome by experience as in any other field of learning to do.

The reader will now see that the technique is based upon the inhibition of the habitual wrong use—i.e., the refusal to react to a stimulus in the usual way, and that the principle of *prevention* is strictly adhered to from the beginning. The habitual wrong employment of the primary control of the pupil's use of himself responsible for his reaction in performing such acts as sitting in and rising from a chair, is *prevented*, and is gradually superseded by a new and improved manner of use which by a reconditioning procedure is associated with new reflex activity.

By steps more or less slow, according to the difficulties to be overcome, the pupil passes from the stage of preventing the repetition of the wrong employment of the primary control of the general use in such acts as sitting or standing, to gaining those new experiences of use in which *the proper relativity* of the parts concerned is brought about. By the repetition of these experiences the pupil develops confidence, and whereas at an earlier stage in these experiences he registered doubt and confusion, little by little the new lines of motor and sensory communication are laid down along which he will sooner or later habitually project his messages.

As long as he inhibits the sending of the old messages the old lines of communication are not used, and as he becomes more and more versed in the procedures of the technique the tendency to make use of them decreases, as does his dependence upon his feeling of rightness associated with them. It was this feeling of "rightness" which in the earlier stages made the pupil feel their employment to be a necessity. Meanwhile the continual communication along the new lines goes on, and day by day the tendency to rely on the new means for sending messages, rather than on the old ones, grows apace. The time ultimately comes when the pupil no longer feels any desire to use the old lines of communication; they fall into disuse, and communicating along the new lines at last comes to feel right and is carried out with confidence.

Up to this point it will be understood that all the pupil has been asked to do is to apply his principle to the circumstances of the lesson, but after some time the pupil can begin the inhibition of the wrong use of the primary control in all the simple and other acts of life, for this is largely a matter of that process of remembering which is involved in "thinking in activity"—a new way of living—and when once he has experienced the joy and satisfaction of this, it is difficult to believe that the old way could be reverted to. The new way of use will have come to feel right while the old way will feel wrong. As we have seen, one of the serious obstacles to be overcome in helping pupils to change their manner of use is that any change from the old wrong use (the known) to the new right use (the unknown) feels wrong to them, and at each stage of change the new improving manner of use has to be experienced for some time before the pupil can feel that it is right and comfortable, and so develop faith and confidence in the employment of it.

Here is the answer to those who work on the principle that if something is wrong with a person's use and functioning, the teacher should tell the pupil as a primary procedure WHAT TO DO to put it right. It can be demonstrated that the one thing we can be certain that such a pupil will not try to do is to employ the right use of himself in carrying out the instructions for the simple reason that to him the right use would feel wrong. *People don't do what they feel to be wrong when they are trying to be right.* That the myth implied in the belief I am here condemning has obtained credence for so long is proof that we do not really think as often as we *feel* we do. Sorry, but it is only too true!

*   *   *   *   *

Inhibition

Different meanings have been given to the word *inhibition*, and this has led to much confusion. According to the report of a conference held in New York last year by members of scientific and other bodies with the aim of encouraging unity of thinking,[30] it was admitted that owing to the departmentalization of human knowledge, language difficulties were encountered among those taking part in the discussions because different groups attached different meanings to the same word.

To make clear, therefore, the sense in which I use the word inhibition, I would refer my readers to my book *Constructive Conscious Control of the Individual* (1923) where I wrote that in the application of my technique the process of inhibition, that is, *the act of refusing to respond* to the primary desire to gain an end, becomes *the act of responding* (volitionary act) to the conscious reasoned desire to employ the means whereby that end may be gained.[31] I have since been interested to learn that in a pamphlet entitled *The Brain and Its Mechanism* (Cambridge University Press, 1937), Sir Charles Sherrington wrote:

> I may seem to stress the preoccupation of the brain with muscle. Can we stress too much that preoccupation when any path we trace in the brain leads directly or indirectly to muscle? The brain seems a thoroughfare for nerve action passing on its way to the motor animal. It has been

[30]See Appendix G.

[31]See page 327; also page 300. [CCCI]

> remarked that Life's aim is an act not a thought. Today the dictum must be modified to admit that, often, to refrain from an act is no less an act than to commit one, because inhibition is co-equally with excitation a nervous activity.

The carrying-out of the procedures in my technique is just this pre-occupation of the brain with the thought responsible for the nervous activity involved in the passing on of messages, whether these result in the prevention or in the carrying-out of an act. The preventive messages projected serve to stop off the misdirection associated with harmful habitual use of ourselves in the performance of an act, and herein we have an activity which is primary to any other activity concerned with the act, and by means of which the way is cleared for the projecting of the new directive messages which bring about a new and improved use of ourselves. As long as the brain is preoccupied with the projection of messages which result in bringing about our habitual manner of use, there is little chance of breaking the vicious circle of the associated reflex activity in "doing." What we feel to be right is wrong, and before this habitual reflex activity can be changed, we need to pass through a series of reconditioning experiences which, because they are previously unknown to us, at first feel wrong, and which must be repeated therefore until the unknown becomes the known and feels right and familiar.

The primary procedure in the technique necessary for gaining these experiences is the inhibition, at a given stimulus, of our habitual reflex activity. To succeed in this means education in the fundamental sense, for it calls for a conscious recognition and understanding of all that is concerned with the formation of habit, and of the means whereby habits can be changed. Our reasoning processes are called upon and, as a result, we must not react at once to a given stimulus, for if we do so react, we merely give consent to a projection of the messages which are responsible for our habitual reflex activity, and we thus make change impossible.

Hence as a result of reasoning on these lines, we, on the receipt of any stimulus to activity, make the important decision *not to give consent to doing anything* in response, as this "doing" would be due to our projection of the habitual messages which have led us into wrongness. If we keep to this decision, we shall have gained the first experience which will in time lead to the control of our habitual reaction.

By this initial inhibition change becomes possible, and we pass on to consider what should be our next procedure. Primarily our concern must be to find out in what way we are interfering with the right employment of the primary control, and decide to prevent this interference by consciously refusing to project the messages which habitually bring it about. Only secondarily are we interested in the projection of the new messages which will in time lead us indirectly, that is, through a change in the employment of the primary control of our use, to the change we desire in our habitual reflex activity.

In this whole procedure we see the new principle at work, for if we project those messages which hold in check the familiar habitual reaction, and at the same time project the new messages which give free rein to the motor impulses associated with nervous and muscular energy along unfamiliar lines of communication, we shall be doing what Dewey calls "thinking in activity." As far as we can judge, mankind has not had the experience of thinking in activity where the projection of messages necessary to the employment of the primary control of his use is concerned. In the ordinary way man has just reacted instinctively to any stimulus to activity, whereas in the new plan which I am suggesting, the messages, preventive and otherwise, must be consciously projected *in their right sequence* throughout the activity.

I wrote in *Constructive Conscious Control of the Individual*:

> The projection of continued, conscious orders, calls for a broad reasoning attitude so that the subject has not only a clear conception of the orders essential ("means-whereby") for the correct performance of a particular movement, but he can also project these orders in their right relationship one to another, the coordinated series of orders resulting in a coordinated use of the organism.

In my experience most people, even those who are recognized as unusually brilliant, find this procedure very difficult. Where they chiefly go wrong is in "forgetting to remember" to inhibit, while the end-gaining habit, which claims most of us as victims, causes them constantly in making a movement to overlook or overrun one or the other in the series of messages they have been asked to project.

This habit of running ahead is the stutterer's difficulty, for when he has several words to say, he invariably tries to say the first word with the formation of lips and use of tongue required for saying the word which follows the one he is trying to pronounce. When movement outruns the messages in this way, it means either that the pupil has ceased to project the new messages, or that he is "doing" them, relying upon the habitual sensory guidance which he has found by experience is constantly misleading him.

Inhibition is a human potentiality of the utmost value in any attempt to make changes in the human self, and my experience has convinced me that it is the potentiality most in need of development. I have found that if a pupil can inhibit his habitual reactions even moderately well when faced with unfamiliar procedures, remarkable changes in his use and functioning can be made in a very short time, changes which judged by ordinary results would seem impossible.

The employment of inhibition calls for the exercise of memory and awareness, the former for remembering the procedures involved in the technique and the proper sequence in which they should be used, and the latter in the recognition of what is happening. In the process both potentialities are developed, and the scope of the use of both gradually increased. Moreover the experiences thus gained, not only help in developing and quickening the recalling and connecting memory, but cultivate what I shall call the motor-sensory-intellectual memory.

My technique is based on inhibition, the inhibition of undesirable, unwanted responses to stimuli, and hence it is primarily a technique for the development of the control of human reaction.

Part III

The Fundamental Approach

In any consideration of means which will meet our needs in changing habit we cannot too often remind ourselves of the demonstrable truth that the nature of a person's reaction is determined by the nature of his use and functioning.

This can be seen clearly enough for instance in the case of a person who reacts to some stimulus by losing his temper, and who immediately assumes the attitude of body and limbs and the facial expression of a person "spoiling for a fight." The same is true of animals. The dog manifests a similar change in use and functioning when reacting to some stimulus which arouses his fighting instinct; the hair on his back is raised, his eyes roll and glare, the lips are contracted to show the teeth, and the angle of his head, attitude of his body and the particular action of his limbs are all manifestations of his desire to quarrel and fight.

Innumerable examples could be given to show that change in a person's manner of reacting is associated with change in the manner of his use and functioning, and when this change is manifested by loss of temper and readiness to quarrel, the desire and intention to quarrel will persist, until some fresh stimulus is received. If he reacts to this by recovering his composure, he will be seen to return to the manner of use and functioning which is associated with his habitual manner of reacting when undisturbed, or if he reacts in yet a different way, this change will again be reflected in the telltale changes in manner of use and functioning associated therewith.

Losing one's temper and the manifestations accompanying this condition amount to loss of control in use and functioning, and it will be observed that in those in whom this tendency to loss of control is habitual, there is also the tendency to react too quickly to the stimuli of their environment and the reactions of their fellows, and to be too much at the mercy of "emotional gusts." No matter in what field of activity we are engaged, or whether the stimuli primarily responsible for our particular manner of reacting are labelled "physical," "mental," or what you will, the same human processes in use and functioning are responsible for the manifestations which constitute our habitual manner of reacting to a particular stimulus, or group of stimuli, and are as characteristic of us individually as is our manner of writing, walking and carrying on our activities generally, and as easily recognizable by those who know us.

We speak of people being in a good or bad mood, and all of us at some time or other have met people who have quite unintentionally irritated us at first sight by some manner of speaking, general behaviour and so on. To the observer all such peculiarities and changes of mood are accompanied by changes in postural attitudes, facial expression, movements of hands and arms, in fact by such movements of parts as we are apt to employ in attempting to express what we feel.

I was with a number of people one evening listening to a broadcast on an important matter given by a well-known man who is recognized as an authority on his subject. In the course of a few minutes one of the listeners exclaimed, "That man irritates me," and it soon became evident that these words conveyed only a mild impression of the nature of his actual reaction.

Later on I had the opportunity to discuss the broadcast with him when he told me that it was the voice and articulation of the speaker that had so irritated him, and this in spite of his deep interest in the subject of the broadcast.

Here then was a man whom I knew to be of more than ordinary intelligence finding it impossible to listen with composure to a talk on a matter of vital importance to himself and others, because of the feeling of irritation aroused in him by certain vocal and other peculiarities in the speaker.

The point of special interest to me in this incident was that my friend's manner of use of himself was so bad that it could well account for the way he reacted to the speaker, and hence I was not surprised by the manner of his reaction. It was just another reminder that probably the greatest problem that is still unsolved in the education and development of mankind is the problem of the control of human reaction, because of the close interdependence between the nature of this control and the nature of the associated manner of use and functioning of the self.

It may be of help here in view of what is to follow if I recapitulate certain points which, as some of my readers may remember, I have already dealt with in my earlier books:

(1) That man tends to become more and more a confirmed end-gainer, one who too often insists on gaining his end by any means, even at the risk of disaster, rather than take time to consider means whereby the end can be gained so as to ensure the best possible result.

(2) That man stumbled along the path which has led by gradual changes to modern civilization from an environment which had probably remained static for thousands of years, and in which all the requirements of his mode of life, as of that of his forebears for countless generations, could be met by an instinctive guidance and control of himself in all of his activities, and by a slowly developing self-adaptation to his environment arrived at through experiences of failure and success. From the outset of civilized life, therefore, man has been handicapped because, by the very nature of the case, his experience in adapting himself to the needs of increasingly rapid environmental changes has been, and still is, inadequate. Furthermore he has not gained that knowledge of the use and functioning of the self which is essential to the maintenance of well-being in an environment where instinctive (automatic) guidance has proved inadequate and too often actually misleading, and where, therefore, an ever-increasing demand is made upon him for quick adaptation to new changes. For want of this knowledge the success of the civilizing plan itself, and of the measures man has taken for the well-being of himself and others, is now in jeopardy. Faced with the unfamiliar, his quick reaction too often leads to results both harmful and unintentional because of his reliance upon instincts which have long since survived their usefulness. At the same time he is fearful of change by reason of his limited experience, his preconceived ideas and habits of thought and action, legacies from an earlier and more static environment, adaptation to which made comparatively small demands upon him. This is true of his reaction to changes within himself, especially such as might adversely affect his

position in the outside world, with what serious results will be obvious when we consider that without change, that is, without coming into contact with the unfamiliar (the unknown) we cannot make those changes in ourselves, and through ourselves in the outside world, which are essential to fundamental growth and development in an advancing civilization.

(3) That this problem of change is made more difficult of solution because man's sensory appreciation of what is happening within himself has gradually become unreliable, and is now demonstrably so, whilst his standard of awareness and observation is being gradually lowered.

I am aware that this does not always apply in activities where the tendency is towards specialism, and where the opportunity for the exercise of these potentialities is narrowed; but even in these cases, so far as my enquiries and observation go, the standard is too often lowered outside the particular specialist sphere.

In consequence of the unreliability of his sensory impressions, man's interpretation of his own and other people's experience in living is too often faulty and illusive, and he is liable to arrive at false conclusions, and to form erroneous judgments, especially where the motives for his own and other people's behaviour and general activities are concerned. These tendencies, combined with that of a too quick and unthinking reaction on his part due to his becoming a confirmed end-gainer, must continue to block his way to success in his attempts to make changes, and to control his reactions. His success in developing his potentialities to a stage where he is able to translate into practice the ideals of good will and peace which he now sees "through a glass darkly," will depend upon whether or not he can reach a plane of living where he substitutes conscious guidance and control of the use of himself for that instinctive (automatic) self-guidance and control that met his needs in primitive life.

The need for the fundamental change in man's guidance and control of himself that I am here postulating has never, so far as I have been able to discover, been recognized by those responsible for methods of training and education until now; indeed, even among so-called "new" methods, I have not found any yet that, in this fundamental respect, differ from those they were intended to supersede.

The advocates of these new plans in every field of reform still seem to think it reasonable to assume that people will be able to make the changes they consider necessary for putting some new ideal into practice, or for substituting new procedures for those which they had previously employed for the gaining of some end, without changing the nature of the guidance and control of the use of the self, the instrument they must employ for carrying out these new procedures.

This misconception comes from failure to recognize that in the majority of people today, misdirection has crept into the automatic working of guidance and control of the use of the self, and that it is necessary as a preliminary to making changes, to restore reliable guidance and control, and to this end to employ a technique by means of which we can bring about that manner of the employment of the primary control which has *an integrating influence* upon the mechanisms of the organism.

And as it can justly be presumed that the automatic working of the human organism was satisfactory in a more or less static environment, but nevertheless went wrong as the demand upon man for quicker adaptation to environment increased, there is no evidence to support the assumption that the original reliability of guidance and control of the automatic working of the organism can be restored by specific means, or that, even if this were possible, this working would be less liable to interference than at any previous period of man's history. No matter in what field of activity it is desired to bring about changes, whether so-called physical, mental or spiritual, the carrying-out of the task demands from us a decision to make that fundamental change in the guidance and control of the working of the mechanisms which is inseparable from change in the manner of use of the self, and unless this is taken into account by those who may be responsible in the future for ideals and plans for individual and social reform, they are not justified in believing that these will prove more beneficial than those which have been found wanting in the past.

To act successfully along new lines of thought means (even after the best "means-whereby" have been selected) the carrying-out of a decision by an unfamiliar use of the self against the impulse to carry it out by the habitual use that feels right, that is, not only in the face of our mental conception of HOW that decision should be carried out, but also in the face of real discomfort and "feeling wrong" in carrying it out. For this reason the person who has hitherto depended in all his "doing" upon an instinctive (automatic) use of himself finds it difficult[32] to adhere to a decision to employ procedures which involve a guidance and control in the use of himself which is not in line with any previous experience either in thought or in action.

[32]This difficulty is continually overlooked by those who pin their faith to the statement of ideological theories, however eloquently put, for converting others to a new point of view, or who put forth plans of reform to help others to make the necessary changes in their reaction in living which correspond to the new ideal they are putting

The new "means-whereby" are unfamiliar, and any attempt on his part to carry them out will be associated with experiences which feel wrong, so that in order to be right in carrying them out, he will have to "do" what he feels wrong—obviously an experience which will be entirely new to him. Hence when the moment comes that he is called upon to employ the new means by a new and unfamiliar use of himself, he finds that in spite of his intellectual acceptance of them as best for his purpose, he is without the necessary sensory confidence to carry out his task, a confidence which would be his if he were asked to carry out "means-whereby" that were familiar to him. Judging by past experience he feels that he is being called upon to take a risk that he should not take, although he is quite willing to take an ordinary risk in familiar situations, as for instance, the risk of falling in learning to skate or ride a bicycle. Going to work in his old trial and error way, he is willing to take early risks although in doing so he has always employed a wrong use of himself, but he is unwilling to run the early risks in this new way of learning, although he has decided with his teacher that this new way will lead to an improving use of himself.

This is a unique situation and one that man, as far as I am aware, has not been previously called upon to face under any method of education, training or scheme of living, and this situation will persist as the greatest stumbling block in the way of making fundamental change until we employ means which provide opportunity for gaining the experiences necessary for passing from the familiar (wrong) to the unfamiliar (right) guidance and control of the psycho-physical organism, the only means which we are justified in concluding make provision for change in the fundamental sense.

A teaching experience of over forty years enables me to affirm that with all the help that can be given them by a teacher experienced in the employment of a technique that provides for change in this fundamental sense, most people are unable to carry out decisions successfully when this implies gaining an end by an unaccustomed use of the self, even in such simple acts as moving an arm, lifting a leg or rising from or sitting down in a chair.

This gives us some idea of the conflicting influences at work when habit is associated with wrong conditions, and it is because this has not been recognized that there is so much confusion and misunderstanding in regard to what is fundamental to success in the carrying out of decisions to make changes. It is also necessary to remember when considering methods for the changing of thought and action and selecting the means whereby this change can be put into practice, that no one can be said to have really accepted a new idea or approved of the "means-whereby" of putting it into practice, until he has actually had the experience himself of employing the procedures necessary for doing this.

According to the conception of change most generally held in the past and which still persists today, "creative power," "willing," and "wishing," as expressed in the words "I will" or "I will not," are means whereby change can be brought about, and those who favour methods based on this conception employ them as an aid to their accomplishment in all fields of activity. In doing this they depend upon instinctive (automatic) guidance and control of themselves on the trial and error plan, without giving consideration to the question of HOW to "do" the "doing" that is inseparable from the practice of "wishing" and "willing."

It is true that more or less success for this method is claimed by those who use it, but when considering how far such claims are justified, it is essential to remember that it is both the psycho-physical experiences of the individual in use and functioning, and those that he gains when he is applying himself as an instrument in his activities in the outside world, which combine to make up his experience in living, and it is this sum total of experience which determines the nature and value of his judgment. Those who claim personal success for their methods must be able to prove that their experience is sufficiently comprehensive to provide a trustworthy basis for sound judgment, before they can expect their judgment to be accepted at face value. All judgment is based upon experience, and a person with limited experience is hardly qualified to judge the reactions of a person whose experiences have been widened by exploring new fields. Man still relies upon an undue proportion of limited and deceptive experiences as a basis for judgment in too many spheres of activity and in regard to too many problems; and this can account in a great measure for the position in which he finds himself today, a position which would seem to show that he has long since been in need of something more than "wishing" or "willing" on the trial and error plan, if he is ever to meet successfully the added demands made upon him by changes in living, let alone those that are likely to be made upon him in the future. He has been "wishing" for continued progress, development and freedom of thought and action, "willing" himself to this end, at one time concentrating upon "physical," at another on "mental" means, and also on "spiritual" means.

But as time goes on his attempts to solve his present day problems by these means have only served to show their limitations,[33] and he is becoming increasingly aware not only of disaster and confusion outside himself, but also of certain growing disabilities *within himself*, in particu-

[33]And never more so than at the present moment. (June, 1940.)

lar of a lowered standard of sensory appreciation and general functioning, and uncertainty in making judgments.

This should have warned him that his means have not, and are not meeting his needs, but notwithstanding he still retains confidence in them. His only idea of "cure" for his disabilities is to concentrate still harder on "wishing" and "willing" on the same old plan as before, and therefore the only kind of change he makes is that which comes from ceasing to concentrate on one point in order to concentrate on another as when, for instance, he claims to be depending more upon "spiritual" than upon "mental," or upon "mental" than upon "physical" means and so forth. Therefore no matter how much people may differ as to the merits of any particular change in his reaction that he may bring about by his concentrating on his will-to-do decision, there can be no divergence of opinion with regard to the fact that not only during, but after the making of the change by this method, he will not have brought about any change in that manner of use of himself which has hitherto tended to lower the standard of his general functioning, and the resultant harmful influence of this will become intensified through any special effort he makes, and remain a retarding and disintegrating *constant*, associated with conditions of disorder and complication which are bound to lead sooner or later to other harmful habits of use, and gradually to the development of organic trouble and disease.

And when we remember that any new change in his reaction is the result of his "doing" in carrying out his will-to-do plan, and that the nature of this "doing" depends upon his particular manner of use, which in its turn determines the nature of his changed reaction, it must surely be clear that change which results from decisions carried out by the direct method of "doing" guided by instinctive (automatic) control can only be of a palliative nature, and will almost certainly be associated with the development of undesired by-products.

It has been found indeed that attempts on these lines to carry out decisions necessary for changing the control of some specific reaction are accompanied by self-repression, even when according to individual judgment the attempts are considered to have proved successful. Now, however, that repression has been recognized on all sides as harmful, its presence as a by-product of such attempts is evidence of failure in the general sense, despite the fact that by means of these attempts some specific control of reaction may have been gained in special instances.

We will now go on to consider the case of a man who decides to try to change his reaction in such a way as to be able to control some habit or defect which troubles him, without the accompaniment of any such harmful by-product as repression.

For our purpose it matters not what the habit or defect may be, whether a tendency to loss of temper, drink, falsehood, drug addiction or to other harmful manifestations, so long as he appreciates the need for change and really desires to gain such control of his reaction as will enable him to effect it.

His problem is to resist the temptation to "do" whenever his "doing" can be shown to be causing his trouble, and this calls for the ability to carry out a decision against great odds. But when it has been demonstrated to him that any specific "doing," such as indulging in a particular habit, is always associated with a particular manner of use of himself, he will appreciate that it is futile to try to control this specific "doing" (habit) *directly*, because this would mean leaving unchanged the manner of use and conditions of functioning associated with this "doing." He does not, therefore, try to suppress his desire to indulge in this habit by sheer force of his will-to-do, but instead learns to approach his problem *indirectly* by inhibiting his habitual manner of use in reacting to the old stimulus. Thus he gives himself the opportunity of making a new decision which calls for new and unfamiliar psycho-physical experiences in the carrying-out of new and unfamiliar procedures, and if he adheres to this decision, and employs the procedures which should be employed for bringing about the required change and improvement in his manner of use, the new reaction he desires is made possible, and the by-product, repression, will not be present.

The training that this presupposes has already been described and has proved to be the means of meeting the problem of making and carrying out decisions such as confront those who are trying to improve conditions of use and raise the standard of functioning in the psycho-physical self, the forerunner of all fundamental change.

The experience involved enables a person in time to carry out decisions which are at variance with his habitual use of himself, and he learns to consciously guide and control his activity in conformity with the new concept he has decided to adopt as best for his purpose, although the sensory experiences associated with the consistent carrying-out of these new means, being unfamiliar, "feel wrong," the crux of the whole matter.[34]

Aldous Huxley, writing from personal experience in his remarkable and enlightening book, *Ends and Means*, speaks of my technique as follows: ". . . no verbal description can do justice to a technique which involves the changing . . . of an individual's sensory experiences. One cannot describe the experience of seeing the colour, red. Similarly one

[34]This applies equally with regard to our reaction in other spheres of activity when we are faced with unfamiliar situations.

cannot describe the much more complex experience of improved physical co-ordination. A verbal description would mean something only to a person who had actually had the experience described; to the mal-co-ordinated person, the same words would mean something quite different. Inevitably, he would interpret them in terms of his own sensory experiences, which are those of a mal-co-ordinated person. Complete understanding of the system can come only with the practice of it." And again, ". . . a technique . . . working (by a kind of organic analogy) to inhibit undesirable impulses and irrelevance on the emotional and intellectual levels respectively. We cannot ask more from any system of physical education; nor, if we seriously desire to alter human beings in a desirable direction, can we ask any less."[35] Finally, he points out that it "is valuable, among other reasons, as a means for increasing conscious control of the body, and, in this way, raising a human being from a condition of physical unawareness to a state of physical self-consciousness and self-control. Such physical self-awareness and self-control leads to, and to some extent is actually a form of, mental and moral self-awareness and self-control."[36]

When all that is important has been said in favour of good thoughts, ideas, systems and methods advanced in theoretical and conceptional form only for helping mankind to change and improve the present deplorable world conditions, and to ensure an era of peace and good will for all men, the real problem—the practical application of the concepts—still remains unsolved. We are by nature creatures of impulse dominated by habitual reaction, and will remain so, more or less, so long as we are content to struggle on, depending upon instinctive guidance and control of our manner of use of ourselves in adapting ourselves to quick environmental changes, economic, social, educational, etc. No matter what method or plan, system of thought or ideas may finally be chosen as the best for dealing with man's shortcomings and difficulties in making changes, in the last analysis, success *will depend upon the individual's capacity to carry out a decision to gain an end by the conscious employment of new "means-whereby," involving unfamiliar psycho-physical experiences which feel wrong, discomfort frequently amounting to irritation, and a sense of unsteadiness in equilibrium.*

* * * * *

[35]In *Ends and Means* (Harpers, N. Y.), Chapter XII, "Education," pp. 258-9.
[36]In *Ends and Means*, Chapter XV, "Ethics," p. 377.

WITHHOLDING ACTION
or
NON-DOING

In connexion with the foregoing discussion on habit the following considerations may be of interest; for although they may appear to emphasize unduly what has already been said, they relate to a question which in these days calls for special consideration. Everyone is familiar with the words "We have left undone those things which we ought to have done; and we have done those things which we ought not to have done; and there is no health in us."

In our work we are concerned primarily with non-doing in the fundamental sense of what we should *not do* in the use of ourselves in our daily activities; in other words, with preventing that habitual misuse of the psycho-physical mechanisms which renders these activities a constant source of harm to the organism.

During recent years a steadily increasing number of people have come to appreciate that the end-gaining and unreasoned procedures inherent in our present plan of civilization have had harmful effects, resulting in an interference with our manner of use and a gradual lowering in the standard of our general functioning; and realizing that the further civilization advances on these lines the greater will be the increase in this interference, they are learning to employ means whereby they will be enabled to prevent such interference with their manner of use of themselves, and so ensure that the standard of their general functioning will be gradually raised instead of lowered in the course of their activities.

In this they are making the greatest contribution the self can make to the self in the direction of restoring or maintaining psycho-physical well-being.

But although they may have become convinced that it is *what they themselves are doing* that is responsible for the wrong manner of use they are anxious to change, and that as a first step in acting on this conviction, they must learn HOW to stop this "doing," there is little to show that in learning their intellectual grasp of the theory furnishes them with the assistance they need for putting it into practice. Nor does it help them to appreciate that in selecting the necessary practical procedures for changing their manner of use, non-doing (in the primary sense of preventing themselves from doing those things which lead to a repetition of their wrong habitual manner of use) is not only of the greatest practical value, but also essential to their purpose.

When to this we add: (1) that they find great difficulty at first in inhibiting their too prompt reaction to a given stimulus, which means that they immediately repeat their wrong habitual manner of use, and (2) that in this too prompt reaction they are guided in their manner of use by unreliable sensory appreciation, the reader can form some idea of what is necessary to the process of changing manner of use, irrespective of the nature of the stimulus and the effect of the new associated experiences at any given moment.

Experience has shown that a person who has had great difficulty in putting into practice the idea of *non-doing* in his attempts to make changes in his own manner of use, will so often be found to be one who consistently advocates the idea of non-doing as practicable for others, as, for instance, when he tries to persuade some one else not to overindulge in drinking, eating, smoking or in any habit he considers harmful. His idea of non-doing leads him to advocate the employment of *direct* "means-whereby" of preventing certain misdirected actions ("doing") that can be observed in a person's behaviour (manner of use). In the application of our technique, on the other hand, the idea of non-doing leads to the employment of *indirect* "means-whereby" of preventing such misdirection. It is the first step in the reconditioning essential to the making of those fundamental changes in functioning which *in process* bring about the desired specific result, but unaccompanied by harmful by-products such as self-suppression.

It is a curious anomaly that acceptance of the theory and practice of non-doing should be comparatively easy in attempts to help the self in external activities, but so difficult in similar attempts connected with internal activities. Such help involves a form of non-doing which must not be confused with passivity, and which is fundamental because it prevents the self from doing itself harm by misdirection of energy and uncontrolled reaction of the self: it is an act of inhibition which comes into play when, for instance, in response to a given stimulus, we refuse to give consent to certain activity, and thus prevent ourselves from sending those messages which would ordinarily bring about the habitual reaction resulting in the "doing" within the self of what we no longer wish to "do." It follows that the putting into practice of the theory of non-doing where the manner of use of the self is concerned is a fundamental experience, and is the most valuable experience to be gained by those who wish to learn to prevent themselves from harmful "doing" in carrying out activities outside themselves. Such prevention is the form of non-doing which is essential to the changing of bad habits, and to the control of human reaction. We have all experienced the difficulty of changing even the simplest habits, and are aware of the comparatively small number of people who succeed in changing what they know to be bad habits however hard they try. The failure in most cases is due to the constant ill effect of the wrong manner of use upon general functioning which makes for misdirection of our energies, and thus causes loss of confidence, disappointment and often distress. By means of the procedures herein described,[37] the constant effect of manner of use upon general functioning will be a more or less good one in accordance with the skill of the teacher and the attitude of the pupil, and even the most difficult cases can be helped to success by the employment of procedures which make for the building up of confidence not only in the pupil's attempts to "do," but—more important still—in his attempts to prevent himself from doing things he knows he should not do, and does not desire to do, first, with regard to his own manner of using himself and then in applying this use through himself to his activities in the outside world. (Non-doing in the fullest sense.)

[37]Experience of this kind has been gained at 16 Ashley Place, London, since 1904 with pupils ranging in age from 2$^1/2$ to over 15 years, and later at the F. Matthias Alexander Trust Fund School at Penhill, Kent, England, with children and young people up to 16 years of age, and the results confirm what I have written here.

CHAPTER VI

PHYSIOLOGY AND PHYSIOLOGISTS

IT has been suggested to me by a friend that it is important that I should try to get what he called: "a physiological explanation for the working of my technique." This interested me so much that I asked him why he considered this of importance. He replied, "Because it would convince medical and scientific men of the soundness of your technique, and enable people to learn to make use of it more easily and quickly."

I pointed out that quite a number of medical, and a few scientific men had become convinced of its soundness after taking lessons and reading my books, while nineteen medical men had put their names to the letter which is reproduced in Chapter II. Hence I considered that I was justified in concluding that what is necessary to bring conviction as to the soundness of my technique is now available.

I then went on to say that I could not understand how he had come to believe that a "physiological explanation" of the working of my technique could make its acquisition easier or speedier for pupil or teacher, and that a study of my books should have made this clear to him. For myself I told him I had yet to meet a physiologist or anatomist whose use of himself could be described as anything but harmful, and for that reason I had long since decided that a knowledge of anatomy or physiology or both does not, and cannot, help a person to rid himself of a harmful manner of use, or indeed to know whether someone else's manner of use is harmful or the reverse.

Apropos of this I remember that the first medical man who gave me valuable support advised me to study anatomy and physiology as an aid to the experimentation I was then engaged in. He interested two of his friends in my ideas and actually persuaded them that it would be worth their while to give me lessons. One was a professor of anatomy, the other of physiology. A meeting was arranged and I received a kindly welcome from the two scientists, but it came as rather a shock to me to observe how badly they were using themselves. Indeed this struck me as most disquieting in men who were so deeply versed in knowledge of physiology and anatomy, the very knowledge that my friend thought would be of value to me in my field of work. I thought the matter over and came to the conclusion that as their knowledge had not brought them to a recognition of the value of a proper use of themselves (let alone the understanding of how to gain such use for their own benefit) it would be a waste of time at the stage I had reached in my career to study subjects which, as they had not been a help to them, seemed hardly likely to be a help to me in my search for a means whereby I could improve my own use and that of others.

I pointed this out to my friend and he agreed with my decision. No doubt the knowledge of physiology and anatomy that these two men possessed was of great value to surgeons and others, but I was concerned with a technique for dealing with the working of the living human organism as a whole, which called for a knowledge of the so-called mental (psychological) and physical (physiological and anatomical) working of the human organism as an indivisible unity.

For over forty-five years my technique has been seen in operation, and it can be seen today by anyone who wishes it. Throughout these years I have been engaged in demonstrating its soundness by the continued employment of experimentally established procedures which are described in "Evolution of a Technique."[38] This being so, I may claim that I am meeting the demands for proof in exactly the same way as an inventor or scientific engineer who points to his machine and shows that it works. There are people who will ask for scientific proof on orthodox lines, although such proof has in the past so often been recognized as untrustworthy, and productive of error. Indeed, it would not be unreasonable to contend that, in the matter of orthodox scientific proof, the initial step should be to demonstrate that the means whereby scientific proof is established are thoroughly sound. The physiological side of my technique has been the subject of friendly discussion between medical men and physiologists, and I am not aware of any physiological findings having been advanced which are at variance with any of its procedures.

* * * * *

The original conception behind the acquisition of the knowledge called physiology was a very narrow one, and those concerned with it became obsessed with end-gaining methods which they believed would ensure for their work in this field the title of "an exact science." The study of physiology as such implies a complete acceptance of the principle of separation in the working of the organism, and this serves to

[38] *The Use of the Self*, Chapter I.

explain why the experiences of the physiologist during the pursuance of his studies have not led him to see that much more than an understanding of the functions of muscles *as such* is necessary, if his fellowmen are to be able to benefit by his findings in their daily activities, or in the field of prevention and "cure." In principle this applies equally to the medical man who applies his knowledge of physiology in diagnosis. In order to meet the need for a full diagnosis and to give adequate treatment, particularly in the field of prevention, the doctor should be versed in the knowledge which Dr. Andrew Murdoch calls "clinical physiology."[39]

Those who have established physiological data after observing the working of the human mechanisms in living subjects had not the knowledge which could have enabled them to assess either the influence of wrong employment of the primary control upon the muscle action, or of the manner of use upon the general functioning of the subjects they were observing, or of the effect of stimuli upon the latter or upon their own reaction during their observations. This would account for the serious errors and misleading information to be found in authoritative works on physiology.

When my book *Constructive Conscious Control of the Individual* was published, I was criticized adversely because of my insistence on the observance of the principle of unity in the study of the working of the human organism, if that study were to yield the best practical results. The subject matter of my last book *The Use of the Self* shows that I had a practical foundation for my theoretical conclusions. My life work has been one of dealing with practical procedures based on the principle of unity, and with the associated theoretical conclusions which flowed from them. There has recently been a more general advocacy of the theory of unity in the working of the human organism, but this does not mean that the principle has gone beyond theory, for, to quote Dr. P. B. Ballard, M.A., when referring to my technique, "It is in fact that education of the 'whole man' about which so much has been said of late and so little has been done."

* * * * *

The physiologist may know the names of the muscles and the particular function of every one of them, but in the matter of employing them to the best advantage in a unified working of the human organism in daily life, this knowledge does not help us very much. The reason

[39]See Appendix B for excerpts from *The Function of the Sub-Occipital Muscles; The Key to Posture, Use and Functioning* by A. Murdoch, M.B., C.H.

is that the way of employing oneself in activity is a matter of the manner of reaction, and the influence of this on the subject being observed is not taken into account by the student of physiology, for reaction means much more than muscle activity in any attempt to discover what constitutes a "normal working of the postural mechanisms." It calls for the unity in action of the psycho-physical processes in:

(1) conceiving what is required or desired to be done; and in
(2) withholding or giving consent to doing it;

in other words, it means either refraining from, or giving consent to, sending the messages to the muscles to be employed in accordance with the subject's manner of employing them, this in turn being determined by his manner of employing the primary control.

As can be demonstrated, most people send messages which initiate overaction of certain groups of muscles, and too often bring into action muscles which should not be brought into action at one and the same time, all indications of *misdirection* arising from that faulty sensory guidance and control which is so common in people today.

May it not be that the concept of separation which led to the study of the organism in parts, as in anatomy, physiology and psychology, is responsible for the failure of the work in these fields to discover the existence of a primary control of the organism, or to recognize the influence of use upon functioning in its fullest sense?

* * * * *

Normality and Complexity. In view of the above, the following admission made by an eminent professor of physiology in a letter written to a medical friend is interesting:

> The underlying basis in anatomy and physiology is a complex business, and personally I am not able to offer a criticism of the theory of the normal working of the postural mechanisms.

If I understand this statement aright, it is a significant admission when viewed in the light of the value now placed on the body of knowledge classed under physiology and anatomy, upon which, for instance, the orthopaedic surgeon depends for his diagnosis and subsequent treatment; for the statement implies that his knowledge does not include an understanding of the "theory of the normal working of the postural mechanisms."

Is not this because the method of experimentation of those who have played their part in the accumulation of anatomical and physiological knowledge has been based upon the principle of separation? They obviously assumed that for their purpose they must *separate* the human psycho-physical organism into parts, and that when they had finished their experimentation they could use the findings that resulted as premises from which to make reliable deductions as to the nature of the working of the mechanisms of the organism *as a whole*.

The separation of the organism into parts by the anatomists and the physiologists is very significant, because it has prevented them from recognizing the importance of trying to gain a knowledge of the normal as well as the abnormal working of the postural mechanisms. Had they done this they would have seen that the psycho-physical controlling part is inseparable from the working of the other parts, and is as responsible for the misdirected use of specific muscles and tendons or groups of muscles, as it is for that co-ordinated working of the postural mechanisms as a whole necessary to the normal use of these mechanisms.

This demands a recognition of the existence of a central (primary) control which influences indirectly the manner of the working of the postural mechanisms both in the person enjoying satisfactory use as well as in those who do not. This influence varies for good or ill according to the trustworthiness or otherwise of the motor-sensory controlling and co-ordinating functioning of the mechanisms in all activity. Unfortunately, the influence of misdirection of the central (primary) control upon the working of the psycho-physical mechanisms has not been recognized, and therefore there has not been due recognition of the harmful influence of this misdirection upon the working of the mechanisms responsible for the normal position at a given time of the head in relation to the neck, and of the head and neck in relation to the torso, etc., upon which the integrated (normal) working of the postural mechanisms depends. Furthermore in this whole matter of the employment of the central (primary) control, the work done by the anatomists and physiologists has not been comprehensive enough to enable them to gain the practical experience necessary for deciding:

(1) when the central control of the postural mechanisms is working normally or abnormally so that they could estimate the influence of this control upon the postural mechanisms,

(2) what constitutes a normal or abnormal employment of the central (primary) control relative to an integrated use of the psycho-physical mechanisms as a whole, and consequently,

(3) what constitutes normal or abnormal working of the postural mechanisms.

I have already pointed out that the opportunity for acquiring the knowledge implicit in the above is not given by orthodox medical training. Consequently, the body of knowledge hitherto known as physiology cannot be said to constitute a "clinical physiology of the human being." Physiology, it is true, does indicate the function of particular muscles, say of the inner or outer intercostal muscles, *but it does not and cannot indicate the means whereby these muscles are operated relatively to the individual's use of his mechanisms as an indivisible unity, so as to ensure that integrated working of the organism which we always find associated with the standard of functioning present in a person in whom the way of employing the primary control is a constant influence for good.*

Hence in attempting to solve their problems, the anatomists and physiologists put their faith in the comparatively limited knowledge to be gained from a study of the nature and relative position of the bony structures and the specific working of the muscles, tendons and the like, which are only the means of motivating the postural mechanisms.

My experience as a teacher of the technique is derived from demonstrating daily to every one of my pupils that there is a primary control of the use of the mechanisms of the self, and that in taking full advantage of the influence for good in correctly employing this primary control, we hold the key to the bringing about of the "normal working of the postural mechanisms" as a whole. Furthermore, the gradual influence for good exerted by the correct employment of the primary control on the general functioning throughout the organism can be readily appreciated by the least attentive observer, and orthodox tests of such functioning have never failed to verify the observer's findings.

Those who laid the foundations of our present knowledge of physiology and anatomy were ignorant of the existence of this primary control. This no doubt accounts in great measure for their conception of what was necessary to a study of physiology, and of the "means-whereby" resulting from this conception upon which they and their disciples were content to depend in "their quest for certainty." Some twenty-eight years after I had discovered this control and employed it in a technique, the late Rudolph Magnus announced his discovery of it and its function, and Sir Charles Sherrington referred to this in his Presidential address to the Royal Society.

Turning again to the statement of the physiologist quoted at the beginning of this section, where he writes that "the underlying basis of anatomy and physiology is a complex business" I would point out that where the employment of the use of the mechanisms is satisfactory, complexity in the working of these mechanisms presents no difficulty. I contend that this would apply equally to the physiologist's inquiries and experimentation if he had had a theoretical and practical knowledge of the use of the primary control of the mechanisms he is concerned with. It is only when the use of the mechanisms is misdirected so that there is interference with the employment of the primary control, that the working of the complex mechanisms becomes complicated and gives rise to difficulties, just as it is the complications in a therapeutic case that increase the difficulties in medical diagnosis and treatment. Small wonder, when we consider that for the reasons already given, the diagnosis upon which the treatment is based cannot be complete.

The ability to estimate the influence of the primary control for good or ill upon the working of the mechanisms in the use of ourselves would enable the diagnostician to recognize the complications due to the misdirection of this use, and to employ means whereby complicated conditions may be changed and gradually become less and less complicated, although the working of the mechanisms would still be complex.

It has not surprised me that physiologists, anatomists, physical culturists and others should not have troubled to examine the facts concerning my discovery of a primary control of manner of use of the self even after I had demonstrated its existence in practical applications, for after all, I am an outsider. But what has surprised me is that the findings of an eminent "insider," the late Rudolph Magnus, should not have aroused sufficient interest in the fields of physiology and medicine to lead to a "re-orientation of the viewpoint"[40] towards the study of physiology, not only in the interests of medical men and physiologists themselves, but also for the sake of those who can benefit by their work, especially as Magnus's findings were the result of the orthodox experimentation to which they are all pledged.

> To take an illustration, Mackenzie showed and proved clinically the disassociated action of auricles and ventricles in fibrillation and the structural basis of this was shown much later.

This quotation from the physiologist's letter touches a matter of great interest. It is not for me to say whether from our standpoint this is a fair illustration or not, but I do wish to point out, however, that the disassociated action of the auricles and ventricles which Mackenzie observed was not really disassociated, any more than any other function can be disassociated from the indirect influence of the use of the primary control. So far as I can judge, Mackenzie was unaware of the existence of a primary control, and of its influence upon the working of the mechanisms of the organism functioning as an indivisible unity.

[40]See Appendix C for excerpts from *Re-orientation of the Viewpoint upon the Study of Anatomy*. A. Murdoch, M.B. (1937).

Consequently, he is not likely to have been aware of the nature of its influence upon the functioning of the auricles and ventricles in the living human being. If I am right in this belief, and I should welcome proof from Mackenzie's writings if I am wrong, the theory of this disassociation in action which Mackenzie worked out from his experimentation and findings is open to doubt, because the data arising from his experimentation and findings cannot be considered other than incomplete.

Another quotation from the physiologist's letter is as follows:

> I wonder if you could not get together a body of clinical observations, showing the disorders, on the basis of Alexander's views, and the results of his treatment? It would provide a definite problem for anatomists and physiologists to work upon.

What I have already written has a distinct bearing upon this point. If the reader will glance once more at the above quotation, and read it in the light of what I have written about separation and the experimentation which I submit has led to a sound theory of the "normal working of the postural mechanisms," he will perceive that the physiologist, in spite of his admissions in the several extracts that I have quoted, was still under the delusion that the clinical and physiological problems he refers to could be solved in the way he suggests. Curious, is it not, that failure or comparative failure to solve important problems in a given sphere has not led physiologists to suspect that in making the deductions upon which they based the means employed for gaining their ends, they had overlooked essential premises? A re-examination on these lines today would surely lead them to admit the existence of the primary control, and that this is the fundamental premise in any deduction on which to base the solving of their problems. All that would then be necessary would be for them to gain the experience of its employment and comprehend the nature of its influence upon use and functioning, by observing their own manner of use and that of others. In this way they would acquire important knowledge which cannot be gained in any other way.[41] In such a case I would invite them to my rooms to apply any tests they suggest when they would very soon be in a position to set down in black and white the very knowledge they have been, and still are, searching for, and I submit that a key to the practical solution of this problem is to be

[41] As John Dewey wrote in his Introduction to my book *Constructive Conscious Control of the Individual*, Introduction p. 223: "With respect to distinctively human conduct, no one, before Mr. Alexander, has even considered just what kind of sensory observation is needed in order to test and work out theoretical principles. Much less have thinkers in this field ever evolved a technique for bringing the requisite sensory material under definite and usable control."

found in the subject matter of *The Use of the Self*, because the results there described came about in the process of employing my technique.

*   *   *   *   *

Unity and Cell Functioning

As bearing upon unity, it may be of value and interest to restate here accepted facts concerned with the unity of activity in cell-functioning involved in the functioning of the sensory mechanisms. The sensory mechanism receives an impression by means of the *cell receptors*, and this impression is a *stimulus* to the *excitors* resulting in a *reaction* in the form of the *production of energy*.

The undue and harmful distribution and misdirection of *energy* for a given need can be prevented by the *inhibitor*, and in such case the energy required will be directed to the proper destination by the *conductor*.

It therefore follows that the standard of receptor, excitor, conductor and inhibitor functioning must not be lowered if the psycho-physical condition associated with the well-being of the individual is to be maintained.

If one studies closely the process involved in the generating and conducting of energy as set forth above, it will be evident that it becomes operative through the receipt of sensory impressions, and that only so long as there is unity, and not separation, between the generating and conducting systems can the process remain operative. I venture to assert that such unified working is characteristic of fundamental life processes, and that every manifestation of activity in living will, if carefully studied in the light of demonstrable knowledge, provide as convincing an example as the foregoing of the impossibility of separating so-called mental, physical or any other processes responsible for human manifestations in living.

*   *   *   *   *

Comparative Biological Evidence Which Reveals Integration as a Working Principle in the Use and Functioning of the Human Organism in Accordance with the "Total Pattern of Behaviour."

I am pleased to be able to print the following words of appreciation from Professor G. E. Coghill, the eminent Biologist and Professor of Comparative Anatomy, formerly of Wistar Institute, Philadelphia.

Gainesville, Florida,
June 4, 1939.

Dear Mr. Alexander:

I am delighted to have the books you sent. . . . . I am reading them with

> a great deal of interest and profit, amazed to see how you, years ago, discovered in human physiology and psychology the same principle which I worked out in the behaviour of lower vertebrates. Yet until now we have never come into personal touch. Possibly this is because we are technically laymen so far as the medical profession is concerned. I am glad to see that the British profession is now recognising your accomplishment and that you are now getting the credit and the hearing which you so richly deserve.
>
> (*signed*) G. E. COGHILL.

I am also permitted to quote the following extract from a letter which Prof. Coghill wrote to Dr. Millard Smith of Boston:

> "Mr. Matthias Alexander owes me nothing in regard to the principle of the 'total pattern,' for he and I worked in total ignorance of each other until the last year or two. That he should discover the principle in the human organism is marvellous, and he deserves all the credit that the medical profession and humanity can give him."

For those interested in biological observations and findings, a comparison between Prof. Coghill's work and mine may be of interest, for his aim was to study the nature, growth and development of the life processes of the lower organisms, functioning in association with conditions considered to be normal. I, on the other hand, was occupied from the beginning with the observation of human material in which abnormality had become established, and it was therefore necessary, in view of my conclusion that it was *what I was doing myself* that was the cause of my throat trouble, to detect the nature of this wrong doing by observation of the working of my own organism. This led me to discover that a particular relativity of the head to the neck and the head and neck to the other parts of the organism brought about a tendency to right or wrong use and functioning of the organism as a whole, and that the motivation for this use was from the head downwards.

This finding corresponds with that of Prof. Coghill who observed that the primary impulses in the lower vertebrates involved in tissue development and behaviour are projected along motor and sensory lines of communication from the head downwards towards the tail, and further, that any interference with the working of the mechanisms associated with the "total pattern" affects adversely the growth and working of the "partial pattern," which means a tendency of the "partial patterns" to gain a more or less dominating influence over the "total pattern" causing interference with growth and development.

These findings furnish again an analogy with observations that I made when dealing with my own problem, for I observed an interference with the working of specific parts of my organism connected with my throat trouble (partial patterns), and found that this was brought about by interference with the working of the organism in general (total pattern). But valuable as these findings were, the essential task still lay before me of learning, first, HOW to prevent myself from continuing to "do," at a given moment, what interfered with the working of my mechanism as a whole (total pattern of behaviour) and brought about wrong working of the specific parts (partial patterns of behaviour) which constituted abnormality, and secondly, how to bring about such changes in my "doing" as would lead to a gradually improving working of the mechanisms as a whole, and finally to a normal working.

Summed up, Prof. Coghill occupied himself with the all-important task of discovering the nature of the processes of normality and the effect of interference with these processes upon general functioning, while, because of the nature of my personal need, I had to try to discover the means whereby I could so change conditions of use and functioning that the trend of the change would be from abnormality to normality, and finally, having reached this desired result, to observe the manner of the working of the mechanisms associated with normality. The experience inherent in the carrying out of this work led as a natural consequence to the evolution of a technique by means of which desirable conditions of normality can be restored and maintained.

A friend of mine in whose judgment I have confidence, and who is familiar with Prof. Coghill's "classical observations," has suggested that the fact that Prof. Coghill and I, working independently, from different standpoints and with different aims in view, should have discovered the same principle in behaviour, he, in observing the lower vertebrates, and I, in observing the human organism beginning with the observation of myself, is striking evidence in observed phenomena from different angles and sources of the working of the principle of integration in the "total pattern" in life's processes and in the development of behaviour. I suggest that those interested should in their survey of data give due consideration to the following extract from Professor John Dewey's introduction to my book *The Use of the Self*:

> The school of Pavloff has made current the idea of conditioned reflexes. Mr. Alexander's work extends and corrects the idea. It proves that there are certain basic, central organic habits and attitudes which condition every act we perform, every use we make of ourselves. This discovery corrects the ordinary conception of the conditioned reflex. The latter as usually understood renders an individual a passive puppet to be played

> upon by external manipulations. The discovery of a central control which conditions all other reactions brings the conditioning factor under conscious direction and enables the individual through his own co-ordinated activities to take possession of his own potentialities. It converts the fact of conditioned reflexes from a principle of external enslavement into a means of vital freedom.

The following extract from a letter written by Dr. Trigant Burrow, Scientific Director of the Lyfwynn Foundation, New York, and well known as a Psychiatrist, to Mr. Walter Carrington, of March 2, 1939, may be of interest in this connexion:

> One cannot fail to recognize in reading his book, *The Use of the Self*, that Alexander has done much in getting at certain physiological reactions, and I was greatly impressed with the originality of his method and the very thorough and precise procedures he developed in the observation of his own behaviour. My own feeling is . . . that his work, expressive of innate scientific endowment, needs no endorsement beyond the objective evidence upon which it is based. To me his patient, painstaking and carefully controlled observations represent an amazing achievement in the field of human behaviour. I myself could not possibly lay claim to having contributed anything of a like nature. . . . Alexander's contribution in the field of behaviour is, as you mention in your letter, a half century old. His thesis has indeed become a commonplace.

Further may I point out that my practice and theory is not affected by the question as to whether or not reflexes are primary and integration of the "total pattern" secondary in behaviour, for the employment of the primary control in my technique is inseparable from the inhibitory procedures necessary to the reconditioning of the reflexes and to integration of the "total pattern," involving the same procedures in a unified process.

The same is true from the practical standpoint of the question as to whether wrong use or wrong functioning is the primary cause of disease. For it can be demonstrated that wrong use, which is always associated with wrong functioning, can be changed indirectly to right use by changing the employment of the primary control, and that in the process wrong functioning is restored to right functioning; whereas any attempt to restore right functioning specifically by direct means can only be palliative, because it still leaves the patient beset with the constant harmful influence of use which will consistently tend to lower the standard of his general functioning.

Note

The MS. of this book was almost ready for the printer when I received from a pupil in England (a medical man), the following extract from Sir Charles Sherrington's recently published book, *Man on His Nature.* In view of the nature of my subject matter I cannot but believe that this passage will be of special interest to my readers, and I will include it in this chapter.

The passage sent me is as follows:

> Take this act of "standing." Suppose my mind's attention be drawn to it, then I become fully aware that I stand. It seems to me an act fairly simple to do. I remember, however, that it cannot be very simple. That to execute it must require among other things the right degree of action of a great many muscles and nerves, some hundreds of thousands of nerve fibres and of perhaps a hundred times as many muscle-fibres. I reflect that various parts of my brain are involved in the coordinative management of all this, and that in doing so my brain's rightness of action rests on receiving and despatching thousands of nerve messages, registering and adjusting pressures, tensions, etc., in various parts of me. Remembering this I am perhaps rather disappointed at the very little that my mind has to tell me about my standing. When it gives its attention to my standing it can make me fully aware that I am standing, but as for telling me how it is that I stand, or as to helping me to analyse my standing, I get extremely little from it. The main thing I get from it seems the unequivocal assertion that it is "I" who stand.
>
> . . . If the standing goes on too long I get similarly an unequivocal assurance that it is "I" who am tired of standing. It seems that this power within me, which identifies itself with me, and calls itself "I," and wills the body to stand upright, and the body does so, or wills the body to sit down and the body does so, does not know how the body does these things. For all its effort, and for all the attention it can give, it does not seem to be able to get inside the act which it yet assumes it does. It cannot think itself into the "how" of the body's doing these things.[42]

As comment on this passage my pupil wrote me:

> This introspective account by a preeminent neurophysiologist is very interesting. . . . What he has discovered about his own "standing" is about as much as anyone would discover if his investigations stopped there. *It is only when an investigation is made into "changing" one's "standing" that any further*

[42]*Man on His Nature* by Sir Charles Sherrington, O.M. (Cambridge University Press, England, Macmillan & Co., New York.) Chapter VI. "A whole presupposed of its parts." Page 174.

> *discoveries are likely to be made.* His statement that we are unaware of how we stand is correct so far as the mechanism of Postural Integration is concerned, but you have shown that we can become aware of how we interfere with that mechanism. My view is as follows: there is a mechanism of Postural Integration which is used by animals unconsciously but efficiently. It is also used by human beings unconsciously, but not efficiently; it is in fact misused. What one becomes aware of in your work is the misuse, and the primary "directions" (orders) are physiologically inhibitory ones. If the mechanism was not already present, even if functioning badly, it could never be discovered and improvement in use consists entirely in not interfering with the mechanism.

I have italicized the point of particular interest in this comment. Sir Charles Sherrington's statement as to what is required for the act of "standing" should be of wide interest, particularly when taken in conjunction with his admission that he is disappointed at the very little that his mind has to tell him about his "standing," despite his knowledge of the intricate working of the central nervous system. The consciousness of this disappointment might have made him conscious that his conception of what was required for a full study of the central nervous system could not have been a comprehensive one, because the knowledge that he had acquired through this study did not help him to meet a need that he had assumed his mind would enable him to meet. He found himself, in his words, "though fully aware that I am standing," unable to tell himself "how it is that I stand"—that is, without that knowledge of the "means-whereby" of the direction and despatching of the messages through the nerve fibres, and the registering and adjusting of pressures and tensions throughout the organism—the "all this"—which results in the act of "standing." These "means-whereby" are all-important, because upon them depends that employment of the primary control of the use of ourselves by means of which we learn to know *how* we do the thing we are doing. Moreover, we come to a standard by which we recognize the "right degree of action" and "co-ordinative management" of the psycho-physical mechanisms in the performance of any act, whether that of "standing" or any other. Further when, for any reason, the integrated and complex working of these mechanisms is interfered with so that this working becomes complicated and disintegrated, it is by the knowledge of the "how" of the conscious employment of the primary control of our use that we are enabled to restore "right degree of action" and "co-ordinative management" to the mechanisms. If Sir Charles's study had led to this knowledge of the use of himself, he could have found out "the how of the body's doing these things," and should he then have become aware of any misdirection of energy and misuse of parts in his way of "standing," sitting or carrying-out any other activity, he would have the knowledge of the "how" of restoring rightness of direction and right degree of action.

CHAPTER VII

THE THEORY OF "THE WHOLE MAN" AND ITS COUNTERPART IN PRACTICE

THE conception of unity, as expressed in such phrases as "The Whole Man" and the "organism-as-a-whole," has become almost a commonplace in scientific and popular discussion; but nevertheless we rarely find that the individual outlook or understanding of those who accept it as a working principle is influenced in such a way that they work consistently to this principle when the opportunity comes to them to do so in attempting to deal with their problems. Indeed, when we give consideration to the activities of those who advocate this principle of unity, we find that the plans of procedure which they suggest or adopt are more in keeping with a belief in the organism as a composite product of which the separate parts can be controlled, affected or examined independently of the rest, than with a belief in the working of the "organism-as-a-whole."

In view of this, I think that it may now prove helpful if I give a number of examples of this inconsistency which have been afforded by a wide diversity of important writings in recent years, together with some comments which may make a small contribution towards a chance of outlook and understanding, and may serve to show what is demanded of the individual in making the change.

As my first example I will quote a sub-leader which appeared in the *Times* of London of May 5, 1938, entitled *The Whole Man*:

> Anyone might be forgiven for feeling hurt or angry if he were told that he is only half a man. But there are smaller fractions of humanity than a half. A distinguished educationist has recently made public confession that in his days of school-mastering he was prone to the error of dividing each boy, Gaul-like, into three parts, and trying to deal with mind, body, and character as if they were separate entities in watertight compartments. He himself looked upon mind as his primary and main preoccupation. In the revulsion from this misleading analysis he sees education as

a process of discovery and development in all three fractions at once. He draws a distinction between education and training. Mind, body and character might be subjected separately to intensive training without securing real education as the result. The mind concentrated, for instance, on obtaining a particular certificate or scholarship; the body put through a rigorous course of drill or gymnastics; and the character thrown, to sink or swim, into the troubled waters of a prefectorial or monitorial system—the trio may easily fail to add up to a truly educated man. It is a big problem. All three factors are essential to the upbringing of the young. They cannot all be in the hands of one and the same preceptor for each boy, and yet, to secure the grand result, there must be somewhere that supervising, guiding influence which will, in the light of some clearly seen ideal, attune the separate treatments to one another and so mix the elements that the final verdict will be "This is a man." It is a great ambition. Like all worthy objects, it has its difficulties. The hopeful sign is a visibly growing impulse to discuss it wherever educational experts are gathered together.

The mistakes against which protest is thus entered flow from the fallacy of treating the results of abstraction and analysis as if they were self-subsisting entities. Body, mind, and spirit are all obviously present in the individual. But the individual is something more than the sum of all three. There is a virtue in their combination which vanishes under dissection. Every man has to admit that if he undertakes an honest self-examination. He may find it pleasant—most of us do—to pay special attention to the needs of his body, that insatiable element whose appetite seems to grow the more it is indulged. Or he may, as some few do, make the claims of mind paramount and become a dry-as-dust highbrow with a starved and withered body. Worst of all, he may fail to see any need to labour at developing the powers and possibilities of that third partner, the spirit, which seems to direct the activity or decree the inactivity of the other two, and to have the mysterious faculty of brooding over thought and deed and passing judgment upon them and upon itself. It is noteworthy that moral verdicts proceed from that third partner. To body and mind things may be pleasant or painful, desirable or undesirable, but it is the spirit which says that they are good or bad. Even that high privilege does not make it independent of its coadjutors. A body wasted and mortified may impair both intelligence and spiritual perception. A misdirected or morbid mind may sap the foundations of right judgment. Each must contribute in its kind of its very best, but always to a common fund. The whole man transcends the addition of his parts as Abt Vogler's three sounds made in combination "not a fourth sound, but a star." It is not for nothing that health means wholeness.

Comment.

Here we have a good example of the inconsistency of which I speak, for although it is pleasing to hear of the conversion of a distinguished educationist to a belief in the principle of unity as the basis for "true education," it is still more disappointing, in view of the "big problem" involved, to find that the only means suggested by the writer for avoiding "the error of trying to deal with mind, body and character as if they were separate entities" is that "there must be somewhere that supervising and guiding influence which will, in the light of some clearly seen ideal, attune the separate treatments to one another and so mix the elements that the final verdict will be 'This is a man.'"

This is indeed to beg the whole question. For even if the means to "attune" and "mix" the products of the three separate treatments were forthcoming (and the subject matter of these pages shows clearly the fallacy in this and like conceptions) the proposal represents an outlook towards change that, while accepting *in theory* the principle of unity in the working of the human organism, leaves the essential task of putting the principle *into practice* to the mercy of disintegrating habits of use of the self which "feel right," and to an associated instinctive sensory guidance that is unreliable.

I would put it to the writer in this article and to the educational experts who, he tells us, show a "visibly growing impulse" to discuss the question, that the unity of THE WHOLE MAN in activity cannot be gained by the means suggested; for before the conception of unity can be put into practice consistently, we need a new understanding, through personal experience, of that manner of use of the self which is an integrating influence upon the working of the mechanisms of the human organism, and therefore a constant and improving influence upon functioning; we need, as Mr. Aldous Huxley has pointed out, "the knowledge of some general principle of right integration and along with it, a knowledge of the proper way to apply that principle in every phase of physical activity."[43]

If, as the writer in the article puts it, "education is to be a process of discovery and development in all three fractions at once (mind, body and character)," it demands from the individual as a "primary and main preoccupation" the education of himself as a consciously-changing integrating entity; and this implies an outlook towards change that welcomes the experiencing of a series of previously unknown psychophysical changes in the manner of use of the self, which, though they may "feel wrong," are fundamental to the process of changing and con-

[43]In *Ends and Means*, pp. 256-7.

trolling the procedures associated with the new conscious sensory guidance (feeling) in use and functioning, which is to supersede the old unreliable instinctive guidance and control.

This applies equally to the task of making changes in dealing with human problems in the outside world. Success in carrying out a new plan to take the place of one which is considered to be a failure must in the last analysis depend upon the nature of the individual human being engaged in the task of carrying out the new plan. Conditions in man which have a disintegrating influence upon his general functioning will render him a disintegrating element in the carrying out of the procedures of any plan or method, and this will militate against success; whereas the opposite is the case when conditions within him have an integrating influence upon his use and functioning, making it possible for him to function in "mind, body and character" as a WHOLE MAN when attempting to put into practice the changes he thinks necessary in carrying out his reforms and other activities.

Two of my pupils who saw the *Times*' sub-leader, and were struck with its relation to my work, thought it called for some comment, and although the letter addressed to the editor by Mr. T. G. N. Haldane was the only one published, and even so, was not published in full, I propose to reproduce his letter together with that of Mr. Eynon Smith, of St. Paul's School, who was the unsuccessful correspondent.

Mr. Haldane's letter was as follows:

THE WHOLE MAN

Sir:

Your extremely interesting sub-leader in last Thursday's issue will have been read by many who have been thinking along similar lines. One need only refer to such distinguished names as those as Mr. Aldous Huxley and Professor John Dewey, and to the review of the work of The Rockefeller Foundation, during 1937, recently published by Dr. Raymond B. Fosdick, who writes: "Just so far as medicine fails to encompass the whole man, it will fail to understand him. Medicine runs the risk of letting synthesis wait too long upon analysis, of ignoring the whole in the knowledge of some parts."

In Mr. Huxley's *Ends and Means* and in the writings of Professor Dewey, similar views are expressed. Although the general public may be interested in this idea, it will naturally ask "How is this idea to be applied in practice?" Your article does not however, give much practical guidance. Mr. Huxley and Professor Dewey, on the other hand, pay tribute and bear witness to the pioneer work of Mr. F. M. Alexander, who for over forty years has applied the principle in practice and has worked out a technique, the success of which can only be described as astonishing. The evidence is, I think, now overwhelming, but it is open to any one who doubts to test the matter by direct personal experience.

The importance of the psycho-physical approach to man can scarcely be exaggerated; it gives that unification, which, in the process of knowledge, the human mind must always seek. In this it is to be compared perhaps with recent developments in physics where, in the theory of relativity, scientists have succeeded in passing from the abstractions of space and time to the unifying conception of four dimensional space. This analogy, although interesting, does not, however, illustrate the enormous practical importance to the human race of the psycho-physical approach and the technique which has been developed by Mr. Alexander.[44]

Yours faithfully,

(signed) T. G. N. HALDANE.

Letter from W. H. Eynon Smith, Esq., of St. Paul's School.

Sir:

Your leading article, "The Whole Man," gives a much needed emphasis to the most difficult problem in education. Over-specialization has led to a disastrous division of function between teachers of "body," "mind," and "spirit." Clearly, if the organism is a unity, a specific change in one part requires a general adjustment of the whole and cannot be satisfactorily made by a teacher who is not equipped to make such a general adjustment. If attempts are made at specific changes without reference to the whole, as is bound to happen with present methods owing to the complexity of the organism, they may appear to succeed, but will in fact, because they are not based on a general coordination, lead to tension and disorder in the organism as a whole. This is most readily seen in "physical" education, where, while it is easy to secure outward conformity to arbitrary standards of posture and movement, there is no means of observing or communicating the deeper coordination essential for efficient activity. Hence the frequent failure in performance of the fine stylist and the success of many who appear to break every law. Hence also the uselessness of "physical training" in imparting the correct bodily functioning so important in activities not obviously "physical"—for example, problem-solving and spiritual meditation. The same argument applies to the training of "mind" and "spirit."

The fact is that neither teacher nor pupil knows with precision what he is doing. Since our judgment of the correctness of what we are doing depends on feeling, and since there are no adequate means of communi-

[44]This paragraph was not printed in the *Times*.

cating the sensory experience of the performance of a given act by the whole man, the pupil is in the position of being unable to perform an act correctly until he has had the experience, and unaware of the experience until he has performed the act. The accepted way out of this impasse is to lay down the end to be achieved and trust to luck that the infinitely complex means will be learned by trial and error. The sort of result produced by this method will be familiar to any teacher who has ever watched a class consciously "concentrating." It is not surprising that we appear to many to be physically deteriorating and spiritually bankrupt and that there is in the average mind a growing impression that life has "got out of control."

I believe that a solution of this problem is to be found, as your correspondent Mr. T. G. N. Haldane maintains, in the work of Mr. F. M. Alexander, whose technique provides a means of access to the whole man and, in your own words, "that supervising and guiding influence which will . . . so mix the elements that the final verdict will be 'This is a man.'" As a schoolmaster, I think that little further progress can be hoped for in education until this technique has received the widest and fullest consideration.

Yours faithfully,
(signed) W. H. EYNON SMITH.

The next quotations are from a *Six Year Review 1930-1936 of the Josiah Macy, Jr., Foundation* of New York, of which Dr. Ludwig Kast is the president. In his Foreword[45] to this journal Dr. Kast writes:

> (1) (The Foundation) does urge, however, that within any comprehensive or systematic plan for providing medical services in the health-care of a nation, it will be necessary to allocate responsibilities and functions under a division of labour that will preserve the unity of the patient as a psychosomatic being.

Elsewhere in the journal we find:

> (2) . . . additions to medical knowledge and equipment . . . have shifted the attention of the physician more and more from the patient as an individual to the disease as an entity, or to some particular organ or tissue as the seat of the disease. (p. 16)
>
> (3) . . . the extension of scientific research brought about a rapid increase in technical knowledge in medicine . . . and created a bewildering multiplication of specialties. Although all these specialties originate from and depend upon common scientific principles, they have become separated in medical education and in

[45]The italics in this and the following quotations are mine.—F. M. A.

> practice, and therefore the specialist often subordinates the *patient as a whole* to his preoccupation with an organ or symptom. (p. 23)
>
> (4) There is an increasing need, therefore, for the integration of these techniques and findings both in diagnosis and treatment. Such a synthesis requires not only a clear conception of the patient as a *total organism* but also a concern for the patient as an *individual personality*. . . . (p. 17)
>
> (5) The advantages which may come from a greater appreciation by the public of progressive medical schools can be realized only through a closer co-ordination of medical practice and medical education, graduate and undergraduate. Such organized medicine requires the greater concern for the personality development and emotional maturity of medical students, for the goals can be realized only by those who, in addition to their intellectual and technical training, sense social values. *Only integrated personalities can deal effectively with those patients in whom disturbance of integration is a part of the problem they bring to their physician.* (pp. 25 and 26)

Comment.

The fundamental problem to be solved in the psychosomatic plan is that which is stated in the sentence which I have italicized in paragraph 5 above. No suggestion is made however as to any solution, nor reference to any means by which the medical student can be helped to acquire the knowledge of the integrated working of his own psychophysical mechanisms or that of others, which is surely the basis upon which an integrated personality must be built up.

> (6) . . . the Foundation has . . . aided several experiments in the hope of revealing leads to new ways for the integration of thinking, or, what is more important, for discovering ends capable of synthesis. (p. 28)
>
> (7) Investigation of these problems can best be conducted through integrated clinical, physiological and psychological studies within the various clinical branches; for until the family physician, the pediatrician and the surgeon, as well as the various specialists, understand and deal with psychosomatic problems, no real advance can be made. When they do so, the term itself will be obsolete, for the practice of medicine will have become the practice of psychosomatic medicine. (p. 32)
>
> (8) Analytical methods are indispensable tools for the observation and study of the human organism and have been of unparalleled fruitfulness but for understanding man as an

> active and responsive being in his "life-space," as an individual personality immersed in his culture, a "symbolic" or integrated concept is necessary; for the *totality of an organism cannot be represented by merely adding up what is found by taking it apart.* (p. 21)

Comment.

The matter in this paragraph (8) is of special interest to me because all that is suggested as means to an end, both in relation to methods of analysis employed as "tools for the observation and study of the human organism," and also to methods of synthesis in the linking-up of observed facts "for understanding man as an active and responsive being" has for many years been used in my work. The reasoned procedures employed for this purpose are described in my books, together with a detailed account of the discovery that the primary procedure in activating the integrating and reconditioning process throughout the human organism (total pattern) was a certain employment of the primary control of the manner of use of the self.

My life's work has demonstrated that by means of this reconditioning process conditions in man can be changed gradually from the abnormal to the normal, although at certain times and in certain circumstances he will have to surmount impeding experiences in his psycho-physical activities. Over and above this he can reach a standard of self-awareness and self-confidence which is denied to those who still continue to depend upon the guidance of instinct in living.

In view of this, how can we expect that until man has reached a stage of development by means of reasoned procedures, where he can depend upon conscious guidance in the control of his psycho-physical self, he can possess that knowledge of himself which is essential for the eradication of undesirable reactions, and thus transcend the limitations which are characteristic of the creature on the animal plane of evolution?

One more point, if it is true that "the totality of an organism cannot be represented by merely adding up what is found by taking it apart," then it is difficult to understand the significance of the word "integrated" in this paragraph in view of the method adopted in practice, and this applies equally to the use of this word in paragraph 9.

I will now go on to quote from a journal entitled *Psychosomatic Medicine,* Vol. I, No. I., January, 1939 (Published quarterly with the sponsorship of the Committee on Problems of Neurotic Behaviour Division of Anthropology and Psychology, National Research Council, Washington, D.C.). In their Introductory Statement the editors write:

> (9) Psychosomatic Medicine is an expression which has not

> yet obtained citizenship. . . . Like all new expressions, the term . . . may lead to misconception and misunderstanding unless a definition is provided. . . . Its object is to study in their interrelation the psychological and physiological aspects of all normal and abnormal bodily functions and thus to integrate somatic therapy and psychotherapy. (p. 3)
>
> (10) In recent years an increasing number of observations have been made concerning the correlation of psychological and physiological processes in the human organism. . . . In the interests of unity and of further progress this journal aims to correlate contributions from the special fields. (p. 4)
>
> (11) . . . (psychosomatic medicine) is an essential approach to every medical specialty in so far as it is *fundamental in all diagnosis and treatment.* (p. 5)

Comment.

With regard to the words I have italicized in extract 11 above, "fundamental in all diagnosis and treatment," I would refer my readers to the letter on page 16 signed by nineteen medical men in which the signatories support my contention that "an unsatisfactory manner of use, by interfering with general functioning, constitutes a predisposing cause of disorder and disease, and that diagnosis of a patient's troubles must remain incomplete unless the medical man in making the diagnosis takes into consideration the influence of use upon functioning."

I fail to find in the pages of the psychosomatic journal even a casual indication that might lead one to believe that those responsible took into their survey the constant influence for good or ill of manner of use upon the function of the self when they formulated their plans of procedure for diagnosis and treatment.

> (12) Reading the expression "psychosomatic medicine," he (the medical reader) may be reminded of scientific or philosophic writings, which were so common in the last century, devoted to new, theoretically postulated, scientific disciplines . . . which were essentially non-existent. . . . A malicious critic of much of the nineteenth century psychology and philosophy might have justifiably observed that the main occupation of psychologists and philosophers consisted in writing introductions to scientific disciplines that did not yet exist. (p. 3)

Comment.

The quotations already given in this chapter will have shown that this "occupation" is that of too many people today, and this statement on the part of the editors of *The Journal of Psychosomatic Medicine* may well prove to be rather nearer the truth than the writers perhaps suspected or intended. Unless they themselves are able to demonstrate the existence of the "scientific discipline" which is "theoretically postulated" and described as "psychosomatic medicine," it will not be the "malicious critic of nineteenth century psychology," but the gentle reader of the present day who will be left wondering whether, after all, they also are not engaged in "writing introductions to scientific disciplines which do not exist."

In his article, *Psychological Aspects of Medicine* in the same issue of *The Journal of Psychosomatic Medicine*, Dr. Franz Alexander writes:

> (13) It belongs to the paradoxes of historical development that the greater the scientific merits of a method, or scientific principle, the greater will be their retarding influence in a later more advanced period of development. . . . With the introduction of the microscope the localization of the disease became even more narrowed down: the cell became the seat of disease. No one was more responsible for this particularistic concept in medicine than Virchow to whom pathology owes more than to any one else. He declared that there are no general diseases, only diseases of the organs and of the cells. His great achievements in the field of pathology and his great authority made of cellular pathology a dogma, which has influenced medical thinking up to the present day. Virchow's influence upon etiological thought is the most classical example of the above mentioned paradox of history. *The greatest accomplishments of the past become later the greatest obstacles against further development.*

Comment.

If it is true, as Dr. Alexander states in this paragraph, that "the greater the scientific merits of a method, or scientific principle, the greater will be their retarding influence in a later more advanced period of development," then it is certain that the principle upon which the method is based must be a false one; otherwise the employment of a method could not prove a "retarding influence," but would help towards a "more advanced period of development."

Dr. Alexander seems to believe that this paradox is inevitable, for while he states that Virchow is more responsible than anyone else for a concept that he describes as one "of the greatest obstacles against further development," he intimates at the same time that pathology owes more to him than to anyone else. I would point out that this inconsistency on Dr. Alexander's part could not have come about if in his consideration of diagnosis and treatment he had taken into account the effect of harmful use and lowered functioning *as a forerunner of cell and organic disease*. Having failed to recognize this, he has also failed to see that when put into practice, Virchow's "particularistic concept in medicine" has been responsible on Dr. Alexander's own admission for a method which limits the scope of both diagnosis and treatment, and is characterized by a narrowing down of the localization of the disease. It is therefore unscientific, and furnishes still another instance of the danger of the *direct* method of approach to the acquisition of knowledge in medicine or in any other field of man's activity. Further on in his article Dr. Alexander writes:

> (14) Not less impressive is the statement of Dr. Allen Gregg ("The Future of Medicine," *Harvard Medical Alumni Bulletin*, Cambridge, October, 1936), a man who views the past and future of medicine from a broad perspective. "The totality that is a human being has been divided for study into parts and systems; one cannot decry the method but one is not obliged to remain satisfied with its results alone. What brings and keeps our several organs and numerous functions in harmony and federation? And what has medicine to say of the facile separation of 'mind' from 'body'? What makes an individual what the word implies—not divided? The need for more knowledge here is of an excruciating obviousness. But more than mere need there is a foreshadowing of changes to come. Psychiatry is astir, neuro-physiology is crescent, neuro-surgery flourishes, and a star still hangs over the cradle of endocrinology. . . . Contributions from other fields are to seek from psychology, cultural anthropology, sociology and philosophy as well as from chemistry and physics and internal medicine to resolve the dichotomy of mind and body left us by Descartes." (Page 9)

Comment.

I do not think I can do better than quote here some notes on this passage which were sent to me by one of my students, Mrs. Alma M. Frank, of New York.

> The quoted statement of Dr. Allen Gregg presents the essential problem. The procedure he suggests however, requires consideration. It requires serious consideration, for on all sides today as well as throughout this issue of this new publication, we find the following conviction: *correlation* of accumulated data *in all fields* will solve the problem.
>
> Here is the rub: can we get rid of the dichotomy of mind and body

through the so-called sciences, when the very sciences themselves and their development rest upon that same dichotomy? Is it not that the dichotomy is the parent of "psychology" and "physiology" as separate sciences? In reality they are dependent for their existence as separate sciences upon this dichotomy inherited from Descartes. It stands to reason, therefore, that we cannot see anything in this direction that will rid us of the dichotomy, and it is obvious that we may expect greater accumulations of data which defy correlation.

What then do we need if not the correlation of more and more data from all "sciences"? The answer is: new principles to be applied in all fields of research, principles which will not only deny the dichotomy of mind and body (which all are now eager to do), but will free us from continuing our research with the same concepts, labels and separatistic tools that were born of the dichotomy we wish to be rid of.

Mrs. Frank's contention here is well supported by the following extract from Dr. L. K. Frank's paper *Structure, Function and Growth*[46] (page 233):

> These criticisms of analytic procedures and of the use of time concepts are associated with the organismic conception, which has been developed as a protest against this parceling out of an organism according to the variety of data which it may yield; it marks a movement toward the explicit recognition of the idea that an existent such as an organism will yield as many different kinds of data as the investigator has the technique for discovering and recording, and that among these data there will be certain relationships arising from the very nature of an organism as an energy complex in a four-dimensional universe, with multiple "fields" in various stages of development. This does not mean that these different data must or should be correlated, since within an organism, especially when growing or developing, the process of change and adjustment and the interactions of "fields" occur with varying degrees of lags and efficiency. The study of individual organisms as they grow and develop is still so new that little is actually known of development.
>
> The analytic tradition of science that insists upon breaking down an organic whole into discrete parts and attempting to correlate two variables is the chief obstacle to the study of organisms. Many investigators assert that the study of an organism instead of the restricted problem of two variables is not scientific, probably because they prefer the abstractions of anatomy and physiology and creating methods for obtaining data and establishing their meaning, which are of course primary to

[46]Published in *Philosophy of Science*, Vol. 2. No. 2, April, 1935.

the study of organisms. Here again we see how the study of organic growth and development is impeded by the conceptual framework of contemporary science.

I will next quote some excerpts from the *Review* of the work of the Rockefeller Foundation for 1937, by President Raymond B. Fosdick.

> (15) Just so far as medicine fails to encompass the whole man it will fail to understand him. Medicine runs the risk of letting synthesis wait too long upon analysis, of ignoring the whole in the knowledge of some parts. With all its wisdom, if medicine neglects what integrates and harmonizes the functions and organs, its picture will be out of focus and its comprehension incomplete.
>
> (16) The average layman, observing the more scientific aspects of the practice of medicine, and reading almost daily accounts of new scientific discoveries, is perhaps tempted to conclude that man knows nearly everything there is to know about the constitution and behaviour of the human organism. As a matter of fact, of all the things that man really knows, he knows least about himself. His knowledge of the stars is probably more complete and more reliable than his knowledge of his own body.

My friend, Mr. Michael March, has made the following comments on this *Review*. In the *Brooklyn Citizen* of March 28, 1938, he wrote as follows:

> In the *Review* of the work of the Rockefeller Foundation for 1937, just published, President Raymond B. Fosdick has occasion, during his discussion of the work being done in the fields of psychiatry and medicine, to lay bare one of the important dilemmas currently facing mankind, to wit: How can science deal with individual man as a whole? The dilemma is implied in the attempts made to integrate the essentially unrelated techniques of medicine with those of psychiatry, or, in other words, to fuse two techniques which had their origin in the wholly false assumption that mind and body are separate entities.

Mr. March then quotes the statement (15) above and continues:

> And by adding that "psychiatry is a headland of medicine and not an island of speculation," Mr. Fosdick believes that psychiatry, which is being heavily backed financially by the Foundation, is the potential integrating factor, an attitude which is certainly not very sound in the light of the fact, as I have implied, that it is sheer folly to try to fuse two techniques, each

> of which originated in the false theory that mind and body are separate entities.
>
> It is interesting to find such statements in the pages of a publication by the Rockefeller Foundation, whose funds are devoted to the advance of knowledge. But the dilemma which gives rise to such speculation is widespread. An impasse has been reached in science's approach to man, and the need for dealing with the individual as an integrated whole is imperative. "The need," says Mr. Fosdick, "is so great that there is little danger at the moment of overstressing it." In the face of this it is curious that the Foundation remains unaware of the existence of a technique which actually employs an integrating principle that is demonstrably practical and scientific. For with a knowledge of the principles and technique of F. Matthias Alexander it is not likely that Mr. Fosdick would ascribe to psychiatry the function of integrating man's "functions and organs." In place of psychiatry, which is at best only a speculative technique, he would have reported enthusiastically upon Alexander's principle of the primary control and his technique for employing it in the integrated action and reaction of the human organism as opening up new avenues into the future well-being of humanity.

In his book, *Man, the Unknown*, Alexis Carrel of the Rockefeller Institute has dealt with this dilemma by the suggestion that the mass of knowledge which is now "disseminated in technical reviews, in treatises, in the brains of men of science"[47] should be correlated by some superman or supermen who will be able to study this mass of acquired and unrelated knowledge, weld it as it were together, and make it applicable to the practical need for which it is intended. In this connexion Dr. Carrel writes:

> (17) . . . is it possible for a single brain to assimilate such a gigantic amount of knowledge? Can any individual master anatomy, physiology, biological chemistry, psychology, metaphysics, pathology, medicine, and also have a thorough acquaintance with genetics, nutrition, development, pedagogy, esthetics, morals, religion, sociology, and economics? It seems that such an accomplishment is not impossible. In about twenty-five years of uninterrupted study one could learn these sciences. At the age of fifty, those who have submitted themselves to this discipline *could effectively direct the construction of the human being* and of a civilization *based upon his true nature.*[48]

[47] *Man, the Unknown*, by Alexis Carrel (Harpers), p. 282.

[48] *Man, the Unknown*, by Alexis Carrel (Harpers), p. 285. The italics are mine.—F. M. A.

To me this is a remarkable statement. Dr. Carrel asks whether it is "possible for a single brain to assimilate such a gigantic amount of knowledge," or whether any individual could "learn these sciences." Strangely enough he does not appear to think this impossible, but what is still more strange he does not seem to question whether such a person will be able to link up the different data he has acquired into a connected whole. Yet in my experience people who have studied and accumulated knowledge in a number of different fields are too often unable to connect up the different data they acquire in this way. They thus miss the opportunity of collecting all the premises possible before making the deductions upon which to build their constructive plans. If those who have spent so much time in accumulating a mass of unrelated knowledge had linked up new knowledge as it came to them with the knowledge they already possessed, they would not now be faced with the task of selecting and then correlating contributions from the special fields in "the interests of unity and of further progress."

Dr. Carrel also believes that those who "could learn these sciences" and "have submitted themselves to this discipline could effectively direct the construction of the human being and of a civilization based upon his true nature." In reply to this I would point to the subject matter of this book as evidence that the knowledge most fundamental to this great task is not mentioned among the "sciences" he has named. This fundamental knowledge is that of the integrated working of the psycho-physical mechanism involved in the use of the self, and the experience necessary for the acquisition of this knowledge cannot be gained by workers in any or the whole of the sciences on Dr. Carrel's list.

I submit, therefore, that this all-important premiss was not taken into consideration by Dr. Carrel when he made the deductions which led him to indicate the means whereby his superman could be fully equipped with what he needed for "the construction of the human being and of a civilization based upon his true nature," and also for diagnosis and treatment of this human being as a "total organism and an "individual personality."

I can assure Dr. Carrel that unless his superman has a conscious knowledge of the procedures which activate the integrating and reconditioning process involved in bringing about that relationship in the working of the parts of the organism which constitutes the employment of the primary control, he will be without the fundamental knowledge essential in preparing himself for his task of effectively directing "the construction of the human being and of a civilization based upon his true nature."

Only when human beings are in possession of this knowledge and are able to put it into practice, can Dr. Carrel expect as a result a civilization which will show any fundamental change for the better; only then can we hope for the coming, not of one superman, but of a large proportion of men and women who, profiting by change in their outlook and approach to the conception of the unity of the living organism and the philosophy of truth, would refuse to bolster up any plan (or examine the results of its practical working) unless they were convinced that their deductions were made from complete premises. Neither could they continue to adhere to methods of acquiring knowledge which, being evolved to meet the needs of investigators working only upon a part or parts of the organism, have led to differentiation and specialization in the past, and have effectively prevented them from acquiring the knowledge that would enable them so to treat the organism that it may be changed *in the process* of reconditioning from a disintegrated to an integrated whole.[49]

[49]See Appendix G.

CHAPTER VIII

AN OSTEOPATH'S IDEA OF A NEW TECHNIQUE

I HAVE been much interested in an article entitled "*Re-education in Technic*" by Mr. Paul Van B. Allen, D.O., published in the *Journal of the American Osteopathic Association of Chicago*, not only because of its generous reference to my work but also because it illustrates in a remarkable way the difficulty experienced even by those who accept my principle in theory, in appreciating the full implication of this principle when they start to put it into practice. As I have tried to make clear throughout this book, the point of issue is of such importance in any consideration of the control of human reaction, that I ask Mr. Allen to believe that in making the following criticism I desire only to clear up what must inevitably tend to confuse and mislead the colleagues he is so anxious to help.

Mr. Allen starts his article by describing at some length certain deficiencies in the osteopathic technique as generally practised. He says:

> . . . We propose to show that in almost every instance our technic falls far short of what it should be, both as to the skill with which we apply our own methods, and as to our ability to broaden and increase the scope of those methods by the adoption of new technic. This is true, first, because we are constantly concerned with the end to be gained to the almost total exclusion of any consideration of the means whereby that end is to be obtained; second, because we have followed the process of intuitive imitation both as we began to learn technic, and later in any effort to add new methods to our armamentarium; third, because we have followed the trial and error method rather than that of reason and fourth, and quite inclusively, because of the very nature inherent in the methods by which we learned and continue to learn technic.
>
> . . . It follows that no matter how much we seek to improve and polish our technic, no matter how skillful it becomes, it is conditioned by the necessity for making it "feel right," in terms of this habitual familiar sen-

sory impression which because of its genesis is almost certain still to be incorrect and misleading. Hence, however much we will to incorporate new and better methods into our habitual procedures, we fall far short of what we ought properly to expect of ourselves unless we analyze the subjective factors of our technic in a critical and objective manner.

At this point Mr. Allen refers to what I have written in my book *The Use of the Self* about the difficulty I experienced at first in correcting certain bad habits in the use of my voice, and proceeds to deal approvingly with the theory and practice of my technique, and not only to recommend it to his colleagues, but to outline a way of employing it. He specially commends to their attention my "basic contention that man living under modern conditions, possesses a distorted sensory appreciation that is thoroughly inadequate and unreliable" so that what is wrong in the use of ourselves has come to "feel right." He goes on to show how "sensory appreciation pertains in the case of osteopathic technic both to the sensing of what is to be done . . . and the sensing of our own muscle and nerve activity in response to the mental commands," and that in whatever he does, the osteopath is faced by a serious problem when he tries to make the change in the use of himself that he considers necessary, because the end-gaining methods adopted in osteopathy tend constantly to perpetuate any bad habits in the use of the self that had already become established and which "carry over from the old to every successive attempt at self-improvement." He writes:

> Our mind is so fixed upon the end which we have in view, that we disregard the means whereby that end is to be gained, and intuitively, fall into the habitual wrong use of our organism, the while having the sense of right feeling and of satisfaction with our work. The result of this process is that the harder we try, the more fixed is our attention upon the end to be gained and the more we revert to the habitual and wrong use of our organism.

And he concludes his analysis thus:

> . . . we seem to be left running in circles in a blind alley, except that the same Alexander comes to our rescue with a means of extricating us from our predicament.

I have quoted Mr. Allen thus fully because, in view of his very careful and clear-sighted diagnosis of this "predicament," when he goes on to discuss the practical application of my technique to osteopathy, he does not give his colleagues any help in solving the problem that confronts them in their attempts to make the changes in the *use of ourselves* which he advises. He gives descriptions of my procedures and certain general verbal directions as to what should be done to put these into practice, but it seems to have escaped his notice that those who may try to carry out his suggestions will in so doing be trusting to the same sensory guidance upon which they had previously relied, and as he does not make any provision in his plan for restoring sensory reliability, it is difficult to understand why he should believe that they would be more successful in carrying out his suggestions as to procedure than they had been hitherto in carrying out those which they attempted in their osteopathic training and in their other efforts to improve themselves. Mr. Allen writes:

> Alexander faces this impasse with the principle of *inhibition*[50] of the *immediate response* . . . one gives the mental order, and then consciously inhibits or holds in abeyance the active response to that order, consciously reviews and senses again in detail what the body must do. . . .

But how can those in the predicament Mr. Allen so graphically describes put this principle successfully into practice? For on his own admission their problem (which is no different from that of others whose sensory appreciation of what they are doing is untrustworthy), is that in their attempts to improve themselves, the moment they get the stimulus to act they rely for guidance upon feeling which Mr. Allen admits is unreliable, and thus, by immediately responding through the instinctive habitual use of themselves which "feels right," continue to indulge in the same bad habits of use they are trying to correct. This is precisely where their predicament lies. The same misunderstanding of their problems underlies Mr. Allen's advocacy of "visualizing" and "sensing," both of which activities he appears quite mistakenly to include in my technical procedure as, for instance, in the passage just quoted or when he writes "every detail of the lesion must be visualized," and again, "He (one) senses in advance the feel of his own muscles as he expects them to act to accomplish his purpose," and "he (one) visualizes the smooth acceleration of force, etc., etc." Such "visualizing" or "sensing" would necessarily be dependent on the same unreliable sensory appreciation (feeling) which had led to the errors it is desired to eradicate. It is therefore curious that Mr. Allen, who is so definite in his warning against trusting to unreliable sensory impressions during attempts to make changes in the use of the self, should not see that if a person whose sensory appreciation is untrustworthy places reliance upon a picture he "visualizes" or a feeling he "senses," he is depending, in Mr. Allen's own words, on "an illusory basis of rightness." Unless then some provision can be made for changing and improving this con-

[50]The italics in this and following quotations from Mr. Paul Van B. Allen's article are mine.—F. M. A.

dition of unreliable sensory appreciation (and of this Mr. Allen makes no mention), in what way can these procedures be of benefit to him?

It is, moreover, unfortunate that in his description of my technique, he does not refer even in passing to the essential part played by the right employment of the primary control in bringing about an improving use of the self, together with a gradual restoration of sensory trustworthiness. In the first chapter of my book, *The Use of the Self*, I related how attempts which were made with the aim of correcting certain defects by *direct* control led through their failure to the discovery of the existence of a primary control of the use of the self, and then to the further discovery that when once the habitual wrong response to the stimulus to activity was inhibited, the right employment of this primary control led *indirectly* to the gradual disappearance of the defects; that, indeed, these defects were found to be by-products of a wrong employment of the primary control.

The discovery of this control made possible the evolution of a technique, and the understanding of the right employment of this control is fundamental therefore to the application of my technique, or indeed to that of any other that could meet the needs outlined by Mr. Allen. Much of the misapprehension in his description of my technique undoubtedly arises from his having apparently missed this connexion in reading my book, together with the further point which proceeds directly from it, that the changes in the manner of use of the self brought about through my technique emerges as an indirect result of means which are conditioned by, and dependent upon, the right employment of the primary control.

From this it follows that the inhibition of the "immediate response" which Mr. Allen quotes as my solution of the "predicament" in which his colleagues find themselves, is *primarily the inhibition of the habitual response to any activity which results in the wrong employment of the primary control.* This point has been missed by Mr. Allen else he would surely have recognized that if those who have no knowledge of the working of the primary control try to follow out my procedures from his verbal descriptions, they can only be said to be making one more trial and error attempt to gain an end regardless of the right "means-whereby," and one which is bound to land them still further in their predicament.

When once he has gained this knowledge of the working of the primary control and has learned to put it into practice, the osteopath, like any one else, will be able to use himself to the best advantage in the carrying out of the technique, or in anything else which he may wish to do, and this knowledge is essential to his success in any attempt to put the technique into practice in his osteopathic work or any other occupation.

For in order to carry out any new idea or instruction given to him with the aim of bringing about a new use of himself, he would at first have to do what "feels wrong" to him, and experience has shown that however much he might desire or decide to carry out the new instructions for improving his use, *in practice* he would almost certainly be unable to abide by his decision, but the moment he started to carry on his osteopathic work would do what he felt was "right," and instinctively relapse into the wrong use associated with his habitual reaction to any stimulus to activity which would bring with it the satisfaction of "feeling right."

Here again Mr. Allen is under a serious misapprehension as to what is fundamental in the application of my technique, for he writes:

> In applying his [Alexander's] method to this problem, the first emphasis is laid upon the fact that the new and better technique contemplated must be worked out step by step, in detail, *first* as to the precise conditions of the lesion and the mechanics of the correction; and *second*, as to each successive step the particular and correct use of our own bodily mechanism in such a way as adequately to meet the requirements placed upon it by the nature of the lesion.

And again:

> Let us outline very briefly a few of the factors to be considered in such an analysis of a procedure of technic. It is assumed that one has already visualized the mechanics of the lesion which determined the direction and the distance through which the corrective force must move. . . . One, *then* considers the use of his own body, etc.

This is indeed to put the cart before the horse. Throughout my writings I have tried to make it clear that in my technique the emphasis is laid *first* and always on the consideration of the right manner of use of the self, and that only on having reached a point where one is able to command the "means-whereby" of a satisfactory use of the self, can one safely go on to apply this satisfactory control of use to an outside occupation. Mr. Allen appears also to have missed the significance of what was set down in the chapter on Golf in *The Use of the Self*, otherwise it is difficult to understand how he failed to appreciate that if he is to help himself and his colleagues to carry out the new procedures in my technique which call for a manner of use that is unfamiliar, the education in this new technique should *begin* with the re-education of their manner of using themselves; better still, that if possible, this re-education should be carried out before beginning their training in osteopathy, starting their osteopathic work only when they had reached the point where they could maintain a constantly improving use of themselves whilst putting their osteopathic technique into practice, or indeed during any other activity they may desire to carry on.

This applies to every field of activity. Let us take as an example the case of a singer or actor who has been taught—say, deep breathing or some other "breathing exercises" as a preliminary to singing and acting, regardless of the effect the performance of the exercises will have upon the manner of use of either the breathing or vocal mechanisms. I am able to write from a very wide experience in this field.

The artist trained in this way goes on to the stage or platform with a definite specific idea of "how to breathe" whilst singing or acting. The bad results of this method are too much in evidence today to need enlarging upon, and where they are present they make it impossible for the singer or actor to maintain his highest standard of functioning as an artist. The idea underlying such methods of training arises from the belief that it is possible to give specific help to separate parts of the organism, as if the breathing mechanisms of the artist for instance functioned separately and apart from his vocal mechanisms or his general use of himself, and what is more to the point as if the use and functioning of these mechanisms could be separated from the use and functioning of the organism as a whole, whereas they are as closely associated and as dependent upon one another as are the parts of our mental and physical make-up. It can be demonstrated that the person who learns to use himself properly by relying upon the correct employment of the primary control of his use of himself will breathe to the best possible advantage in singing or speaking, as well as in all the other activities of life. He will not need the help of specific "breathing exercises" for doing anything that is necessary in carrying out his activities, even though these may include the task of putting into practice the procedures of a technique such as is employed, or may in the future come to be employed, in osteopathy or the like.

The generous appreciation of my technique that Mr. Allen expresses led him to advocate it to his colleagues as a contribution of value to osteopathic method and treatment, but he has missed the point that in the recognition and conscious employment of the primary control lies the fundamental difference between the theory and practice of my technique and that of osteopathy, and that the two methods of approach, the direct method of osteopathy as described by Mr. Allen, and the indirect method as exemplified in my procedures, cannot be combined or brought into line with each other as they are based on principles of working that are irreconcilable. The confusion of ideas which has caused him to overlook this is, I suggest, foreshadowed in the title of his paper *Re-education in Technic.*

It is possible to re-educate a person who is to carry out a technique, but I am at a loss to see how he or she can be re-educated in a new technique. That would surely imply education, not re-education. Re-education means a gradual restoration of something that has been previously experienced; something which we have been educated in, but for some reason have lost, as for instance when a person whose use of the self has been gradually interfered with over a period of years manifests, as time goes on, more and more harmful effects of this interference in his general use and functioning. *Re-education is not a process of adding something but of restoring something.* It was to meet the need of restoring actual conditions of use and functioning which had been previously experienced and afterwards lost, that my technique for the re-education of the use of the self was evolved. But when Mr. Allen offers this technique as a contribution to osteopathy he is offering something new to his colleagues, something not previously experienced (the unknown) by them, and as so often happens when a person versed in a theory and practice based on a principle which is familiar is led to consider and approve a theory and practice based upon a principle which is unfamiliar, he was misled in his conception of the "means-whereby" that were required for the successful adoption of this new technique.

He gives his reasons for believing that he and his colleagues could not be certain whether or not they were doing their work in the way best suited to their individual make-up, and that because of the deceptive guidance of their sensory appreciation, they were likely to become less rather than more proficient as they continued to practise their manipulative work. He believed he could free them from this predicament by passing on to them knowledge he believed he had gained through reading my books. His practical suggestions however fit in, not with my practice and theory as set forth in my books, but with his own interpretation of it. For as I have already pointed out he has overlooked the important—the all-important—part played in the practice of my technique by the primary control of use, and has not seen that if the influence of the right employment of this primary control is unrecognized or ignored in the practical working out of my theory, my technique cannot prove more useful than any other in extricating his colleagues from their "predicament."

His diagnosis of cause and effect in considering my technique as an aid in helping his colleagues or patients was, therefore, incomplete. This however is not to be wondered at, seeing that his previous experience and training did not enable him to realize, any more than did that of the original founder of the method of osteopathy, the far reaching influence of use upon the functioning of the human organism, nor the impeding and harmful effect of the constant lowering of the standard of general functioning in a patient by reason of the bad habits of use of the self which are responsible for this lowered standard of functioning. This applies equally to his diagnosis of the manipulator's shortcomings, defects and individual peculiarities in his use of himself during each manipulative act, for without a knowledge of the right employment of the primary control in the use of himself, a reliable diagnosis of the manipulator's defects or those of his patient is not possible.

Neither the training of the osteopath nor that of the doctor includes that knowledge of the influence of use upon functioning which is necessary to full diagnosis if changes made in structural and functional conditions are to be permanent and unaccompanied by any harmful by-products. Osteopathic treatment, like all other forms of treatment, is impeded by the fact that the patient who is being treated is beset by a constant influence for ill, because of the harmful effects of his wrong habitual use of himself upon his general functioning—harmful effects which osteopathic treatment not only cannot change, but, if I may judge by my experience with pupils who have been treated by osteopathy, tends to exaggerate. No treatment given under the osteopathic method includes the "means-whereby" of restoring that right employment of the primary control which is associated with a manner of general use of the self that ensures a constant influence for good upon the patient's general functioning. To put the position in accordance with Mr. Allen's viewpoint and contention: If what he says is true about the theory and practice of osteopathy and of the method of training students, then I think it can justly be concluded that their method both of diagnosis and treatment was based upon premises that were incomplete, and that judged by the by-products, i.e., by the harmful effects upon practitioner or patient and the consequent lowering of the standard of the work of treatment, the demands of scientific method have not been met.

I have a keen appreciation of Mr. Allen's attempts to help his colleagues, and hence it is with reluctance I am forced, in justice to my work, to try to correct the impression of my practice and theory conveyed to his colleagues in his article. Above all, I am anxious to impress on them that in trying out procedures which are new to them, they have to depend upon the guidance of their sensory appreciation which Mr. Allen points out is too prone to be defective, and that it is through trusting to this guidance that they have been led into the errors in the use of themselves that they desire to change.

As the result of many years of teaching experience I would warn all those who, like Mr. Allen, are endeavouring to help others to make the changes in the use of themselves that they desire, that both they and the people they wish to help must face the fact that the very essence of change demands coming into contact with the unknown, and that therefore, their past experiences (the known) will not help but rather impede them. Unless those who are attempting to change their habitual reactions in the use of themselves can obtain from experienced teachers, or from such long study as I gave to it, the means whereby they can gain the new sensory experiences that are associated with such process of change, they are not likely to solve the problem which is inherent in the process of substituting conscious for instinctive control of human reaction, whether for "effecting lesion correction" or for any other end desired.

CHAPTER IX

THE TEST OF PRINCIPLE IN NEW WAYS FOR OLD

THOSE who are desirous of drawing up new plans of action to supersede plans they have followed in the past but now find wanting, should be careful to include in their preliminary survey the experiences that came to them in the course of following out their earlier plans. Especially should they take note of the principle on which the earlier plans had been based and which accounted for these experiences, and compare it with the principle on which they propose to base their new plan. By this means they can apply a test, the test of principle, to any plan they formulate. If, when tested in this way, the new plan is found to be based on the same principle as the plan they have decided to discard, then it should be rejected, as it can only lead to experiences as disappointing as those which were associated with the old plan. If on the other hand the principle underlying the new plan is found to be different, then it should be welcomed as one with possibilities and be put to the test in its turn. This test of principle, when applied generally, will be found to be a dependable means whereby the value of new plans can be gauged, and the formulators of new plans for the reform of conditions, whether educational, social or otherwise, who fail to apply the test of principle to the plans they advocate, are devoid of a due sense of responsibility to those they wish to help and are untrue to themselves.

Even if they succeed in their advocacy of a new plan which is based on the same principle as the one which it is to supersede, they will be putting back the clock of civilization for a further term while it is being tried out, thus increasing the difficulties in the future for those who are not satisfied with such trial and error attempts to solve their problems.

Too many people develop a mania for assuming the role of one to "show the way" without first developing the mania for gaining the knowledge and experience which would justify them in assuming the role. Too many people want to teach others that which they are not prepared to learn themselves; and hence we have a gradual increase in the numbers of the blind leading the blind. For these to teach or to lead others is too often an end to be gained, not a "means-whereby" to an end which their experience and training has justified them in trying to achieve. Such people are little concerned with the consideration of principle as a test of value in such an undertaking or as a guide or aid in arriving at decisions. It is doubtful whether it has ever occurred to them to work to principle in anything they have decided to teach or to reform.

For instance, if we study the technique that those employ who claim that by their method they succeed in changing conditions in others and are working for the progress and development of the individual and the mass, we shall find that in their plan of procedure no provision, in the fundamental sense we are interested in, has been made for bringing those they are desirous of helping into contact with what is unfamiliar and unknown. Yet progress and development depend upon the making of this contact, not only by the acceptance in theory of the new and the unfamiliar, but also by facing the unknown in the consistent carrying out of the procedures which are demonstrably the practical counterpart of the theory. If we do not continue to gain new experiences, or if the same conditions are present in our organism next year as obtained this year, then we can conclude that we have not succeeded in making progress, or in furthering our growth and development. Unfortunately, in most of us, the impediment which blocks the way to our acceptance of facts which do not fit in with our beliefs and theories is a deeply-rooted subconscious reaction, amounting to what might almost be described as an obsession for clinging blindly to the orthodox or the familiar, and is due to habits of thought which orthodox methods of education do little to correct and much to encourage. If anyone should doubt this, let him mention something which his listeners have not heard before and await their reaction. It will almost certainly be one of doubt, scepticism and too often a sudden emotional reaction revealing unreasoning resistance and prejudice, particularly if the acceptance of what is put forward would be likely to affect adversely in any way the interests and desires of his listeners. This would not be so if we really stood for progress, development and truth, for then the mention of something unknown to us would immediately stimulate our interest. The unorthodox would be welcomed and investigated with the same sense of responsibility as is aroused by any great opportunity for service, for opportunity is a great thing.

For years now the technique described in my book *The Use of the Self* has made possible the gaining of previously unknown experiences by reasoning from known to unknown experiences in the process of bringing about changes in manner of use. By this means any harmful influences associated with the habitual manner of use are changed to influences for good by becoming associated with a new and previously unknown manner of use which ensures the raising of the standard of general functioning.

The thought and action necessary for the establishment of these influences for good call for the discarding of cherished beliefs, the giving up of familiar ways and the learning of unfamiliar ways of doing things. Hence the need for a technique which enables us to put into practice new beliefs in new ways of doing things in the process of making changes in the habitual use of the self, and it is necessary for us to gain the experiences involved in this before we can possibly understand the significance of change in the working of a *constant* (use) which can influence for good or ill the general psycho-physical functioning of the individual. The acceptance of the need of new "means-whereby" for the carrying-out of the desired "doing," the inhibition of familiar ways and all that is necessary for the new way of doing things call for thinking along unfamiliar lines, and for a wide range of human experiences which I believe to be indispensable to man's growth and development.

But except in rare instances man has chosen to think along familiar lines, and his enthusiasm for end-gaining methods has always been in striking contrast to his reluctance to undertake the difficult task of providing the best means whereby he could carry out consistently the decisions necessary to the success of the plan of civilization. In face of any situation demanding a reasoned decision as to the best line of action to adopt, he has the habit of reacting more in accordance with his unreasoned fears than with any balanced appreciation of his fundamental needs and requirements, and in this respect he has been no more successful in the sphere of religion than elsewhere.

Past and present teachers in the field of religion as in other fields offer us in their writings and instructions theoretical help, good thoughts and advice as to what we should or should not do to realize their ideals, but their methods are on the trial and error plan and do not provide those they wish to help with adequate "means-whereby" for the gaining of their end; especially in the matter of making changes in the self, these people, with all their stimulation of our will-to-do, provide no means whereby we are enabled to carry out consistently the well-intentioned decisions which result from this stimulation, leaving us in the dilemma in which St. Paul found himself when he made his agonized exclamation:

> "For the good that I would I do not; but the evil which I would not, that I do." (Rom. VII:19.)

Here we have an indirect admission by St. Paul that the "means-whereby" at his disposal did not meet his needs in enabling him so to control his reactions that he could consistently put into practice his well-intentioned decisions for self-help, and this is not surprising in view of all we now know of the influence of use upon functioning, and of the effect of unreliable sensory guidance upon our attempts to gain ends which conflict with our habitual reaction.

The plan of putting forward ideas, good thoughts and the like have persisted from early times, but that this plan profiteth little is shown by the terrible state of world affairs today, the result of man's reactions and of his attempts to carry out decisions on the trial and error plan in the myriad fields of his activities.

The effect of this habitual manner of reacting upon the individual has been noticeable in the people who have come to me for lessons and to whom I have tried to explain the nature of the errors it involves. For although my teaching experience is a large one, and I have numbered among my pupils a great variety of types, I have so far failed to discover any difference in their capacity to carry out a decision demanding an unfamiliar manner of reacting to a given stimulus in the use of themselves, a capacity which only becomes possible when, in the course of the lessons, the habitual reaction is inhibited while experience is gained in reconditioning the requisite reflex activity for the new reactions desired.

The disquieting fact is that the originators of good ideas, and the adherents of religious and other sects, such as Christian Science and the Oxford Group, all rely upon feeling for guidance in putting their ideas into practice, as well as upon the emotional reaction of both converter and converted in judging the value of results. Their wish is not only "father to their thought" but also to their judgment.

As the Oxford Group has been much to the fore of late, it may be both helpful and interesting to relate some experiences I have actually had with friends and pupils connected with the group who have come to me for lessons. I have found them particularly difficult to teach because of their over-excited fear reflexes and of their habit of instinctively seeking the easy way, even when admitting that it is not the best for their purpose. They are self-hypnotic to a high and harmful degree, and find the inhibition of habitual reaction much more difficult than most other pupils. Until their manner of use has been improved, which means that some reconditioning has been effected, it is almost impossible to get them to use their reasoning processes in trying to understand new "means-whereby" to their ends. One of them actually said: "I don't want to understand what I am doing." He really meant that he had no desire to use his will-to-do in carrying out consciously the new procedures he had decided were to his advantage.

The projection of messages necessary to the carrying out of new procedures is inseparable from previously unknown sensory experiences of use and functioning, and tend to excite unduly the fear reflexes in all people who are faced with the difficulties of the pupil we are discussing. As we all know fear is the most fundamental source of human frailty, and in this connexion I have just received from a friend who wishes to remain anonymous an Open Letter which gives a most interesting and pertinent instance of the effect of fear development.

Dear Mr. Alexander:

At this present time, there are many people searching for security and peace, for some means for restoring stability and order, and of coping with all the sudden, unforeseen, disruptive and revolutionary influences which are upsetting the course of life, and in this search many are turning once more to that ancient consolation of the human spirit—religion. People have always been ready to pay lip-service to religion as the time-honoured custodian of morality[51] and social order, and this trend will therefore no doubt be applauded by many, but it occurs to me that it may involve great dangers, and for this reason I venture to write to you in the hope that you will deal with this problem in your next book.

The need for solving it was brought home to me recently when talking with a friend whom I have known for a considerable number of years. He had always seemed especially interested in religion and punctilious about religious observances. We had often talked about these things, our general outlook apparently being almost identical; but it was not until this occasion that I realized we differed in one fundamental respect.

As you know I have always taken some part in formal religious activities myself; but while I cannot pretend to have gone into my motives very deeply, I should say that, apart from upbringing, I do so because I like it and because it is a way of responding to an inner need which I appreciate. If I may judge by what my friend told me, this was not so in his case, but he spoke of a constant, semi-rationalized fear. Since early childhood, the fear of an unknown after-life with its possibilities of retribution and punishment had been held over him, until this had become the mainspring of his religious activity and indeed of much of his general behaviour. Prayer and other religious exercises were for him duties which it was necessary for him to perform on pain of severe penalties. His conception and practice of prayer, in particular, was restricted to the repetition of requests for some sort of divine intervention and as a means of evading personal responsibility for his actions.

[51]An eminent friend of mine has pointed out to me that the word "morality" is not to be found in the Bible.

This outlook was so foreign to my own feelings and experience that while I knew that fear of the unknown is supposed to be the basis of all religion, it had never occurred to me that this might be true of the religion of civilized man today, still less of anyone whom I thought I knew so well, but what my friend told me presented the question of religion in a new light, and I realized for the first time that its practice may involve great dangers.

You have pointed out in your books that fear paralyses growth and development in us and it seems to me that such a religious outlook as I have described would not only arouse fear but even stimulate it. Such people as my friend, of course, can be under no illusion that a more fervent practice of religious exercises will enable them to cope with life as they desire; all their experience of failure and frustration in this connexion points to the contrary, and it is because I am anxious to prevent others from disillusionment, who may turn to religion for help in like difficulties, that I think if you could find space to say a few words about this matter in your new book it might be of great interest and value to a number of your readers.

Yours sincerely,

In reply to my friend's request I will point out that in this and my other books I am offering a psycho-physical approach to the problem of translating ideals, theories and beliefs into practice, and have shown that this calls for that fundamental change in the use of the self by means of which the standard of general functioning is raised and psycho-physical defects and ills, whether fears or any other emotional reactions, are overcome. This means psycho-physical reconditioning, and such reconditioning cannot be effected by means of ideals alone, any more than man can live by bread alone.

The appeal to what John Dewey calls "emotional gusts," and reliance upon feeling as a guide both to manner of reaction and to judgment of results, have always been the basic principle in all revivalist movements, and the fact that both orthodox and unorthodox religious bodies still think it necessary to make a special effort to rouse interest in the revivalist method as a "means-whereby" is surely an admission that the results of this method in the past could not have been what they were claimed to be, and hence have failed to secure lasting results in the desired direction. What greater proof could there be of the need for test of principle?

Emotional appeal is always more or less dangerous for, no matter what its immediate specific result may be at any particular time, experience has shown that this result cannot be permanent and that judgment of results by the guidance of feeling can be deceptive, and can too often lead to dangerous and even harmful perversions. Furthermore, it is to be condemned because, in dealing with their problems, it encourages people to rely more and more upon instinct and ever less and less upon thinking and reasoning. Where this method is used there is an increasing tendency to react as creatures of impulse, and to become ever less capable of developing that fundamental control and that understanding of the self and of others, which in this world of crises is the most pressing need of the moment. Throughout the ages the rousing of mass emotion has been the means employed, whenever it has been thought desirable or profitable to induce people to do what it would never have occurred to them to do under the guidance of thinking and reasoning.

Until something is done to help mankind to evolve beyond this point, which is too close to the animal plane of evolution, and to get a better control of his reactions, it is difficult to see how we can expect any improvement in mass reaction to any potent emotional stimulus. At present man is at the mercy of any individual or people who may think out some means of playing upon his emotions, no matter for what purpose. In the past few years we have seen some startling and terrible results gained in this way and used in an attempt to destroy all that is best in men and women. People have been robbed of their most priceless heritage—freedom of thought and action—despite all the suffering, and bloodshed by which these sacred rights have been won in the past.[52] It must be obvious that too many of the individuals prominent in world affairs today are "creatures of impulse," and it is in countries where the masses have in their reaction been for centuries more influenced by impulse than by thinking and reasoning, or have chosen the "easy way" of allowing others to think for them, that the irresponsible individuals to whom I refer are able by the imposition of their demoralizing regimen to rob people of all that makes life worth living, and force upon them a way of life which is nothing more than a degrading and devastating form of slavery.

One of our most vital problems is concerned with the changing of thought and action, so essential to the successful carrying out of any plan for individual self-help that calls for the acceptance of new ideas involving unorthodox beliefs and attitudes. But the urgency of the subject does not lessen the difficulties to be overcome in dealing with it, and for the very reason that the problem, from our point of view, has not yet been understood, let alone solved, in the fundamental sense. Many people will contend that they can change their habitual thought and action,

[52]What has happened will not be a surprise to those who read the chapter "Evolutionary Standards Before the War" in my book *Man's Supreme Inheritance.*

others that it has been done by the individual and the mass and so on. But the viewpoint of such people is that of those who claim that change has been made, for instance, when at a revival meeting someone states that he has been "saved" and will henceforth renounce his past beliefs and give up his bad habits, or when the peoples of a country are forced by ruthless individuals, backed up by an armed minority, to live under debasing conditions imposed on them by brute force and murder. These are not changes of thought and action such as we are here concerned with, and it is because such changes in the past have not been fundamental in meeting man's needs, that conditions in human beings are as we find them today: the individual, incapable of making changes in his thought and action without the accompaniment of harmful by-products within the self, whilst change and reform in the masses has been made too often by brutal methods of suppression, especially of those ideas and beliefs for which men and women have fought and died in the past, and which today are still the mainspring of their longing for freedom of thought and action.

CHAPTER X

A NEW PATTERN AND WORKING TO PRINCIPLE

FEW people will deny that the affairs of the world today are "out of shape," and that the pattern of the parts which go to make up the whole in the scheme of civilization is a bad one. Yet it is demanded by the "powers that be" that any new pattern, no matter how valuable, must fit into the old pattern if it is to receive even the smallest consideration.

The skilled artisan and craftsman on discovering that a pattern is either bad or unsatisfactory would at once discard it and replace it by a new one no matter how valuable for its purpose it may have been, and this is indeed the only rational course. In these pages a new pattern is offered to enable man, as an adventurer in the task of putting forward the clock of civilization, to deal with the new and unfamiliar situations that are now confronting him. This pattern provides him with the means of changing and controlling his reaction in face of the difficulties which are inevitable in his attempts to pass from the known (wrong) to the unknown (right) experiences essential for the making of fundamental change.

This new pattern is designed both for the youth and the adult, but it cannot be fitted into any present pattern orthodox or unorthodox, and if it is to be used, the pattern that it is to replace must be discarded. For young children the adoption of the new pattern is a comparatively simple and easy matter, and the system of work in the F. Matthias Alexander Trust Fund School, at Penhill, near Bexley, Kent, an undertaking made possible by the foundation of the Alexander Trust Fund, has been modelled upon it. This pattern takes shape and form through the application of the "means-whereby" of the technique, and we now know that it meets the primary need in the education of the child by providing not only new situations, but also the opportunity of developing the potentialities of the child, so as to help him to gain the experience of dealing with the unfamiliar and unknown as the adult adventurer does.

Let us then consider the situation of the child, youth or adult about to begin the "great adventure" involved in the adoption of a new pattern which calls for change in the fundamental sense from an instinctive to a conscious and reasoned way of living, and it will be seen that the principle upon which the "means-whereby" of change is based will be the same, whether the object be to gain new experiences in the development of potentialities, or to prevent the development of some functional trouble by learning *how not* to interfere with that working of the primary control which restores a manner of use associated with a satisfactory standard of functioning.

In the case of children and most youths, the decision to try to benefit by means of the technique will be made by the parent or guardian. But the necessity for the step will be brought to the child's notice and his interest gradually quickened by explanation and demonstration on simple lines. This interest will be further increased when he discovers that by not giving consent to the gaining of an end along familiar lines, he can prevent any wrong use of himself that he is led to recognize is habitually impeding him in his attempts to carry out some action in which he wishes to excel, and that this makes possible the employment of new means whereby a desired end can be gained by an improving use of himself. His interest will be further aroused when it is made clear to him that not giving consent in the foregoing circumstances is analogous to not giving consent in those circumstances when he refuses to "do" some act he does not feel inclined to do, is afraid to do, or for some reason of his own decides not to do. The same psycho-physical processes are at work in these cases, but the difference in the benefit to be derived is that in the one case he is consciously improving his use during his employment of new procedures, whilst in the other cases the benefit is limited to that which results from the prevention of a repetition of his harmful habitual use. Children are naturally interested in the working of machinery, and this interest can be turned to most valuable account.

In the case of the adult, the decision to benefit from the technique is usually made independently, and since it presupposes the recognition of a need, where need is so rarely recognized, the decision implies a full recognition of responsibility for the care of the self in the sense indicated in these chapters. "To thine own self be true and it must follow as the night the day thou canst not then be false to any man."

The recognition of the responsibility to which I refer is the essence of all that is indicated in these words—for it is being true to the self in this fundamental sense which alone makes possible the end which Shakespeare indicates. Furthermore, it means the acceptance of an individual responsibility which, so far as I am aware, has never been accepted by man before; one which has been unthinkingly left to the "curative" agency of Nature with all the consequences which are now causing distress, pain, discontent and disorder within and without man's organism. Being true to oneself in the sense advocated here presupposes being true to others, and if this had once been established not merely as an ideal but as an habitual reaction for several generations, the resultant sense of responsibility might, I believe, lead to a consideration for others and their well-being, such as has never yet, except in isolated instances, resulted from educational, religious or other means for the cultivation of desirable human qualities.

In therapeutics the effect would be just as fundamental. For being true to the self implies an acceptance of the unfamiliar idea of individual responsibility for that manner of use of our ourselves which makes for the preservation of the highest standard of functional well-being, the natural antidote to all individual shortcomings and defects, disease and organic troubles.

But the stumbling block in the way of those who wish to help towards such ideals as this are the habits of thought, the preconceived ideas, inherited beliefs and prejudices which have formed in most people in the process of becoming dominated by orthodox methods of training and education, causing many people whose reactions are reasonable and just in familiar situations, to react, when they are faced with the unfamiliar, as if they were suddenly bereft of their ordinary judgment, common sense, self-control, sense of justice and reasoning.

The pages of man's history are full of such blots as the persecution of people with foresight like Galileo who did no more than confront his fellow men with a new belief subsequently recognized as a great truth. It is only necessary to read of the treatment meted out by orthodox thinkers, including men of science and religion, to the discoverers of other epoch-making truths—such men as Jenner, Semmelweiss, Pasteur, Lister, Simpson, Hunter and others—to appreciate the importance of so educating the child, the youth, and the adult that their reaction to the unfamiliar will be one of enquiry, tolerance and sympathy, rather than hostility. Only in this way can they be given the opportunity for examining the unfamiliar and for employing all possible means for finding out whether or not another valuable discovery may not have come to light.

Those who have read the account of the evolution of my technique in *The Use of the Self* will be aware that I was continually led into unknown experiences, and when employing new "means-whereby" found myself in unfamiliar situations, and experiencing impeding and illuminating adventures in dark places.[53] This was appreciated by the late Joseph Rowntree when he said of my technique that it was "reasoning from the known to the unknown, the known being the wrong and the unknown being the right."

This experience of passing from a "known" to an "unknown" manner of use of the self is the basic need in making a fundamental change in the control of man's reaction, and he will remain impotent in meeting it, unless it is possible to give him the opportunity of accepting an unfamiliar theory, and of acquiring the experience of employing consistently the unfamiliar procedures which are its practical counterpart, by means of an integrating process of reconditioning associated with experiences of use and functioning previously unknown to him. Although these experiences feel wrong at first, they will gradually replace the old experiences which felt right, and in time the new experience becomes established as a *Constant* in the use of the self in daily activity.

The professional golfer, footballer, cricketer or other expert in games, artist or craftsman, who remains dependent upon instinctive guidance and control in his activities, will not have had the benefit of these experiences, and therefore it is almost certain that the constant influence of his use of himself will be a more or less impeding one in his games and other activities. This can account largely for the fact that professional athletes can and do play at times like second-class amateurs, and so often fail to do their best when the occasion most demands it. It is probable that anyone with a knowledge of what constitutes interference with the employment of the primary control of use, would be able to observe in these players such varying interference with this control as could account for the variation in the standard of their play at different times. The manner of interference varies with the different ways of using the self, and the degree of interference tends to increase with repetition.

This is not surprising seeing that experts in games, as in arts and craftsmanship of all kinds, do not recognize the existence of a primary control of their use nor that the manner of the employment of this control is indirectly responsible for the manner of working of all the other parts of the organism. This means that in each attempt to gain an end in learning or playing their games or in pursuing their art or craft, they are doing a great deal to lessen their chance of success by cultivating undesirable habits of use in their trial and error efforts to gain their end.

---

[53]As a medical friend wrote to me after reading *The Use of the Self*: "The only criticism that I can offer of your new book is that it is just about the most interesting that I have ever read. It beats the usual explorer's yarn into a cocked hat, because you wandered through a much darker country than any of them did."

We are all aware that a person performing acts under different circumstances can be subject to varying influences leading to different results, in one set of circumstances to a good result, and in different circumstances to another. For instance, there is the influence of the wind, or of rain-sodden ground, whether in golf, cricket or football. Emotional strain and health conditions may affect artistic production, craftsmanship or even the simplest acts of life. Even routine actions, like sitting down or rising from a chair, may under the unusual conditions of being watched by others become altered and complicated. In cricket the effect of some unexpected happening, such as the failure of the first two batsmen, upon the rest of the team is notorious.

In such circumstances the people concerned will be aware of impeding influences, but will be unaware that they are the result of their harmful interference with the employment of the primary control of their use of themselves. In their attempts to counter these influences, they instinctively react to their desire to be as successful under the unusual and adverse circumstances as at any other time. This too often results in comparative failure, because it is simply another trial and error attempt to achieve success under circumstances of emotional stress and undue anxiety.

An analogy from the world of machinery would be found in the experiences of a driver struggling to get his car moving over ground that is unsuitable, particularly if the controls and adjustments of the car were interfered with as if by magic as the wheels met unfamiliar and more and more difficult ground. In such circumstances, the functioning of the car and driver would not be up to the standard that would be present if the controls and adjustments of the car had not been interfered with, and this applies to the human being who depends upon instinctive guidance and control, when reacting to unusual circumstances in games and other activities. A degree of composure and confidence is essential to success in unfamiliar situations, and particularly in those which allow us only one opportunity of scoring a success, as is the case with games and examinations.

Compare the chances of success enjoyed by the human machine working as an integrated whole, with that of a person in whom energy is being more or less misdirected, as it must be in all those who do not have a knowledge of the employment of the primary control of the use of themselves. Think of the different effect upon the self of a plan which makes for a maximum of successes, instead of a maximum of failures. The one is a builder of confidence, satisfaction, happiness and conscious control of the self, while the other places us more and more at the mercy of the vagaries of emotion and habit, and tends to undermine our confidence in ourselves and in our manner of doing things, and to make for dissatisfaction, irritation and discontent.

I read the following in a newspaper (*Sunday Pictorial*, Jan. 9, 1938):

> In his reply to the toast of "Our Guests" at a Golf Club Dinner at Galway, the Bishop of Galway, Dr. Brown, said that golf developed in most men a deep and profound sense of humility. . . . "In fact," he added, "there is one thing I have noticed about golf, and that is that I have never heard of it being played by dictators."

If the good bishop had been speaking of my technique with the same knowledge of it as he has of golf, he would have substituted the word "all" for "most" in his first sentence. But while the trial and error experiences which develop that valuable quality of humility in the playing of golf lead to increased uncertainty, loss of confidence, loss of temper and irritation, the experiences to be gained in employing consciously directed "means-whereby" lead to the development of humility by reason of the fuller understanding of relative values which follows expanding experience in the employment of any technique.

The chapter on golf in *The Use of the Self* and all that has been written on the subject in my other books reveals the why and the wherefore of the golfer's difficulties. I have shown that these arise chiefly from bad manner of use, and are too often increased by his attempts to improve his play by the adoption of practical procedures based on a wrong principle, his own preconceived ideas and those of the professional teacher. Working to this principle, the golf pupil attempts to gain his ends by direct means, without taking into consideration the influence of his manner of use upon the means he employs, a use which in the case of most golfers will be an impeding influence. It may be said that he knows of no better plan than this, but from personal touch with such golfers one finds that hardly one in a hundred would take the trouble to go through the process necessary to change his habit of use even if he were convinced that it would improve his game. The majority prefer to go on with their trial and error attempts, and in consequence fail to make a success of their game (their end).[54] This would not be serious but for the fact that it brings about a condition of affairs which causes emotional disturbance and disappointment.

And what is true of games is true of man's activities in life in general. If the thousand and one activities involved in the business of living are

[54]It would sometimes seem as if the experiences of golfers and others in their efforts to improve their game or other activities bring them to the point in Shakespeare's words, when they would rather "bear those ills they have than fly to others that they know not of."

to be performed without exerting unknowingly a constant harmful influence upon the organism, there is just as much need for the average modern person to change his habits of use of himself as for the golfer, tennis star or any other skilled player of games. The time has come for realizing that by means of a conscious employment of the primary control of use we can with confidence ensure the best possible manner of use of ourselves at all times and in all circumstances, and that by this indirect means our psycho-physical self can be energized and controlled to the best advantage, no matter what our activities may be.

In this way "trying to do our best" becomes a practical reality instead of a pious hope; it amounts to no more or less than putting the psycho-physical machinery of the self in order on the lines of the scientific engineer who overhauls his engine so that the particular individual machinery shall be constantly capable of optimum functioning.

Learning to "do" by this procedure is not learning to "do" exercises on a trial and error plan, but learning to work to a principle, not only in using the self but in the application of the technique outside the self. A person who learns to work to a principle in doing one exercise will have learned to do all exercises, but the person who learns just to "do an exercise" will most assuredly have to go on learning to "do exercises" *ad infinitum*.

However resourceful, for instance, a man may be who has learnt to play cricket in the orthodox way, any interference with the working of the primary control that was present when he began, will have tended to increase as time went on. Any success therefore he may have achieved will have been because of his natural gift for the game and *in spite* of the constantly impeding influence of any interference which will have tended to lower the standard of his functioning not only in cricket but in all his other activities.

On the other hand, if he had known how to employ the primary control of his use so that it would tend to raise the standard of his general functioning in his game, he would have shown a constant tendency to improve in his manner of employing it, and his success would have been the greater because of this. Most important of all he would have learned to be able to work to a principle, and to take advantage of this when learning to play any other game, or in learning to "do" in any sphere of individual activity.

CHAPTER XI

STUPIDITY IN LIVING

MR. (now the Rt. Hon.) Herbert Morrison, when speaking at a public dinner recently, is reported to have said: "It is an irony that man, so skilled in learning, should be so stupid in living."[55]

He might also have referred to the irony that man is so skilled in the nature and working of the machines he has invented, but is so very unskilled in the nature and working of the mechanisms of his own organism; he knows all about the means whereby he can keep the inanimate machine in order, and considers it his duty to make proper use of these, but he knows little or nothing about the means whereby he can keep in order that animate human machine—himself.

The great majority of people are, in Mr. Morrison's words, "so stupid in living" that they have not yet awakened to the great and growing need of such "means-whereby," and so have not yet appreciated that these are essential to the art of living healthily, happily and in harmony with one another.

Even among those people today who accept the ideal of "wholeness," there are few who are sufficiently skilled in the art of living to put the ideal into practice, and their failures may be ascribed to the fact that knowledge of the use of themselves, as it affects the guidance and control of their reaction, is not part of the foundation on which present civilization has been built, nor is this knowledge part of the equipment of those who undertake to teach and rule humanity. In my own case, the experiences which preceded my attempt to work out a technique, as well as those which were gained in the process of working it out, led me to a gradual realization that man's most tragic mistake has been his failure to acquire knowledge of himself as an individual functioning as a psycho-physical whole in his daily activities, for this has deprived him of

[55] I regret that being out of my own country at this time (September, 1940) I am unable to refer to my papers to give particulars of date, etc., of Mr. Morrison's speech as reported.

the key to knowledge which could give him a new technique in living. It is useless to urge people to live the full life without the "means-whereby" to wholeness in the motivation and activation of the human self.

So far man has been content to occupy himself in acquiring relatively unimportant miscellaneous, and in many respects unrelated, knowledge concerned with his activities outside himself, never having seemed to appreciate that accurate and full knowledge and control of the integrated working of his own self was essential to success in making use of that other knowledge upon which he relied for carrying on his activities in the outside world, or that a knowledge of himself was actually necessary to prevent him from gradually becoming more and more mal-coordinated and maladjusted as a result of his increasing misuse of himself in applying the knowledge he had acquired in meeting his needs in living.

Had he given due attention to the study of himself, and had he turned this study to good effect, he would have gained the experience in the guidance and control of his mechanism in activity, which would have led him to appreciate the unity in the working of his organism in use and functioning. Then if he had brought the result of this study of his individual self to his study of the wonders of the universe, and had postulated unity instead of separation as a working principle, he would inevitably have studied everything as a whole and not piecemeal.

The fact that the opposite has been done until now, both in the science of man and of the world outside, has resulted in many people now beginning to wonder whether if there be a creative principle, it had any other purpose than destruction. In recent years, however, a small minority have come to see further than their fellows in this matter, but this minority is still tied down to orthodox methods of procedure in their attempts to gain the new ends indicated in their new theories, because they have not the means of putting into practice the principle of unity in the carrying out of educational procedures. Educators themselves are bewildered by a situation which grows worse in proportion to the increase of theories advanced to cope with it. Recognition is widespread that something must be wrong with a system that sets youth adrift in a chaotic world in a state of confusion which, as I shall show, can be attributed to a want of knowledge of the self, and of the guidance and control of that self in daily activity.

This, which is too often the tragedy of modern youth, is strikingly typified in a recent article by Miss Dorothy Thompson,[56] who recounts the case histories of four young men who graduated from college with high

[56] *On the record*: A Footnote, by Dorothy Thompson, New York *Herald Tribune,* October 4, 1940

scholastic honors, but whose stories concerning the effect of their education upon their lives were very distressing to Miss Thompson, as they must have been to all who read her very moving article. These stories comprise a serious indictment of American education, so serious in fact, and so pertinent to the whole theme of this book, that I feel justified in quoting at some length from Miss Thompson's article:

> . . . For they testified that what their education had done had been to break down their belief in any *positive values*,[57] to weaken their faith in their country, in its history, in its traditions, and in its future; to put them, themselves, into *intellectual and psychological confusion*, and into inner despair out of which they had sought refuge in various ways at various times: one through casting his lot, temporarily, in with Young Communists, because "they alone seemed to be perfectly clear in their minds where they were going"; another, and for a period, into complete skepticism and cynicism; another into "the only thing that seemed solid—my own egotism and self-interest."
>
> One of them had come near to the edge of a nervous breakdown. He had left college in the midst of his course, and gone home to be pampered, on the ground that he had "been working too hard." His solicitous family had sent him to a psychiatrist. "Then one day I had it out with myself, and I knew that unless I pulled myself together, I should be in the hands of a psychiatrist forever. Somehow I managed to tell myself the truth: that I had not been overworking, but underworking: and that the real truth was that I didn't have any guts."
>
> This was the same boy who said, "When I went to college I was full of enthusiasm, particularly interested in history and philosophy. I wanted to find out what made the wheels go round in this world. I wanted to prepare myself to do something—not just make money—not just be a 'success' but achieve something—something bigger than I am—I wanted to be part of something. But by my junior year I had become convinced that there wasn't anything that could be believed. Everything was relative. And *I was swimming around in space.* I was like the guy in that rhyme of Gelett Burgess's: 'I wish that my room had a floor. I don't so much care for a door. But this floating around without touching the ground is getting to be quite a bore!'"
>
> Another of the boys—the most articulate and thoughtful one—took it up. "We were told to maintain the critical attitude. We were soaked in historic relativism. I tried to maintain a 'healthy skepticism.' The trouble was that I observed, in reading history, that the people who moved this

[57]The italics in this and the following quotations from Miss Thompson's article are mine. F. M. A.

> world were people animated by a passion for something. I could see that you couldn't write off faith as one of the prime molders of history, and that when there wasn't any faith, pure gangsterism and piracy broke loose. I could see that if I and my generation were going to mean anything in this world and not just be dots and specks pushed around by forces we couldn't control we had to find out what our convictions were. But meanwhile I had lost my moorings."

In the light of all I have written concerning the unity in working of the human organism, and the influence of use upon functioning, it should, I think, be clear to the reader wherein the educational system had failed to equip Miss Thompson's four young men for success in living. In spite of their scholastic achievements, their high degree of intelligence and, as Miss Thompson says, "their fine physical type," it is all too tragically clear that these young men were not in a condition of psycho-physical well-being and had reached a point where the standard of their general psycho-physical functioning had become seriously lowered. They had, although they were unaware of it, become the victims of a constant influence for ill, which adversely conditioned their reaction to their education as well as to all their activities of life.

I have always found in persons afflicted with "nervous breakdown" and so-called mental disorders who have been sent to me for help by their medical advisers, harmful conditions of use and functioning associated with "intellectual and psychological" (and it should be added, "physical") "confusion," which, in my experience, lead ultimately to reactions that are concomitants of "inner despair." The serious element in the situation of such "emotionally and spiritually unemployed youth" as Miss Thompson describes is that although they recognize that they have "lost their moorings" through the breakdown of "positive values" in the pursuit of their academic studies, they remain completely unaware of a much more serious, because fundamental, breakdown in connexion with the working of the self, as manifested in the use and functioning of mechanisms, organs and processes of thinking and reasoning. The knowledge of the integrated working of the organism in use and functioning which alone establishes and maintains well-being within the self, has not been an integral part of the educative process. It has had no place in the educational curriculum and hence has been no part of their preparation for life, so that these youths have actually been deprived of the study that could have led to belief in the one "positive value" which their academic education could not have broken down, namely, knowledge of the working of the self in its application to living. Thus deprived, it followed as the night the day, that while they were acquiring a variety of external knowledge, the influence of harmful use was a *Constant*, lowering the standard of the general functioning of the instrument of learning, and therefore lowering the standard of their judgment of "positive values."

It is this which is at the root of the dilemma facing modern education. For if, in the education of these boys, they had first been taught to appreciate the value of the principle of the unity in working of the psycho-physical organism, and had been given the means of maintaining this unity in working in all their daily activities, they would have gained experience in assessing the value of the changing conditions accruing at the different states of development leading to psycho-physical health, that basic experience which could have given them a standard of judgment of the subject matter submitted to them. Without this knowledge they were bound from the very outset of their education to drift into a danger zone, to "lose their moorings." Small wonder, then, that they developed "mental" and "nervous" disorders.

So much then for the education of these four young men. But there is an epilogue, which Miss Thompson calls "a happy ending," and which concerns the vastly important subject of re-education, or fundamental change. Miss Thompson continues:

> Fortunately, this particular story has a happy ending. These young men came into contact with one professor, a remarkable teacher, who *bucked them up*, and told them they had power in them and beauty. He opened their eyes to the real world; he taught them something about the survival values of history; he brought to them some intellectual convictions regarding character, and thus *he saved their souls*. And a very good job he made of it, too, and the immediate response indicated that this generation is by no means lost, even though so clever as to be on the verge of limbo. I concluded that it would not take a great deal to undo much of the harm that has been done. *But it would take a new orientation in education—and there one is up against the system.*

One is up against the "system" indeed, for one is up against those habitual reactions to stimuli by which human beings are so often enslaved. Fundamental change, as I have shown in Chapter V, involves the re-education and the readjustment of the individual *as a whole*. A mere change of "mind" or of belief does not change the habitual manner of psycho-physical use and the associated conditions of general functioning. And without in any way wishing to question Miss Thompson's estimate of the professor's methods or of his good intentions, I must put one or two questions. Firstly, in what way does the means that she tells us the professor employed, embody a "new orientation" in outlook and education? Secondly, in what way does the method employed by the professor differ from those employed by "remarkable teachers" throughout the history of civilization? Religion, philosophy, ethics, and education have always sought to inculcate such ideas as cheerfulness, confidence, courage, altruism, justice, compassion, etc. Thirdly, if such methods were any more than palliative, why such widespread intellectual and psychological confusion, such prevalent "jitters" today? There has been no dearth of good advice, no lack of wise precept. Most of us know *what* we ought to do (ends), but are sadly lacking in knowledge of *how* to do ("means-whereby"), and unfortunately seem to be unaware of the dangers incurred by palliative methods which attempt to inspire enthusiasm and belief in ideals which, however admirable in theory, are not based upon knowledge of the self as the instrument of the "doing" required for putting them into practice.

Miss Thompson's "remarkable teacher" bucked up these misguided young men, but in the light of my experience in teaching people who were said to have been "changed" by such methods, I cannot find any reason, for instance, for supposing that despite the change brought about in his "intellectual convictions" for the time being, the one young man will not again "come near to the edge of a nervous breakdown," because the general working of his organism and the associated conditions remain unchanged.

It is just in this failure of the professor to take into consideration the influence of use upon functioning in "bucking up" the depressed young men that we may appreciate the inadequacy of the educational system itself, and in another paragraph Miss Thompson adds, quite unintentionally, to her indictment of the educational system where she writes:

> It was out of just such a generation of emotionally and spiritually unemployed youth—youth whose "dynamic and historic relativism" had left *utterly rudderless*—that Hitler made the leadership of a movement that has plunged a large part of the earth into destruction. I knew just such youth fifteen years ago in Germany and with fascinated and horrified eyes I saw how easy it was for the first leader, *appealing to their confused unconscious longing for a faith*, to sweep them with him, *merely by affirming the barbaric standard of blood and soil.* Our colleges are full of youths who think that Hitler or Stalin . . . are great men. Why should they not, since *they have no measuring rods* by which to test greatness.

Here we get a remarkable parallel between the method of the professor in dealing with the four confused youths, and the method of Hitler in dealing with the "rudderless" youths of Germany, a parallel that should be clear to those who have followed my thesis through the earlier chapters of this book. For the two methods (and I write *methods* not *ends*, please bear in mind), are alike in principle however much they may differ in aim, and this principle is the antithesis of the principle of psycho-physical unity in the working of the human organism in the making of fundamental change, as advocated in these pages. Whereas Hitler, according to Miss Thompson, appealed to "their confused unconscious longing for faith merely by affirming the barbaric standard of blood and soil," the professor appealed to the same "unconscious longing for a faith" merely by affirming the loftier standards of "power and beauty," "intellectual convictions regarding character" and "the survival values of history," and the fact that the objectives (ends) of the dictator and those of Miss Thompson's teacher are as the poles apart does not alter the fundamental point, to wit: *that in neither case were the youths given any standard of self-judgment.* In Miss Thompson's words, "they have no measuring rods by which to test greatness." Certainly there is no evidence that the young men who came under the influence of the inspiring teacher, any more than those who came under the influence of Hitler, were given any means by which they could confidently evaluate the ideas, convictions, standards, etc., presented to them, and therefore, in making their judgement, they were forced to rely upon their obviously unstable emotions and untrustworthy feeling characteristic of their habitual reaction which in all such situations had tended to block off the operation of the processes we call reasoning. Ideas and ideals were merely affirmed and believed, but the underlying psycho-physical use and functioning, I must repeat, remained unaltered, so that fundamental change affecting the whole man could not have taken place. The world just now is overridden by conflicting ideologies, plans, ways of life, all "ends" which lie in ambush to trap the confused and rudderless youths of the world. Millions, the highly endowed and the average alike, are left to find their way out of "utter confusion" the best way they can by drifting to which ever leader appeals most to their organic instability.

"Out of this youth," Miss Thompson writes further, "should come the intellectual, spiritual, and political leadership of tomorrow. . . . But if the intellectually gifted, the naturally superior, and the relatively privileged, *are rendered impotent of leadership by their education*, then the power will certainly pass into the hands of those whom Whitman called 'powerful uneducated persons,' who have, at least, the realistic education of the shops and the gutters, the discipline of the factories and the farms, who have learned that you can't debate with hurricanes or hunger, or with tanks, or guns, or machines."

A disturbing analysis indeed! And it is because of my awareness of the tendencies which result from our present educational systems that I have for so long advocated a new orientation in education. My work is in the wide sense educational, but it cannot by any stretch of the imagination be labelled a "system," for that implies something limited, complete, calling for the employment of direct means in the gaining of ends; whereas in my technique the procedures are carried out by indirect means which lead the pupil from the known (wrong) to the unknown (right) in experience, the first imperative in the employment of these procedures being to provide for the child, adolescent or adult the "means-whereby" or standard, by which, first, to judge and direct his own psycho-physical mechanisms in the activities of life, and then, in accordance with this standard, to judge the value of ideals and suggestions proposed to him in experience. Individuals who are equipped with this knowledge of their own psycho-physical tendencies towards unduly depressed or excited emotional reactions, together with that of the means whereby they can hold such tendencies in check, cannot easily be influenced by others to the extent of becoming mere puppets, a danger to themselves and to their fellows.

Working in accordance with the principle underlying these procedures obviously brings one, as Miss Thompson says, "up against the system" of both orthodox and unorthodox education, as that word is at present understood. But the individual so educated (or re-educated in the case where something lost needs to be restored), can be developed to the point where he will be able without confusion to inhibit his tendency to be "carried away" by his desire to gain his "end," before he has set in motion conscious impulses in the laying down of new lines of communication in the use of the self (his instrument). In this way he will learn how to "think in activity" even at moments of greatest stress. This new knowledge of himself in use and functioning will give the modern youth a firm basis for the acquisition of other knowledge, and for putting that knowledge into practice, enabling him to make those endless adjustments to his environment which life in civilization demands of its members if they are to survive.

A typical example of the effort that is being made by professional educators to adapt the educational system to what has come to be known as "a changing world" is to be found in a recent pamphlet[58] by Dr. William Heard Kilpatrick of Columbia University. Dr. Kilpatrick discusses his subject very learnedly, beginning with the nature of behaviour and ending with the theoretical objective, to wit: Education of *The Whole Child*; but his discussion does not advance beyond the academic stage, as with so many other of the tentative and experimental remedi-

[58]*A Reconstructed Theory of the Educative Process*, by William Heard Kilpatrick, Bureau of Publications, Teachers College, Columbia University, New York City, N.Y.

al ideas which have made their appearance.

Dr. Kilpatrick's pamphlet interests me because he advocates the concept of "the whole organism in each learning act," and employs such phrases as: "Integration of the Self," "Conscious Direction," "Conscious Action," and "Re-making of the Self," and declares that the term "self is a very convenient one with which to treat certain manifestations of behaviour." Such statements are especially interesting because in *The Use of the Self*, published in 1932, I made a statement of technique which was wholly concerned with the use and development of the self as a manifestation of all, not merely certain, kinds of behaviour. This technique, moreover, was shown to have been based upon the principle of unity in the integrated working of the psycho-physical organism, whether in the act of "learning" or in any other activity, and to have provided the practice which makes possible the "conscious direction" without which there can be no "remaking of the (psycho-physical) self" and, therefore, no sound education. From this practice emerged the theoretical conception put forward in all my books. Yet here we find Dr. Kilpatrick, in 1935, advocating similar concepts applied to the "educative process," but apparently without considering it necessary to go beyond mere theory.

Certainly a reading of the pamphlet makes it difficult to believe that Dr. Kilpatrick fully understands the nature of the practice required to support the concepts he advocates. Let us, for example, examine the following passage quoted from the pamphlet:

> Where the organism faces a sufficiently novel situation, old responses will not suffice. A new response is called for or failure confronts. If fortunate, the organism will contrive a response new to it and adequate to cope with the novel difficulty. Such a contriving we call "learning." A dog is upset at being shut up in an enclosure. He finds or contrives a way out. It works. Therefore, if shut in, he uses his new-found exit (or, more exactly, his newly contrived response). He has "learned" how to meet the situation.

Dr. Kilpatrick's conception in the matter of *response* to the stimulus to carry out the activity or activities necessary for "contriving" is open to serious question. Upon the attitude towards the nature of response rests the success or failure of any educational process, for the simple reason that the primary response to the stimulus to any activity in animal or human being is, in fact, the motivation of the mechanisms that leads to activity within the organism—activity which makes "contriving" possible in the gaining of some end, such as the satisfaction of a desire or need.

The word "motivation" is here used to convey that which takes place within the self immediately before the mechanisms are activated. It is the primary response that *leads to* activity; the process that, in a sense, mobilizes the organism as a whole at the instant of the receipt of a stimulus. To consider the word in the usual sense as a "mental" act or influence would not be correct, since, as always, the whole organism is involved even though activity of the mechanisms has not yet taken place. It is interesting to find the following quotation from J. Martineau in Webster's *New International Dictionary*: "There are but two varieties of *motive* (i.e., of influence tending to volition); a blind impulse from behind, and a conceived good before us." The first kind can be attributed to Dr. Kilpatrick's dog, whose motivation is the outcome of a "blind impulse from behind," and the second also, in so far as it "conceives good" in gaining its ends by making its escape; but only the second can be attributed in any fundamental sense to the person who "conceives good" in that use and functioning of the self as the instrument of learning and learning to do, which is the outcome of experience in conscious guidance and control of the psycho-physical mechanisms of the self.

I join issue with Dr. Kilpatrick when he contends that it is a "new" response (or "newly contrived response") to a novel situation when the organism of the dog "contrives a way out." Anyone who has had experience with wild or tame animals knows that they are the victims of habitual response. It is for this reason that the hunter and the bushman arrange "novel situations" for the animal they are trying to capture, for they know quite well that it will respond in the new situation as it has always done in familiar situations, become confused and render itself the more easily captured. Wherever or whenever a dog is enclosed, it will repeat its habitual tactics (response) of smelling, pressing, nosing, on the trial and error plan, with the end in view of trying to find a weak spot which it can tear down or squeeze through or jump over in order to achieve its freedom (end). In these activities the habitual motivation of its mechanism will be repeated as a *primary* response to its desire or need to "contrive a way out" from an enclosure, or to meet any other need. How then can its response to a novel situation be termed a "new" one, when in fact it is responding as it always does new in accordance with inherited instinct, repeating the means to its end which have been the dog's habit through countless ages of experience in "finding a way out"? One of the most striking instances of the persistence of habit is that of the tame bird which, after picking up each seed, instinctively looks around in self-preservation, although in a situation that has become familiar and in which it has never experienced danger, just as it did in the "novel situation" in which it found itself in the early days of the taming process.

I assume that Dr. Kilpatrick employs the illustration of the dog to support the theory upon which he proposes to reconstruct the educational process. With the utmost desire to analyze his theory at its full value, I must point out that whether he is aware of it or not, he in his pamphlet is advocating the automatic trial and error method while, at the same time, stressing the importance of "conscious direction" and the necessity for "conscious action." This inconsistency is further revealed in the lack of any concrete knowledge to support his plea for "remaking the self," and, when referring to behaviour (response to stimuli), in such statements as: "Rather does each new way of behavior mean in some degree a remaking of the whole organism," or "learning builds structure," or "correlative with all said above is the effect of the self as it lives," and again, "we must think always of the self." The point of course is that nowhere in the pamphlet is to be found any knowledge of that use and functioning of the self which determines the nature of "each new way of behavior," and ensures "desirable structure building" through the "remaking of the self" in living by gradual change and improvement in manner of use of the self.

If the manner of use is a harmful one, as it is in most people today, it is a constant influence for ill upon the whole organism, and therefore, in each "new way of behavior" or in "the remaking of the whole organism," it will be one that is constantly lowering the standard of general functioning, impeding and undermining the "structure building" within the organism in learning and learning to do, bring in about those functional disorders which precede organic disorders and disease.

Dr. Kilpatrick's illustration shows that he is only interested in the dog's behaviour in gaining its end in "contriving, a way out," *not in the use it makes of itself as the instrument in gaining it.* In other words, he is concerned with the end, not with the "means-whereby." And this is exactly what is wrong with the existing educational system, under which it is generally considered that a child has made a good response when it gains the end set for it by the teacher, although it can be demonstrated that the primary response in that motivation of the child's mechanisms which leads to a certain manner of use of itself in the gaining of the end, is having a constantly harmful influence upon the general functioning of its organism. One is forced to conclude that Dr. Kilpatrick does not take into consideration the influence of manner of use, harmful or otherwise, upon the functioning of those who may be subjected to his educational process. Therefore no matter what benefit he may claim can accrue, he cannot escape the serious charge that he is allowing his pupils to remain the victims of a constant impeding influence upon their general functioning, and one that will continue gradually to undermine their psycho-physical energy and potential development in the employment of their thinking and reasoning processes in learning and learning to do, as well as in all other responses to the stimuli of living.

"If we who deal with children," he writes, "will bring ourselves to understand both the possibilities of the situation and the dangers of going astray, we can the better help those under our care to grow in clear-eyed vision of things as they are and in the use of the means appropriate to change them—not mere wishful thinking, or spineless acceptance of injustice, or rash insistence on our way." To which I would reply that in this book I hope I have shown why they cannot be made "to grow in clear-eyed vision of things as they are" (and, I would add, as they should be) unless they are given that knowledge of the use of the self which includes the means whereby (means appropriate) they are enabled to inhibit the habitual (automatic) reaction to the stimuli of daily living, which, as I have been teaching since the beginning, must be inhibited before any such fundamental change can be brought about in the psycho-physical organism as would make possible the change in educational procedure that is Dr. Kilpatrick's objective.

In view of this it is interesting that John Dewey, a colleague of Dr. Kilpatrick, writing of my technique in the Introduction to *The Use of the Self* in 1932, said:

> The technique of Mr. Alexander gives to the educator a standard of psycho-physical health—in which what we call morality is included. It supplies also the means whereby this standard may be progressively and endlessly achieved, becoming a conscious possession of the one educated. It provides therefore the conditions for the central direction of all special educational processes. It bears the same relation to education that education itself bears to all other human activities.

CHAPTER XII

IN CONCLUSION

In this unparalleled crisis, characterized by almost unthinkable human manifestations, there is evidence of a burning desire in the great majority of people to fix the blame for the mistakes or wrongdoing inseparable from such a crisis, upon some individual or individuals, some government or governments.

I have listened to the charges made against some of these and have questioned others who have done the same, but I have failed to meet or hear of a person who, when making these charges, realized that he should take his share of the blame for the mistakes or wrongdoing attributed to individuals or governments. This particularly applies to those who have been active participants in fostering the outlook, intent and misunderstanding which, taken all together, have made possible the present recrudescence of barbarity, rendered more and more hideous by the means of destruction and disaster that are now placed within the reach of the irresponsible through the labours of scientific man, who, in gaining his ends, has been little concerned with the solution of the problem of how man could be prevented from making harmful use of the products of his research, although only too well aware that without these, the present devilish orgy of murder and cruelty, unprecedented during man's long and chequered career,[59] would certainly not have been possible.

The desire in man to fix blame upon another is on a line with his innate resistance to self-accusation, as revealed in his habit of attributing any personal ills and shortcoming to Nature or some other cause, when he is not prepared to shoulder the responsibility. For instance, when the idea of universal suffrage came to him, he believed that he welcomed it because of the greater opportunity for freedom of thought

[59]See Appendix A for excerpts from the Presidential Address entitled *Some Accomplishments of the Chemist* given by Thomas D. Hall, Esq., B.A., M.Sc., before The South African Chemical Institute.

and action that it brought to him and to others, but even if we admit this, there is no getting away from the fact that the influence of that fundamental desire in man to be relieved of responsibility caused him to see just this relief in the act of voting for his member of Parliament and henceforth holding him responsible for the nature of all national and international happenings. Hence his member and members of the Cabinet are specially selected by him for recrimination and too often abuse, as soon as something happens which, from his point of view, is the result of an error of judgment, of neglect or of some other cause; but not for a moment does he suspect that he is in any way responsible, although he is well aware that he chose as his member one of the men who made up that Parliament, and that from the members of that Parliament come the Cabinet Ministers who carry out the measures enacted in Parliament. Whether or not their combined efforts are good or bad, every voter is more or less responsible, and a recognition of this would stop much useless and unjust criticism, and thus prevent the bitterness as well as the hatred which is so often engendered by it.

This failing in man's reaction was in evidence in recent happenings, when there was a genuine desire for peace by the "powers that be," strongly supported by the great majority of voters. The measures taken to this end where generally approved, and I well remember the scene in a large cinema house in London when the announcement was made that Mr. Chamberlain had returned with a signed document for peace. The enthusiasm manifested in that house was general throughout the British Isles, but strangely enough when it became known that one of the signatories had defaulted, as it was known he had done before, the enthusiasts, though well aware of the reputation of the defaulter, became denouncers of the very man whose act they had originally approved. The attitude revealed in making one signatory responsible for the honesty and decency of the other is just another instance of the blind instinctive shortcoming in man's make-up which enables him to try to escape from his obvious responsibility without any recognition of the injustice which is involved in this.

If we face the facts, every honest man and woman on this earth today must admit that each and every one of us is more or less responsible for what is happening at this moment. Should any person join issue with me in this, I would ask how Hitler or Mussolini or any such could be in the position they occupy today unless on the one side they had had the necessary support, and on the other that the ideas and principles they stood for were acceptable to the people who supported them? And again I ask how could these men have built up an armed force greater than that of the total forces of their opponents in this war unless the peoples of the rest of the world were foolish and shortsighted enough to allow them to do it? Neither the resources of Germany or Italy or both embraced the necessary sinews of War. So many essentials for the making of armaments had to be purchased from other countries and stored in quantities greater, as was well known, than was necessary for their home consumption, and yet the free supply of these essential materials was permitted until War was declared, and even after. The cutting-down process was unbelievably slow, and even supposing for the sake of this discussion we admit, as some people contend, that these nations could not be prevented from building up a gigantic war machine, surely in such case sanity demanded that the rest of the world should have seen to it that they defeated them in the armaments race at any rate, as a necessary preliminary to defeating them when they plunged the world into war as they were certain to do. I know many people will try to explain all this away by telling us that we wanted peace. No one will disagree, but the trouble lay in the nature of the "wanting" which was too closely allied to the attitude of "willing" and "wishing" as such. What, I wonder, is wrong with the letter W? I ask this because it is the first letter in these three words, and it is rare that either of these are found to be brothers or sisters of responsibility. If this were not so, surely those "wanting" peace would have accepted the responsibility of the carrying-out of the only reasonable means to that end—the prevention of the importation of essential materials into Germany and Italy in quantities necessary for the creation of a gigantic war machine greater than was possible with the combined resources in material of these countries alone.

Most of the peoples of the world are now concerned with the effort necessary to bring this conflict to an end, to a quick end if possible. Their thoughts are bent upon this and rightly so, but I want if I can to direct the thoughts of every person to the great problem to be solved if, after the War is ended, history is not to be repeated. This solution is to be found, as is that of all fundamental problems, in the development of the potentialities of the individual by means which make for improvement in and control of human reaction, and the speed of this improvement and control must more than keep pace with man's progress and advancement in the outside world. As John Dewey put it in his Introduction to my book *Constructive Conscious Control of the Individual*:

> Through modern science we have mastered to a wonderful extent the use of things as tools for accomplishing results upon and through other things. The result is all but a universal state of confusion, discontent and strife. The one factor which is the primary tool in the use of all these other tools, namely ourselves, in other words, our own psycho-physical

disposition, as the basic condition of our employment of all agencies and energies, has not even been studied as a central instrumentality. Is it not highly probable that this failure gives the explanation of why it is that in mastering physical forces we have ourselves been so largely mastered by them, until we find ourselves incompetent to direct the history and destiny of man?

Man has not complied with the basic demands in living, and this could account in the wide view for his innate objection to taking responsibility wherever and whenever he can escape from it, and also for his many errors of judgment and want of foresight. These characteristics have been manifested in a too tardy response to urgent demands for prompt action in the upholding of the principles and protection of the rights for which mankind has striven, in the face of strong opposition and at great sacrifice, during his experiences in civilization, and the non-compliance with these demands have resulted in the serious situation in human affairs we are face to face with today.

In this matter of taking responsibility and the laying of blame, much has been written and spoken as to the relative responsibility of leaders and people of the nation that fired the first shots in this War. One of the most common arguments is that the people of that nation are to be freed from blame because they were led into it by specious arguments and the personal influence of an unscrupulous man. But in my opinion they are not the less to blame on this account, rather the more, for it is an admission that the reaction of these people can be so easily influenced by evil forces that they remain a menace to the peace and safety of the rest of the world. Their outlook towards life, their innate egotism and their astounding misunderstanding of the outlook and disregard of the welfare of the peoples of other nations has always been characteristic of them. Add to this their mania for shelving individual responsibility on to the shoulder of some leader or leaders, their desire to be told what to do and what not to do, and the instinctive self-hypnotic docility, too firmly associated with barbarity, which they have for so long manifested, and who can then be surprised that this nation, claiming as it does a highly civilized outlook and *Kultur*, is guilty in the manner of waging war of the most criminal outrage upon human society that can be recorded in history?

The improvement and control of man's reaction, and the bearing of its influence upon the matter of taking responsibility is the premiss that calls for first consideration in any survey of man's experiences, and of the "means-whereby" upon which he has depended for progress and development in every field of his activity up to the outbreak of war. When this premiss is examined in the light of man's reaction to the events which have led us to this world conflict and to those which have occurred since, how can we come to any conclusion but one? Namely, that if past experiences are not to be repeated, and man is to gain a better understanding of the nature of the aims and characteristics of the peoples of other nations as well as his own, he must have new "means-whereby" for living in the future. There must be a reorientation of our viewpoint upon education, culture, religion, politics, economics, medicine, science, industry, and last but not least, upon class and social relations and intercourse. Such reorientation as I envisage is not possible without that fundamental change in guidance and control of the self which is the theme of the subject matter of this book. This will demand a radical change in the methods of education of the young child right on to adolescence, and also in the methods to be adopted by man in his future intercourse with his fellow men in his social, business, and other activities in the outside world. Essential to this will be his realization of the need for accepting responsibility for all that has made for troubles and difficulties within himself, and of the need of some means for ridding himself of these. If and when he accepts this primary responsibility, existing as it were on his own doorstep, the experience will be the best possible preparation for the acceptance of responsibility in his contacts with the outside world, that sense of his own personal responsibility which includes being true to himself, and equally so to his fellow men.

* * * * *

In the midst of the conditions prevailing today, people are being driven to a revaluation of the "means-whereby" of all that has made up the way of life called democracy, for in the view of most people it is the "means-whereby" that is at fault, not the democratic way of life. This very viewpoint should in its turn lead to a revaluation of all that man has depended upon as the "means-whereby" of progress and development within and without himself. If those who do this are not prejudiced by past beliefs and ideas and take the wide view, they will find that man's educational plan for the development of the potentialities of the individual self has been a meagre one as compared with his plan for development outside himself. His accumulated knowledge of the world outside himself, more or less unrelated to his meagre knowledge of himself, has become a Frankenstein, and has made possible the very activities which today are menacing his democratic way of life. He adopted this ideal as the way to freedom of thought and action, but he failed to understand that its realization can only come through full development of man's potentiality not only for individual freedom *of* thought and action, but for that individual freedom IN thought and action in the general use and functioning of the self, which gives in process control of individual and therefore collective reaction in the way of life essential to the practice of the theory of democracy.

* * * * *

My teaching experience has shown me that a person who has accepted the idea of freedom of thought and action, and has consistently advocated it in daily life, is not any the more capable on this account of freedom in thought and action, when it comes to holding to a decision to employ procedures, the carrying out of which involves a use of the self which is not in keeping with his habitual reaction in thought and action.

F. M A.

APPENDICES

Appendix A

Extract from the Presidential Address entitled *Some Accomplishments of the Chemist* by Thos. D. Hall, B.A., M.Sc., and delivered to the members of the South African Chemical Institute.

After describing "Chemistry's Bewildering Possibilities" and its various benefits to industry and living generally in the modern world, Mr. Hall continued:

> We have added to the material wealth of the world and increased its tempo by many beats. There is, too, enough for all, but the majority do not get enough as the materialistic and mechanised world has outrun its social and economic development. Nature has warned us throughout geological ages that one-sided or unbalanced development always ends in disaster. It truly seems as if the world might be better off if the chemists, for some time to come, made no more new discoveries with which further to embarrass our economists and social workers. . . .
>
> The wizard workings of the chemist have changed life in all aspects and altered the habits of man, but unfortunately not always for the better. There are indications that despite the achievements of medical science in saving life, particularly in its younger years, and thus increasing the average span, more diseases of the mind and body are developing in later life. Various remedies for the ills of the world have been suggested by as many prophets in the fields of religion, economics, social welfare and politics.

The Deterioration of Man and its Remedy.

Hamlet's words seem most appropriate to our age and ourselves:

> The time is out of joint; O cursed spite,
> That ever I was born to set it right.

I am not even going to try but I've found a scapegoat, or rather I should say a philosopher and teacher who has new precepts and teachings, and, despite his wonderful and original discoveries, more modesty than the chemist. Quietly and thoroughly he has pursued his studies scientifically for over thirty years and has proved his theories step by step. He has been studying man not as dead bones or a physical body only or mentally only, but as a co-ordinated, psycho-physical living being and has come to the conclusion that man has developed so fast mentally and changed his material environment so rapidly that his instinctive or subconscious control is no more reliable in guiding him in the correct use of his body.

So quite unbeknown to himself man is using his body wrongly, even in the simplest acts of life, and doing himself untold functional harm. This is quite unlike the animal or the savage, whose instincts guide them aright in a fairly stable environment.

This deterioration he thinks has proceeded most quickly during the past hundred years. I should like to quote the opinion of the eminent American philosopher, Professor John Dewey. He states:

> Mr. Alexander has demonstrated a new scientific principle with respect to the control of human behaviour, as important as any principle which has ever been discovered in the domain of external nature. Not only this, but his discovery is necessary to complete the discoveries made about non-human nature, if these discoveries and inventions are not to end by making us their servants and helpless tools.

From what I have gathered from Alexander's writings he has little hope of the world improving its condition until these fundamental wrongs are appreciated and corrected. When around the council tables of the nations sit men with slumped and shortened spines, contracted thoracic regions, crowded vitals, unhealthy paunches, with poor circulation and breathing wrongly, monuments to the instinctive incorrect use of their bodies and of which they are blissfully unaware, how can the world hope for any solutions of its problems from such sources?

He further explains that the present physical exercise revival, which is an acknowledgement that something is seriously wrong with man, will not help matters, because it is a case of the blind leading the blind, and that while these exercises will correct some physical faults they will only accentuate others, as no exercise can benefit a body as a whole in which instinctive control is wrong and where there is a lack of proper co-ordination. He has, however, in his thirty years' work discovered a method by which man can obtain the conscious control of his psycho-physical being and bring about perfect co-ordination of all his bodily acts. "His procedure and conclusions meet all the requirements of the strictly scientific method," says Professor John Dewey. When our instincts are unreliable, what seems correct to us is often wrong and Alexander states that we have to relearn the simplest acts and obtain a new sensory appreciation of ourselves before these faults can be remedied. Unfortunately this new sensory appreciation and correction comes slowly as each person needs individual attention from a properly trained teacher for a month or more and at present there are few of these available. More efficient results are obtained by training children in school or at an early age in these methods as more individuals can be handled in this way.

Those of you who would like to know more about this remarkable system, which has already received some recognition in the *British Medical Journal*, are referred to the books by F. Matthias Alexander, *Man's Supreme Inheritance*, *Constructive Conscious Control of the Individual* and *The Use of the Self*. . . .

Some of you will no doubt be thinking, "Well, what has all this to do with chemistry?" We have seen enough, I hope, to realise that the wonderful achievements of the chemist are perhaps not all as beneficial to the human race as we should like to imagine. As I have nothing personally to offer you, I think it is only intellectually honest to tell you about the man whom I do sincerely believe has the best remedy so far evolved. Again I shall quote Professor Dewey in substantiation:

> "In the present state of the world it is evident that the control we have gained of physical energies, heat, light, electricity, etc., without having first secured control of ourselves is a perilous affair. Without control of ourselves our use of other things is blind; it may lead to anything. Moreover, if our habitual judgments of ourselves are warped because they are based on vitiated sense material—as they must be if our habits of managing ourselves are already wrong—then the more complex the social conditions under which we live the more disastrous must be the outcome. Every additional complication of outward instrumentalities is likely to be a step nearer destruction; a fact which the present state of the world tragically exemplifies."

Alexander believes that man's evolution will never be complete until conscious control of himself has replaced the instinctive or subconscious. He has given a new outlook and a new hope to the harassed human race. I truly believe that when his teachings are properly appreciated and put into effect for a generation or more it will then be realized that they have done more good even than the wonderful work of Pasteur, which had the advantage that it could be applied impersonally and in the mass, whereas this system is most personal and will thus take longer to produce visible effects on a national scale.

That Alexander . . . will one day be among the immortals along with Pasteur I do not doubt. When once the human race has achieved this proper conscious control of itself and is able to adapt itself advantageously to the rapid changes brought about by chemistry and other sciences in its environment, then the future discoveries of the chemist will be a blessing, but in the present state of the world there are many who think that they are a blight.

Appendix B

Excerpts from *The Function of the Sub-Occipital Muscles. The Key to Posture, Use and Functioning*, by A. Murdoch, M.B., C.M. Paper read at the Hastings Division of the British Medical Association, May 5, 1936.

. . . When I was elected President of the Sussex Branch of the British Medical Association I used the occasion of the Presidential Address to refer to Alexander's work, and as a result of the publication of a Synopsis of it, I received a request from the Editor of the *Journal of Massage and Medical Gymnastics* to write a paper on Posture with special reference to Alexander's Theory.

While searching for fresh material for this paper, I examined the dissection of the Sub-Occipital region as shown in the Edinburgh Stereoscopic Atlas of Anatomy, since which time I have also examined the dissected specimen in the Royal College of Surgeons' Museum. With the idea dominant in my mind of the head being a weighty mass, poised on the summit of the vertebral column, the peculiar and distinctive arrangement of the muscles seen in the Sub-Occipital space seemed to me to be such as might have been designed purposely for holding the head securely on the joint, and for giving it the necessary movements in the delicate function of balancing. The muscles in the group are the following: Rectus Capitis Posticus Major and Minor, Superior and Inferior oblique (posteriorly), Rectus Lateralis (one each side), Rectus Capitis Anticus Major and Minor (anteriorly). They all arise from the Atlas or Axis, and their function would appear to be that of moving the head at the Atlanto Occipital and Atlanto Axial joints and are the *intrinsic* muscles of these joints. The large neck muscles are outside this ring of muscles, their insertions being chiefly posterior to the Atlanto Occipital joint, while their origins are so wide-spread as to enable them to function as head and neck and body muscles. They are not purely head muscles like the Sub-Occipital group. The appearance in the photograph as well as in the dissected specimen is as if the head were poised on the tips of so many fingers, represented by the Sub-

Occipital muscles which act as so many muscular ties between the head and the first two Vertebrae.

I sought the opinion of the Assistant Curator of the Museum and Dr. Cave kindly wrote me this letter:

> "In reply to your queries, the head (skull) and first two vertebræ are associated intimately on grounds of development, gross anatomy (human and comparative) and function. The name I coined for this apparatus (Arris and Gale Lecture, unpublished, 1932) was Cervico-Cranium, a term of convenience if not of strict Etymology. Both Atlas and Axis suffer the profoundest modifications in their structure and development in consequence of their being handmaids of the Cranial Globe as functionally they are through life. Special ligaments and specially differentiated muscles serve to maintain this close association and the upper Cervical Pole of the X-ray is simply a manifestation of this anatomic physiological entity—the Cervico-Cranium."

Here then is an association of parts—Cranial Globe, Atlas and Axis and Sub-Occipital muscles, related in development, in structure and function, but the function of the combination has never been alluded to, much less defined.

My observations and Dr. Cave's views of the relationship between the Cranial Globe and the Vertebrae and the Sub-Occipital muscles raise the following questions:

Has this system, "this apparatus," any special function?

Does it contain a mechanism which we can direct and use to control ourselves?

Has it any relation to Alexander's theory of the Primary Control and his technique for re-educating it?

The function of balancing requires a co-ordinating apparatus. Wright says "the vestibular apparatus serves to adapt the position of the trunk and limbs to that of the head and it supplies afferent impulses which enable the erect position of the head and the normal attitude of the body to be maintained."

An extract from Dr. B. Kinnear Wilson's *Modern Problems in Neurology* (page 130), is most explicit as to the influence of the head in determining every attitude of the body, but like every other authority gives no indication as to what muscular mechanism causes the "displacements" or movements of the head. This is the extract: "The apparatus for the auto regulation of attitude must be in being if cortical excitations are to effect movements and acts. Winekler expresses the same idea when he says *that with each displacement of the head a given attitude of the whole body is determined* and it follows that for *each voluntary movement* the body finds itself in such a position as to enable the appropriate contraction of the muscles to be attained at the movement of production of that voluntary movement."

This is Alexander's theory in a nutshell, as this dominating influence of the head was discovered by Alexander more than 30 years ago and was called by him "The Primary Control," but "the apparatus" and its mechanism were unknown to him. By means of the Primary Control it is possible *to condition* all the known reflexes discovered by Magnus and others, as well as those still to be discovered regarding the inter-relations between the vestibule and the nerve-muscle systems of the body, whenever a change of posture or a complex muscular movement has to be executed. But the neural paths, and the means whereby these inter-relations are affected must be left to be worked out by the anatomist and the physiologist.

This co-ordinating apparatus—the Vestibular apparatus—is situated in the substance of the Petrous portion of the Temporal bone and in close proximity to the Atlanto Occipital joint, so that the slightest movement of the head at this joint would be communicated to the delicate media in the Vestibular apparatus through the action of the Sub-Occipital muscles, and it is my suggestion that it is the delicate movements of the Sub-Occipital group at the Atlanto Occipital joint which activate the media in the Vestibule; that although the movements at this joint are limited (30 degs. backwards and 20 degs. forwards) they are enough for balancing and maintaining our muscular co-ordinations, which are constantly changing, because of our constantly changing postures and require movements that are as sensitive and delicate as those of the needle of the compass.

The question might be asked at this point: Why is the Vestibular apparatus situated in bone and not in the soft substance of the brain, if it be not to prevent it from being affected by any other stimulus than its own normal stimulus, from the delicate movements of the head, at the Atlanto Occipital joint, as otherwise the delicacy of the movements of the fluid in the canals would be interfered with, by the varying pressures, from the varying conditions of the circulation, in the brain.

The Cranial Globe containing the Vestibular apparatus is a passive agent and requires some muscular agency to move it for its special function, and my suggestion is that the Sub-Occipital group is the obvious and appropriate mechanism as they are handmaids of the Cranial Globe according to Dr. Cave. These muscles are voluntary muscles and are, therefore, capable of being used voluntarily, and as they have the special function of moving the Cranial Globe at the Atlanto Occipital and Atlanto Axial joints, I suggest that these muscles are the primary movers of the Cranial Globe and constitute the primary mechanism used in the control of ourselves. I submit that these movements should be primary, and being due to the action of voluntary muscles are, therefore, under control so that their use establishes a mechanism, man can use for conditioning his muscular reflexes through the medium of the Vestibular apparatus. The neural control of the mechanism may be considered as the *Muscular Control Centre* and is comparable to the centres governing other systems of the body, e.g., the Cardiac, the Respiratory, the Vaso motor centres, etc., but with this vital and important difference, that according to the manner in which we use this Primary Control, we are actually imposing the external conditions under which all our vital organs and systems function.

The limited movement at the Atlanto Occipital joint contrasts with the wide range of movement of the Cervico-Cranium at the middle of the neck through the action of the large neck muscles. This again points to a difference in function of the two groups of muscles. The first is a comparatively small movement, within another very large movement, and I submit it has been overlooked in experiments carried out on the functions of the labyrinth, and that the significance of the Sub-Occipital system as the primary mover of the Cranial Globe has been missed—attention having been given solely to the larger, freer, wider movements which take place at the middle of the neck, when the Cranial Globe with the Atlas and Axis move together. The smaller movement is the all important one of maintaining a proper balance of the Cranial Globe and so allowing the co-ordinating and regulating apparatus—the labyrinth, to maintain proper and correct relationships between the Cranial Globe and the body. Such bringing of the whole of the muscular apparatus into correct co-ordination, creates the correct conditions in our external body wall for the functioning of the vital organs, and constitutes the Primary Control which Alexander has postulated and taken advantage of and which Magnus described, but did not locate, many years after.

The control of this function of the Cranial Globe through the action of the Sub-Occipital muscles in the great majority of people has been lost—it never has been consciously learnt—and with it our power to maintain a proper poise and posture, and from this loss come many of the disabilities from which man suffers.

From the nature of the arrangement of the parts and the fact that man is the only erect mammal, it has been impossible to investigate the function of these muscles in their relation to the Cranial Globe, in the usual experimental manner, but Alexander, by a long series of experiments on himself, has been able to devise a technique to re-educate these muscles and bring back their original function with the result of an alteration in poise, posture and functioning as a whole. Invariably this re-education is accompanied by the disappearance of maladjustments and usually of their associated symptoms of disease.

In order to understand the importance of Alexander's discovery and its significance, together with the perfection and simplicity of his technique, one has to remember that in no text-book of Anatomy or Physiology, or Physical Culture, is there any hint of using the Cranial Globe as the organ or key to play such an important part as the apparatus for rectifying defects of posture as such, or to connect such widely differing conditions as Asthma and Flatfoot, or even Neurasthenia, with the manner in which the Cranial Globe is poised relatively to the Vertebral Column.

In estimating the importance of Alexander's discovery of the Primary Control and his manner of directing it to restore better use and functioning throughout the body, one should contrast it with the barren results as regards the practical application to our daily needs of the discovery of the Central Control by Magnus through experiments on animals. The different results are due to the fact that Alexander's experiments were done on a human being with all his critical faculties alert, and with the object of finding out the cause of the recurring hoarseness and inflammatory conditions of his vocal organs, which medical treatment had failed to prevent and which threatened to ruin his career as an elocutionist.

On the other hand the physiologist's experiments were made on animals whose postural conditions were always normal and whose use of themselves would always, be correct, i.e., they would always do the same things in the same way. They could not be made to use themselves wrongly for lengthy periods as man has done, and so create bad postural conditions with their accompanying disabilities which might be investigated as to cause and effect as in Alexander's case.

Appendix C

Excerpts from *Reorientation of the View Point Upon the Study of Anatomy* by Mungo Douglas, M.B. (1937).

Two important discoveries in the last thirty years have led to vantage points from which anatomy can be re-viewed. Firstly, the late Rudolph Magnus of Utrecht revealed that the use of the head and neck in relation to the torso conditioned uses throughout the body. Written anatomically this would be thus—that groups of muscles in their working as well as adjusting the relation of parts to parts do work which is, in fact, a linking in a chain without which assumedly specific action in more ultimate parts could not occur.

Secondly, and more important than Magnus, F. Matthias Alexander of London, studying living men and women in use, observed that, although all human beings were provided with the same mechanism, divisible into anatomical elements, these elements in use showed a diversity of structure as elements and as a means to produce human edifices of bewildering variation. The observation was not of similars varying in magnitude for that was an observation to be expected and accepted as in the course of things; but of similars directed without law to utter dissimilarity.

From his studies Alexander was able to deduce certain conclusions which anatomically may be written thus, that there were certain functions certain groups of muscles could not be considered to perform, although human beings so used them, and for the reason that, firstly, from such use obvious hurt resulted to the mechanism in part or whole, or, secondly, functions in ultimate parts were hindered or stopped.

Proceeding further he discovered that by using that function of the central nervous system called inhibition, certain usages of groups of muscle could be stopped, whereupon the remaining usages of these groups could be used both to produce movements of parts about joints, and maintain relations of parts with least friction.

Essentially he discovered that these usages of groups of muscles lying in the neck posterior to the spine were those that first must be inhibited before it was possible to permit all groups of muscles to perform movements of parts about joints, and maintain relations of parts to parts, with least friction.

Viewing anatomy in the light of these discoveries it is seen that the function of muscles is two-fold, namely, movement of parts about joints, and directive of part to part. . . .

Basically it becomes essential that anatomy shall recognise that the relationing function of muscle is the primary function of muscle, and that movements of parts upon parts is secondary.

Secondly, it must be recognised that the primary relation upon which all more ultimate relations depend is that relation established by the small group of muscles which comprise the atlas-occipital, axis-occipital, atlas-axis system.

The stupendous importance of this relationing function of muscles cannot be realised by the mere description of its existence. The failure to recognise the conception is charged with a heavy responsibility since it means the approach to all living, and human endeavour with but an imperfectly formed knowledge of physiological means.

Appendix D

Excerpts from an Address delivered by John Hilton, M.A., Professor of Industrial Relations, Cambridge University, England, at a Conference of the Institute of Labour Management held at Buxton, England, October 17, 1936.

Smooth Rhythms or Shocks

. . . Now a word on the physique of the worker of the new generation. The children that are coming forward are being better cared for, better fed, better housed, better looked after medically, than those of our immediately preceding generations. In that respect you will have more promising material. But in another respect they are going to be more difficult, more fragile than their predecessors. They are going to be more highly strung. Their nerves are going to be still more on edge. You had better be aware of that.

Why should it be so? In great part because of the stress under which we live our lives in these days, and, more than anything else, because of the extent to which we use or are used by racing, throbbing, vibrating machinery.

I wonder has it ever occurred to you that through the hundreds and thousands of years of his history, man knew no vibration, more rapid or sustained than the jolt of a wheel on the rough road, or the whimper of a taut sail or the murmur of a scudding hull—no more than that, until as lately as a hundred years ago. The physical frame of man is matched to smooth rhythms. In this last infinitesimal phase of our development we have been subjecting that frame to sustained shocks and vibrations of the most intense kind. Do you wonder that our nerves go wrong; that our controls get out of order. And not only vibrations. Also speeds. Have you ever thought, I wonder, that our physical and nervous systems have developed through hundreds and thousands of years, attuned not only to gentle rhythms but also to smooth movements at low speeds, quickened only in moments of stress and danger.

In the last hundred years we have come to have the power-driven machine by us, under our hands, in our service. Almost without our knowing it, the machine has been setting a new pace for our bodily motions. We ape the machine. Our bodies were not made for such movements.

The result of this fantastic mimicry is movements of sharp jerks, plucking wrenching movements of the limbs. See the overstrung man or woman, child indeed, with the tense rapid jerking walk. See what the novelist calls the "quick nervous gestures." Every movement destructive

of nervous tranquillity. But vastly more destructive, the quick jerky movements of head and body—of the head relative to the body, of the body relative to the head.

Unknown to ourselves, by unconscious mimicry, we set our pace by the machine; and the pace destroys us by destroying our most sensitive and delicate co-ordinations and controls.

Do you wonder we have so many nervous wrecks? Do you wonder that our madhouses are ever filling? We are the descendants of four generations of machine mimics. Will you wonder if the workers of the new generation are touchy, apt to fly off the hinge, apt to go down with mysterious disorders and leave you in the lurch. Will you wonder if you yourselves get more rattled, more inclined to daily exhaustions and annual breakdowns than your forefathers were.

Among you are medical men. I'm going to talk to you like an uncle—and make no apology for doing so. All this that I am saying, about the co-ordination of the controls of the body that are being dislocated and deranged—thrown out of flunter we say in Lancashire—by almost all of us at almost every moment of our waking lives—in our striding, and stretching, and reaching, and bending, and sitting down, and standing up, and looking, and speaking—all this that comes to us from the unconscious mimicking of machine speeds—and is daily destroying our poise and our power and our health and our sanity—all this has been explored and expounded by a quiet genius of whose immensely important discoveries your medical authorities have decided, in their organised professional capacity, to take no notice.

These things of which I speak are not, alas, of my discovering, though I have been hunting them all my life, they are the discoveries of F. Matthias Alexander. If you don't know about the work of Alexander, and of his technique for neutralising the errors into which we have fallen for re-educating ourselves and for restoring the co-ordinations of the body so lately disastrously lost by civilised man, I beg you do so at once.

Shortly you will be hearing of the confirmatory discoveries of distinguished men of your profession who have stood out against the ban upon any serious notice being taken of Alexander's work. If you want F. M. Alexander's own account of his researches, his discoveries, and his technique, read his book "The Use of the Self," or his book "The Conscious Control of the Individual." If you want a philosophical elaboration of the principles underlying Alexander's discoveries and of their significance to the future of mankind, read Aldous Huxley's latest book, "Eyeless in Gaza."

If you want to know what effect a series of jerks can have upon the nervous system, jerks that shake the head relative to the trunk, try filing out with vigour and in haste a rough round hole with a file that jams at every other stroke. Try it. You'll know better than any words of mine can tell you the effect upon the physical and nervous structure of shocks to the sub-cranial controls of the body. Or if you would like a demonstration of the extreme effects of a displacement of the head get Max Schmelling or Joe Louis to hit you under the jaw, slightly sideways, just once.

When you come round, go into the works, and watch the workpeople who are under your medical guardianship or managerial charge. You will see right and left one and another doing to himself or herself, by his overstrained, overtense, and jerky physical movements, exactly what the blow under the chin did to you. In a milder degree, of course; but doing it perhaps sixty times to the hour for eight or more hours a day.

The workers of the new generation will come to you with already ingrained bad habits in poise, in movement, and in co-ordination. If you don't know these things that Alexander has brought to light you will not only let him keep his bad uses of his limbs and head and body; you will set him tasks that will aggravate them, and then you won't know why he goes sour and goes sick, you won't know why he can't stand a day's work.

Ah, some of you say, we're up to all that. We encourage our youngsters to join physical culture classes and do exercises. Do you? I'll only say that the exercises prescribed and taught by most of our physical culturists are popularly known as "Physical Jerks." I make no comment: "Physical *Jerks*." I'll add that only the strongest can survive an orthodox course of physical culture. I have seen, and read, the Report of the Physical Education Committee of the British Medical Association. I have looked for any mention in it of the crucial matters I am putting to you now. None. Not a word. You say it isn't true; it can't be true. I tell you, not a mention, not one word.

The Report of the Physical Education Committee of the British Medical Association is not merely the play of Hamlet without the Prince of Denmark. It is the play of Hamlet with only two characters: Rosencrantz and Guildenstern. They are a bad lot, you remember, and die in the middle act.

Will you medical men here make amends. Go into this thing. If you will, collectively, I'll work in with you. Alexander has not a hundred years to live. We'd better learn from him, get his knowledge and technique, while we can.

I've covered man the citizen, and man the being of flesh and blood, living in a machine world for which he was never meant. One last word on Man the creature of imagination, of passion, of honour, of dignity.

I'll say again, what I said to some of you not very long ago. There are four needs of the human spirit, which must somehow be satisfied even at our work. To be looked on as a somebody. To use our faculties. To feel that we belong. To respect ourselves for the work we do.

There are those who say: we can't be bothered with all that. Tell them, you who know better, that if they can't be bothered with all that, their schemes, however well built and apparently sea-worthy, will run on the rocks, for the most dangerous of all rocks is frustrated human nature.

I remind you again of what the Prince of Denmark said. You will remember how old Polonius, when told to take the players in and use them well, said he would use them according to their desert; and I hope you always remember Hamlet's reply: "Od's bodykins, man, much better: use every man after his desert and who should 'scape whipping? Use them after your own honour and dignity." I think the secret is there. Not only for the employer to the workman but for the workman to the employer. Let each use each after his own honour and dignity. Only so, I think, will the whole race of mankind, and the whole industrial process that it is building up "'scape whipping."

Appendix E

Tic Douloureux. The following letters were received from this pupil:

August 4, 1938

"I have been home a week. . . . I am feeling decidedly better and the pain is gradually lessening in the daytime. I have eaten several meals without having to mop my eyes—a great improvement! The pain is still rather tiresome at night. . . . I am doing my best to carry out your instructions and have not had so much as a sniff of coffee!"

August 12, 1938

"Here is another good report:

(1) The pain is not nearly as bad in bed now, and I am having much better nights.

(2) My left eye is now as wide open as the other one.

(3) I am beginning to feel a new woman.

(4) Friends keep telling me how much better I am looking. I hope you will consider this satisfactory."

August 20, 1938

"I came up here yesterday by car taking nearly three hours, and with the exception of about one minute did not have a scrap of pain all the way—it was the best day I have had. Miss M. says the difference in me, since we parted at Euston is amazing and that I am looking better than she had ever seen me.

"I do not think that I could send you a better report."

August 27, 1938

"I am very pleased to send you another good report. I am having comparatively little pain now, and it seems to have quite gone from the back of my head. It is just the left side of my forehead that is tender and sore and very painful when touched by anything; but the pain only lasts for about a minute or so and is soon over. I'm sure you will open your eyes at my improved appearance. Miss B. thinks the change in me is marvellous."

October 3, 1938

"I do not know how to express my thanks for all you have done for me . . . everyone I meet is amazed at the tremendous difference in me."

October 22, 1938

"Here is a very good report for you. That bruised place in my forehead has greatly improved this last week. I can scarcely feel it at all now. It is a joy to be able to wash my face all over and powder my nose! without pain. I am carefully carrying out your instructions and still being complimented on my altered looks."

Appendix F

In Number 20 of *Bulletins From Britain* for the week ending January 15, 1941, published by The British Library of Information, 50 Rockefeller Plaza, New York, N.Y., will be found the following "damning series of reports prepared by German medical officers" concerning the mental and physical results of youth training in Germany:

> On the mental qualities produced we have the following: "When the young cadets present themselves for the officers' examination they usually excel in a remarkable lack of logic. Logic and disciplined thinking are usually replaced by an incredible tendency to using meaningless claptrap."
>
> (*Militar-Wochenblatt*, December 10, 1938)
>
> "The psychological examination of the cadets has become necessary because the candidates today exhibit very grave lack of knowledge and, to a very great extent, have a rather faulty point of view in regard to men-

tal work. Stupidity and laziness of mind are always defects of character."
(*Dr. Simoneit* (Head of the Psychological Laboratory at the War Ministry) in a lecture at Hanover, November 23, 1937).

This is not surprising when we read in *Deutsche Wehr* (periodical of the German Officers' Corps, August 9, 1936) that "the next war will require the highest degree of brutality"; in May 1934 Goebbels demanded that the high schools should produce "tough guys" and stated that "the intellect is a danger to the shaping of character."

FLAT FEET AND DISEASE

One might have thought that with this "exaggerated physical training" at least the bodies of German youth might have benefited. Here, however, is the Army's verdict on the health of the young men of Germany:

"Military examinations indicate that an alarming number of conscripts are incapable of service in the army because of flat feet."
(*Munich Medical Journal*, April 2, 1937)

"More than 50% of those on worker's duty and liable to military service suffer from foot weakness and weakened spines."
(*Report on examination of "Jungvolk,"* May, 1937)

"Inflammatory conditions, which were formerly found principally among apprentices and in the years of adolescence, now often appear among school children, at an age when they never used to appear. The reason for this is that too much is demanded of the feet of these boys and girls through marches on hard roads, carrying heavy burdens besides—in other words, exerting them to tasks beyond their strength."
(*Munich Medical Journal*, April 2, 1937)

Official German figures, too, show progressive increases in children's diseases:

	Scarlet Fever	Diphtheria	Infantile Paralysis	Dysentery	Meningitis
1933	79,830	77,340	1,318	2,685	617
1935	112,509	133,843	2,153	3,430	1,362
1937	117,544	146,733	2,723	7,545	1,574

(*Statistisches Jahrbuch*, 1937)

Appendix G

My attention has been drawn to an article in the *New York Times* of Sept. 30, 1940, entitled:

UNITY OF THINKING TERMED BIG TASK
But It Is Possible And Vital
To Democracy, Philosophers
Agree After Conference.

In this article a report is given of a 3-days' "Conference on Science, Philosophy and Religion in their relation to the Democratic Way of Life" at which "500 leaders" in these fields "concluded a first attempt to unify the thought of democracy," in "an effort to bring together the various compartments into which human knowledge has been separated by specialization during the past century," an effort which, as the writer of the article truly says, "was long overdue." My special interest is in what the writer gives as the statement of the special group of thinkers who had the task of communicating to the press the achievement of the Conference so far, namely, that "it had found it possible to engage in 'corporate thinking,'" and that the first product of the corporate thinking in the last week was as follows:

> The conference was unanimous in its conviction that modern civilization can be preserved only by a recognition of the supreme worth and moral responsibility of the individual human person.

I quote this with great satisfaction because of my persistent crusade, in the face of much opposition, on behalf of the individual person, and because, as readers of my books are aware, I have not only persistently contended that the realization of this ideal implied the need for a new technique in living, but have succeeded in demonstrating that the "means-whereby" of the new technique I have evolved will enable the individual to consistently develop his potentialities in his "doing" in daily life. I would suggest, therefore, to the leaders of this conference that if they wish to accomplish their aim they should, at least, take into their survey the evidence accumulated during a lifetime by a fellow worker, who has employed personally the technique he has advocated in teaching others to employ it, and in this way has gained for himself, and enabled others to gain, the personal experience and realization of a new way of living in the fundamental sense.

Another point of interest to me in view of what I have written regarding human reaction is the following (again quoted from the article):

> In their (the Group's) judgment, the greatest achievement of this first conference was the demonstration that they could come together not merely for the purpose of expressing their individual minds but also in a willingness to change their minds, at least their attitude towards each other. . . . There was some delicacy as to whether the sessions should be labelled "Conference of Science, Philosophy and Religion" or "Conference of Religion, Philosophy and Science." Happily (the writer goes on), both sides were satisfied when the scientists accepted first mention on the principle that leaders come first; while the theologians accepted last mention because in religious processions the highest dignitary brings up the end.

Accepting this as stated, I venture to point to the significant fact that the general satisfaction did not come from what the order of the words signified, but from an arrangement which in the carrying out did not call for any change in the habitual reaction of anyone present to the stimulus of individual interest or belief.

F. M. A.

INDEX OF NAMES